Essentials of Exercise and Sports Medicine

Essentials of Exercise and Sports Medicine

Editor: Ellis Baker

Callisto Reference
www.callistoreference.com

Callisto Reference,
118-35 Queens Blvd., Suite 400,
Forest Hills, NY 11375, USA

Visit us on the World Wide Web at:
www.callistoreference.com

ISBN: 978-1-63239-947-2 (Hardback)

Printed in China.

Cataloging-in-Publication Data

Essentials of exercise and sports medicine / edited by Ellis Baker.
p. cm.
Includes bibliographical references and index.
ISBN 978-1-63239-947-2
1. Exercise. 2. Sports medicine. 3. Physical education and training. I. Baker, Ellis.
GV461 .E87 2018
613.71--dc23

Table of Contents

Preface

Exercise enhances and helps in maintaining physical fitness. It helps in improving athletic performance. Sports medicine helps in dealing with physical fitness and in treating the injuries caused during sports or exercise. Some of the primary injuries treated under this branch are ligament tear, muscle cramp, ankle sprat, etc. The topics included in this book on exercise and sports medicine are of utmost significance and bound to provide incredible insights to readers. It strives to provide a fair idea about this discipline and to help develop a better understanding of the latest advances within this field.

Various studies have approached the subject by analyzing it with a single perspective, but the present book provides diverse methodologies and techniques to address this field. This book contains theories and applications needed for understanding the subject from different perspectives. The aim is to keep the readers informed about the progresses in the field; therefore, the contributions were carefully examined to compile novel researches by specialists from across the globe.

Indeed, the job of the editor is the most crucial and challenging in compiling all chapters into a single book. In the end, I would extend my sincere thanks to the chapter authors for their profound work. I am also thankful for the support provided by my family and colleagues during the compilation of this book.

Editor

Evaluation of an Exercise Field Test Using Heart Rate Monitors to Assess Cardiorespiratory Fitness and Heart Rate Recovery in an Asymptomatic Population

Crystal L. Coolbaugh[1], **Ivan B. Anderson**[2], **Machelle D. Wilson**[3], **David A. Hawkins**[1,4]*, **Ezra A. Amsterdam**[2]

1 Biomedical Engineering Graduate Group, University of California Davis, Davis, California, United States of America, **2** Division of Cardiovascular Medicine, Department of Internal Medicine, University of California Davis, Sacramento, California, United States of America, **3** Division of Biostatistics, Department of Public Health Sciences, University of California Davis, Davis, California, United States of America, **4** Department of Neurobiology, Physiology, and Behavior, University of California Davis, Davis, California, United States of America

Abstract

Purpose: Measures of cardiorespiratory fitness (CRF) and heart rate recovery (HRR) can improve risk stratification for cardiovascular disease, but these measurements are rarely made in asymptomatic individuals due to cost. An exercise field test (EFT) to assess CRF and HRR would be an inexpensive method for cardiovascular disease risk assessment in large populations. This study assessed 1) the predictive accuracy of a 12-minute run/walk EFT for estimating CRF ($\dot{V}O_{2peak}$) and 2) the accuracy of HRR measured after an EFT using a heart rate monitor (HRM) in an asymptomatic population.

Methods: Fifty subjects (48% women) ages 18–45 years completed a symptom-limited exercise tolerance test (ETT) (Bruce protocol) and an EFT on separate days. During the ETT, $\dot{V}O_{2peak}$ was measured by a metabolic cart, and heart rate was measured continuously by a HRM and a metabolic cart.

Results: EFT distance and sex independently predicted $\dot{V}O_{2peak}$. The average absolute difference between observed and predicted $\dot{V}O_{2peak}$ was 0.26±3.27 ml·kg^{-1}·min^{-1} for our model compared to 7.55±3.64 ml·kg^{-1}·min^{-1} for the Cooper model. HRM HRR data were equivalent to respective metabolic cart values during the ETT. HRR at 1 minute post-exercise during ETT compared to the EFT had a moderate correlation ($r = 0.75$, $p < 0.001$).

Conclusion: A more accurate model to estimate CRF from a 12-minute run/walk EFT was developed, and HRR can be measured using a HRM in an asymptomatic population outside of clinical settings.

Editor: Vincenzo Lionetti, Scuola Superiore Sant'Anna, Italy

Funding: This project was supported by the National Center for Advancing Translational Sciences (NCATS), National Institutes of Health (NIH), through grant #UL1 TR000002, and by an institutional K30, 2 UL1 RR024146-06 in Davis, CA, USA. The funders had no role in study design, data collection and analysis, decision to publish, or preparation of the manuscript.

Competing Interests: The authors have declared that no competing interests exist.

* E-mail: dahawkins@ucdavis.edu

Introduction

Risk assessment is the foundation for primary prevention of future cardiovascular disease, yet attempts to evaluate the large population of asymptomatic individuals are limited [1,2]. Clinical exercise tolerance tests (ETTs) to quantitatively assess cardiorespiratory fitness (CRF) and heart rate recovery (HRR) post-exercise can improve risk stratification [3–5], but the expense of testing large populations [6,7] and low primary care utilization rates in young adults [8] limits clinical efforts for early risk detection. Exercise field tests (EFTs) completed while wearing commercial heart rate monitors (HRMs) may provide an inexpensive alternative for risk assessment in large populations, but improved CRF prediction models and validation of HRR measures are needed. A regression model, developed by Cooper in 1968 [7], has been widely used to estimate CRF (peak oxygen uptake ($\dot{V}O_{2peak}$)) for a 12-minute run/walk EFT, but the predictive accuracy of the model is dependent on the population being tested. In the original study, 115 male, military officers with an average age of 22 years (range 17 to 52) and a moderate range of $\dot{V}O_{2peak}$ values (31–59 ml·kg^{-1}·min^{-1}) and 12-minute run/walk distances (1770–3218 m) were tested [9]. Application of the Cooper model in similar populations of moderately fit men has yielded accurate estimates of CRF [10–13]; however, CRF predictions are often underestimated when the model has been used for women or subjects with lower fitness levels [11,14,15]. Development of a model based on a diverse range of fitness levels that includes subject characteristics (e.g. age, sex, and body composition) [16,17], therefore, may improve CRF estimates. In addition, use of a HRM during the EFT affords continuous and accurate measurement of heart rate in response to exercise and during recovery. The validity of HRR measured by a HRM outside of clinical settings, however, has not been examined. The purposes of this study were to 1) develop a CRF (peak oxygen uptake ($\dot{V}O_{2peak}$)) prediction model applicable to both men and women with a greater fitness range than the Cooper model [9] and 2) evaluate the accuracy of HRR during a 12-minute run/walk EFT in an asymptomatic, low-risk population.

Methods

Ethics Statement

The University of California, Davis Institutional Review Board approved the protocol, and all subjects gave written informed consent.

Participants

Participants, age 18–45 years were screened and were excluded if a moderate or high risk for a cardiovascular event during exercise was identified [18]. This population was considered because it includes a portion of the people we hope to be able to screen in large numbers to identify those warranting physician consultation and possible additional risk stratification. A total of 26 men and 24 women were enrolled (Table 1). No specific criteria were used ensure a diversity in fitness levels of the subject population, but efforts were made to enroll subjects with an even distribution of activity levels ranging from sedentary to very active. Sample size was based on the desired width of confidence intervals for parameters in the regression model to predict $\dot{V}O_{2peak}$. In this approach, the probability, Υ, that the confidence interval (at level α) will be no wider than twice a desired half-width w was specified [19]. We selected $\Upsilon = 0.8$, $\alpha = 0.05$, and $w = 0.3$. We assumed the highest correlation between predictor variables did not exceed 0.7, and the final R^2 of the model would be approximately 0.7, a conservative estimate compared to previous correlations [9]. A minimum sample size of 45 subjects was required to achieve these specifications for any given parameter estimate. Additional subjects were recruited to account for subject drop-out.

Protocol

Each subject completed an ETT and then an EFT on separate days with at least a 48 hour interval and no more than 2 weeks between sessions. The ETT was conducted first to allow investigators to continuously monitor the subject in a controlled environment and ensure that the subject could safely complete the subsequent EFT without any adverse events. Subjects were instructed to not vary their physical activity levels between sessions. Subjects were asked to refrain from eating or drinking food or caffeine within three hours of testing. Physical exercise and use of alcohol were prohibited on the day prior to and the day of testing. Prior to testing, age predicted maximum heart rate (HR_{max}) was calculated for each subject [20]. Subjects' height and mass were measured to the nearest 0.5 cm and 0.1 kg, respectively, and body mass index (BMI) was calculated as mass (kg) divided by height (meters, [m]) squared. Before each session, subjects were fitted with a commercially available HRM (Polar Coded 31 Transmitter and OEM module, Polar Electro Oy, Kempele, Finland), and resting blood pressure and heart rate were assessed to screen for contraindications to ETT.

Participants performed a symptom-limited ETT by the Bruce protocol [21] on a motorized treadmill until volitional exhaustion. Symptoms, heart rate, and blood pressure (measured by arm-cuff sphygmomanometry) were recorded during the last minute of each exercise stage, at test termination (peak exercise), and 1 and 2 minutes into recovery, which comprised a controlled walk at 3.2 km per hour and a 0 percent grade. Ventilation and gas exchange were measured (TrueOne 2400 Metabolic Measurement System, Parvo Medics, Sandy, UT) and reported as the mean value per 15-second epoch. Criteria for maximal oxygen consumption rate ($\dot{V}O_{2peak}$) (i.e. respiratory exchange ratio > 1.1 and HR_{max} within 10 beats of age-predicted reference value) were achieved in most subjects; however, a plateau of oxygen consumption rate was not observed in all cases [22]. Therefore, the highest 15-second mean value of oxygen consumption ($\dot{V}O_{2peak}$) was determined and used in subsequent analyses. Respiratory exchange variables were used to estimate energy expenditure per minute and metabolic equivalents (METs) [23]. Heart rate was measured continuously by the HRM and as a mean value per 15-second epoch by a Polar receiver module connected to the metabolic cart. HR_{max} was defined as the heart rate value obtained at peak exercise. HRR at 1- and 2-minutes were defined as the reduction in heart rate from HR_{max} to 1 minute and 2 minutes after cessation of exercise, respectively.

Subjects completed an EFT outdoors on either a rubberized running track or hard dirt trail. They were instructed to run the maximum tolerated distance in 12 minutes. Most subjects completed the test while running; however, two subjects walked intermittently. Verbal cues of the remaining test time were called out after the first lap, halfway, and with one minute remaining. Upon test completion, total distance to the nearest 100 m mark was recorded, and the subject walked at a self-selected pace for at least 5 minutes in recovery. HRM data were used to determine HR_{max} and HRR values.

Statistical Analysis

All statistical analyses were performed in SAS (version 9.3, SAS Institute, Cary, NC). Means and standard deviations were calculated for subject demographics and exercise parameters. Differences between sexes were assessed using t-tests with significance defined as $p<0.05$. A general linear model was fit by using the EFT data and the SAS software procedure GLM to predict $\dot{V}O_{2peak}$. Hypothesized predictors of $\dot{V}O_{2peak}$ included distance, sex, HR_{max}, age, and BMI. Backward selection was conducted with the goal of minimizing the prediction error as measured by the predicted residual sum of squares (PRESS) statistic. Significance was defined at $p<0.05$. The model was validated using leave-one-out cross validation, and the PRESS statistic was calculated to compare prediction accuracy between models. As Cooper's model was not derived from our sample, two approaches were used to obtain an estimate of the prediction error. First, the sum of squared prediction errors was calculated for Cooper's model. Second, we re-fit Cooper's model to our sample (i.e. only distance was used to predict relative $\dot{V}O_{2peak}$) to obtain a PRESS estimate. The PRESS statistic or sum of square prediction errors, root mean square error (RMSE), and Pearson correlation coefficients for the new model, the re-fit model, and Cooper's model were compared. Predictions from the new model were compared to those produced using Cooper's model to assess bias (under- or over-estimation), prediction error (observed – predicted), and the associated standard deviation. The degree of agreement between HR_{max} and HRR values obtained by (1) the metabolic cart and HRM during the ETT and (2) the HRM during the ETT and EFT were assessed. The difference in means was used to estimate bias, and Pearson correlation coefficients were calculated as a measure of relative reliability. To obtain objective measures of agreement, equivalency tests were conduct-

Table 1. Demographic, resting, and exercise parameters of participants.

	Men	Women	p
Age (years)	28.9±7.6	31.0±7.4	=.3335
Height (m)	1.78±0.62	1.63±0.65	<.0001
Mass (kg)	78.0±8.8	59.4±8.2	<.0001
BMI ($kg \cdot m^{-2}$)	24.5±2.1	22.2±2.4	=.0008
Resting			
Heart Rate (bpm)	68.4±13.3	71.3±12.9	=.4429
Systolic Blood Pressure (mmHg)	119.0±9.7	110.5±8.7	=.0020
Diastolic Blood Pressure (mmHg)	74.2±8.9	72.4±11.8	=.5398
Exercise Tolerance Test			
Exercise Time (min)	13.5±1.9	11.2±1.7	<.0001
$\dot{V}O_{2peak}$ ($L \cdot min^{-1}$)	4.38±0.72	2.68±0.64	<.0001
$\dot{V}O_{2peak}$ ($ml \cdot kg^{-1} \cdot min^{-1}$)	56.3±8.2	45.1±7.4	<.0001
Total METs	16.1±2.3	12.9±2.1	<.0001
Exercise Field Test			
Distance (m)	2700±400	2200±400	<.0001

Mean ± one standard deviation are reported.
BMI body mass index, *bpm* beats per minute, *METs* metabolic equivalents, $\dot{V}O_{2peak}$ peak oxygen uptake.

ed using the SAS software procedure TTEST with the two one-sided tests (TOST) option with upper and lower bounds specified at ±6 beats per minute (bpm). These equivalency limits were based on a previous study reporting that heart rates measured by a Polar HRM and electrocardiogram equipment were within 6 bpm [24]. The validity of the normality assumption was assessed using histograms and QQ plots of the residuals.

Results

The general physical and physiological characteristics of the subjects tested were unremarkable. There were significant differences between men and women in height ($p<.0001$), body mass ($p<.0001$), BMI ($p = 0.0008$), and resting systolic blood pressure ($p = 0.0020$) (Table 1). There was no difference in age ($p = 0.33$) between the sexes. Men achieved greater performance than women during the ETT and EFT as indicated by the exercise time ($p<.0001$), $\dot{V}O_{2peak}$ ($p<.0001$), total METs achieved ($p<.0001$), and distance completed ($p<.0001$).

Prediction of $\dot{V}O_{2peak}$ from a 12-Minute Run/Walk Exercise Field Test

Our final model that minimized the prediction error of $\dot{V}O_{2peak}$ from a 12-minute run/walk included distance ($p<.0001$) and sex ($p = 0.0281$) and had lower prediction errors than the re-fit Cooper model and the Cooper model (Table 2). There was insufficient evidence that HR_{max} ($p = 0.96$), age ($p = 0.42$), and BMI ($p = 0.30$) improved the performance of our model. Our model (expressed by two equations, one for men and one for women), the re-fit Cooper model, and the original Cooper model are reported in Equations 1-4 and Table 3).

Our model for men (Equation 1):

$$\dot{V}O_{2peak} = (1.82X10^{-2}) \bullet \text{distance} + 7.514$$

Our model for women (Equation 2):

$$\dot{V}O_{2peak} = (1.82X10^{-2}) \bullet \text{distance} + 4.998$$

Re-fit Cooper model (Equation 3):

$$\dot{V}O_{2peak} = (1.97X10^{-2}) \bullet \text{distance} + 2.703$$

Original Cooper model (9) (Equation 4):

$$\dot{V}O_{2peak} = (2.23X10^{-2}) \bullet \text{distance} - 11.288$$

$\dot{V}O_{2peak}$ and distance are expressed in $ml \cdot kg^{-1} \cdot min^{-1}$ and meters respectively.

Predicted $\dot{V}O_{2peak}$values determined from our model and the Cooper model were compared with observed $\dot{V}O_{2peak}$ values (Figure 1). The Cooper model demonstrated a consistent downward bias and underestimated $\dot{V}O_{2peak}$ by an average of 7.55 ± 3.64 $ml \cdot kg^{-1} \cdot min^{-1}$. The underestimation of $\dot{V}O_{2peak}$ was most pronounced at the lower levels of CRF (Figure 1). The average absolute differences between observed and predicted

Table 2. PRESS statistic, RMSE, and correlation coefficients for our model, the re-fit Cooper model, and the Cooper model.

	PRESS	RMSE ($ml \cdot kg^{-1} \cdot min^{-1}$)	Correlation (r)
Our Model	595.6	3.45	0.88
Re-fit Cooper Model	636.4	3.57	0.87
Cooper Model	3498*	8.36	0.90

The correlation coefficient reported for the Cooper model was based on the original study [7].
PRESS predicted residual sum of squares, *RMSE* root mean square prediction error.
* Sum of squared prediction errors was used rather than PRESS for Cooper's model as the error was not based on a fitted model.

$\dot{V}O_{2peak}$ values using our model indicate a slight underestimation of 0.26 ± 3.27 $ml \cdot kg^{-1} \cdot min^{-1}$.

Comparison of Heart Rate Recovery between an Exercise Tolerance Test and a 12-minute Run/Walk Exercise Field Test

HR_{max} and 1- and 2-minute HRR measured by the metabolic cart demonstrated a strong relationship and were equivalent within 6 bpm of the same values measured by the HRM (Table 4). HR_{max} at the time of the ETT and EFT both measured by the HRM were equivalent (Table 5). HRR at 1- and 2-minutes were outside the specified equivalency limits; however, correlation coefficients demonstrate a moderate relationship between the ETT and EFT values (Table 5).

Discussion

Traditional methods for risk stratification for cardiovascular death are improved with inclusion of measures of both CRF and HRR [4], thus, low-cost methods to assess CRF and HRR in large populations outside of clinical settings may enable early risk detection for cardiovascular disease and identify asymptomatic individuals in need of additional clinical risk evaluations. In this study, we developed a CRF ($\dot{V}O_{2peak}$) prediction model applicable to both men and women with a greater fitness range than the Cooper model [9] and evaluated the accuracy of HRR during a 12-minute run/walk EFT in an asymptomatic, low-risk population. Our linear model includes sex and distance achieved during a 12-minute run/walk EFT to predict $\dot{V}O_{2peak}$. Our model improved accuracy for women and subjects with low CRF compared to the Cooper model (Figure 1) suggesting that it may be a useful method for screening for cardiovascular disease risk. We also demonstrated that a HRM is a valid tool to assess HRR. Lastly, we found that there was insufficient agreement of HRR values for ETT and EFT obtained by a HRM for interchangeable use. These differences, however, may be attributable to variations in test conditions and day-to-day variations in HRR and highlight a need to determine the effect of this variability on HRR prognostic criteria.

Prediction of $\dot{V}O_{2peak}$ from a 12-Minute Run/Walk Exercise Field Test

The improved predictive accuracy of our CRF model over the Cooper model [9] is likely due to differences in the populations studied. While the mean of $\dot{V}O_{2peak}$ for our study population was above average (> 90th percentile based on the average age) [25], there was sufficient variability in fitness to expand the range of $\dot{V}O_{2peak}$ (31–72.7 $ml \cdot kg^{-1} \cdot min^{-1}$) and 12-minute run/walk distances (1561–3798 m) compared to the Cooper study [9]. As our population included not only a wider range of fitness levels, but also both sexes, it is not surprising that Cooper's model underestimated $\dot{V}O_{2peak}$ values in our population, a finding consistent with previous studies [11,14,15]. CRF is known to be greater in men than women due to differences in cardiac output and arterial-venous oxygen difference [26,27]. Therefore, the inclusion of sex as an independent predictor of $\dot{V}O_{2peak}$ is an important improvement to the CRF prediction model to control for this source of variability. The clinical utility of an EFT is the identification of patients with low CRF and autonomic dysfunction as evidenced by low HRR, a population at increased cardiovascular risk [4]. Given that our model differentiates between sex and improved predictive accuracy in women and those with low CRF, it has the potential to be a useful tool for screening of pre-clinical cardiovascular disease.

Table 3. Standard errors and p values for our model and the re-fit Cooper model developed to predict relative $\dot{V}O_{2peak}$ ($ml \cdot kg^{-1} \cdot min^{-1}$) from a 12-minute run/walk EFT.

	Our Model		Re-fit Cooper Model	
	SE	p	SE	p
Intercept	2.788	=.0795	2.707	=.323
Distance	1.981	<.001	1.753	<.001
Sex (male/female)	1.110	=.0281	-	-

SE standard error.

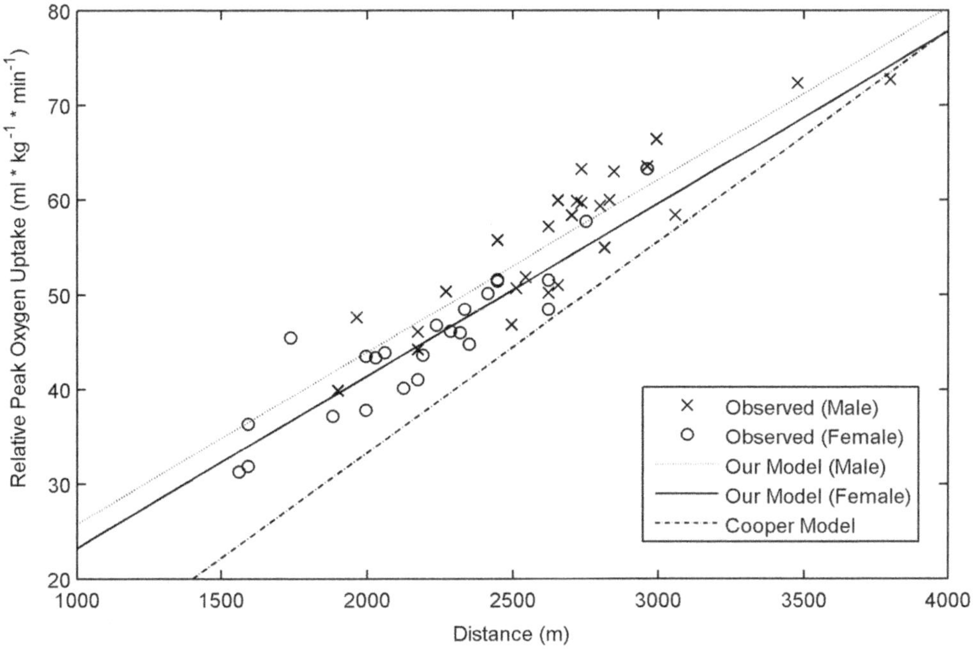

Figure 1. Comparison of observed $\dot{V}O_{2peak}$ values to our model and the Cooper model. Our model was plotted for males and females. The Cooper model underestimated observed $\dot{V}O_{2peak}$ in all but one male subject and demonstrated increased error with decreased 12-minute run/walk distance.

Comparison of Heart Rate Recovery between an Exercise Tolerance Test and a 12-minute Run/Walk Exercise Field Test

HRR values for ETT and EFT obtained by a HRM had insufficient agreement for interchangeable use. Preference for a slower recovery speed following the EFT may have increased HRR values in some subjects. HRR cut-off values have been demonstrated to vary by 6 bpm between active and passive recoveries [28]. Standardization of recovery in the resting supine position in our protocol, therefore, could have improved the equivalency of HRR values between the ETT and EFT. Further, variation in HRR between successive symptom-limited exercise tests is not well established, and the equivalency bounds may have been too restrictive. This concept is supported by a previous HRR reliability study that reported standard errors of approximately 10 bpm for two maximal exercise tests completed within 72 hours [29]. Variation in day-to-day HRR may result from external factors known to affect heart rate (e.g. time of day, ambient temperature, mental stress, and hydration status) [30], but it is difficult to minimize the effect of these variables during exercise testing.

The ease of administering an EFT with a commercial heart rate monitor may improve accuracy and precision of HRR measurement to alleviate some of these issues. Imai and colleagues [31] demonstrated that parasympathetic reactivation is greatest in the first 30 seconds of recovery with rapid declines observed in athletes. The continuous measurement ability of the HRM can assess this rapid change and could increase the sensitivity of HRR calculations compared to clinical systems that use data averaging or smoothing algorithms. Further, the low-cost nature of an EFT permits the test to be performed serially. An average of multiple HRR values could mitigate the effect of day-to-day variations on HRR prognostic reliability.

Limitations

Testing a population with greater diversity than tested here and in previous studies (e.g. age, BMI, health status) is a logical next step to refine and increase the applicability of an EFT CRF model

Table 4. Heart rate parameters obtained by the metabolic cart and HRM during the ETT (means ± SD), correlation between metabolic cart and HRM, bias, and two one-sided test (TOST) equivalency limits.

Parameter	Metabolic Cart	HRM	Correlation (r)	Bias	TOST 95% Equivalency Limits	Equivalent
HR_{max} (bpm)	187±8.6	190±8.9	0.99 (p<.001)	−2.50	−2.17 to −2.82	Yes
HRR1 (bpm)	23±8.4	27±9.4	0.92 (p<.001)	−4.34	−3.49 to −5.19	Yes
HRR2 (bpm)	44±13.1	48±12.5	0.97 (p<.001)	−3.86	−3.06 to −4.66	Yes

Upper and lower equivalency bounds were defined as 6 bpm.
Bias: Difference between metabolic cart and HRM parameters.
BPM beats per minute, *HRM* heart rate monitor, HR_{max} maximum heart rate, *HRR1* heart rate recovery at 1 minute post-exercise, *HRR2* heart rate recovery at 2 minutes post-exercise, *TOST* two one-sided test.

Table 5. Heart rate parameters obtained by the HRM during the ETT and EFT (means ± SD), correlation between ETT and EFT, bias, and two one-sided test (TOST) equivalency limits.

Parameter	ETT	EFT	Correlation (r)	Bias	TOST 95% Equivalency Limits	Equivalent
HR_{max} (bpm)	190±8.9	193±9.2	0.74 (p<.001)	−3.13	−4.68 to − 1.59	Yes
HRR1 (bpm)	27±9.4	33±10.1	0.75 (p<.001)	−6.12	−7.75 to −4.49	No
HRR2 (bpm)	48±12.5	52±12.7	0.68 (p<.001)	−3.90	−6.31 to −1.49	No

Upper and lower equivalency bounds were defined as 6 bpm.
Bias: Difference between ETT and EFT parameters.
RPM beats per minute, *EFT* exercise field test, *ETT* exercise treadmill test, HR_{max} maximum heart rate, *HRR1* heart rate recovery at 1 minute post-exercise, *HRR2* heart rate recovery at 2 minutes post-exercise, *TOST* two one-sided test.

and to assess the prognostic value of EFT HRR. The population tested in this study was more diverse than Cooper's but otherwise had little variance in age and BMI, or other variables that are known to affect CRF [32,33] and are significant in prediction models developed for shorter field tests [16,17]. Expansion of this study's testing protocol to a more diverse population is necessary to adequately distinguish the influence of these variables on $\dot{V}O_{2peak}$ in the EFT. It should also be appreciated that a 12-minute run/walk EFT is not appropriate for all individuals. We believe that persons with functional limitations that impair their ability to walk or run, or with poor exercise capacity, or symptoms of cardiac ischemia would be poor candidates for an EFT. Such patients could be identified by a tool such as the Duke Activity Status Index as is the case for pre-operative surgical evaluation [34,35]. For people with sufficient exercise capacity, the EFT may provide a valuable screening alternative for some clinical populations due to the ability of our model to predict exercise capacity (i.e. $\dot{V}O_{2peak}$) better than previous models in subjects with low CRF. HRR assessments were made using intra-individual comparisons thereby reducing population effects; however, selection of a healthy population rather than patients referred for clinical indications limited assessment of the prognostic value of HRR.

Conclusions

A 12-minute run/walk EFT completed while wearing a HRM was demonstrated as an effective method to estimate CRF and measure HRR. Linear regression models for men and women were developed to predict $\dot{V}O_{2peak}$ from 12-minute run/walk distance in an asymptomatic population between 18–45 years of age. These models are more accurate than the commonly used Cooper model. In addition, HRMs capable of continuously measuring heart rate were shown to accurately assess HRR compared to clinical equipment. Use of this technology with the completion of multiple EFTs could improve the accuracy and precision of HRR measurements. Collectively, these findings indicate that field-based evaluations of CRF and HRR are feasible and warrant further investigation as an inexpensive approach to screen and monitor cardiovascular disease risk in large asymptomatic populations.

Acknowledgments

The authors would like to thank the study participants. We would also like to express our gratitude to Barbara Gale, MS, Brent Twiford, Kody Simpson, Kendra Sellers, and Christine Finnigan for their assistance with data collection.

Author Contributions

Conceived and designed the experiments: CLC IBA MDW DAH EAA. Performed the experiments: CLC IBA DAH. Analyzed the data: CLC IBA MDW DAH EAA. Contributed reagents/materials/analysis tools: CLC IBA MDW DAH. Wrote the paper: CLC IBA MDW DAH EAA.

References

1. Pasternak RC, Abrams J, Greenland P, Smaha LA, Wilson PW, et al. (2003) Task force# 1—identification of coronary heart disease risk: is there a detection gap? J Am Coll Cardiol 41: 1863–1874.
2. Greenland P, Smith SC Jr, Grundy SM (2001) Improving Coronary Heart Disease Risk Assessment in Asymptomatic People Role of Traditional Risk Factors and Noninvasive Cardiovascular Tests. Circulation 104: 1863–1867. doi:10.1161/hc4201.097189.
3. Shetler K, Marcus R, Froelicher VF, Vora S, Kalisetti D, et al. (2001) Heart rate recovery: validation and methodologic issues. J Am Coll Cardiol 38: 1980–1987. doi:10.1016/S0735-1097(01)01652-7.
4. Mora S, Redberg RF, Sharrett AR, Blumenthal RS (2005) Enhanced risk assessment in asymptomatic individuals with exercise testing and Framingham risk scores. Circulation 112: 1566–1572.
5. Kokkinos P, Myers J, Doumas M, Faselis C, Pittaras A, et al. (2012) Heart rate recovery, exercise capacity, and mortality risk in male veterans. Eur J Prev Cardiol 19: 177–184. doi:10.1177/1741826711398432.
6. Fowler-Brown A, Pignone M, Pletcher M, Tice JA, Sutton SF, et al. (2004) Exercise tolerance testing to screen for coronary heart disease: a systematic review for the technical support for the US Preventive Services Task Force. Ann Intern Med 140: W–9.
7. Lauer M, Froelicher ES, Williams M, Kligfield P (2005) Exercise Testing in Asymptomatic Adults A Statement for Professionals From the American Heart Association Council on Clinical Cardiology, Subcommittee on Exercise, Cardiac Rehabilitation, and Prevention. Circulation 112: 771–776. doi:10.1161/CIRCULATIONAHA.105.166543.
8. Cherry D, Lucas C, Decker S (2010) Population aging and the use of office-based physician services. NCHS data brief. Hyattsville, MD: National Center for Health Statistics. Available: http://www.cdc.gov/nchs/data/databriefs/db41.htm#fig1. Accessed 2013 September 13.
9. Cooper KH (1968) A means of assessing maximal oxygen intake. Correlation between field and treadmill testing. JAMA 203: 201–204.
10. Burke EJ (1976) Validity of Selected Lab and Field Tests of Physical Working Capacity. Available: http://www.eric.ed.gov/ERICWebPortal/detail?accno=ED100839. Accessed 2013 June 27.
11. McCutcheon MC, Sticha SA, Giese MD, Nagle FJ (1990) A further analysis of the 12-minute run prediction of maximal aerobic power. Res Q Exerc Sport 61: 280–283.
12. Grant S, Corbett K, Amjad AM, Wilson J, Aitchison T (1995) A comparison of methods of predicting maximum oxygen uptake. Br J Sports Med 29: 147–152.
13. McNaughton L, Hall P, Cooley D (1998) Validation of several methods of estimating maximal oxygen uptake in young men. Percept Mot Skills 87: 575–584.
14. Katch FI, McArdle WD, Pechar GS, Czula R (1973) Maximal Oxygen Intake, Endurance Running Performance, and Body Composition in College Women. Res Q Am Assoc Health Phys Educ Recreat 44: 301–312. doi:10.1080/10671188.1973.10615208.

15. Maksud MG, Cannistra C, Dublinski D (1976) Energy Expenditure and VO2 Max of Female Athletes during Treadmill Exercise. Res Q Am Alliance Health Phys Educ Recreat 47: 692–697. doi:10.1080/10671315.1976.10616730.
16. Cahalin LP, Mathier MA, Semigran MJ, Dec GW, DiSalvo TG (1996) The six-minute walk test predicts peak oxygen uptake and survival in patients with advanced heart failure. CHEST J 110: 325–332. doi:10.1378/chest.110.2.325.
17. Cureton K, Sloniger M, O'Bannon J, Black D, McCormack W (1995) A generalized equation for prediction of VO2peak from 1-mile run/walk performance. Med Sci Sports Exerc 27: 445–451.
18. Balady GJ, Chaitman B, Driscoll D, Foster C, Froelicher E, et al. (1998) Recommendations for Cardiovascular Screening, Staffing, and Emergency Policies at Health/Fitness Facilities. Circulation 97: 2283–2293. doi:10.1161/01.CIR.97.22.2283.
19. Kelley K, Maxwell SE (2003) Sample Size for Multiple Regression: Obtaining Regression Coefficients That Are Accurate, Not Simply Significant. Psychol Methods 8: 305–321. http://dx.doi.org/ doi:10.1037/1082-989X.8.3.305.
20. Gellish RL, Goslin BR, Olson RE, McDonald A, Russi GD, et al. (2007) Longitudinal Modeling of the Relationship between Age and Maximal Heart Rate. Med Sci Sports Exerc 39: 822–829. doi:10.1097/mss.0b013e31803349c6.
21. Bruce RA, Kusumi F, Hosmer D (1973) Maximal oxygen intake and nomographic assessment of functional aerobic impairment in cardiovascular disease. Am Heart J 85: 546–562.
22. Howley ET, Bassett DR Jr, Welch HG (1995) Criteria for maximal oxygen uptake: review and commentary. Med Sci Sports Exerc 27: 1292–1301.
23. Weir JB de V (1949) New methods for calculating metabolic rate with special reference to protein metabolism. J Physiol 109: 1–9.
24. Godsen R, Carroll T, Stone S (1991) How well does the Polar Vantage XL heart rate monitor estimate actual heart rate. Med Sci Sports Exerc 23: 14.
25. American College of Sports Medicine (2010) ACSM's guidelines for exercise testing and prescription. 8th ed. Philadelphia, PA: Lippincott Williams & Wilkins, Philadelphia.
26. Cureton K, Bishop P, Hutchinson P, Newland H, Vickery S, et al. (1986) Sex difference in maximal oxygen uptake. Effect of equating haemoglobin concentration. Eur J Appl Physiol 54: 656–660.
27. Hutchinson PL, Cureton KJ, Outz H, Wilson G (1991) Relationship of cardiac size to maximal oxygen uptake and body size in men and women. Int J Sports Med 369: 373.
28. Vivekananthan DP, Blackstone EH, Pothier CE, Lauer MS (2003) Heart rate recovery after exercise is apredictor of mortality, independent of the angiographic severity of coronary disease. J Am Coll Cardiol 42: 831–838. doi:10.1016/S0735-1097(03)00833-7.
29. Bosquet L, Gamelin F-X, Berthoin S (2008) Reliability of Postexercise Heart Rate Recovery. Int J Sports Med 29: 238–243. doi:10.1055/s-2007-965162.
30. Valentini M, Parati G (2009) Variables Influencing Heart Rate. Prog Cardiovasc Dis 52: 11–19. doi:10.1016/j.pcad.2009.05.004.
31. Imai K, Sato H, Hori M, Kusuoka H, Ozaki H, et al. (1994) Vagally mediated heart rate recovery after exercise is accelerated in athletes but blunted in patients with chronic heart failure. J Am Coll Cardiol 24: 1529–1535. doi:10.1016/0735-1097(94)90150-3.
32. Hossack KF, Bruce RA (1982) Maximal cardiac function in sedentary normal men and women: comparison of age-related changes. J Appl Physiol 53: 799–804.
33. Buskirk E, Taylor HL (1957) Maximal Oxygen Intake and Its Relation to Body Composition, With Special Reference to Chronic Physical Activity and Obesity. J Appl Physiol 11: 72–78.
34. Fleischmann KE, Beckman JA, Buller CE, Calkins H, Fleisher LA, et al. (2009) 2009 ACCF/AHA Focused Update on Perioperative Beta Blockade. J Am Coll Cardiol 54: 2102–2128. doi:10.1016/j.jacc.2009.07.004.
35. Nelson CL, Herndon JE, Mark DB, Pryor DB, Califf RM, et al. (1991) Relation of clinical and angiographic factors to functional capacity as measured by the Duke Activity Status Index. Am J Cardiol 68: 973–975. doi:10.1016/0002-9149(91)90423-I.

2

Activity Monitor Intervention to Promote Physical Activity of Physicians-In-Training: Randomized Controlled Trial

Anne N. Thorndike[1]*, Sarah Mills[1], Lillian Sonnenberg[2], Deepak Palakshappa[1], Tian Gao[1], Cindy T. Pau[1], Susan Regan[1]

1 Department of Medicine, Massachusetts General Hospital, Boston, Massachusetts, United States of America, **2** Food and Nutrition Services, Massachusetts General Hospital, Boston, Massachusetts, United States of America

Abstract

Background: Physicians are expected to serve as role models for healthy lifestyles, but long work hours reduce time for healthy behaviors. A hospital-based physical activity intervention could improve physician health and increase counseling about exercise.

Methods: We conducted a two-phase intervention among 104 medical residents at a large hospital in Boston, Massachusetts. Phase 1 was a 6-week randomized controlled trial comparing daily steps of residents assigned to an activity monitor displaying feedback about steps and energy consumed (intervention) or to a blinded monitor (control). Phase 2 immediately followed and was a 6-week non-randomized team steps competition in which all participants wore monitors with feedback. Phase 1 outcomes were: 1) median steps/day and 2) proportion of days activity monitor worn. The Phase 2 outcome was mean steps/day on days monitor worn (≥500 steps/day). Physiologic measurements were collected at baseline and study end. Median steps/day were compared using Wilcoxon rank-sum tests. Mean steps were compared using repeated measures regression analyses.

Results: In Phase 1, intervention and control groups had similar activity (6369 vs. 6063 steps/day, $p = 0.16$) and compliance with wearing the monitor (77% vs. 77% of days, $p = 0.73$). In Phase 2 (team competition), residents recorded more steps/day than during Phase 1 (Control: 7,971 vs. 7,567, $p = 0.002$; Intervention: 7,832 vs. 7,739, $p = 0.13$). Mean compliance with wearing the activity monitor decreased for both groups during Phase 2 compared to Phase 1 (60% vs. 77%, $p < 0.001$). Mean systolic blood pressure decreased ($p = 0.004$) and HDL cholesterol increased ($p < 0.001$) among all participants at end of study compared to baseline.

Conclusions: Although the activity monitor intervention did not have a major impact on activity or health, the high participation rates of busy residents and modest changes in steps, blood pressure, and HDL suggest that more intensive hospital-based wellness programs have potential for promoting healthier lifestyles among physicians.

Trial Registration: Clinicaltrials.gov NCT01287208.

Editor: Naoyuki Hayashi, Tokyo Institute of Technology, Japan

Funding: Dr. Thorndike is supported by the grant K23 HL93221 from the National Institutes of Health/National Heart Lung and Blood Institute. The funders had no role in study design, data collection and analysis, decision to publish, or preparation of the manuscript.

Competing Interests: The authors have declared that no competing interests exist.

* E-mail: athorndike@partners.org

Introduction

A growing body of evidence suggests that poor physician health is associated with suboptimal patient care. [1–4] "Physician wellness" has typically been described in the context of mental health, [5–7] with less attention to the positive aspects of health promotion. [8,9] Physicians are expected to serve as role models for healthy lifestyles, [10] and evidence suggests that physicians are more likely to counsel when they practice these behaviors themselves. [11–14] However, many physicians do not take the time to care for themselves, [6,15–19] and long work hours reduce time for healthy behaviors. [6,17,20,21] Lack of sleep, stress, and intense interactions with patients contribute to burnout, substance abuse, and depression [2,6,22].

Regular physical activity helps prevent obesity and chronic disease [23] and is associated with reduced psychological symptoms, including depression, anxiety, and burnout symptoms. [24–27] Residency is a period when time-constraints are particularly acute, and symptoms of burnout and depression are high. [2,28,29] One survey of residents found that self-care activities, including exercise, were associated with the absence of burnout. [30] However, residents are less likely to exercise regularly than medical students or attendings, [21,31] and a survey of radiology residents found that only 37% engaged in recommended guidelines for physical activity. [20] A study of military physicians found that physical fitness declined and weight increased during residency training, [32] and a study of 375 residents from two academic medical centers found that third year medical residents were more likely to be overweight than first year residents [33].

Promoting physical activity among residents could help establish a pattern of healthy lifestyle during and after residency [34] as well as reduce depression and burnout. Physical activity interventions that use pedometers or activity monitors can be effective among healthy, working populations. [35–37] We conducted a 2-phase study over 12 weeks to determine if use of an activity monitor as part of a resident wellness program would result in increased physical activity levels. We hypothesized that 1) residents who were randomly assigned to an activity monitor with visual feedback would have higher physical activity levels as measured in steps per day compared to residents assigned to a blinded monitor and 2) conducting a team-based steps competition would increase activity levels of residents compared to the non-competition phase. Phase 1 was a randomized controlled trial, and Phase 2 was a team-based steps competition.

Methods

Ethics Statement

This study was approved by the Partners Healthcare Institutional Review Board on June 28, 2010. Written informed consent was obtained from all study subjects upon enrollment. The authors confirm that all ongoing and related trials for this intervention are registered. This study is registered at Clinicaltrials.gov NCT01287208. The study was registered after all subjects were enrolled but prior to the intervention. The registration delay was due to a misunderstanding by the investigator. The study protocol that was registered was exactly the same as the study protocol approved by the Institutional Review Board prior to subject enrollment. Subjects were recruited starting in July 2010 and follow-up was completed in May 2011. The protocol for this trial and supporting CONSORT checklist are available as supporting information; see Checklist S1 and Protocol S1.

Setting and Participants

Massachusetts General Hospital (MGH) is a 907 bed teaching hospital in Boston, Massachusetts. Since 2005, the hospital has offered a ten week team-based, worksite wellness program called "Be Fit" at no cost to employees, [38,39] but medical residents have not been able to participate because of their intense work schedules. The current study was developed as a wellness program for residents that would be both convenient and fun and therefore not perceived as burdensome.

During the academic year from July 2010 through June 2011, there were 169 Internal Medicine and Medicine/Pediatric residents employed at the hospital. From July through November 2010, 127 medicine residents participated in a required ambulatory rotation during which the study team conducted a one-hour session as part of the ambulatory curriculum to describe the exercise and nutrition program.

Exercise and Nutrition Program

During the 12 week study period from January through March 2011, all residents were given access to the on-site fitness center and could complete a one hour personal training session weekly at no cost. To address nutrition, a "Be Fit" lunch prepared by the MGH Food and Nutrition Services was substituted once a week for one of the daily catered resident lunches at their noontime conference. Residents could schedule up to two individual appointments with one of the Be Fit staff nutritionists during the study period.

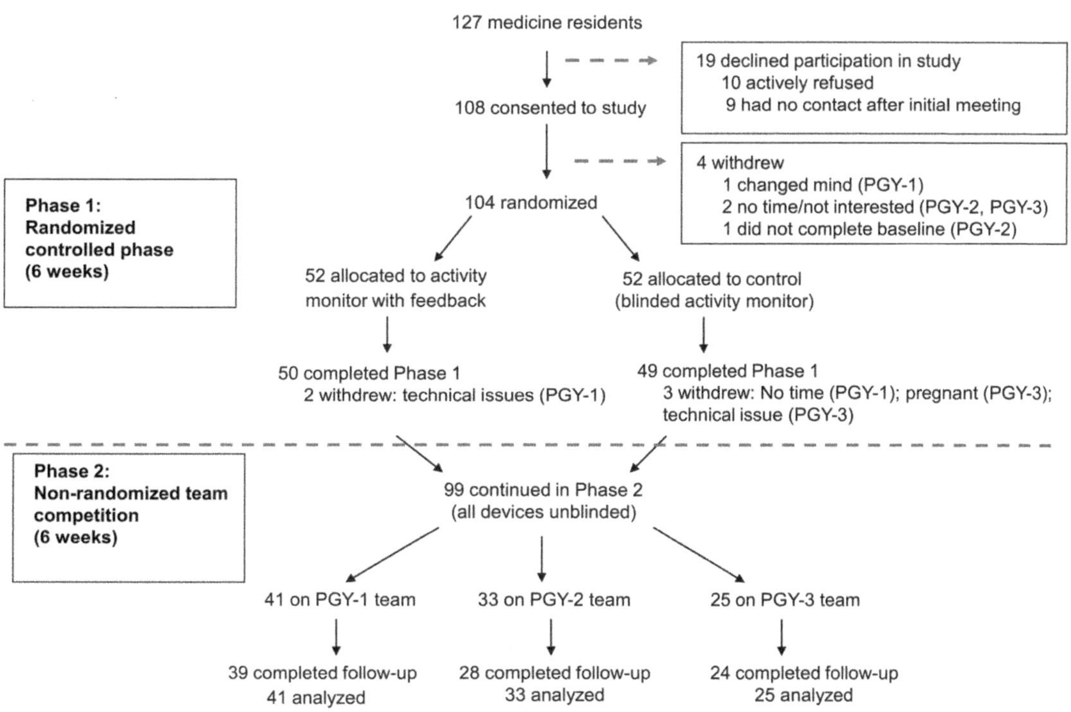

Figure 1. Study flow diagram.

Table 1. Baseline characteristics of residents.

	Total	Intervention	Control	P value
	(N = 104)	(N = 52)	(N = 52)	
Age, mean (range)	29 (23–37)	29 (23–36)	9 (25–37)	0.45
Sex, female, %	54	51	56	0.69
Race, white, %	66	66	65	0.95
Married/living with significant other, %	52	46	58	0.24
Body mass index, kg/m^2, mean (range)	24.1 (17.8–35.6)	23.7 (19.4–34.9)	24.6 (17.8–35.6)	0.23
Non-smoker, %	95	92	98	0.16
Reported gaining weight in past year, %	50	52	46	0.49

Activity Monitor

All study participants were provided with an activity monitor (Fitbit) that tracked daily activity and wirelessly uploaded the data to a website (http://www.fitbit.com). The Fitbit monitors are valid and reliable devices for monitoring step counts in healthy young adults. [40] The device was lightweight (11 grams) and could be worn clipped to the clothing or in a pocket. The monitor displayed steps, energy consumed, and distance traveled, and it also displayed an activity "avatar" that would grow larger with increasing activity and smaller with more sedentary behavior. The website allowed users to track their data over time, log daily weights, and enter dietary information to calculate daily caloric intake.

Phase 1 Intervention: Randomized Trial

Phase 1 of the intervention started at the beginning of January 2011 and lasted for six weeks. Half of residents were assigned to the activity monitor with visible data (intervention) and half were assigned to an identical activity monitor that was blinded and did not display data (control). Prior to Phase 1, all participants were simultaneously randomized to the intervention or control arm, stratifying by year of training. A random number was assigned to each subject using the built-in random number function in Microsoft Access. A list was created in which subjects were grouped by year of training and then sorted by the random number within each year. Study arm assignments were made by alternating allocation of the listed subjects to intervention or control. The study statistician generated the random allocation sequence. All participants were given a unique anonymous email address that was not connected to their work email and could be used to log on to the Fitbit website to set up an account and provide information on gender, age, height, and weight. Residents randomized to the intervention could log on to the website throughout Phase 1, but residents randomized to control were not able to log on to the website after the account was set up.

Study staff sent weekly emails to remind residents to charge the device and to offer an incentive for wearing it. Residents who wore the monitor at least five of seven days of the week were included in a lottery for a $10 gift card, and two winners were announced in the following week's email. Study staff monitored the Fitbit website to determine if the blinded monitors were functioning properly. Individual technical assistance was provided to residents as needed.

Phase 2 Intervention: Non-randomized Team Competition

At the end of Phase 1, residents in the control group were given instructions to unblind their devices so that the steps, calories, and distance would be visible and they could utilize the Fitbit website. Residents were divided into three teams based on year of training: post-graduate year one (PGY-1), post-graduate year two (PGY-2), and post-graduate year three or four (PGY-3). All participants were notified that their team would be competing for the highest average number of steps per week for six weeks. Each week, two residents from the winning team received a $10 gift card.

Measures and Outcomes

All residents participated in an assessment before and after the 12 week study. Baseline assessments were conducted between July and November 2010, and final assessments were conducted in April and May 2011. We offered four baseline and three follow-up assessment dates so that residents could choose a morning that they would not be post-overnight call. Assessments were performed between 6:30 am and 8:00 am so that subjects could

Table 2. Median steps per day and compliance with wearing activity monitor during the 6-week randomized phase.

	Intervention*	Control†	Difference	P value
	(N = 50)	(N = 49)		
Steps/day, median (IQR)	6369 (1999–8796)	6063 (1299–8723)	306	0.16
Number of days activity monitor worn, mean (%)	33.2 (77%)	33.0 (77%)	0.2	0.73
Steps/day on days monitor worn, mean (SD)	7886 (3622)	7600 (3492)	286	0.63

IQR = interquartile range; SD = standard deviation.
*Residents in intervention group wore an unblinded monitor (with visual activity feedback) during both Phase 1 (randomized) and Phase 2 (team competition).
†Residents in the control group wore a blinded monitor (no feedback) during Phase 1 and an unblinded monitor during Phase 2.

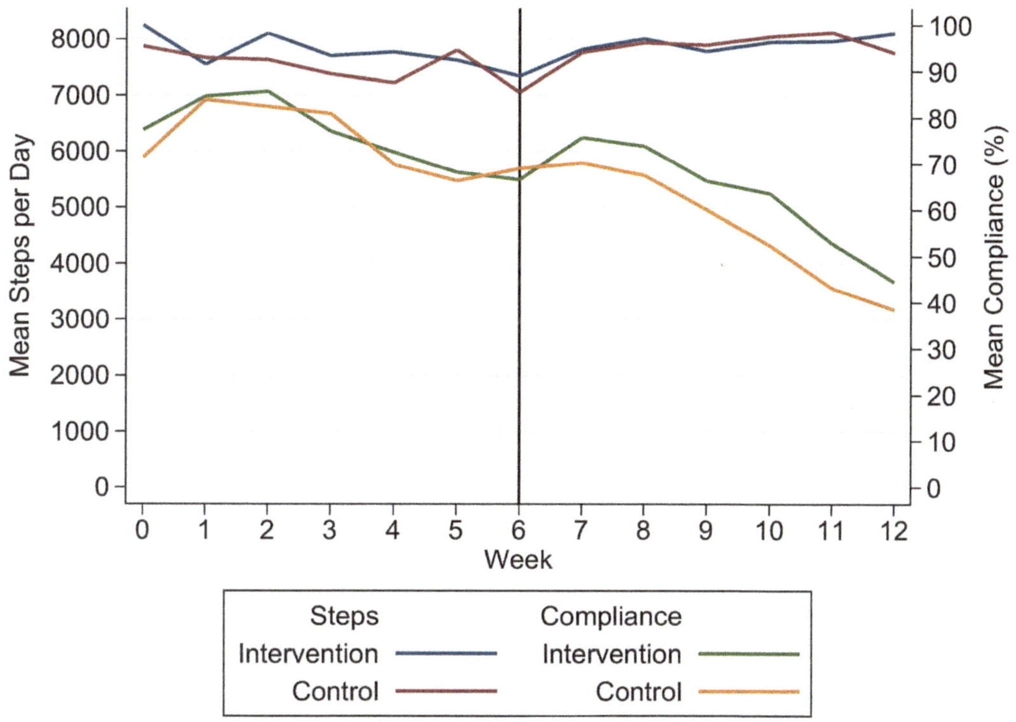

Figure 2. Resident activity levels and compliance with wearing activity monitor by study arm over 12 weeks. Activity levels are the number of steps taken on days when steps were recorded (>500 steps/day). Compliance is the mean percentage of days residents wore the activity monitor per week.

fast overnight. Height was recorded at baseline, and weight, waist circumference, blood pressure, and fasting lipids were measured at baseline and the final assessment. Residents completed a survey with questions about demographics, living with a significant other, smoking status, and weight gain or loss over the previous year.

Compliance with wearing the activity monitor was defined as the percentage of days the activity monitor was worn (500 or more steps recorded in a day) during each phase. We defined inpatient and outpatient weeks for each resident by reviewing the electronic resident scheduling system to determine whether the resident was on an inpatient or outpatient (ambulatory) rotation for each week of the study. If the resident switched rotations in the middle of a week, they were assigned to the rotation on which they spent the most number of days for that week.

Analysis

The baseline differences between the intervention and control groups were assessed with chi-squared and t-tests. An intention-to-treat analysis of steps for the randomized phase was performed using median steps per day because steps were not normally distributed. Days with no steps recorded were counted as 0 steps per day. Compliance was assessed on a daily basis; participants were considered compliant on days when the monitor recorded at least 500 steps. We report the percentage of days that participants were compliant. We tested differences in compliance using logistic regression models adjusted for clustering within participant.

The median steps per day were compared using Wilcoxon rank-sum tests. Analyses of the team competition phase were performed to compare mean steps per day on days when the activity monitor was worn, defined as 500 or more steps recorded in a day. For the analysis of inpatient and outpatient weeks, we excluded vacation days. We used repeated measures regression analyses to assess the effects of study group and rotation (inpatient vs. outpatient) on steps per day when the monitor was worn. We compared physiologic measurements and self-reported minutes of activity at baseline and end of study for all residents who had a measurement from both assessments using t-tests and Wilcoxon rank-sum tests. All analyses were conducted using Stata statistical software (StataCorp, 2008. Stata Statistical Software: Release 10. College Station, TX: Stata Corporation). We calculated a sample size of 50 per group would have 84% power to detect a difference of 1200 steps assuming that the common standard deviation is 2000 steps using a two group t-test with a 0.05 two-sided significance level.

Results

A total of 108 of 127 (85%) internal medicine residents enrolled in the study between July and November 2010 (Figure 1). Four residents withdrew from the study prior to randomization, and 104 (82%) were randomized in January 2011. Five residents withdrew during Phase 1, and 99 continued participation in Phase 2. At baseline, the mean age of residents was 29, 54% were female, 66% were white, and 52% were living with a significant other. The mean body mass index was 24.1 kg/m^2, and most residents were non-smokers. Half of residents reported that they had gained weight in the previous year. The intervention and control group did not differ significantly in any of these characteristics (Table 1).

Table 2 shows the intention to treat analyses with median steps per day and compliance with wearing the activity monitor during the randomized phase (Phase 1). During this phase, there was no difference in the median steps recorded or compliance with wearing the monitor between the intervention (unblinded) and control (blinded) groups. Table 2 also shows a secondary analysis including only days that the monitor was worn, and there was no

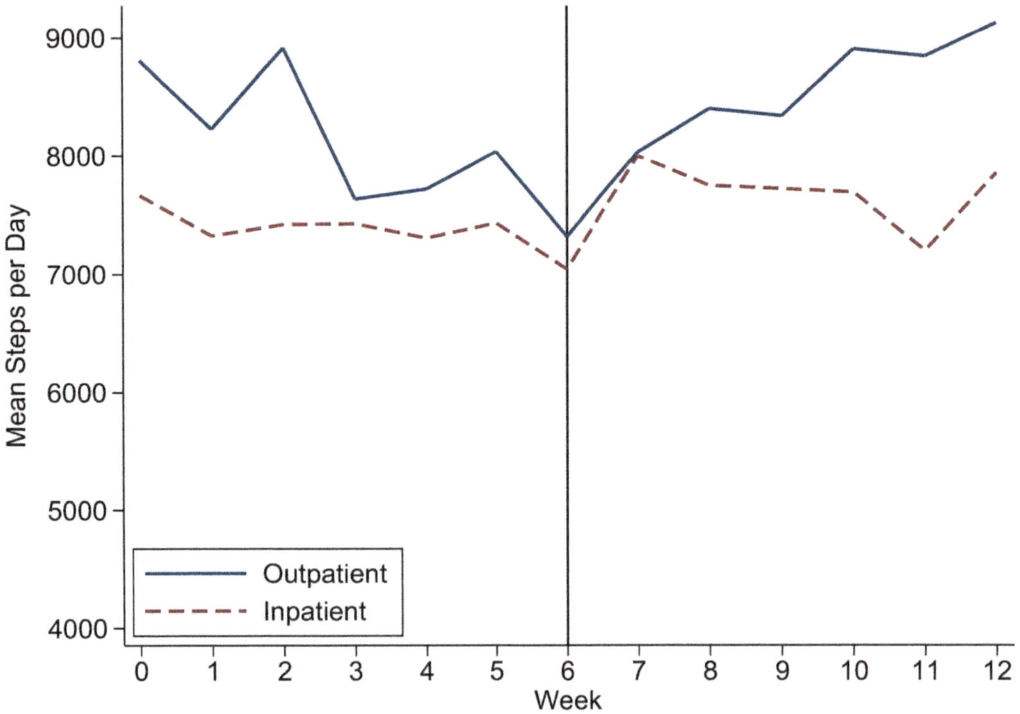

Figure 3. Activity levels during inpatient and outpatient rotations over 12 weeks. Activity levels are the number of steps taken on days when steps were recorded (>500 steps/day) when residents were on inpatient or outpatient rotations.

significant difference in mean steps per day between the intervention and control groups.

Figure 2 shows the mean steps per day for days when the activity monitor was worn (>500 steps recorded in a day). More steps were recorded during the team competition phase compared to the randomized phase; this was statistically significant for residents assigned to the control group for Phase 1 (7,971 vs. 7,567, $p = 0.002$) but not for residents assigned to the intervention group (7,832 vs. 7,739, $p = 0.13$). Mean compliance with wearing the activity monitor decreased for both groups during Phase 2 compared to Phase 1 (60% vs. 77%, $p < 0.001$).

Figure 3 shows mean steps per day on inpatient or outpatient rotations. Residents recorded a higher mean number of steps per day during outpatient rotations compared to inpatient rotations during the entire study (difference of 648 steps/day, $p < 0.001$).

Table 3 shows the change in body composition, blood pressure, and lipids from baseline to the end of the 12-week study for all residents. At study end, mean systolic blood pressure decreased ($p = 0.004$) and HDL cholesterol increased ($p < 0.001$), but there were no significant changes in weight, BMI, diastolic blood pressure, or total and LDL cholesterol.

We assessed residents' utilization of the on-site fitness center, personal training, and individual nutrition appointments offered during the 12 week study. From July–December 2010 (prior to intervention), 3 residents (3%) had used the fitness center. During the study when residents were given a free membership and

Table 3. Change in body composition, blood pressure, and lipids at baseline and end of the study.

	Baseline	End of study	P value
Weight, lbs, mean (SD)*	154 (27.9)	155 (29.8)	0.59
Body mass index, mean (SD)*	23.8 (3.9)	23.9 (4.2)	0.67
Waist, inches, mean (SD)†	30.2 (3.9)	30.2 (3.8)	0.83
Systolic BP, mm Hg, mean (SD)‡	121 (15.4)	117 (12.6)	0.004
Diastolic BP, mm Hg, mean (SD)‡	76 (11.2)	77 (8.3)	0.13
Total cholesterol, mg/dL, mean (SD)§	169 (20.7)	172 (26.5)	0.19
LDL cholesterol, mg/dL, mean (SD)§	94 (22.0)	92 (26.7)	0.44
HDL cholesterol, mg/dL, mean (SD)§	57 (14.7)	61 (15.7)	<0.001

SD = standard deviation; IQR = interquartile range.
*Weight and BMI data available at baseline and end of study for 91 residents.
†Waist and self-reported exercise available at baseline and end of study for 87 residents.
‡Blood pressure available at baseline and end of study for 81 residents.
§Fasting cholesterol available at baseline and end of study for 67 residents.

personal training, 54 residents (55%) used the fitness center at least once (mean visits = 6.7, range 1 to 21), and of these, 42 (76%) went to at least one personal training session (mean sessions = 4.4, range 1 to 10). Twenty-three residents (23%) met with the nutritionist individually.

Discussion

This is the first randomized study to test an activity monitor to promote physical activity among physicians. Despite their busy schedules, we found that medical residents were motivated to participate in a physical activity program, as evidenced by high consent, participation, and follow up rates. However, wearing an activity monitor with real time feedback did not result in increased activity compared to wearing a blinded monitor. Adding the team competition had a modest effect on increasing activity levels of residents. For all residents, there were significant improvements in systolic blood pressure and HDL cholesterol at the end of the study. Although this activity monitor intervention did not have a major impact on activity or health, the high participation rates of busy residents and modest changes in steps, blood pressure, and HDL suggest that more intensive hospital worksite wellness programs have potential for promoting healthier lifestyles among health care professionals.

The rate of burnout among physicians, especially residents and primary care providers, is higher than for other professions. [41] Although duty hour restrictions will likely contribute to some improvement, [28,28,42] strengthening physician resilience to burnout, depression, and illness also requires attention to the positive aspects of wellness. Physicians report physical exercise as one of the coping strategies for avoiding burnout and maintaining wellness, [43–45] but many physicians do not adequately incorporate regular exercise into their lives. [17,19–21] Our study demonstrates that a wellness program using activity monitors to promote physical activity had a high rate of participation and was feasible to incorporate into a busy internal medicine residency schedule. Future research will be needed to determine whether increasing physical activity and other healthy lifestyle habits of will lead to lower rates of burnout and better health.

This study has limitations. Two factors may have contributed to increased activity levels of both groups, resulting in the finding of no difference in steps during Phase 1. First, we were not able to measure baseline steps per day, and it is possible that the residents in both the intervention and control groups increased their steps because they knew steps were being monitored. Second, free access to the fitness center was provided to residents assigned to both groups. This study included residents from a single residency program in an urban setting, and therefore the results may not be generalizable to all residents and physicians.

Physicians spend a majority of their time at work, and therefore hospital or office-based worksite wellness programs could provide an opportunity to initiate and reinforce healthy habits. Our results clearly show that this young, healthy population of medical residents had activity levels below the recommended 10,000 steps per day, [46] and therefore more intense interventions will be needed for clinically significant health benefits. Although using an activity monitor with real time and on-line feedback did not result in a statistically significant increase in activity, adding a team steps competition did result in a small increase. Residents utilized the on-site gym more frequently during the 12-week program, and there was some evidence of improvement in systolic blood pressure and HDL cholesterol at the end of the study. Despite the perception that residents on inpatient rotations are on their feet walking for extended hours, a secondary analysis revealed that residents recorded more steps when they were on outpatient rotations and had more time for leisure-time physical activity. Increasing opportunities for residents to be physically active during outpatient rotations will promote exercise during training as well as provide a model for maintaining healthy habits post-training.

Promoting healthy lifestyle habits of physicians will not only create better role models for patients but will also improve physician health. Hospitals, residency programs, and other healthcare institutions should consider ways to integrate wellness programs into medical training and practice. The Institute of Medicine suggests that "health care organizations and providers serve as models for the incorporation of healthy eating and active living into worksite practices and programs". [10] Potential opportunities for increasing physical activity among physicians, especially in the inpatient setting, might include encouraging structured physical activity breaks, allotting space for on-site exercise equipment, and creating team competitions among physicians and other health care professionals. These types of interventions are relatively low cost and may ultimately increase work efficiency and contribute to a healthier and happier physician workforce.

Acknowledgments

We thank Dr. Dennis Ausiello, Chairman, Department of Medicine, Massachusetts General Hospital at the time of the study, and Mr. Jeff Davis, Vice President, Human Resources, Massachusetts General Hospital, for their support in developing this project.

Author Contributions

Conceived and designed the experiments: ANT LS SR. Performed the experiments: ANT SM LS DP TG CTP . Analyzed the data: ANT DP TG CTP SR. Contributed reagents/materials/analysis tools: SR. Wrote the paper: ANT. Interpretation of data and approval of final manuscript: ANT SM LS DP TG CTP SR.

References

1. Shanafelt TD, Bradley KA, Wipf JE, Back AL (2002) Burnout and self-reported patient care in an internal medicine residency program. Ann Intern Med 136(5): 358–67.
2. Thomas NK (2004) Resident burnout. JAMA 292(23): 2880–9.
3. West CP, Tan AD, Habermann TM, Sloan JA, Shanafelt TD (2009) Association of resident fatigue and distress with perceived medical errors. JAMA 302(12): 1294–300.
4. Fahrenkopf AM, Sectish TC, Barger LK, Sharek PJ, Lewin D, et al. (2008) Rates of medication errors among depressed and burnt out residents: Prospective cohort study. BMJ 336(7642): 488–91.
5. Taub S, Morin K, Goldrich MS, Ray P, Benjamin R, et al. (2006) Physician health and wellness. Occup Med (Oxf) 56(2): 77–82.
6. Wallace JE, Lemaire JB, Ghali WA (2009) Physician wellness: A missing quality indicator. Lancet 374(9702): 1714–21.
7. Firth-Cozens J (2001) Interventions to improve physicians' well-being and patient care. Soc Sci Med 52(2): 215–22.
8. Shanafelt TD, Sloan JA, Habermann TM (2003) The well-being of physicians. Am J Med 114(6): 513–9.
9. Millstine D (2011) Wellness for physicians. SGIM Forum 34(8): 14.

10. Institute of Medicine (2012) Accelerating progress in obesity prevention: Solving the weight of the nation, recommendations. Available: http://www.iom.edu/Reports/2012/Accelerating-Progress-in-Obesity-Prevention.aspx.
11. Lewis CE, Clancy C, Leake B, Schwartz JS (1991) The counseling practices of internists. Ann Intern Med 114(1): 54–8.
12. Abramson S, Stein J, Schaufele M, Frates E, Rogan S (2000) Personal exercise habits and counseling practices of primary care physicians: A national survey. Clin J Sport Med 10(1): 40–8.
13. Frank E, Breyan J, Elon L (2000) Physician disclosure of healthy personal behaviors improves credibility and ability to motivate. Arch Fam Med 9(3): 287–90.
14. Lobelo F, Duperly J, Frank (2009) Physical activity habits of doctors and medical students influence their counselling practices. BJSM online 43(2): 89–92.
15. Gross CP, Mead LA, Ford DE, Klag MJ (2000) Physician, heal thyself? regular source of care and use of preventive health services among physicians. Arch Intern Med 160(21): 3209–14.
16. Arnetz BB (2001) Psychosocial challenges facing physicians of today. Soc Sci Med 52(2): 203–13.
17. Bazargan M, Makar M, Bazargan-Hejazi S, Ani C, Wolf KE (2009) Preventive, lifestyle, and personal health behaviors among physicians. Acad Psychiatry 33(4): 289–95.
18. Wallace JE, Lemaire J (2009) Physician well being and quality of patient care: An exploratory study of the missing link. Psychol Health Med 14(5): 545–52.
19. McNerney JP, Andes S, Blackwell DL (2007) Self-reported health behaviors of osteopathic physicians. J Am Osteopath Assoc 107(12): 537–46.
20. Collins J, Hinshaw JL, Fine E, Albanese MA (2008) Diagnostic radiology resident compliance with recommended health guidelines: Effect of resident work environment. Acad Radiol 15(8): 1046–57.
21. Hull SK, DiLalla LF, Dorsey JK (2008) Prevalence of health-related behaviors among physicians and medical trainees. Acad Psychiatry 32(1): 31–8.
22. Rosen IM, Gimotty PA, Shea JA, Bellini LM (2006) Evolution of sleep quantity, sleep deprivation, mood disturbances, empathy, and burnout among interns. Acad Med 81(1): 82–5.
23. Warburton DE, Nicol CW, Bredin SS (2006) Health benefits of physical activity: The evidence. CMAJ 174(6): 801–9.
24. Jonsdottir IH, Rodjer L, Hadzibajramovic E, Borjesson M, Ahlborg G Jr (2010) A prospective study of leisure-time physical activity and mental health in Swedish health care workers and social insurance officers. Prev Med 51(5): 373–7.
25. Lucas M, Mekary R, Pan A, Mirzaei F, O'Reilly EJ, et al. (2011) Relation between clinical depression risk and physical activity and time spent watching television in older women: A 10-year prospective follow-up study. Am J Epidemiol 174(9): 1017–27.
26. Ahola K, Pulkki-Raback L, Kouvonen A, Rossi H, Aromaa A, et al. (2012) Burnout and behavior-related health risk factors: Results from the population-based Finnish health 2000 study. J Occup Environ Med 54(1): 17–22.
27. Toker S, Biron M (2012) Job burnout and depression: Unraveling their temporal relationship and considering the role of physical activity. J Appl Psychol 97(3): 699–710.
28. Gopal R, Glasheen JJ, Miyoshi TJ, Prochazka AV (2005) Burnout and internal medicine resident work-hour restrictions. Arch Intern Med 165(22): 2595–600.
29. West CP, Shanafelt TD, Kolars JC (2011) Quality of life, burnout, educational debt, and medical knowledge among internal medicine residents. JAMA 306(9): 952–60.
30. Eckleberry-Hunt J, Lick D, Boura J, Hunt R, Balasubramaniam M, et al. (2009) An exploratory study of resident burnout and wellness. Acad Med 84(2): 269–77.
31. Rye PL, Reeson ME, Pekrul CM, Asfour NA, Kundapur R, et al. (2012) Comparing health behaviours of internal medicine residents and medical students: An observational study. Clin Invest Med 35(1): E40–4.
32. Arora R, Lettieri C, Claybaugh JR (2004) The effects of residency on physical fitness among military physicians. Mil Med 169(7): 522–5.
33. Leventer-Roberts M, Zonfrillo MR, Yu S, Dziura JD, Spiro DM (2013) Overweight physicians during residency: A cross-sectional and longitudinal study. Journal of Graduate Medical Education 405–11.
34. Rogers LQ, Gutin B, Humphries MC, Lemmon CR, Waller JL, et al. (2005) A physician fitness program: Enhancing the physician as an "exercise" role model for patients. Teach Learn Med 17(1): 27–35.
35. Bravata DM, Smith-Spangler C, Sundaram V, Gienger AL, Lin N, et al. (2007) Using pedometers to increase physical activity and improve health: A systematic review. JAMA 298(19): 2296–304.
36. Chan CB, Ryan DA, Tudor-Locke C (2004) Health benefits of a pedometer-based physical activity intervention in sedentary workers. Prev Med 39(6): 1215–22.
37. Freak-Poli R, Wolfe R, Backholer K, de Courten M, Peeters A (2011) Impact of a pedometer-based workplace health program on cardiovascular and diabetes risk profile. Prev Med 53(3): 162–71.
38. Thorndike AN, Healey E, Sonnenberg L, Regan S (2011) Participation and cardiovascular risk reduction in a voluntary worksite nutrition and physical activity program. Preventive medicine 52: 164–6.
39. Thorndike AN, Sonnenberg L, Healey E, Myint-U K, Kvedar JC, et al. (2012) Prevention of weight gain following a worksite nutrition and exercise program: A randomized controlled trial. Am J Prev Med 43(1): 27–33.
40. Takacs J, Pollock CL, Guenther JR, Bahar M, Napier C, et al. (2013) Validation of the fitbit one activity monitor device during treadmill walking. Journal of Science and Medicine in Sport. Available: http://dx.doi.org/10.1016/j.jsams.2013.10.241.
41. Shanafelt TD, Boone S, Tan L, Dyrbye LN, Sotile W, et al. (2012) Burnout and satisfaction with work-life balance among US physicians relative to the general US population. Arch Intern Med 172(18): 1377–85.
42. Fitzgibbons SC, Chen J, Jagsi R, Weinstein D (2012) Long-term follow-up on the educational impact of ACGME duty hour limits: A pre-post survey study. Ann Surg 00: 1–5.
43. Shanafelt TD, Novotny P, Johnson ME, Zhao X, Steensma DP, et al. (2005) The well-being and personal wellness promotion strategies of medical oncologists in the north central cancer treatment group. Oncology 68(1): 23–32.
44. Lemaire JB, Wallace JE (2010) Not all coping strategies are created equal: A mixed methods study exploring physicians' self reported coping strategies. BMC Health Serv Res. 10: 208.
45. Meldrum H (2010) Exemplary physicians' strategies for avoiding burnout. Health Care Manag (Frederick) 29(4): 324–31.
46. Tudor-Locke C, Bassett DR Jr (2004) How many steps/day are enough? preliminary pedometer indices for public health. Sports Med 34(1): 1–8.

3

Bank of Standardized Stimuli (BOSS) Phase II: 930 New Normative Photos

Mathieu B. Brodeur[1]*, Katherine Guérard[2], Maria Bouras[3]

1 Douglas Mental Health University Institute and Department of Psychiatry, McGill University, Montréal (Québec), Canada, **2** Department of Psychology, Université de Moncton, Moncton (New Brunswick), Canada, **3** Department of Education, University of Sheffield, Sheffield (South Yorkshire), United Kingdom

Abstract

Researchers have only recently started to take advantage of the developments in technology and communication for sharing data and documents. However, the exchange of experimental material has not taken advantage of this progress yet. In order to facilitate access to experimental material, the Bank of Standardized Stimuli (BOSS) project was created as a free standardized set of visual stimuli accessible to all researchers, through a normative database. The BOSS is currently the largest existing photo bank providing norms for more than 15 dimensions (e.g. familiarity, visual complexity, manipulability, etc.), making the BOSS an extremely useful research tool and a mean to homogenize scientific data worldwide. The first phase of the BOSS was completed in 2010, and contained 538 normative photos. The second phase of the BOSS project presented in this article, builds on the previous phase by adding 930 new normative photo stimuli. New categories of concepts were introduced, including animals, building infrastructures, body parts, and vehicles and the number of photos in other categories was increased. All new photos of the BOSS were normalized relative to their name, familiarity, visual complexity, object agreement, viewpoint agreement, and manipulability. The availability of these norms is a precious asset that should be considered for characterizing the stimuli as a function of the requirements of research and for controlling for potential confounding effects.

Editor: Kevin Paterson, University of Leicester, United Kingdom

Funding: This study was funded by the Natural Sciences and Engineering Research Council of Canada #388752-2012 (www.nserc-crsng.gc.ca/index_eng.asp). The funders had no role in study design, data collection and analysis, decision to publish, or preparation of the manuscript.

Competing Interests: The authors have declared that no competing interests exist.

* Email: mathieu.brodeur@douglas.mcgill.ca

Introduction

Stimuli are the key component of experiments. They must therefore be of outstanding quality and be selected meticulously as a function of specific criteria, which explains why they need to be normalized. Normalization is the process through which a representative sample of individuals evaluates images and their names according to specific variables. Normative data characterizes the images and provides a thorough description of their basic features. For instance, by discerning the name given to concepts depicted in images by the majority of individuals, it is possible to determine the level of consensus in naming the specific concepts. The name given by a majority of individuals is the modal name and the consensus is called the name agreement. Through an analysis of the different names given to each image, it is also possible to explain the variability in the given names and to determine how accurately concepts are identified [1]. Other norms commonly tested in sets of pictures include conceptual familiarity, visual complexity, and the typicality of the object. These variables are often normalized because they have a strong influence on many cognitive performances (e.g. object naming) and on the strategies used during image processing.

The need for normative sets of pictures in research is unequivocal and the number of normative studies has rapidly increased in the past years. Indeed, at least 12 new normative sets of pictures, including 2 sets intended to complement older sets [2,3], were developed between 2000 and 2009 [2–13] and 9 new normative sets of pictures were published since 2010 [14–22]. Each set is unique about the features of the visual stimuli it includes and the normative dimensions it provides. For example, in Viggiano and colleagues [13]'s dataset, stimuli were normalized in color and in greyscale tones. Op de Beeck and Wagemans [11]'s dataset includes multiple exemplars of each object. Adlington and colleagues [4]'s set includes concepts and images with a broad range of item difficulty and semantic subcategories. Finally, the sets of Barbarotto and colleagues [5] and Magnié and colleagues [10] present imaginary objects, created by combining different objects together. Some sets also offer stimuli normalized for specific visual attributes of the images (e.g. luminosity as opposed to familiarity or visual complexity). For example, the Amsterdam Library of Object Images (ALOI) is a color image set with a large number of images varying in angle, illumination and color. Other sets, such as that of Verfaille and Boutsen [23], use objects in 3-dimensional space instead of line drawings or 2-dimensional images.

The choice between sets of stimuli is made based on each set's distinctive character and stimulus type. Researchers must first decide whether line drawings or photos of objects are to be used as stimuli. An increasing number of researchers opt for photos of stimuli, highlighting the need for more ecological stimuli. Photos offer a more realistic depiction of everyday concepts. They provide great depth and richness, which potentially influences the way in which the stimulus is attended, memorized and acted upon [24–27]. Using photos as the experimental stimuli increases the chances of activating the same neuronal circuits that are activated in daily tasks. Line drawings, such as those created in 1980 by Snodgrass and Vanderwart [28], may also be privileged depending on the researchers' objective. Line drawings offer a simple and prototypal depiction of concepts, free of details (e.g. color, texture, or 3D cues) that could influence their naming and visual processing. Moreover, line drawings are easier to modify than photos of real objects in order to create additional experimental conditions. They can be made more difficult to recognize by fragmenting their line contours [29] and imaginary and impossible objects can easily be drawn [5,10].

Once researchers have chosen the type of stimuli they want to use, they have to decide which dimensions they want to control or manipulate in order to determine the set that best suits the needs of the experiment. The number of stimuli available is certainly an important feature that researchers must consider. Experiments often require hundreds of stimuli, especially those including multiple testing sessions, such as memory tasks and experiments involving recording of electrophysiological brain activities. The number of stimuli can be even more crucial for experiments requiring specific types of concepts, such as experiments including specific semantic categories. For example, if the selection of stimuli is limited to the category of fruits and vegetables, only 24 out of the 260 concepts from the Snodgrass and Vanderwart [28]'s set can be used. This issue is usually overcome by combining stimuli from different sets [2–3,30]. However, this practice increases the heterogeneity of the visual parameters and norms.

To our knowledge, the Bank of Standardized Stimuli (BOSS) [15] is the set offering the highest number of normative stimuli (see http://sites.google.com/site/bosstimuli/). It currently includes 538 normative photos of high quality color resolution. In Brodeur and colleagues (2010), stimuli that had a name agreement below 20% or were unrecognized by at least 20% of the participants were excluded from the analyses. Norms presented in this article were thus limited to 480 stimuli. These norms were for the name, familiarity, visual complexity, manipulability, object agreement and viewpoint agreement. Norms are described in more details below. The BOSS, however, does not include some categories that might be useful to researchers, such as animals, vehicles, and buildings. Moreover, a set of 538 images might still be insufficient for some experiments.

The present project further developed the BOSS by adding 930 normative photos. These photos increased the number of stimuli in the existing categories, and offer new categories including animals, building infrastructures, body parts, and vehicles. Differences of norms across categories as well as differences between males and females were also examined. Intrinsic (e.g. biological, neuropsychological, etc.) and extrinsic (e.g. social activities, exposure to specific stimuli, etc.) characteristics of men and women could indeed influence the way they name and rate the concepts. Surprisingly, this has not yet been examined in normative studies.

Materials and Methods

Participants

Participants, whose first language is English, were recruited through ads published in journals and newspapers, and via online classifieds such as Craigslist and Kijiji. A total of 141 participants between the ages of 18 and 55 participated in the project. They each participated in one of four normative studies. The subgroups participating in studies 1, 2, 3, and 4 respectively included 42 participants (22 female, mean age: 25.2, SD: 7.5), 33 participants (15 female, mean age: 30.7, SD: 9.3), 32 participants (17 female, mean age: 28.3, SD: 9.9), and 34 participants (15 female, mean age: 30.5, SD: 10.0).

Ethic Statements

This project was approved by the Research Ethics Board of the Douglas Institute and all participants gave their written consent. Their names were not written anywhere in order to secure confidentiality. Prior to the normative session, participants were told that they were free to interrupt their participation at any time and for any reason. Participants were compensated for their time.

Stimuli

The 930 new colored photos are all concepts that were not in the original BOSS, except for the cork, ice cube, kiwi, lollipop, mug, and recorder. These concepts were re-normalized by presenting new photos that were considered of better quality than those used in the original BOSS. The new photos depicted concepts of categories that were lacking in the original BOSS, including animals, building infrastructures, body parts, and vehicles. The number of concepts for other categories was significantly increased such as musical instruments, furniture, and weapons. The new set of 930 photo stimuli was created through a 5-step procedure, identical to the procedure used to generate the images for the first phase of the project [15]. Some objects were gathered, cleaned and digitally photographed one at a time in a box that uniformly diffused the light provided by two projectors. Other objects however, were photographed as part of a bigger scene and were then cut out of their backgrounds. These photos were taken in many locations. Consequently, the environmental conditions of the photos were not always uniform. The majority of animal photos were taken in museums and zoos. Few photos were taken from the internet and were generously donated to the project by their authors. Adobe Photoshop (Adobe Systems Inc., San Jose, U.S.A.) was used for image editing, including lighting adjustments and the cutting out of the objects. Examples of photos are presented in Figure 1.

General Procedure

Stimuli were presented using the software E-Prime 2.0. Participants were tested individually in a room equipped with one desktop computer and one laptop. The desktop was set up with E-Prime and the experiment's instructions. This computer was used for the stimuli presentation. The photos were presented in 500×500 pixels, centered on the computer screen. On the laptop screen, a blank response sheet was shown in which subjects recorded their responses by writing the name, selecting a category among a list, or entering a value between 1 and 5 on the keyboard. The response sheet was anonymous. The order of the stimuli in each study was random and differed across participants.

Study 1. The goal of this study was to normalize the new 930 photo stimuli for name, familiarity and visual complexity. Prior to the experiment, instructions were given orally and a written version was given to each participant. The first task was to "Identify the object as briefly and unambiguously as possible by writing only one name, the first name that comes to mind. The name can be composed of more than one word". Participants were told to write DKO (don't know object) if they had no idea what the object was. If they knew the object but not the name, they wrote DKN (don't know name) and if they knew the name but were

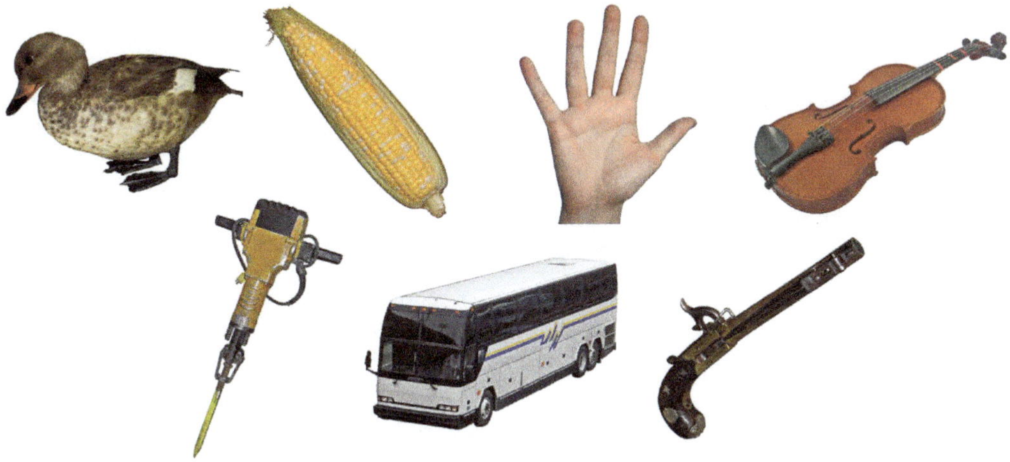

Figure 1. Examples of stimuli from the animal, food, body part, musical instrument, hand labour tool and accessory, vehicle, and weapon and war related item categories.

unable to retrieve it at that moment, they wrote TOT (tip-of-the-tongue).

For familiarity, participants were asked to "Rate the level to which you are familiar with the object". Responses were provided on a 5-point rating scale with 1 indicating very unfamiliar and 5 very familiar. Participants were asked to rate the concept itself and not the picture of the object. Responses were not required for the objects for which they responded DKO.

For visual complexity, participants were asked to "Subjectively rate the level to which the image appears to be complex in terms of the quantity of details and the intricacy of the lines". on a 5-point scale with value 1 indicating a very simple image and 5, a very complex image.

Images were presented one at a time and participants could change to the next image at their own pace, meaning that there was no set amount of time for the participants to see each image. Participants were unable to go back to previous images. For each concept, participants first wrote the name in one column and then provided their rating for familiarity and visual complexity rating in the two next columns of the response sheet. For both familiarity and visual complexity, participants were reminded to use the entire 5-point rating scale and not only its end points.

Study 2. The goal of this study was to normalize the photo stimuli for category agreement, which is the extent to which they are representative of their category. In the 2010 normative study (original BOSS) [15], participants classified each object within the most appropriate of 18 categories. This proved problematic when objects fell under more than one category heading. For example, a toy tank could be classified either within the weapon and war related category or within the games, toys and entertainment category. To avoid this problem, the participants in the present study had the possibility to classify the concept within two categories. Considering the change of instructions for this study, the categorization was performed for the 930 new photos as well as for the original 538 normative photos summing to 1468 categorizations.

Categories were created in a drop down box in an excel sheet in alphabetical order. The instructions read, "Determine to which category the concept belongs". Participants were asked to make a choice among the following five categories: animal, body part, building infrastructure, object, and vehicle. When they chose animal or object, participants were presented with a list of more specific categories allowing them to refine their selection. The list of animals included bird, canine, crustacean, feline, fish, insect, mammal, reptile, and sea mammal. The list of objects included building material, clothing, decoration and gift accessory, electronic device and accessory, food, furniture, game toy and entertainment, hand labour tool and accessory, household article and cleaner, jewel and money, kitchen item and utensil, medical instrument and accessory, musical instrument, natural element, outdoor activity and sport item, skincare and bathroom item, stationary and school supply, weapon and war related item.

Study 3. The goal of this study was to normalize the photo stimuli for image agreement, which is the degree to which the mental image generated from the modal name (the name most commonly used), matched the object stimulus. Image agreement was separated into object and viewpoint agreement, meaning that participants had to decide to which extent the mentally generated concept was structurally similar to the photo concept (image agreement) and the extent the two concepts had comparable positions (viewpoint agreement).

For each concept, its name was first presented in black 14-point Times New Roman, centered on the computer screen. This name featured the modal name, which is the name that reached the greatest name agreement, as determined by the results from study 1. Only the 464 stimuli for which at least 21 participants (50%) gave the modal name in study 1 were normalized for object and viewpoint agreement. Following the appearance of the name, participants had to generate a mental image of the concept related to the name, after which, they pressed the space bar and the photo appeared. Participants were then asked to rate image agreement and viewpoint agreement. For object agreement, participants were asked "How closely does the picture of the BOSS resemble the mental image you had for the object name, independently from its position?" For viewpoint agreement, participants were asked to determine "How closely does the object of the BOSS match the position of the object you imagined?" In both tasks, participants had to provide a rating from 1 to 5, 1 corresponding to a low agreement and 5 corresponding to a high agreement. An example of low and high object and viewpoint agreements were presented before the session began.

Study 4. In the last study, all 930 stimuli were presented to participants at their own pace in order to rate the manipulability of the concept. Participants were instructed to determine "Could you easily mime the action usually associated with this object so that any person looking at you doing this action could decide which object is associated with this action?" Responses were provided on a 5-point rating scale where 1 was a definite "no" response and 5 was a definite "yes" response. Participants were instructed to use the entire scale and not only its end points.

Data analyses

Modal name and name agreement. For each image, the names provided by participants were analyzed after first excluding the data for which participants had responded DKN, DKO, or TOT. The name given by the highest percentage of participants was considered the modal name. The percentage of participants who agreed on the modal name is the name agreement. In the case where two names had the same percentage of responses, the most specific name for the object was used (e.g. plastic cup as opposed to cup). Composite names in which the order of the words was rearranged (e.g. ham slice or slice of ham) were considered to be the same name.

H value. The H value for each object was computed. The statistic H is a value sensitive to the number and weight of alternative names. It is computed with the following formula [28]:

$$H = \sum_{i=1}^{k} P_i \log_2(1/P_i)$$

Where k refers to the number of different names given to each picture and excludes the DKN, DKO, and TOT responses, and P_i is the proportion of participants that gave a name for each object. This proportion varies across pictures because of the exclusion of the DKN, DKO, and TOT responses. The H value of a picture with a unique name and no alternative is 0. The H value of a picture with two names provided with an equivalent frequency is 1.00. This value is smaller for an alternative that is provided to a lower frequency rate. On the other hand, the H value increases as a function of the number of alternatives. For instance, one picture with its modal name provided by 50% of participants and two alternative names each with a frequency of 25% would have an H value of 1.50.

Modal category and category agreement. The modal category and category agreement were computed following the same procedure used for the names. These statistics were computed on the first category selected by the participants. A second category was rarely selected by participants and was considered only when two or more categories were selected at the same frequency for a stimulus. However, the second response was not added to the percentage of agreement.

H_{cat} value. An H value for the category, referred to as a H_{cat} value, was measured following the same procedure used for the names.

Variables rated on a 5-point scale. Familiarity, visual complexity, object agreement, viewpoint agreement, and manipulability were computed by averaging the scores on the 5-point rating scale and by calculating the standard deviations.

Statistical analyses. Means and standard deviations were analyzed using independent sample t-tests, with the stimuli as for the participants and the categories as for the between-"stimulus" variables. Comparisons of categories were limited to the most commonly used and studied categories in cognitive science. The categories included animal, food, tool, musical instrument, weapon and vehicle. Tool, musical instrument, weapon, and vehicle are typically used as non-living or man-made concepts and are generally opposed to food and animal that are used as living or natural concepts. Because many food items of the BOSS are non-living (e.g. bottle of wine), a second category of food was created for the analyses which included only fruits, vegetables, and nuts. Categories analyzed thus consisted of animal (i.e. all animals collapsed together, except for the mussel, the seashell, and the fish skeleton), food, hand labour tool and accessory, musical instrument, vehicle, and weapon and war related item, as well as a seventh category including fruit/vegetable/nuts. Category comparisons were done for all norms except H value, H_{cat} value, and TOT, in order to reduce the number of comparisons. Alpha threshold was Bonferroni corrected to .00003 for multiple (189) comparisons.

Comparisons between genders were also performed with independent sample t-tests. Samples opposed stimuli responded by males and by females. Gender differences were examined for the mean norms and within each of the seven categories retained for the analyses. Alpha threshold was Bonferroni corrected to .0042 for multiple (12) comparisons.

Results

Norms

Table 1 summarizes the agreement and ratings obtained for each normative dimension. The stimulus-specific norms are presented in supporting Tables S1 and S2. In these tables, photo stimuli are sorted as a function of their filename, which at times, differs from the modal name and is more precise. All norms except those related to category are listed in Table S1. Categories, category agreements and H_{cat} for all stimuli, including the 538 photos of phase I, are presented in Table S2.

Norms per categories

The norms for each category, computed for all 1468 photos of the BOSS, are presented in Table 2. The first comparisons of categories, carried out on the categories in the upper part of Table 2, were conducted to determine whether some types of concepts were more difficult to recognize or name than others. DKO was significantly higher for tools ($t(201) = 5.150$, $p < .00001$) and weapons ($t(201) = 5.150$, $p = .00003$) than for animals. Tools were more difficult to name than all categories (all $p < .00003$) except musical instruments.

The next comparisons looked at differences of modal name and category agreement. Animals and fruits/vegetables/nuts were named with a relatively similar consensus and their modal name agreement was significantly higher (all $p < .00003$) than that for tools and vehicles, which yielded more inconsistent names. The modal name agreement for fruits/vegetables/nuts was also significantly higher than for foods ($t(166) = 5.326$, $p < .00001$). The lower name agreement for tools was contingent to the lowest category agreement. Tools were classified more inconsistently than animals, foods, fruits/vegetables/nuts, and musical instruments (all $p < .00001$). In contrast, fruits/vegetables/nuts were classified more consistently than all other categories (all $p < .00001$), except musical instruments.

The least familiar category was that of weapons. They were significantly different from vehicles, foods, and fruits/vegetables/nuts (all $p < .00001$). The most complex stimuli were animals which were rated significantly higher than all other categories (all $p < .00001$). Vehicles were also more visually complex than foods, fruits/vegetables/nuts, and weapons (all $p < .00001$). Finally, musical instruments were more complex than foods ($t(211) = 5.907$, $p < .00001$) and fruits/vegetables/nuts ($t(117) = 5.127$, $p < .00001$).

Object agreement was the highest for fruits/vegetables/nuts, meaning that the photos in this category matched the mental image evoked by the concepts to a larger extent than the other

Table 1. Norms.

	Male (n = 20)			Female (n = 22)		Gender
Normative dimension	Mean	SD	SD	Mean	SD	comparison
Modal Name Agreement*	58%	25%	25%	61%	26%	t = 2.240***
H value*	1.89	1.06	0.97	1.53	0.09	t = 4.255***
DKO	3%	7%	6%	4%	10%	t = 4.903***
DKN	5%	8%	8%	6%	9%	t = 4.115***
TOT	3%	4%	3%	4%	7%	t = 12.458***
Category Agreement*	76%	21%	21%	77%	22%	t = 0.450
H_{cat} value*	0.97	0.75	0.72	0.87	0.75	t = 0.590
Familiarity	4.16	0.50	0.51	4.16	0.55	t = 0.147
Visual Complexity	2.43	0.54	0.52	2.49	0.59	t = 4.905***
Object Agreement**	3.69	0.52	0.54	3.57	0.57	t = 4.799***
Viewpoint Agreement**	3.60	0.44	0.45	3.45	0.51	t = 8.240***
Manipulability	2.57	0.78	0.84	2.67	0.76	t = 4.527***

*The modal name and category of males and females were not systematically the same, thus explaining why the norms of all subjects do not correspond to the averages of the two subgroups.
**Statistics for 464 stimuli.
***p<.0001.

stimuli. Object agreement for foods was significantly higher than all other categories except for musical instruments (all $p<.00001$). Viewpoint agreement was also the greatest for fruits/vegetables/nuts and for foods in general. These categories had a viewpoint agreement significantly higher than animals and vehicles (all $p<.00001$).

Finally, large differences were found with respect to manipulability. Foods, fruits/vegetables/nuts, and animals had manipulability ratings that were significantly smaller than all other categories (all $p<.00001$). In addition, musical instruments, which had the highest rating, were significantly more manipulable than vehicles ($t(107) = 7.789$, $p<.00001$).

Norms per sex

Norms of males and females and the statistics resulting from their comparisons are presented in Table 1. Modal name agreement, DKO, DKN, and TOT were all significantly higher in females than in males. Females also rated visual complexity and manipulability with higher scores than males. In contrast, males provided significantly higher scores for object and viewpoint agreement than females. No differences were denoted for category agreement and familiarity.

Table 3 presents the norms of males and females within seven categories. Although they were not systematically significant, differences between genders were consistent with those described in Table 1, except for the tool category. Tools were more familiar to males and named with a higher agreement. Tools were the items that females recognized and named with the greatest difficulty, compared to males. Those difficulties also occurred for weapons, despite a greater modal name agreement for females.

Correlations

As is generally done in normative studies, the relation between the different normative dimensions was examined using correlational analyses. The alpha threshold was Bonferroni corrected and lowered to .0014. Results, which are presented in Table 4, show that the strongest correlations were between the agreement (name and category) and their respective H value. Name agreement correlated with all other norms except for visual complexity. In Brodeur and colleagues [15], modal name agreement did not correlate with category agreement however, in the present study there was a weak but significant correlation.

Object agreement and viewpoint agreement also exhibited a pattern of results very similar to that found in Brodeur and colleagues [15]. These ratings correlated with name dimensions and familiarity but not with category dimensions and visual complexity. The normative dimensions that differ the most between the present study and Brodeur and colleagues [15] are familiarity and visual complexity, which negatively correlated with each other in the present study. Moreover, familiarity no longer correlated with category agreement whereas visual complexity did. Finally, these two normative dimensions strongly correlated with manipulability.

Discussion

This project proposes 930 new normative photos of concepts from different categories to be added to the 538 photos that already compose the BOSS [15]. The norms for the new set are very similar to those collected for the initial set, except for name agreement, which is slightly lower than in the initial set. This difference is essentially due to the use of more stringent criteria for keeping stimuli in Brodeur and colleagues [15], where only photos with a DKO below 20% and a name agreement above 20% were included in the analyses.

Some norms also differ from those of other normative sets of photos. For instance, Moreno-Martinez and Montoro [20] and Adlington and colleagues [4] had name agreement of 72% and 67%, respectively. The lower name agreement of the BOSS mostly pertains to its high number of stimuli and the inclusion of concepts that are necessarily more difficult to name. As argued in Brodeur and colleagues [15], adding new stimuli is generally associated with a reduction of name agreement. Rating for familiarity was higher than in Moreno-Martinez and Montoro [20] and Adlington and colleagues [4] as well as in most normative

Table 2. Norms as a function of categories.

Category	Nb BOSS 2010	Nb BOSS 2014	Total Nb	DKO	DKN	TOT	NA	*H*	CA	Hcat	Fam	VC	OA	VA	Manip
Food	93	75	168	4%	4%	1%	63%	1.68	92%	0.38	4.24	2.25	4.05	3.89	1.96
- Fruit, vegetable & nut*	59	15	74	3%	5%	2%	74%	1.19	97%	0.20	4.28	2.25	4.27	3.99	1.66
Hand labour tool & accessory	49	46	95	7%	14%	4%	53%	2.15	70%	1.20	4.03	2.37	3.85	3.67	2.85
Musical instrument	5	40	45	4%	9%	4%	62%	1.65	89%	0.52	4.07	2.60	3.97	3.74	3.58
Vehicle	3	61	64	1%	5%	3%	56%	2.02	76%	0.97	4.24	2.74	3.60	3.40	2.59
Weapon & war related item	1	35	36	6%	6%	2%	59%	1.90	76%	1.04	3.73	2.24	3.65	3.56	2.90
Animal**	1	141	142	1%	5%	2%	71%	1.23	89%	0.49	4.02	3.09	3.77	3.50	1.89
- Bird	0	32	32	1%	5%	1%	72%	1.22	97%	0.18	4.01	3.16	3.74	3.46	1.85
- Canine	0	8	8	1%	6%	1%	63%	1.65	82%	0.70	4.20	3.00	3.46	3.45	2.38
- Crustacean	2	6	8	5%	7%	4%	54%	1.81	68%	1.32	3.88	3.13	3.57	3.69	1.88
- Feline	0	10	10	0%	2%	2%	62%	1.64	78%	0.93	4.27	3.10	3.83	3.58	2.06
- Fish	0	16	16	2%	7%	1%	75%	1.14	78%	0.94	3.71	3.02	3.44	3.49	1.74
- Insect	0	13	13	1%	1%	1%	73%	1.12	92%	0.40	4.18	3.06	3.86	3.38	1.82
- Mammal	0	42	42	1%	4%	2%	76%	1.00	93%	0.31	4.15	3.07	3.98	3.64	1.94
- Reptile	0	9	9	0%	3%	1%	60%	1.34	95%	0.29	3.98	3.21	3.31	3.34	1.98
- Sea mammal	0	7	7	2%	5%	2%	67%	1.49	76%	0.96	4.03	2.86	4.10	3.36	1.67
Body part	0	18	18	0%	0%	0%	69%	1.29	82%	0.78	4.67	2.57	4.01	3.64	3.14
Building infrastructure	0	96	96	3%	7%	4%	54%	2.17	67%	1.36	4.23	2.26	3.48	3.65	2.21
Building material	15	12	27	6%	11%	4%	49%	2.13	57%	1.64	4.35	2.18	3.81	3.60	2.19
Clothing	33	31	64	2%	3%	1%	63%	1.70	83%	0.70	4.13	2.18	3.65	3.56	2.93
Decoration & gift accessory	31	49	80	3%	6%	2%	56%	1.99	68%	1.24	4.05	2.52	3.45	3.61	2.21
Electronic device & accessory	44	47	91	4%	5%	2%	50%	2.30	68%	1.28	4.13	2.64	3.77	3.62	2.64
Furniture	3	32	35	1%	2%	2%	58%	1.87	78%	0.91	4.49	2.06	3.39	3.66	2.95
Game, toy & entertainment	27	40	67	3%	7%	2%	52%	2.15	76%	0.94	4.24	2.32	3.78	3.66	2.72
Household article & cleaner	38	21	59	2%	6%	2%	57%	2.02	55%	1.77	4.26	2.21	3.81	3.62	2.70
Jewel & money	7	1	8	2%	1%	1%	77%	1.07	60%	1.34	4.37	2.57	3.75	3.75	3.09
Kitchen & utensil	71	46	117	3%	8%	2%	53%	2.19	80%	0.88	4.23	2.23	3.86	3.78	2.62
Medical instrument & accessory	12	2	14	5%	9%	3%	57%	1.99	67%	1.38	4.24	2.41	3.94	3.73	3.11
Natural element	9	31	40	2%	3%	2%	65%	1.52	82%	0.74	4.14	2.61	3.56	3.66	2.02
Outdoor activity & sport item	19	75	94	4%	5%	3%	61%	1.73	72%	1.14	4.19	2.29	3.86	3.74	3.26
Skincare & bathroom item	34	11	45	2%	4%	2%	65%	1.60	74%	1.11	4.16	2.25	3.90	3.57	3.38
Stationary & school supply	42	18	60	1%	5%	3%	59%	1.87	75%	1.05	4.29	2.12	3.98	3.62	2.63

Nb = Number of stimuli, DKO = Don't know object, DKN = Don't know name, TOT = Tip-of-the-tongue, NA = Modal name agreement, H = H value, Fam = Familiarity, VC = Visual Complexity, CA = Category Agreement, Hcat = H value for category, OA = Object Agreement, VA = Viewpoint Agreement, Manip = Manipulability.

*Fruit, vegetable, and nut category was statistically compared with the other categories.

**All animals were collapsed together and compared statistically with the other categories. Subgroups of animals were not statistically compared.

Table 3. Norms as a function of gender.

Category	Gender	DKO	DKN	TOT	NA	*H*	CA	Hcat	Fam	VC	OA	VA	Manip
Food	Male	5%	3%	1%	54%	1.82	89%	0.46	4.29	2.23	3.81	3.86	2.08
(n = 75)	Female	4%	4%	2%	57%	1.63	92%	0.32	4.28	2.23	3.68	3.61	2.30
Fruit/vegetable/nut	Male	5%	5%	1%	52%	1.85	94%	0.28	4.27	2.21	3.91	4.18	1.86
(n = 15)	Female	4%	5%	4%	63%	1.43	98%	0.12	4.30	2.28	3.66	3.58	2.06
Tool	Male	3%**	8%**	1%**	62%*	1.67	74%	1.01	4.11*	2.24	3.84	3.84*	3.00
(n = 46)	Female	13%**	14%**	8%**	52%*	1.86	72%	1.07	3.72*	2.42	3.69	3.53*	2.83
Musical instrument	Male	4%	7%	2%**	64%	1.46	90%	0.46	4.01	2.47	4.09	3.89**	3.63
(n = 40)	Female	4%	10%	6%**	62%	1.41	91%	0.38	4.03	2.68	3.81	3.41**	3.62
Vehicle	Male	0%	5%	1%**	57%	1.82	75%	0.88	4.24	2.69	3.73*	3.59**	2.46
(n = 61)	Female	2%	7%	5%**	63%	1.52	79%	0.83	4.21	2.80	3.42*	3.21**	2.69
Weapon	Male	2%*	3%*	1%**	55%	1.87*	77%	0.98	3.86	2.18	3.88*	3.76*	3.05
(n = 35)	Female	10%*	9%*	4%**	65%	1.37*	77%	0.88	3.60	2.22	3.47*	3.34*	2.77
Animal	Male	1%	5%	1%*	70%	1.22	89%	0.45	3.94**	2.90**	3.88**	3.64**	1.70**
(n = 141)	Female	2%	4%	2%*	72%	1.06	89%	0.44	4.11**	3.24**	3.66**	3.37**	2.13**

DKO = Don't know object, DKN = Don't know name, TOT = Tip-of-the-tongue, NA = Modal name agreement, H = H value, Fam = Familiarity, VC = Visual Complexity, CA = Category Agreement, Hcat = H value for category, OA = Object Agreement, VA = Viewpoint Agreement, Manip = Manipulability.
*The agreement or rating is significantly different (.05< p <.0042) from the agreement or rating of the other gender.
**The agreement or rating is significantly different (p<.0042) from the agreement or rating of the other gender.

Table 4. Matrix of correlations.

	NA	H	Fam	VC	CA	Hcat	OA	VA
H	−.952*							
Fam	.340*	−.384*						
VC	.046	−.056	−.338*					
CA	.166*	−.194*	.081	.247*				
Hcat	−.172*	.203*	−.113	−.270*	−.960*			
OA	.288*	−.352*	.354*	−.034	.095	−.096		
VA	.176*	−.168*	.168*	−.097	.006	−.006	.323*	
Manip	.198*	−.223*	.445*	−.349*	.019	−.033	.183*	0.124

NA = Modal Name Agreement, Fam = Familiarity, VC = Visual Complexity, CA = Category Agreement, OA = Object Agreement, VA = Viewpoint Agreement, Manip = Manipulability.
*Significant correlation.

sets using line drawings. The BOSS includes a higher proportion of familiar everyday life objects (e.g. binder, pencil, toaster, etc.) than in these two other studies which, in contrast, offer a greater proportion of categories such as animals. Moreover, Adlington and colleagues [4] included concepts in their set that were intended to cover high, medium, and low familiarity ranges. Object and viewpoint agreements were very similar to the rating of typicality reported in Moreno-Martinez and Montoro [20] and visual complexity was only slightly smaller in the present study. Moreno-Martinez and Montero [20] also reported a higher rating for manipulability but the instructions were significantly different from those used in the present study.

The addition of animals, furniture, vehicles, weapons, musical instruments, and of many other types of concepts has not affected the mean ratings relative to Brodeur and colleagues [15] but it has slightly affected the pattern of correlations between norms. For instance, in contrast to Brodeur and colleagues [15], familiarity was negatively correlated with visual complexity. This negative correlation is consistent with most of the existing sets of images including a wide range of categories [28]. Moreover, manipulability was negatively correlated with visual complexity in the present study whereas this correlation was not significant in Brodeur and colleagues [15]. This new pattern of relationships is likely due to the addition of new categories in the present set. For instance, animals and vehicles, which were not in the original set, are amongst the most complex and the least manipulable concepts of the set. Moreover, the category of furniture was highly familiar but rated as visually simple, a pattern of correlation that contributes to the negative correlation found between familiarity and visual complexity. Overall, correlations found in this study are very similar to those reported in most previous studies using line drawings, likely because the present set includes animals, vehicles, furniture, and additional concepts also used in these other studies. For instance, like in other studies, name agreement correlated with familiarity [2,8,31–32] and norms of image agreement [2,31,33] but not with visual complexity [30–31,33–37]. Accordingly, correlations between norms must thus be examined cautiously as they highly depend on the categories included in the set of stimuli and they may be relatively independent from the stimulus format.

By adding new categories of concepts and by increasing the number of stimuli per category, the present study demonstrated how the norms vary across different categories of concepts. Overall, it was found that animals are easily recognized and named and that they are consistently categorized within their specific sub-categories (i.e. bird, reptile, mammal, etc). Animals are also the most visually complex, most likely due to furs and feathers that represent a rich texture. Most animals in the present set are common but there are also unfamiliar animals such as a fennec, a cuttlefish, and a horseshoe crab. This contributed to increase DKO responses and decrease the familiarity rating. Moreover, some animals were confounded with similar animals, such as the alligator which was recognized as a crocodile, the caribou as a moose, and the falcon as an eagle.

The food category also has distinctive features. Food, and more particularly fruits, vegetables, and nuts are among the concepts that are the easiest to recognize and name, along with the fact that they are also among the most familiar concepts. Fruits, vegetables, and nuts are also the least manipulable in the sense that they are not associated with specific manipulations that allow distinguishing among them. Finally, foods obtained the highest object agreement, which suggests that the BOSS pictures were very consistent with the way people imagined these concepts. This is probably due to the fact that most food items, including fruits, vegetables, and nuts are not man-made, and therefore, are less subject to various designs.

The tool category includes concepts with heterogeneous features which led to a large variability along the different dimensions. There are familiar tools (e.g. leaf rake) which are easily named, categorized, and associated to specific uses and there are unfamiliar tools, such as professional tools (e.g. flooring stapler) which are difficult to name and use. Moreover, category agreement was lowered because some tools can be used for multiple purposes that can be related to another category (e.g. ice scrapper, metal brush, etc.). This heterogeneity across tools calls for caution when interpreting norms and reminds that a mean is not warrant of the individual components of some categories.

For some categories, differences between genders were to be expected. For instance, previous studies showed a naming advantage for females with living things and a naming advantage for males with non-living things [38–39]. Comparisons of genders indicate that females had more difficulty recognizing and naming tools and weapons than males. Tools and weapons were also less familiar to females, although this difference was significant only for tools. This can be explained by a lower interest or use of these types of objects by females in general. Tools and weapons were the only categories with an atypical pattern of gender differences. The typical pattern, found in most categories, consisted in a greater use of the DKO, DKN, and TOT by females, in addition to a higher modal name agreement and a lower H value. Instead of reflecting a naming difficulty, the higher rate of DKO, DKN, and TOT in females could indicate that they tend to avoid giving a name when they think this name is incorrect. This tendency necessarily reduces the variability of names and increases the modal name agreement. Females also rated visual complexity and manipulability with higher scores. The two genders reach comparable agreement when categorizing concepts and rate familiarity similarly. On the other hand, object and viewpoint agreements were higher in males. This could simply be explained by the fact that most photos were selected and taken by a male (i.e. first author).

Norms are fundamental not only to characterize stimuli but also to measure variables that could introduce confounding effects. Confounding effects were demonstrated several times. For instance, Laws and Neve [40] compared living and non-living stimuli and showed that the disadvantage in naming living stimuli was reversed after controlling for familiarity, visual complexity, and name frequency. Similar findings were replicated with other categories and stimulus dimensions [12,41], which led Laws [42] to conclude that: "it is necessary to examine the performance of controls on sets of living and nonliving stimuli that are not confounded by these and other potential artefactual variables" (p. 842). In another study, Fillitier and colleagues [43] reported shorter response times for non-manipulable items compared to manipulable items. When they controlled for familiarity by including only familiar items in their analyses, they obtained the opposite effect. These confounding effects do not discard the existence of an effect inherent to the categories but they underline the importance of fully characterizing the stimuli before drawing conclusions on an effect.

Conclusion

Norms are a precious asset that should be considered when creating experimental conditions in order to control for potential confounding effects. The BOSS now includes 1,468 normative colored photos of various concepts from multiple categories. The BOSS also offers 1,179 non-normative photos depicting other exemplars of the normative concepts, and the normative concepts photographed from different viewpoints. In addition, 275 photos are also available in a black and white line drawing version. Norms collected thus far for the BOSS include those described in the present study as well as norms related to symmetry [44]), color diagnosticity (unpublished), and different actions afforded by the objects including those for grasping, using, and moving the object [45–47]. There are yet no norms on the names of the concepts, such as frequency and age-of-acquisition, but they may be collected in the future. Finally, norms were collected from English native speakers [15] and French native speakers [48]. More information about the BOSS can be found at http://sites.google.com/site/bosstimuli/.

Acknowledgments

We are grateful to Lara Berliner, Sébastien Lagacé, Frédéric Downing-Doucet, and Samantha Burns for having edited a number of stimuli.

Author Contributions

Conceived and designed the experiments: MBB KG. Performed the experiments: MB. Analyzed the data: MBB KG MB. Contributed reagents/materials/analysis tools: MBB KG MB. Contributed to the writing of the manuscript: MBB KG MB.

References

1. O'Sullivan M, Lepage M, Bouras M, Montreuil T, Brodeur MB (2012) North-american norms for name disagreement: pictorial stimuli naming discrepancies. PLoS One 7: e47802.
2. Bonin P, Peereman R, Malardier N, Meot A, Chalard M (2003) A new set of 299 pictures for psycholinguistic studies: French norms for name agreement, image agreement, conceptual familiarity, visual complexity, image variability, age of acquisition, and naming latencies. Behav Res Methods InstrumComput 35: 158–167.
3. Nishimoto T, Miyawaki K, Ueda T, Une Y, Takahashi M (2005) Japanese normative set of 359 pictures. Behav Res Methods 37: 398–416.
4. Adlington RL, Laws KR, Gale TM (2009) The Hatfield Image Test (HIT): a new picture test and norms for experimental and clinical use. J Clin ExpNeuropsychol 31: 731–753.
5. Barbarotto R, Laiacona M, Macchi V, Capitani E (2002) Picture reality decision, semantic categories and gender. A new set of pictures, with norms and an experimental study. Neuropsychologia 40: 1637–1653.
6. Cuetos F, Alija M (2003) Normative data and naming times for action pictures. Behav Res Methods InstrumComput 35: 168–177.
7. De Winter J, Wagemans J (2004) Contour-based object identification and segmentation: stimuli, norms and data, and software tools. Behav Res Methods InstrumComput 36: 604–624.
8. Dell'Acqua R, Lotto L, Job R (2000) Naming times and standardized norms for the Italian PD/DPSS set of 266 pictures: direct comparisons with American, English, French, and Spanish published databases. Behav Res Methods Instrum Comput 32: 588–615.
9. Kremin H, Akhutina T, Basso A, Davidoff J, De Wilde M, et al. (2003) A cross-linguistic data bank for oral picture naming in Dutch, English, German, French, Italian, Russian, Spanish, and Swedish (PEDOI) Brain Cogn 53: 243–246.
10. Magnié MN, Besson M, Poncet M, Dolisi C (2003) The Snodgrass and Vanderwart set revisited: norms for object manipulability and for pictorial ambiguity of objects, chimeric objects, and nonobjects. J Clin Exp Neuropsychol 25: 521–560.

11. Op De Beeck H, Wagemans J (2001) Visual object categorisation at distinct levels of abstraction: A new stimulus set. Perception 30: 1337–1361.
12. Rossion B, Pourtois G (2004) Revisiting Snodgrass and Vanderwart's object pictorial set: the role of surface detail in basic-level object recognition. Perception 33: 217–236.
13. Viggiano MP, Vannucci M, Righi S (2004) A new standardized set of ecological pictures for experimental and clinical research on visual object processing. Cortex 40: 491–509.
14. Brielmann AA, Stolarova M (2014) A New Standardized Stimulus Set for Studying Need-of-Help Recognition (NeoHelp) PLoS ONE. DOI:10.1371/journal.pone.0084373.
15. Brodeur MB, Dionne-Dostie E, Montreuil T, Lepage M (2010) The Bank of Standardized Stimuli (BOSS), a new set of 480 normative photos of objects to be used as visual stimuli in cognitive research. PLoS One 5: e10773.
16. Dan-Glauser ES, Scherer KR (2011) The Geneva affective picture database (GAPED): a new 730-picture database focusing on valence and normative significance. Behav Res 43: 468–477.
17. Denkinger B, Koutstaal W (2014) A set of 265 pictures standardized for studies of the cognitive processing of temporal and causal order information. Behav Res Methods, DOI:10.3758/s13428-013-0338-x.
18. Janssen N, Pajtas PE, Caramazza A (2011) A set of 150 pictures with morphologically complex English compound names: norms for name agreement, familiarity, image agreement, and visual complexity. Behav Res Methods 43: 478–490.
19. Migo EM, Montaldi D, Mayes AR (2013) A visual object stimulus database with standardized similarity information. Behav Res Methods 45: 344–354.
20. Moreno-Martinez FJ, Montoro PR (2012) An ecological alternative to Snodgrass &Vanderwart: 360 high quality colour images with norms for seven psycholinguistic variables. PLoS One 7: e37527.
21. Nishimoto T, Ueda T, Miyawaki K, Une Y, Takahashi M (2010) A normative set of 98 pairs of nonsensical pictures (droodles) Behav Res Methods 42: 685–691.
22. Salmon JP, McMullen PA, Filliter JH (2010) Norms for two types of manipulability (graspability and functional usage), familiarity, and age of acquisition for 320 photographs of objects. Behav Res Methods 42: 82–95.
23. Verfaillie K, Boutsen L (1995) A corpus of 714 full-color images of depth-rotated objects. Percept Psychophys 57: 925–961.
24. Biederman I, Ju G (1988) Surface versus edge-based determinants of visual recognition. Cogn Psychol 20: 38–64.
25. Brodie EE, Wallace AM, Sharrat B (1991) Effect of surface characteristics and style of production on naming and verification of pictorial stimuli. Am J Psychol 104: 517–545.
26. Leder H (1999) Matching person identity from facial line drawings. Perception 28: 1171–1175.
27. Rhodes G, Brennan S, Carey S (1987) Identification and Ratings of Caricatures: Implications for Mental Representations of Faces. Cogn Psychol 19: 473–497.
28. Snodgrass JG, Vanderwart M (1980) A standardized set of 260 pictures: norms for name agreement, image agreement, familiarity, and visual complexity. J Exp Psychol Hum Learn 6: 174–215.
29. Snodgrass JG, Corwin J (1988) Perceptual identification thresholds for 150 fragmented pictures from the Snodgrass and Vanderwart picture set. Percept Mot Skills 67: 3–36.
30. Cycowicz YM, Friedman D, Rothstein M, Snodgrass JG (1997) Picture naming by young children: norms for name agreement, familiarity, and visual complexity. J Exp Child Psychol 65: 171–237.
31. Alario FX, Ferrand L, Laganaro M, New B, Frauenfelder UH, et al. (2004) Predictors of picture naming speed. Behav Res Methods Instrum Comput 36: 140–155.
32. Pompeia S, Miranda MC, Bueno OF (2001) A set of 400 pictures standardised for Portuguese: norms for name agreement, familiarity and visual complexity for children and adults. Arq Neuropsiquiatr 59: 330–337.
33. Sanfeliu MC, Fernandez A (1996) A set of 254 Snodgrass Vanderwart pictures standardized for Spanish: Norms for name agreement, image agreement, familiarity, and visual complexity. Behav Res Methods Instrum Comput 28: 537–555.
34. Barry C, Morrison CM, Ellis AW (1997) Naming the Snodgrass and Vanderwart pictures: Effect of age of acquisition, frequancy, and name agreement. Q J Exp Psychol 50A: 560–585.
35. Berman S, Friedman D, Hamberger M, Snodgrass JG (1989) Developmental picture norms: Relationships between name agreement, familiarity, and visual complexity for child and adult ratings of two sets of line drawings. Behav Res Methods Instrum Comput 21: 371–382.
36. Sirois M, Kremin H, Cohen H (2006) Picture-naming norms for Canadian French: name agreement, familiarity, visual complexity, and age of acquisition. Behav Res Methods 38: 300–306.
37. Weekes BS, Shu H, Hao M, Liu Y, Tan LH (2007) Predictors of timed picture naming in Chinese. Behav Res Methods 39: 335–342.
38. Laws KR (2000) Category-specific naming errors in normal subjects: the influence of evolution and experience. Brain Lang 75: 123–133.
39. Laws KR (2004) Sex differences in lexical size across semantic categories. Pers Individ Dif 36: 23–32.
40. Laws KR, Neve C (1999) A 'normal' category-specific advantage for naming living things. Neuropsychologia 37: 1263–1269.
41. Laws KR (2001) What is structural similarity and is it greater in living things? Behav Brain Sci 24: 486–487.
42. Laws KR (2005) "Illusions of Normality": a Methodological Critique of Category-Specific Naming. Cortex 41: 842–851.
43. Filliter JH, McMullen PA, Westwood D (2005) Manipulability and living/non-living category effects on object identification (2005) Brain Cogn 57: 61–65.
44. Brodeur MB, Chauret M, Dion-Lessard G, Lepage M (2011) Symmetry brings an impression of familiarity but does not improve recognition memory. Acta Psychol 137: 359–370.
45. Lagacé S, Downing-Doucet F, Guérard K (2013) Norms for grip agreement for 296 photographs of objects. Behav Res Methods 45: 772–781.
46. Guérard K, Lagacé S, Brodeur MB (2014) Four types of manipulability ratings and naming latencies for a set of 560 photographs of objects. Behav Res Methods. DOI:10.3758/s13428-014-0488-5.
47. Guérard K, Brodeur MB (2014) Manipulability agreement as a predictor of action initiation latency. Behav Res Methods. DOI:10.3758/s13428-014-0495-6.
48. Brodeur MB, Kehayia E, Dion-Lessard G, Chauret M, Montreuil T, et al. (2012) The bank of standardized stimuli (BOSS): comparison between French and English norms. Behav Res Methods 44: 961–970.

4

Oxidative Stress in Patients with Type 1 Diabetes Mellitus: Is It Affected by a Single Bout of Prolonged Exercise?

Maria Pia Francescato*, Giuliana Stel, Mario Geat, Sabina Cauci

Department of Medical and Biological Sciences, University of Udine, Udine, Italy

Abstract

Presently, no clear-cut guidelines are available to suggest the more appropriate physical activity for patients with type 1 diabetes mellitus due to paucity of experimental data obtained under patients' usual life conditions. Accordingly, we explored the oxidative stress levels associated with a prolonged moderate intensity, but fatiguing, exercise performed under usual therapy in patients with type 1 diabetes mellitus and matched healthy controls. Eight patients (4 men, 4 women; 49±11 years; Body Mass Index 25.0±3.2 kg·m^{-2}; HbA_{1c} 57±10 mmol·mol^{-1}) and 14 controls (8 men, 6 women; 47±11 years; Body Mass Index 24.3±3.3 kg·m^{-2}) performed a 3-h walk at 30% of their heart rate reserve. Venous blood samples were obtained before and at the end of the exercise for clinical chemistry analysis and antioxidant capacity. Capillary blood samples were taken at the start and thereafter every 30 min to determine lipid peroxidation. Patients showed higher oxidative stress values as compared to controls (95.9±9.7 vs. 74.1±12.2 mg·L^{-1} H_2O_2; $p<0.001$). In both groups, oxidative stress remained constant throughout the exercise (p = NS), while oxidative defence increased significantly at the end of exercise ($p<0.02$) from 1.16±0.13 to 1.19±0.10 mmol·L^{-1} Trolox in patients and from 1.09±0.21 to 1.22±0.14 mmol·L^{-1} Trolox in controls, without any significant difference between the two groups. Oxidative stress was positively correlated to HbA_{1c} ($p<0.005$) and negatively related with uric acid ($p<0.005$). In conclusion, we were the first to evaluate the oxidative stress in patients with type 1 diabetes exercising under their usual life conditions (i.e. usual therapy and diet). Specifically, we found that the oxidative stress was not exacerbated due to a single bout of prolonged moderate intensity aerobic exercise, a condition simulating several outdoor leisure time physical activities. Oxidative defence increased in both patients and controls, suggesting beneficial effects of prolonged aerobic fatiguing exercise.

Editor: Massimo Pietropaolo, University of Michigan Medical School, States of America

Funding: Unconditioned financial support by Bayer Italia S.p.A. (Italy) and the Fondazione Cassa di Risparmio di Gorizia (Italy) allowed the study to be carried out. The funders had no role in study design, data collection and analysis, decision to publish, or preparation of the manuscript.

Competing Interests: Part of this study was funded by unconditional financial support from Bayer Italia S.p.A. (Italy). There are no patents, products in development or marketed products to declare.

* E-mail: maria.francescato@uniud.it

Introduction

Oxidative stress is a condition where the increased formation of free radicals overwhelms the available antioxidant capacity [1] and is involved in many human diseases, such as atherosclerosis, cardiovascular and neurological disease as well as in aging [1,2]. Oxidative stress is also a widely accepted participant in the development and progression of diabetes mellitus (DM) and its complications [2,3]. Indeed, disruption of the physiological free radicals homeostasis has been implicated in the impairment of beta-cell function [4,5].

Regulated production of free radicals, however, participates in several physiological processes, being also beneficial [6]. In fact, free radicals act as a double-edged sword in modulating insulin signaling, being required for insulin to exert its physiological action, but also being implicated in the pathogenesis of insulin resistance [3]. There are multiple likely sources of reactive oxygen and nitrogen species (ROS/RNS), especially in diabetes, including glucose autoxidation, glycation of proteins, consumption of NADPH through the polyol pathway, and activation of protein kinase C [7,8].

In patients with type 2 DM, an increased oxidative stress has been consistently shown [8] using different markers [7]. In contrast, in patients with type 1 DM both increases in oxidative stress [9–11], as well as unchanged levels [7,12,13] compared to healthy controls were reported.

Presently, there is evidence that regular physical activity can reduce the risk of several chronic diseases (e.g. cardiovascular disease, cancer, hypertension, obesity) and premature death, even in patients with diabetes [14]. However, for patients with type 1 DM, the available literature does not provide clear-cut guidance on the intensity, duration or type (aerobic/resistance) of physical activity that will offer the greatest benefits [15]. Notably, several patients perform only occasional outdoors leisure time physical activities (e.g., hiking, hill walking, biking, cross-country skiing), which tend to be prolonged in time, while being light to moderate in intensity. The effects of this kind of physical activity, however, are largely unexplored.

There is indirect evidence, on healthy subjects, that exercise may promote oxidative stress [1,6]. The association of type 1 DM and exercise-induced free radicals production is still understudied [10,16], although it is of great clinical and practical interest. In particular, data are lacking in patients exercising without modifying their usual therapy and/or as a result of a single bout of prolonged fatiguing exercise.

We studied the oxidative stress in a group of patients with type 1 DM at baseline and during a single bout of prolonged (3-h) moderate intensity aerobic exercise performed without modifying patient's usual insulin therapy or forcing a constant glycemia applying a clamp procedure, in comparison with a group of well-matched healthy controls. Lipid peroxidation (an indicator of oxidative stress) and the antioxidant defence were investigated by means of rapid point-of-care systems [2,17].

Materials and Methods

Patients

Eight patients with type 1 DM (4 men and 4 women) and 14 age- and gender-matched healthy subjects (8 men and 6 women) were recruited. All subjects practiced some aerobic physical exercise regularly, but none was highly trained. All participants were informed of the nature, purpose, and possible risks involved in the study before giving their voluntary written consent to participate. The study was approved by the Ethical Committee of the University of Udine and conducted according to the Declaration of Helsinki.

Patients were accepted if they were not affected by other chronic diseases, had no evidence of diabetes complications contraindicating physical activity, and showed glycated hemoglobin (HbA_{1c}) level ≤ 75 mmol·mol^{-1} (i.e. $\leq 9.0\%$) [18,19]. All patients were on a basal-bolus insulin regimen; 5 patients used lispro insulin before meals, 3 used regular insulin. At bedtime, 7 patients used insulin glargine, while 1 used NPH insulin. Physical and clinical characteristics of the two study groups were summarized in Table 1.

Experimental protocol

All the volunteers were asked to refrain from physical activity, alcohol, and caffeine in the 24-h period preceding the experimental session. In addition, patients were advised to maintain their usual diet and insulin regimen and to carefully control their blood glucose levels according to the self-management procedures in order to avoid hypoglycemic events.

All volunteers attended the laboratory early in the morning. At 7:30 AM patients injected themselves with their usual insulin dose (0.08 ± 0.04 IU·kg^{-1}) subcutaneously in the abdomen wall and consumed their usual breakfast, which included ~0.6 g·kg^{-1} of carbohydrates. Healthy control subjects had only a light breakfast at 7:30 AM, which included their usual average carbohydrate intake (~0.7 g·kg^{-1}). Thereafter, all participants rested in an armchair. About 45 min prior to the start of the exercise, an indwelling catheter was inserted into a forearm vein of the subject, patency of which was maintained by intermittent flushing with saline. Volunteers were then equipped with the belt of a heart rate monitoring system (Polar Electro, Kempele, Finland) to acquire heart rate (HR) values every 15 s throughout the exercise; HR data were subsequently downloaded and averaged over 15 min periods.

Volunteers performed a 3-h (from 10:00 AM to 1:00 PM) walk on a treadmill (Saturn, H-P Cosmos, Traunstein, Germany) maintaining HR constant by automatically adjusting speed and/or slope. To minimize dizziness due to the prolonged treadmill exercise, 5 min rest was allowed at the end of each hour of exercise. Work intensity was set to 30% of individual heart rate reserve ($HR_{target} = HR_{rest} + (HR_{max} - HR_{rest}) \times 0.3$), where HR_{max} was estimated using the common equation 220 minus age (expressed in years). Higher work rates would likely increase the risk of hypoglycemia in patients and decrease compliance of volunteers to complete the task.

In patients, to counteract an excessive fall of glycemia, the algorithm of Francescato et al. [20,21] was applied for each half-an-hour exercise to estimate the amount of required carbohydrates. Accordingly, patients were given 13 ± 14 g (range 0–40 g) of fruit fudge about 30 minutes before the start of the exercise. Thereafter, additional amounts of fruit fudge (10 ± 8 g; range 0–32 g) were administered to patients for each of the following 30 min exercise. Control subjects did not receive carbohydrates since there was no risk at all of hypoglycemia. All volunteers were allowed to drink water ad libitum.

Just before the start and at the end of the exercise, a venous blood sample (8.5 mL, and 5.5 mL, respectively) for clinical chemistry analysis and a capillary sample (50 μL) to determine the free oxygen radical defence (FORD tests; Calligari, Parma, IT) were drawn. Additionally, to determine lipid peroxidation (FORT tests; Calligari, Parma, IT), capillary blood withdrawals (20 μL) were taken just before the start of the exercise and, subsequently, at 30 min intervals. At the same times, glycemia was also tested in patients by using reactive strips on capillary blood (ContourLink, Bayer Healthcare Diabetes Division).

At the end of the trials, healthy control subjects were free to leave the laboratory. In contrast, to minimize the risk of late-onset hypoglycemic events [22], patients were kept under supervision of a physician trained in diabetes until the following morning. Patients received their usual insulin doses and meals for lunch and dinner (at 1:30 PM and 7:30 PM, respectively) and were allowed to sit quietly in an armchair (or lay in bed) while their glycemia was tested by means of reactive strips at least hourly. All the glycemic levels were recorded on appropriate forms, the analysis of which confirmed us that late-onset hypoglycemia after the trials was actually avoided in all patients.

Analyses

Venous blood was collected in a tube with gel and clot activator (Vacutainer SST II advance #368965), a tube containing a glycolysis inhibitor (4 mg kalium oxalate +5 mg sodium fluoride; Vacutainer #368920), and a tube containing EDTA (Vacutainer #368856). Immediately after collection, tubes were gently mixed and the hospital laboratory processed the samples within 1 hour from collection.

Plasma glucose concentration was determined by applying a hexokinase based methodology (Olympus Diagnostic Systems AU2700; Olympus America Inc., Miami, FL, USA); our determined coefficient of analytical variation was <2% in the range 3.27 to 11.67 mmol·L^{-1}.

Insulin concentrations were determined by the DxI800 Automated Immunoassay system (Beckman Coulter, Fullerton, CA, USA) (coefficient of analytical variation was <6% in the range 11.08 to 49.13 IU·L^{-1}), which measures all the relevant insulin analogs with a cross-reactivity of about 80% [23].

HbA_{1c} was determined using the G8 HPLC Analyzer (Tosoh Biosience Inc, S. Francisco, CA, USA). Our determined coefficient of variation was 1.06% at an average concentration of 33 mmol·mol^{-1} (5.2%). Samples from two control subjects were unavailable for HbA_{1c} analysis.

Concentrations of uric acid, homocysteine, triglycerides, total cholesterol, HDL cholesterol, ALT, AST, and hs-CRP were

Table 1. Demographic, clinical, and baseline biochemical parameters of the study subjects.

	Patients with type 1 DM	Healthy controls	p
Male/Female	4M-4F	8M-6F	
Age (y)	49.1±10.5	46.8±10.7	NS
Body mass (kg)	74.1±15.4	73.3±14.5	NS
Stature (m)	1.71±0.10	1.73±0.11	NS
Body Mass Index ($kg \cdot m^{-2}$)	25.0±3.2	24.3±3.3	NS
Duration of diabetes (y)	29.4±14.2	-	
Insulin dose ($IU \cdot kg^{-1}$ per day)	0.51±0.08	-	
HbA_{1c} (%)	7.4±1.0	5.7±0.5	<0.001
($mmol \cdot mol^{-1}$)	57.0±10.4	38.3±5.0	<0.001
Creatinine ($mg \cdot dL^{-1}$)	0.86±0.10	0.99±0.19	NS
Uric acid ($mg \cdot dL^{-1}$)	2.7±0.7	4.3±1.4	<0.005
Total cholesterol ($mg \cdot dL^{-1}$)	181.6±32.5	189.2±34.3	NS
LDL-C ($mg \cdot dL^{-1}$)	116.9±24.3	118.6±29.9	NS
HDL-C ($mg \cdot dL^{-1}$)	53.1±12.4	55.6±12.8	NS
Triglycerides ($mg \cdot dL^{-1}$)	58.0±18.2	97.2±37.6	<0.05
ALT ($U \cdot L^{-1}$)[§]	16.5 (10–34)	13.5 (11–40)	NS
AST ($U \cdot L^{-1}$)[§]	30.0 (21–47)	25.0 (15–40)	NS
Homocysteine ($mg \cdot dL^{-1}$)[§]	9.1 (7.3–12.5)	11.0 (7.1–37.3)	NS
hs-CRP ($mg \cdot L^{-1}$)[§]	0.67 (0.39–1.75)	1.00 (0.06–3.21)	NS
Iron ($\mu g \cdot dL^{-1}$)	52.9±33.6	92.1±49.5	NS
Transferrin ($mg \cdot dL^{-1}$)	184.5±21.5	226.5±61.7	<0.05
Tf saturation (%)	44.6±8.4	33.1±16.2	NS
FORT ($mg \cdot L^{-1}$ H_2O_2)	95.9±9.7	74.1±12.2	<0.001
FORD ($mmol \cdot L^{-1}$ Trolox)	1.16±0.13	1.09±0.21	NS

Values are expressed as means ±SD. Parameters failing normal distribution ([§]) are shown as median value and range (in brackets) and the Mann-Whitney U test was used to test their statistically significant differences.

measured on Olympus AU5400 analyzer (Olympus America Inc., Miami, FL, USA) by original reagents. LDL cholesterol was calculated from total cholesterol, triglycerides, and HDL according to the Friedewald equation.

Reactive oxygen species, in the form of lipid peroxides, were determined using a colorimetric assay called FORT test (Callegari, Parma, Italy) [2,24–27]. Results were expressed as FORT units, whereby 1 FORT unit corresponded to 0.26 $mg \cdot L^{-1}$ H_2O_2. Our determined coefficient of analytical variation was <3.6%. Blood antioxidant capacity was determined by the colorimetric FORD test (Callegari, Parma, Italy) [2,24]. The absorbance values of the samples were compared with a standard curve obtained using Trolox, a derivative of vitamin E commonly used as an antioxidant. Coefficient of analytical variation was <5.0%.

Statistical Analysis

All variables were tested for normal distribution. Differences between patients and controls were examined using the Student t test or the Mann-Whitney U test as appropriate.

For multiple comparisons, analysis of variance for repeated measures (MANOVA) was applied with time as within-subjects factor and study group as between-subjects factor, followed by specific contrasts when appropriate. The two-tailed Spearman correlation coefficient for nonparametric variables was used to evaluate associations between the plasma concentrations of FORT with the study parameters. Two-tailed $p<0.05$ was considered significant. Systat version 11 software (Systat Software GmbH, Erkrath, Germany) was used. Values were expressed as means±SD or median and range, as appropriate.

Results

Demographic characteristics and baseline biochemical parameters of the 8 patients and 14 controls were described in Table 1. There were no significant differences between patients and controls for most variables. Eight subjects were overweight but none was obese (Body Mass Index<30 $kg \cdot m^{-2}$). Values of serum biomarkers did not differ significantly between the two groups, with the exception of uric acid, triglycerides, and transferrin, all of which were lower in patients.

Actual exercise intensity, expressed as percentage of individual's heart rate reserve, was not significantly different between patients and controls (p = NS), amounting on average to 28.8±2.3% in patients and 31.4±4.1% in controls, corresponding to a grand-average value of 101±4 bpm. Progression speed was not significantly different between the two groups (group effect, $F=0.43$, p = NS), showing a slight decrease across exercise duration from 5.3±0.6 $km \cdot h^{-1}$ to 5.0±0.7 $km \cdot h^{-1}$ (time effect, $F=1.980$, $p<0.05$). Total traveled distance was 15.7±1.5 km, with no difference between the two groups.

Both at the start and the end of exercise, glycemia was significantly higher in patients than in controls (Figure 1, panel A; group effect, $F=19.04$, $p<0.001$). Glycemia followed a different behavior in the two groups (group × time effect, $F = 11.22$, $p < 0.005$); in controls glycemia did not change significantly throughout the exercises (time effect, $F = 0.01$, $p = NS$) amounting on average to 4.6±0.5 mmol·L^{-1}, whereas in patients glycemia fell significantly from 8.0±2.7 mmol·L^{-1} at the start to 5.9±1.6 mmol·L^{-1} at the end of the exercise (time effect, $F = 7.21$, $p < 0.05$).

Figure 1, panel B, illustrates the significantly higher insulin concentrations of patients as compared to controls before and at the end of the exercise (group effect, $F = 81.87$, $p < 0.001$). In both groups, insulin concentration decreased significantly at the end of the exercise (time effect, $F = 40.88$, $p < 0.001$).

Figure 2 shows that oxidative stress (FORT) values remained constant in both groups of volunteers throughout the 3-h exercise (time effect, $F = 0.21$, $p = NS$). At each time point, oxidative stress was significantly higher in patients than in controls (group effect, $F = 14.67$, $p < 0.001$). On the opposite, in both groups, total antioxidant capacity (FORD) values increased significantly from baseline to the end of the exercise (1.16±0.13 vs. 1.19±0.10 mmol·L^{-1} Trolox in patients and 1.09±0.21 vs. 1.22±0.14 mmol·L^{-1} Trolox in controls; time effect, $F = 6.73$, $p < 0.02$) without any significant difference between the two groups (group effect, $F = 0.11$, $p = NS$).

Average oxidative stress values were positively related to the HbA_{1c} values (Figure 3, panel A; $n = 20$, $R = 0.649$, $p < 0.005$), and a negative relation with serum concentration of uric acid was found (Figure 3, panel B; $n = 22$, $R = 0.621$, $p < 0.005$). No significant correlation was found between oxidative stress and the triglycerides or the transferrin levels.

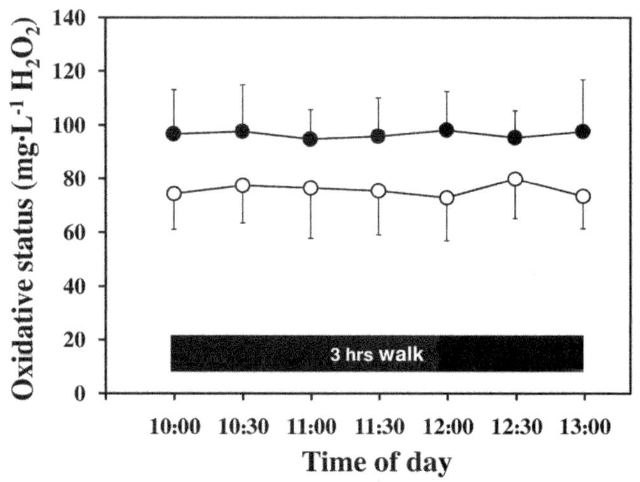

Figure 2. Oxidative stress values throughout the 3-h exercises. Oxidative stress was significantly higher in patients ($p < 0.005$), but remained essentially unchanged in both groups across the exercise ($p = NS$). Full dots = patients with type 1 DM, open dots = healthy control subjects.

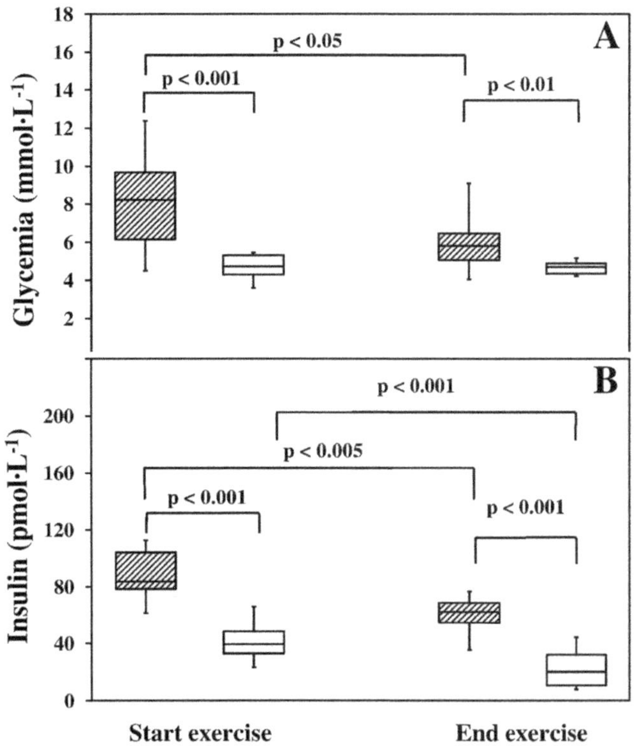

Figure 1. Glycemia and insulin concentration before and at the end of the 3-h exercises. Panel A. Glycemia (mmol·L^{-1}) was significantly higher in patients both before and at the end of the exercise ($p < 0.01$) and decreased significantly in patients with type 1 DM at the end of the trial ($p < 0.05$). Panel B. Insulin concentration (pmol·L^{-1}) was significantly higher in patients both before and at the end of the exercise ($p < 0.001$) and decreased significantly in both groups at the end of the trial ($p < 0.005$). In both panels: shaded boxes = patients, open boxes = healthy control subjects.

Discussion

The present study first showed that a single bout of prolonged moderate intensity aerobic exercise did not increase the lipid peroxidation levels (FORT test, as marker of oxidative stress), in both patients with type 1 DM and healthy subjects, despite higher peroxidation levels were observed throughout in patients. In contrast, an increase in the anti-oxidant defence (evaluated by the FORD assay) was observed at the end of the exercise in both patients and controls.

Physical exercise is strongly recommended in DM patients because of its numerous health benefits [15], but it might also cause oxidative stress [8], resulting in a potentially harmful condition [1]. Indeed, accumulating evidence suggests that oxidative cell injury caused by free radicals contributes to the development of DM complications [3,5], thus patients should avoid situations that might increase oxidative stress. Our results suggest that the 3-h exercise performed in the present study, which simulate several outdoor leisure time physical activities, although fatiguing, were not of sufficient intensity to provoke a large enough increase in free radical production to overwhelm the antioxidant defences [1,6]. Conversely, other authors found that an exercise at higher intensity and/or at exhaustion increased the oxidative stress levels in type 1 DM patients [10,16].

The observed constancy of the oxidative stress during the 3-h exercise provided new information on the effects of a single bout of aerobic exercise both in the general population and type 1 DM patients, which are considered more prone to oxidative stress effects [16]. Indeed, contractile activity is known to cause an increase in ROS generation in muscle, but the factors influencing the magnitude of this response include also the nature and the duration of the contractile activity [28]. Thus, we can speculate that our exercise condition was not able to induce a significant increase in free radicals production. On the other hand, the investigated physical activity resulted in a significant increase in the serum antioxidant capacity, suggesting that the pathways that

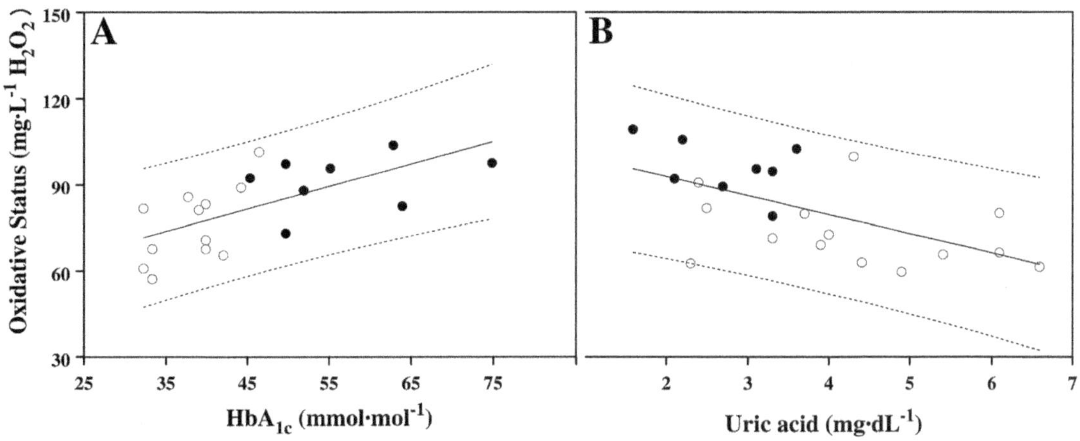

Figure 3. Relationship between oxidative stress and HbA_{1c} or uric acid. Panel A. Relationship between baseline HbA_{1c} values (mmol·mol^{-1}) and oxidative stress (mg·L^{-1} H_2O_2). The relationship is statistically significant (n = 20, R = 0.649, $p<0.005$). Panel B. Relationship between baseline uric acid values (mg·dL^{-1}) and oxidative stress (mg·L^{-1} H_2O_2). The relationship is statistically significant (n = 22, R = 0.621, $p<0.005$). In both panels: full dots = patients with type 1 DM, open dots = healthy control subjects, dotted lines = 95% confidence limits.

generate free radicals and those stimulating the antioxidant defence are in some way unrelated, as recently observed by other authors [24]. Indeed, during moderate exercise, ROS act also as signals resulting in an upregulation of powerful antioxidant enzymes such as superoxide dismutase, glutathione peroxidase and catalase [29,30]. In general, ROS/RNS generated during muscle contraction appear to have a physiological role in the adaptation to exercise, leading to the view that moderate exercise can be considered also an antioxidant with beneficial effects [30,31]. Our results induce to postulate that the same conclusion can apply also to patients with type 1 DM. Main purpose of our study was the investigation of lipid peroxidation; accordingly, only a general test, i.e. the FORD assay, was used to obtain overall information about the anti-oxidant activity. In the future, to depict in greater detail the effects of a prolonged exercise, it will undoubtedly be of great interest to investigate the activity of specific enzymes.

It should be pointed out here that patients with type 1 DM often require some extra carbohydrates before/during the effort to prevent an excessive fall of glycemia [21], even when they reduce the dose of injected insulin in anticipation of exercise [32]. This extra amount of carbohydrates might be considered a caloric load that will be oxidized in mitochondria, resulting in a potential higher production of free radicals and thus constituting a confounding variable in the experimental setup of the present work. Nevertheless, an experimentation similar to the present one [33] showed that the whole-body carbohydrates oxidation rate was not significantly different between patients with type 1 DM receiving appropriate amounts of fruit fudge (to avoid an excessive fall of glycemia) and the control group, who was not given carbohydrates during the exercise. In addition, it was reported by others that increased extracellular glucose availability does not necessarily translate into increased intracellular glucose oxidation during exercise [34,35]. Furthermore, Chokkalingam et al. [36] observed that only patients exercising under high insulin infusion rates showed a slightly increased whole-body carbohydrates oxidation rate. Accordingly, we believe that the administration of fruit fudge to our patients during the 3-h walks had only a negligible effect on their oxidative stress levels.

The positive relationship we observed including all study subjects (patients and healthy controls), between oxidative stress and glycated hemoglobin (HbA_{1c}) levels was unexpected. Our finding, however, is in line with the loose relationship (p = 0.02) between urinary 8-hydroxydeoxyguanosine concentration and HbA_{1c} in patients with type 1 DM reported by others [37]. Indeed, moderate elevations of glucose can potentially affect the oxidative stress [38]. Nevertheless, only rather prolonged periods of improved glycemic control induced a reduction in the oxidative stress in patients with diabetes [18,19], while no similar observations have ever been reported for acute changes of glycemia occurring within a few hours. Thus, the constancy of oxidative stress levels observed in our patients at the end of the 3-h walks, despite a clear fall of their glycemia, is not surprising.

An unexpected finding was also the negative relationship, including all study subjects, between oxidative stress and serum uric acid levels. Indeed, uric acid is a powerful antioxidant and scavenger of singlet oxygen and radicals [39,40]. The lower uric acid levels in patients in comparison to controls were consistent with few previous findings where a significantly reduced level of plasma uric acid amongst subjects with type 1 DM was reported [9,13]. It remains to be clarified whether the low uric acid concentration observed in patients is a consequence or a cause of the high oxidative stress levels observed in these subjects. Although future research is warranted to better evaluate this relationship on a larger number of patients, clinicians should be suggested to carefully monitor uric acid, due to its association with the oxidative stress, in particular in patients with type 1 DM.

In our work, lipid peroxidation was used as marker of ROS [17] because of their interesting association with atherosclerosis and cardiovascular disease [41], but, on the other hand, it might represent a limitation of the present study. In fact, the observed levels of oxidative stress might depend also upon the kind of investigated oxidative stress marker [7], because reactive oxygen species are a vast group of agents, which are usually short lived and often difficult to measure. We choose the FORT and FORD tests because of their simplicity and rapidity of the assays, requiring only a small drop of capillary blood, thus allowing repeated and minimally invasive measuring. According to Kamhieh-Milz et al. [24], we are confident that the FORT and the FORD tests provide actually reliable results. Among others, the FORT test was also used to investigate the association between oxidative stress and C-reactive protein levels among healthy adults [25], to evaluate the effects of an innovative treatment in cancer-related anorexia/cachexia [27] and to investigate oxidative stress in different populations with type 2 diabetes [2,26]. It appears thus that measurement of oxidation markers by means of point-of-care methods may be helpful to assess oxidant activity and to monitor the effectiveness of the antioxidant system in several different physiological conditions including exercise.

The rather small number of investigated patients might represent a further limitation. This was the consequence of the challenging protocol, especially for patients who had to be monitored for several hours following the exercise for the high risk of severe late-onset hypoglycemia. To partially compensate for this small number, we recruited a number of controls almost twice the patients. Furthermore, the small number of examined subjects did not allow us to investigate eventual gender differences [42].

Conclusions

Results of the present study showed that the 3-h walking exercise did not worse the oxidative stress levels, suggesting that a single bout of prolonged moderate intensity aerobic exercise can be performed as leisure time outdoors activity also by patients with type 1 diabetes, despite they show a baseline oxidative stress higher than healthy controls. In the mean time, oxidative defence increased in both patients and controls, suggesting beneficial effects also of prolonged fatiguing but not exhausting exercise. Finally, the role of uric acid and chronically elevated glycemia in patients with type 1 DM in relation to oxidative stress should be investigated in greater detail.

Acknowledgments

We gratefully thank all the volunteers who accepted to participate to the study.

Author Contributions

Conceived and designed the experiments: MPF MG SC. Performed the experiments: MPF MG GS. Analyzed the data: MPF MG SC. Contributed reagents/materials/analysis tools: GS SC. Wrote the paper: MPF SC.

References

1. Powers SK, Nelson WB, Hudson MB (2011) Exercise-induced oxidative stress in humans: Cause and consequences. Free Radic Biol Med 51: 942–950.
2. Pavlatou MG, Papastamataki M, Apostolakou F, Papassotiriou I, Tentolouris N (2009) FORT and FORD: two simple and rapid assays in the evaluation of oxidative stress in patients with type 2 diabetes mellitus. Metabolism 58: 1657–1662.
3. Bashan N, Kovsan J, Kachko I, Ovadia H, Rudich A (2009) Positive and Negative Regulation of Insulin Signaling by Reactive Oxygen and Nitrogen Species. Physiol Rev 89: 27–71.
4. West IC (2000) Radicals and oxidative stress in diabetes. Diabet Med 17: 171–180.
5. Drews G, Krippeit-Drews P, Dufer M (2010) Oxidative stress and beta-cell dysfunction. Pflugers Arch 460: 703–718.
6. Vollaard NBJ, Shearman JP, Cooper CE (2005) Exercise-Induced Oxidative Stress: Myths, Realities and Physiological Relevance. Sports Med 35: 1045–1062.
7. VanderJagt DJ, Harrison JM, Ratliff DM, Hunsaker LA, Vander Jagt DL (2001) Oxidative stress indices in IDDM subjects with and without long-term diabetic complications. Clin Biochem 34: 265–270.
8. Golbidi S, Badran M, Laher I (2012) Antioxidant and Anti-Inflammatory Effects of Exercise in Diabetic Patients. Exp Diabetes Res 2012: 941868.
9. Marra G, Cotroneo P, Pitocco D, Manto A, Di Leo MAS, et al. (2002) Early Increase of Oxidative Stress and Reduced Antioxidant Defenses in Patients With Uncomplicated Type 1 Diabetes: A case for gender difference. Diabetes Care 25: 370–375.
10. Laaksonen DE, Atalay M, Niskanen L, Uusitupa M, Hanninen O, et al. (1996) Increased Resting and Exercise-Induced Oxidative Stress in Young IDDM Men. Diabetes Care 19: 569–574.
11. Domìnguez C, Ruiz E, Gussinye M, Carrascosa A (1998) Oxidative Stress at Onset and in Early Stages of Type 1 Diabetes in Children and Adolescents. Diabetes Care 21: 1736–1742.
12. Reis JS, Veloso CA, Volpe CM, Fernandes JS, Borges EA, et al. (2012) Soluble RAGE and malondialdehyde in type 1 diabetes patients without chronic complications during the course of the disease. Diab Vasc Dis Res 9: 309–314.
13. Vessby J, Basu S, Mohsen R, Berne C, Vessby B (2002) Oxidative stress and antioxidant status in type 1 diabetes mellitus. J Intern Med 251: 69–76.
14. American Diabetes Association (2004) Physical activity/exercise and diabetes. Diabetes Care 27: S58–S62.
15. Chimen M, Kennedy A, Nirantharakumar K, Pang T, Andrews R, et al. (2012) What are the health benefits of physical activity in type 1 diabetes mellitus? A literature review. Diabetologia 55: 542–551.
16. Davison GW, George L, Jackson SK, Young IS, Davies B, et al. (2002) Exercise, free radicals, and lipid peroxidation in type 1 diabetes mellitus. Free Radic Biol Med 33: 1543–1551.
17. Garelnabi MO, Brown WV, Le NA (2008) Evaluation of a novel colorimetric assay for free oxygen radicals as marker of oxidative stress. Clin Biochem 41: 1250–1254.
18. Sharma A, Kharb S, Chugh SN, Kakkar R, Singh GP (2000) Evaluation of oxidative stress before and after control of glycemia and after vitamin E supplementation in diabetic patients. Metabolism 49: 160–162.
19. Berg TJ, Nourooz-Zadeh J, Wolff SP, Tritschler HJ, Bangstad H-J, et al. (1998) Hydroperoxides in Plasma Are Reduced by Intensified Insulin Treatment: A randomized controlled study of IDDM patients with microalbuminuria. Diabetes Care 21: 1295–1300.
20. Francescato MP, Carrato S (2011) Management of Exercise-induced Glycemic Imbalances in Type 1 Diabetes. Curr Diabetes Rev 7: 253–263.
21. Francescato MP, Geat M, Accardo A, Blokar M, Cattin L, et al. (2011) Exercise and Glycemic Imbalances: a Situation-Specific Estimate of Glucose Supplement. Med Sci Sports Exerc 43: 2–11.
22. Tamborlane WV (2007) Triple Jeopardy: Nocturnal Hypoglycemia after Exercise in the Young with Diabetes. J Clin Endocrinol Metab 92: 815–816.
23. Owen WE, Roberts WL (2004) Cross-Reactivity of Three Recombinant Insulin Analogs with Five Commercial Insulin Immunoassays. Clin Chem 50: 257–259.
24. Kamhieh-Milz J, Salama A (2014) Oxidative Stress Is Predominant in Female but Not in Male Patients with Autoimmune Thrombocytopenia. Oxid Med Cell Longev 2014: 9.
25. Abramson JL, Hooper WC, Jones DP, Ashfaqe S, Rhodes SD, et al. (2005) Association between novel oxidative stress markers and C-reactive protein among adults without clinical coronary heart disease. Atherosclerosis 178: 115–121.
26. De Cosmo S, Lamacchia O, Rauseo A, Viti R, Gesualdo L, et al. (2006) Cigarette Smoking Is Associated With Low Glomerular Filtration Rate in Male Patients With Type 2 Diabetes. Diabetes Care 29: 2467–2470.
27. Mantovani G, Madeddu C, Macciò A, Gramignano G, Lusso MR, et al. (2004) Cancer-Related Anorexia/Cachexia Syndrome and Oxidative Stress: An Innovative Approach beyond Current Treatment. Cancer Epidemiol Biomarkers Prev 13 1651–1659.
28. Powers SK, Jackson MJ (2008) Exercise-Induced Oxidative Stress: Cellular Mechanisms and Impact on Muscle Force Production. Physiol Rev 88: 1243–1276.
29. Takahashi M, Miyashita M, Kawanishi N, Park J, Hayashida H, et al. (2013) Low-volume exercise training attenuates oxidative stress and neutrophils activation in older adults. Eur J Appl Physiol 113: 1117–1126.
30. Gomez-Cabrera M-C, Domenech E, Viña J (2008) Moderate exercise is an antioxidant: Upregulation of antioxidant genes by training. Free Radic Biol Med 44: 126–131.
31. Viña J, Sanchis-Gomar F, Martinez-Bello V, Gomez-Cabrera M (2012) Exercise acts as a drug; the pharmacological benefits of exercise. Br J Pharmacol 167: 1–12.
32. Grimm JJ, Ybarra J, Berné C, Muchnick S, Golay A (2004) A new table for prevention of hypoglycaemia during physical activity in type 1 diabetic patients. Diabetes Metab 30: 465–470.
33. Geat M, Stel G, Poser S, Driussi C, Stenner E, et al. (2013) Whole-body glucose oxidation rate during prolonged exercise in type 1 diabetic patients under usual life conditions. Metabolism 62: 836–844.
34. Jenni S, Oetliker C, Allemann S, Ith M, Tappy L, et al. (2008) Fuel metabolism during exercise in euglycaemia and hyperglycaemia in patients with type 1 diabetes mellitus—a prospective single-blinded randomised crossover trial. Diabetologia 51: 1457–1465.
35. Stettler C, Jenni S, Allemann S, Steiner R, Hoppeler H, et al. (2006) Exercise capacity in subjects with type 1 diabetes mellitus in eu- and hyperglycaemia. Diabetes Metab Res Rev 22: 300–306.
36. Chokkalingam K, TzinTzas K, Norton L, Jewell K, Macdonald IA, et al. (2007) Exercise under hyperinsulinaemic conditions increases whole-body glucose disposal without affecting glycogen utilisation in type 1 diabetes. Diabetologia 50: 414–421.
37. Goodarzi MT, Navidi AA, Rezaei M, Babahmadi-Rezaei H (2010) Oxidative damage to DNA and lipids: correlation with protein glycation in patients with type 1 diabetes. J Clin Lab Anal 24: 72–76.
38. Menon V, Ram M, Dorn J, Armstrong D, Muti P, et al. (2004) Oxidative stress and glucose levels in a population-based sample. Diabet Med 21: 1346–1352.

39. Lippi G, Montagnana M, Franchini M, Favaloro EJ, Targher G (2008) The paradoxical relationship between serum uric acid and cardiovascular disease. Clin Chim Acta 392: 1–7.
40. Ames BN, Cathcart R, Schwiers E, Hochstein P (1981) Uric acid provides an antioxidant defense in humans against oxidant- and radical-caused aging and cancer: a hypothesis. Proc Natl Acad Sci 78: 6858–6862.
41. Peluso I, Morabito G, Urban L, Ioannone F, Serafini M (2012) Oxidative stress in atherosclerosis development: the central role of LDL and oxidative burst. Endocr Metab Immune Disord Drug Targets 12: 351–360.
42. Di Santolo M, Banfi G, Stel G, Cauci S (2009) Association of recreational physical activity with homocysteine, folate and lipid markers in young women. Eur J Appl Physiol 105: 111–118.

5

Effects of Different Types of Jump Impact on Trabecular Bone Mass and Microarchitecture in Growing Rats

Yong-In Ju[1]*, Teruki Sone[2], Kazuhiro Ohnaru[3], Kensuke Tanaka[2], Hidetaka Yamaguchi[4], Masao Fukunaga[5]

1 Department of Health and Sports Sciences, Kawasaki University of Medical Welfare, Kurashiki, Okayama, Japan, **2** Department of Nuclear Medicine, Kawasaki Medical School, Kurashiki, Okayama, Japan, **3** Department of Orthopedic Surgery, Kawasaki Medical School, Kurashiki, Okayama, Japan, **4** Department of Sports Social Management, Sports Health Course School of Social Science, KIBI International University, Takahashi, Okayama, Japan, **5** Kawasaki Medical School, Kurashiki, Okayama, Japan

Abstract

Substantial evidence from animal studies indicates that jumping increases bone mass and strength. However, most studies have focused on the take-off, rather than the landing phase of jumps. Thus, we compared the effects of landing and upward jump impact on trabecular bone mass and microarchitecture. Male Wistar rats aged 10 weeks were randomly assigned to the following groups: sedentary control (CON), 40-cm upward jumps (40UJ); 40-cm drop jumps (40DJ); and 60-cm drop jumps (60DJ) (n = 10 each). The upward jump protocol comprised 10 upward jumps/day, 5 days/week for 8 weeks to a height of 40 cm. The drop jump protocol comprised dropping rats from a height of 40 or 60 cm at the same frequency and time period as the 40UJ group. Trabecular bone mass, architecture, and mineralization at the distal femoral metaphysis were evaluated using microcomputed tomography. Ground reaction force (GRF) was measured using a force platform. Bone mass was significantly higher in the 40UJ group compared with the DJ groups (+49.1% and +28.3%, respectively), although peak GRF (−57.8% and −122.7%, respectively) and unit time force (−21.6% and −36.2%, respectively) were significantly lower in the 40UJ group. These results showed that trabecular bone mass in growing rats is increased more effectively by the take-off than by the landing phases of jumps and suggest that mechanical stress accompanied by muscle contraction would be more important than GRF as an osteogenic stimulus. However, the relevance of these findings to human bone physiology is unclear and requires further study.

Editor: Luc Malaval, Université Jean Monnet, France

Funding: This study was supported by Kawasaki University of Medical Welfare Scientific Research Fund. The funder had no role in study design, data collection and analysis, decision to publish, or preparation of the manuscript.

Competing Interests: The authors have declared that no competing interests exist.

* Email: jyi.k@mw.kawasaki-m.ac.jp

Introduction

Although exercise is considered one of the best strategies for enhancing bone mass and strength, not all types of exercise are beneficial. Numerous studies over the last few decades have investigated which types of exercise are more effective for increasing bone mass and strength. High-impact and weight-bearing activity are generally accepted as being beneficial for strengthening skeletal bone. Among various types of exercise in rats, high-impact loading such as jumping seems to be most beneficial for increasing bone mass and strength rather than low-impact loading such as running [1,2,3].

The impact transmitted to hindlimb bone during jumps can be divided into take-off and landing phases. Peak ground reaction force (GRF) is generally considered greater during the landing, than the take-off phase [4,5,6]. Thus, landing impact is considered more beneficial for building bone mass and increasing strength than take-off impact. The effects of landing (free-fall landing) on bone mass and strength have been investigated in growing rats [7,8,9]. Welch et al. [9] found that free-fall landing produced significantly larger increases in strength, geometry, and density in the forelimbs of growing rats. However, upward jump exercise in the form of vertical jumps from the bottom to the top of a board, without GRF at landing has been most widely applied as an exercise model for promoting bone mass, strength, and structure in rodents [10,11,12,13,14]. Welch et al. [9] also showed that free-fall landing imparts greater osteogenic effects to the bones of the forelimb than the hindlimb in rats [1]. Their report suggested that the type of landing could increase bone mass more effectively than take-off, but the effects of the two jump phases have not been directly compared in the same bone.

We postulated that GRF would be higher at the landing, than at the take-off phase of jumps and that bone mass and quality in the exercised limb would be more effectively improved by the landing, than the take-off impact. We tested this hypothesis by comparing the effects of upward and drop jumps on trabecular bone mass and the microarchitecture of the distal femur in growing rats.

Materials and Methods

Ethics statement

This study proceeded in strict accordance with the recommendations described in the Guide for the Care and Use of Laboratory Animals of the National Institutes of Health. The Committee for the Ethics of Animal Experiments at Kawasaki University of Medical Welfare approved the experimental protocol (Permit Number: 10-010). The rats were anesthetized with intraperitoneal pentobarbital sodium (0.1 mL/100 g of body weight) and sacrificed by exsanguination from the abdominal aorta at the end of the experiment.

Animals and experimental design

Nine-week old male Wistar rats (CLEA Japan, Osaka, Japan), weighing 200–250 g at the start of the experiment, were singly housed in 20×33×14-cm cages in a sanitary ventilated animal room under a controlled temperature (22°C±1°C) and a 12 h/12 h light-dark cycle. The rats were acclimated to the environment, and were given a diet of standard MF laboratory rodent chow (Oriental Yeast Co. Ltd., Chiba, Japan) and water ad libitum for one week before starting the experiment. The rats were weighed and food intake was measured daily before exercise. After one week of acclimation to the diet and new environment, the rats were randomly assigned to the following groups (n = 10 per group): sedentary controls reared in the breeding cage (CON), rats that jumped upwards to a height of 40 cm (40UJ), and rats that fell from a height of 40 (40DJ) or 60 (60DJ) cm. After sacrifice, the right soleus and gastrocnemius muscles were collected from each rat and immediately weighed. Excised femora from each rat were cleaned of soft tissue and then the femoral length was measured using digital calipers. Right femora were stored at −40°C until analysis using micro-computed tomography (micro-CT) and left femora were fixed in 70% ethanol for histomorphometric analysis.

Exercise conditions

Upward jumps proceeded according to our previous publications [11,12,13]. Briefly, rats in the 40UJ group were placed individually at the bottom of a wooden box (Figure 1A) and then an electric stimulus was initially provided to force them to jump and grasp the top of one of the sides of the box with the forepaws, climb up onto it and remain there for 11 seconds. A technician then gently placed each rat back on the floor of the box to repeat the procedure without generating GRF above the body weight at landing. Since the rats rapidly became conditioned to jump voluntarily, the electrical stimulus was not required after the first few days. The rats jumped upwards 10 times daily at a frequency of once per 11 seconds, 5 days per week for 8 weeks. The initial height of the box was 25 cm and this was progressively increased to 40 cm during the first week.

Drop jumps proceeded as described with slight modification [9]. In brief, rats were dropped through the inside of a transparent plastic cylinder (internal diameter: 14.5 cm, outside diameter: 15.0 cm) that formed part of a device designed in-house (Figure 1B). The device was fashioned such that the rats would land hindlimb-first on the ground. A preliminary experiment confirmed that the rats indeed landed mostly with hindlimb first when dropped through this device. Rats in the 40DJ and 60DJ groups were dropped 10 times daily onto a bare floor from a height of 40 and 60 cm at the same frequency and duration as the 40UJ group. The 40-cm drop height was selected for comparison with the 40UJ group. Since the 40UJ group grasped the top of the board set at 40 cm with their forelimbs and then climbed onto it, the position in which the drop started was adjusted so that their forelimbs were located 40 cm above the ground. The 60-cm drop height was selected to exceed the impact produced by the 40DJ group. The initial drop height was 25 cm like the 40UJ jump group and progressively increased to 40 cm and 60 cm during the first week. The rats were monitored and jumps were periodically

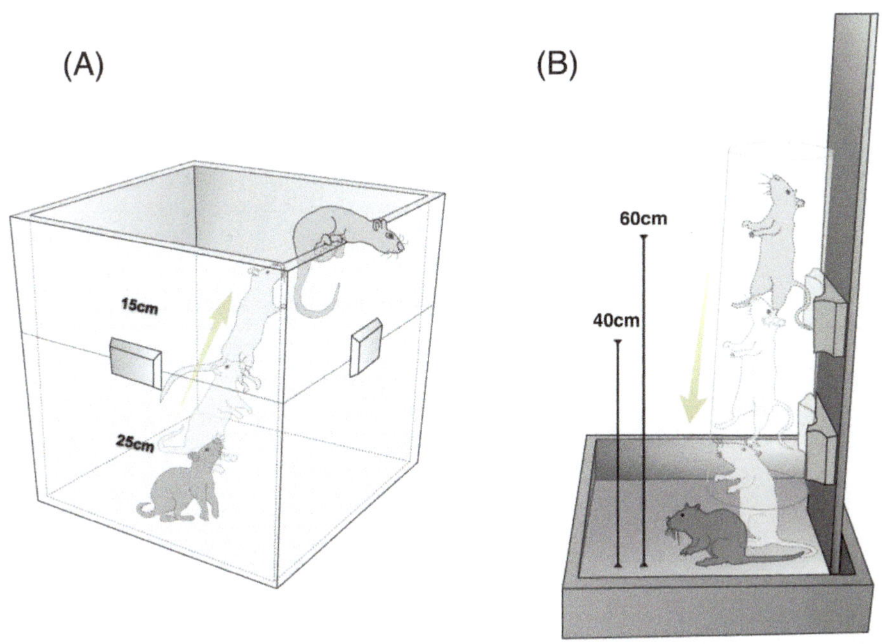

Figure 1. Schematic representation of upward (A) and drop (B) jumps. (A) Rats jumped vertically upward 40 cm from the bottom to the top of a box 10 times per day without landing. (B) Rats landed after being dropped 10 times per day through a 40- or 60-cm-high transparent plastic cylinder without take-off.

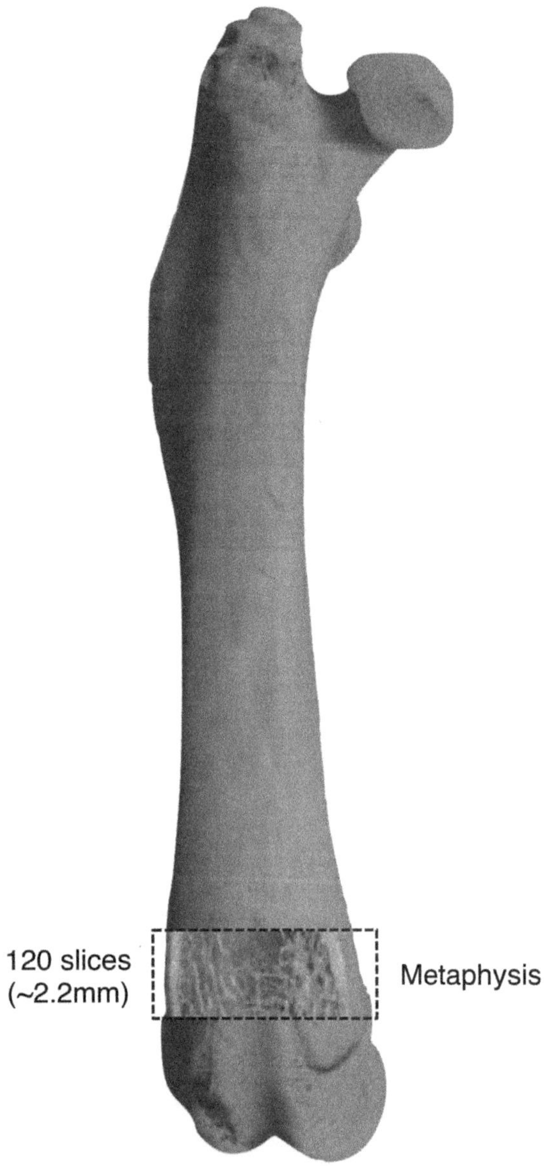

Figure 2. Location of volume of interest in distal femoral metaphysis for micro-CT analysis of trabecular bone.

recorded using a high-speed video camera to verify correct and safe landings.

Determination of GRF

The GRF during take-off or landing for each jump exercise was measured using a Type 9286A multicomponent force platform with dimensions of 40×60 cm (Kistler, Winterthur, Switzerland). Analog voltage signals from each force plate sensor were recorded at a sampling rate of 1000 Hz and sent to a 9865E1Y28 force plate amplifier (Kistler), where they were converted to digital data using a Powerlab 16/30 ML880 system and analyzed using LabChart 7 software (ADInstruments, Nagoya, Japan). The GRF was measured four weeks after the jump program was started. The upward and drop jump devices were installed above the force platform. Rats in the 40UJ group were placed on the force platform from which they jumped 10 times upward to the top edge of the box. The 40DJ or 60DJ rats were dropped 10 times each from a height of 40 or 60 cm onto the force platform using a drop-jump training device. Impulse, peak GRF, contact time, and impulse per contact time (unit time force) from 10 jumps were averaged and the GRF was normalized by body weight (GRF/body weight). Peak GRF was determined as the highest GRF achieved during take-off and landing for each jump.

Measurement of 3D architectural indices and mineralization density of cancellous bone

Trabecular bone microarchitecture and mineralization were evaluated using an Ele Scan mini micro-CT system (Nittetsu Elex, Tokyo, Japan) that has an X-ray tube with a microfocus (spot size, 6×8 μm) and a maximum resolution of 4 μm (pixel size) [11,12,13]. All specimens were scanned at a source energy of 45 kVp and 90 μA to maximize contrast between bone and soft tissue. A 0.1-mm copper plate served as the X-ray filter. The right femur was positioned 2.8–3.0 mm proximal from the distal end of the femur, including the border between the distal metaphysis and the growth plate. We acquired 300 consecutive 18.11 μm (approximately 5.4 mm)-thick tomographic slices and reconstructed CT images with a pixel size of 18.11 μm in 512×512 matrices.

The microstructural indices and the mineralization density of the trabecular bone were calculated using TRI/3D-BON bone structural analysis software (Ratoc System Engineering, Tokyo, Japan). A volume of interest (VOI) for each femur was defined as 120 slices above the most proximal portion of the growth plate (Figure 2). The resulting gray-scale images were segmented using a 3×3 median filter to remove noise, and a threshold was fixed to

Table 1. Body weight, hindlimb muscle weight, and femoral length in experimental rats.

	CON (n=10)	40DJ (n=10)	60DJ (n=10)	40UJ (n=10)
Body weight before experiment (g)	291.79±09.57	292.41±08.63	292.29±17.11	295.21±08.78
Body weight after experiment (g)	421.56±09.68	421.04±22.89	420.01±24.67	420.55±14.88
Calf muscle weight				
Soleus (g)	0.74±0.01	0.73±0.02	0.73±0.01	0.74±0.01
Gastrocnemius (g)	2.48±0.09	2.43±0.20	2.48±0.16	2.47±0.08
Total muscle weight (g)	3.22±0.09	3.16±0.21	3.22±0.17	3.20±0.08
Femoral length (mm)	37.61±0.86	37.46±0.60	37.63±0.68	38.16±0.53

Values are shown as means ± SD. n, number of rats in each group; CON, sedentary control group reared in breeding cage; 40DJ, rats that jumped downwards from a height of 40 cm; 60DJ, rats that jumped downwards from a height of 60 cm; 40UJ, rats that jumped upwards to a height of 40 cm.

Table 2. Peak GRF, impulse, contact time and unit time force produced by upward and drop jumps.

	40DJ	60DJ	40UJ
	(n = 10)	(n = 10)	(n = 10)
Peak GRF ($N*N^{-1}$)	$9.94 \pm 0.46^{\ddagger}$	$14.03 \pm 0.54^{\ddagger\|\|}$	6.30 ± 0.31
Impulse (Nms)	1.099 ± 0.047	$1.163 \pm 0.092^{*}$	1.042 ± 0.082
Contact time (ms)	$0.110 \pm 0.011^{*}$	$0.104 \pm 0.009^{\dagger}$	0.127 ± 0.011
Unit time force (N)	$10.01 \pm 0.668^{\dagger}$	$11.21 \pm 1.278^{\dagger\S}$	8.23 ± 0.343

All values are shown as means ± SD. 40DJ, rats that jumped downwards from a height of 40 cm; 60DJ, rats that jumped downwards from a height of 60 cm; 40UJ, rats that jumped upwards to a height of 40 cm. GRF, ground reaction force. Significant difference vs. 40UJ group: $^{*}p<0.05$, $^{\dagger}p<0.01$, $^{\ddagger}p<0.001$. Significant difference vs. 40DJ group: $^{\S}p<0.05$, $^{\|\|}p<0.001$.

extract the mineralized bone phase. Isolated small particles in the marrow space and isolated small holes in bone were removed using a cluster-labeling algorithm. Cortical and trabecular bone were subsequently separated by semi-automatically drawn contours and then structural indices were calculated. The following 3D morphometric parameters were calculated by measuring distances in 3D directly in the trabecular network [15]: total bone marrow volume including trabeculae (TV; mm^3), trabecular bone volume (BV; mm^3), trabecular bone volume fraction (BV/TV; %), mean trabecular number (Tb.N;/mm), mean trabecular thickness (Tb.Th; μm), and mean trabecular separation (Tb.Sp; μm). Degrees of trabecular bone mineralization (mineralization density; mg/cm^3) were measured as described [16]. The CT number was converted into bone mineralization density using a calibration curve obtained from bone mineral density (BMD) measured using a hydroxyapatite phantom (6×1 mm; 200 to 800 mg/cm^3; Kyoto Kagaku, Kyoto, Japan) and the average degree of mineralization was measured in the region of interest. The BMD phantoms were assessed by CT under the same conditions as actual bone.

Bone histomorphometry

One and five days before dissection, 8 mg/kg body weight of fluorescent calcein (Dojindo Laboratories, Kumamoto, Japan) in 2% sodium hydrogen carbonate was subcutaneously administered to all rats. The left femur were fixed in 70% ethanol and stained with Villanueva bone stain for six days, dehydrated in graded concentrations of ethanol, and embedded in methyl-methacrylate (Wako Pure Chemical Industries, Osaka, Japan) without bone decalcification. Seven random specimens per group were histomorphometrically analyzed. Fluorochrome-based dynamic histomorphometric parameters were determined in the frontal plane, 5-μm thick sections of the distal metaphysis cut using a RM2255 rotary microtome (Leica, Wetzlar, Germany). A region of interest was positioned 0.9–3.5 mm proximal to the distal femoral growth cartilage/metaphyseal junction, and 0.9 mm from the endosteal border of the cortices. The sections were analyzed at 320× magnification using a semiautomatic image analyzing system (System Supply, Nagano, Japan), linked to a BX-53 light/epifluorescent microscope (Olympus, Tokyo, Japan). Sections were histomorphometrically assessed at the Ito Bone Histomorphometry Institute (Niigata, Japan). The following indices for cancellous bone were determined: BV/TV (%); Tb.Th (μm); Tb.N (/mm); Tb.Sp (μm); osteoclast surface/bone surface (Oc.S/BS, %); eroded surface/BS (ES/BS, %); osteoblast surface/BS (Ob.S/BS, %); mineral apposition rate (MAR, μm/day); mineralizing surface/BS (MS/BS, %); and bone formation rate/BS (BFR/BS, $\mu m^3/\mu m^2$/day) [17].

Statistical analysis

All data were statistically analyzed using the IBM SPSS Statistics 22.0 software (IBM, Armonk, NY, USA). Categories were compared by a one-way analysis of variance followed by Tukey's post hoc analysis. All data are expressed as means ± SD. The level of statistical significance was set at $p<0.05$.

Results

Body weight, calf muscle weight, and bone length

Table 1 shows body weight before and after the experiment, the weight of the soleus/gastrocnemius (calf) muscles, and the femoral length of the rats in each group. Body weight did not significantly differ throughout the study between the sedentary controls and the three groups of exercised rats. Calf muscles were weighed to confirm the effect of drop and upward jumps on skeletal muscle. The weight of the calf muscles and the length of the femur were similar among the four groups of rats at the end of the experiment. Thus, drop and upward jumps did not affect either skeletal muscle weight or femoral length.

Ground reaction force

Table 2 shows the outcomes of comparisons of peak GRF, impulse, contact time, and unit time force between each group after 4 weeks. Peak GRF, impulse, and unit time force were significantly greater in 40DJ and 60DJ groups than in 40UJ group, except for impulse in the 40DJ group. Peak GRF and unit time force were also significantly greater in the 60DJ, than in the 40DJ group. In contrast, contact time was significantly greater in 40UJ, than in the 40DJ and 60DJ groups.

Trabecular microstructure and mineralization

Figure 3 shows the 3D microstructural parameters in the distal femur. Among trabecular bone parameters, BV/TV and Tb.Th were significantly higher in the 40UJ, than the CON, 40DJ, and 60DJ groups and Tb.N was significantly higher in the 40UJ and 60DJ groups than in the CON group. However, Tb.Sp did not significantly differ among the four groups. The degree of trabecular bone mineralization was significantly higher in the 40UJ, than in the CON group.

Histomorphometry

Table 3 shows the results of histomorphometric analysis of cancellous bone in the distal femur. Both BV/TV and Tb.Th were significantly higher in the 40UJ, than in the CON and 40DJ groups. With respect to bone resorption, both Oc.S/BS and ES/BS were lower in all jump groups than in the CON group, although the differences were statistically significant only in the

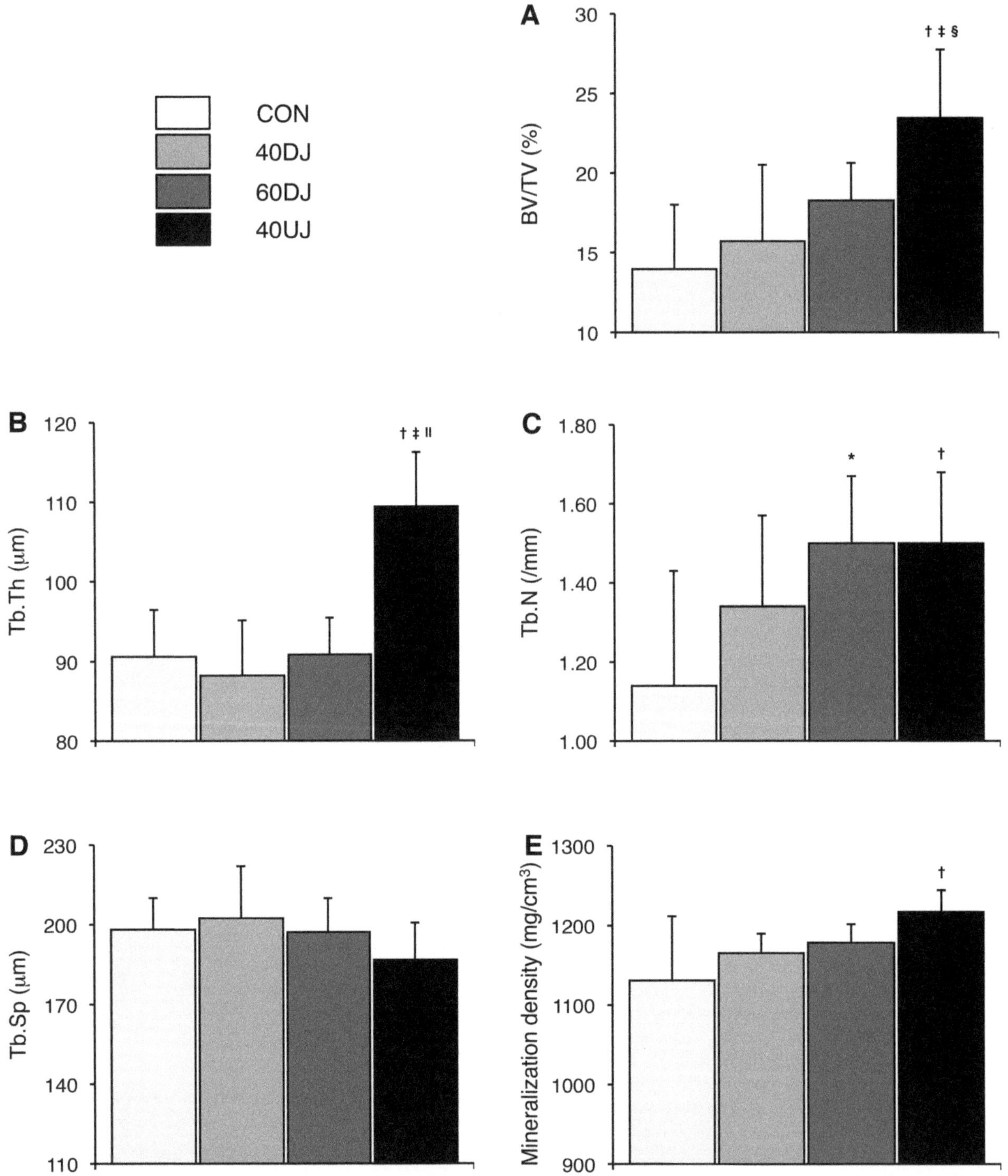

Figure 3. Microstructural parameters in the femoral metaphysis of rats that jumped downwards from a height of 40 (40DJ) or 60 (60DJ) cm, or upwards to a height of 40 cm (40UJ) or remained sedentary (CON) measured by micro-CT. A, Trabecular bone volume fraction (BV/TV); B, trabecular thickness (Tb.Th); C, trabecular number (Tb.N); D, trabecular separation (Tb.Sp); E, degree of trabecular bone mineralization. Significant differences: $^{*}p<0.01$ and $^{\dagger}p<0.001$ vs. CON; $^{\ddagger}p<0.001$ vs. 40DJ; $^{\S}p<0.05$ and $^{\|}p<0.001$ vs. 60DJ.

40DJ and 40UJ groups for Oc.S/BS and ES/BS, respectively. Values for Ob.S/BS and MS/BS reflecting bone formation were highest in the 40UJ group and significantly differed from those in the 60DJ group. In addition, MS/BS was also higher in the 40UJ, than in the CON group, whereas MAR and BFR/BS did not differ significantly among the four groups.

Discussion

The main purpose of this study was to empirically test the hypothesis that a higher GRF produced during landing would be more effective for stimulating an elevation in trabecular bone mass compared with take-off. However, although landing was associated with a higher GRF, its ability to increase trabecular bone

Table 3. Static and dynamic histomorphometry at distal femoral metaphysis of growing rats.

	CON	40DJ	60DJ	40UJ
	(n = 7)	(n = 7)	(n = 7)	(n = 7)
BV/TV (%)	17.7±5.0	16.4±2.3	19.1±4.8	24.7±5.0*†
Tb.Th (μm)	67.7±11.4	67.7±7.2	74.1±6.3	82.3±3.0*†
Tb.N (/mm)	2.6±0.5	2.4±0.2	2.6±0.4	3.0±0.6
Tb.Sp (μm)	330.7±84.7	348.7±39.1	327.1±78.6	262.9±76.9
Oc.S/BS (%)	15.5±2.1	11.2±2.3*	12.7±2.1	12.1±2.3
ES/BS (%)	21.3±2.6	17.5±3.3	19.6±4.3	15.9±2.1*
Ob.S/BS (%)	29.3±3.5	27.7±2.7	25.6±2.3	30.5±3.1‡
MAR (μm/day)	2.4±0.2	2.5±0.1	2.4±0.2	2.3±0.2
MS/BS (%)	34.7±4.9	35.3±4.0	31.3±1.6	41.1±3.6*§
BFR/BS ($\mu m^3/\mu m^2$/day)	0.81±0.1	0.89±0.1	0.75±0.1	0.97±0.1

Values are shown as means ± SD. n, number of rats in each group; 40DJ, rats that jumped downwards from a height of 40 cm; 60DJ, rats that jumped downwards from a height of 60 cm; 40UJ, rats that jumped upwards to a height of 40 cm. BFR/BS, bone formation rate/BS; BV/TV, trabecular bone volume fraction; CON, sedentary control group reared in breeding cage; MAR, mineral apposition rate; ES/BS, eroded surface/BS; MS/BS, mineralizing surface/BS; Ob.S/BS, osteoblast surface/BS; Oc.S/BS, osteoclast surface/bone surface; Tb.N, trabecular number; Tb.Sp, trabecular separation; Tb.Th, trabecular thickness. Significant difference vs. CON group: *$p<0.05$. Significant difference vs. 40DJ group: †$p<0.05$. Significant difference vs. 60DJ group: ‡$p<0.05$; §$p<0.0$.

mass was weaker than that of take-off in this rat model of jump exercise. Our results showed that GRF alone cannot account for the impact of jumps on limb bone and suggest that local impact by muscle contraction serves an important role in increasing bone mass.

The effects of exercise on bone mass and strength depend on the loading magnitude, frequency and duration of stimulation, and the loading direction applied to the bone during the activity. High strain rates positively affect bone formation [18,19]. Several published animal studies have found that jumping yields greater increases in bone mass and strength than running due to imposing greater anabolic stimulus upon the bone [1,2,3]. Human studies of high-impact activity have shown that exercise involving jumping elicits greater bone gain than repetitive high-frequency activities such as running or walking [20,21]. Jumping impacts lower limb bones and is an essential athletic feature of many sports such as volleyball, basketball, gymnastics, triple jumping, dance, and figure skating. Ground reaction force is generated by the acceleration of all segments of a body that contact the ground. The actions of take-off and landing during jumps involve different magnitudes of GRF [22]. Reports indicate that the magnitude of the GRF during jumps in terms of athletic performance is greater during landing than during the take-off phase [5,6]. Therefore, we postulated that the landing impact would result in more pronounced stimulation than the take-off impact. To the best of our knowledge, the effects of take-off and landing during jumps on bone mass and structure in rats as well as in humans has not been directly compared.

The effects of exercise on bone mass, strength, and structure of rodents have commonly been assessed using upward jumps [10,11,12,13,14], but also in rats dropped from specific heights [7,8,9]. One study has found that voluntary jump exercise including both upward jumps and landings produced significant increases in bone formation rates and BV/TV in cancellous bone of long-bone metaphyses [23]. It remains unclear, however, which phase of jumping is more effective for the increasing bone mass. Welch et al. [9] found that 10 free-fall landings per day produced significantly larger increases in the strength, geometry, and density of the forelimbs of growing rats without obvious changes in the hindlimbs. They also found that the cross-sectional area and breaking force were 20% and 40% higher at the ulnar diaphysis in free-fall, compared with control rats. Umemura et al. [1] found that upward jumps increased femoral cross-sectional area and breaking force by 14–15% and 13–18%, respectively. However, the present study found that bone mass and mineralization significantly increased only in the 40UJ, compared with the CON group. Drop jumps did not significantly improve trabecular bone mass except in Tb.N despite a higher GRF. These results suggested that trabecular bone mass at the distal femur is enhanced more effectively by forces generated on bone at take-off, than at landing. Wu et al. found similar results in female rhythmic sports gymnasts [24], in whom bone mass at the proximal femur was higher on the take-off (left) than the landing (right) leg. The apparent discrepancy between the results reported by Welch et al. [9] and the present findings might be explained by a difference in study design including the type of landing on the forelimbs instead of the hindlimbs. We designed a specific device to ensure that the rats landed on their hindlimbs during drop jumps to compare the effects of upward- and drop-jump impact at the same skeletal site.

Reports indicate that high-impact jumps with a GRF of 5–16 times body weight effectively increase bone mass in rats [9,10,14]. Here, the peak GRF was 9.94 and 14.03 times body weight in the 40DJ and 60DJ groups, respectively, which was higher than that of 6.30 in the 40UJ group. The range of peak GRF in the 60DJ group was similar to those of a previous study [9] that examined GRF during free-fall landing from a height of 60 cm. Drop jumps resulted in more than twice the peak GRF compared with upward jumps, but little affected trabecular bone mass, microarchitecture, and mineralization in the distal femur. The reason that drop jumps exerted less effects might be that GRF does not sufficiently reflect mechanical stress on trabecular bone at the femur. The notion that muscles and tendons absorb (dissipate) mechanical energy while eccentrically lengthening during the landing phase of jumps is generally accepted [25,26,27,28]. Therefore, the transmission of GRF produced during landing might be attenuated by eccentric muscular action. On the other hand, during the take-off phase of jumps, stored elastic energy is used to enhance force production, which acts on the lower limb bone and could induce substantial local stress on bone. Both GRF as well as forces generated by muscular contraction should contribute to the loading of limb bones. Biomechanical analyses suggest that muscle contraction generates larger forces than body weight *per se* [29]. Moreover, the results of a human study *in vivo* by Lu et al. [30] showed that >70% of bending moments on a bone during gait are transmitted by force generated from muscle than from external reaction. Similarly, direct muscle contraction force on a bone during upward jumps might contribute to a substantial portion of the mechanical stress at the distal femur in addition to GRF.

Bone histomorphometry confirmed the positive effect of upward jumps on bone mass and dynamic histomorphometry showed that bone formation was stimulated more by upward, rather than drop jumps. Bone resorption parameters did not significantly differ between upward and drop jumps. Taken together, these results show that more osteogenic effects are generated by upward, rather than drop jumps.

One limitation of this study is that we did not measure the magnitude and rate of strain in femoral bone during the take-off and landing phases of jumps. Further studies are needed to define the mechanism(s) involved in skeletal responses to take-off and landing impact. Another limitation is that mechanical stress might be differently transmitted by muscle contraction at lower limb bones between humans and smaller animals, in which the relative contribution of muscle contraction to the impact on bone might be substantially higher. The specific effects of the upward phase of jumps on human bone have not yet been defined. Controlled studies of drop jumping in children have found positive effects on bone gain [20,31]. Nonetheless, the present findings suggest that muscle contraction plays a key role in improving the trabecular bone mass and structure of limb bones.

Conclusion

The present findings did not support the hypothesis that a higher GRF exerted by the landing phase would increase trabecular bone mass of the distal femoral metaphysis more than the take-off phase of jumps in growing rats. The results suggest that local impact accompanied by muscle contraction during jumps plays an important role in enhancing trabecular bone mass compared with impact expressed as GRF.

Acknowledgments

The authors thank Hak-Jin Choi for assistance with taking care of the rats.

Author Contributions

Conceived and designed the experiments: YIJ TS MF. Performed the experiments: YIJ KO KT HY. Analyzed the data: YIJ HY. Contributed to the writing of the manuscript: YIJ. Data interpretation: YIJ TS MF. Revising manuscript content: TS. Responsibility for integrity of data analysis: YIJ TS. Approving final version of manuscript: YIJ TS KO KT HY MF.

References

1. Umemura Y, Ishiko T, Tsujimoto H, Miura H, Mokushi N, et al. (1995) Effects of jump training on bone hypertrophy in young and old rats. Int J Sports Med 16: 364–367.
2. Notomi T, Okazaki Y, Okimoto N, Saitoh S, Nakamura T, et al. (2000) A comparison of resistance and aerobic training for mass, strength and turnover of bone in growing rats. Eur J Appl Physiol 83: 469–474.
3. Notomi T, Lee SJ, Okimoto N, Okazaki Y, Takamoto T, et al. (2000) Effects of resistance exercise training on mass, strength, and turnover of bone in growing rats. Eur J Appl Physiol 82: 268–274.
4. Adrian MJ, Laughlin CK (1983) Magnitude of ground reaction forces while performing volleyball skills. In: Matsui H, Kobayashi K, eds. Biomechanics VII-B. Champaign, IL: Human Kinetics 903–914.
5. Kato T, Terashima T, Yamashita T, Hatanaka Y, Honda A, et al. (2005) Effect of low-repetition jump training on bone mineral density in young women. J Appl Physiol 100: 839–843.
6. Richards DP, Ajemain SV, Wiley JP, Zernicke RF (1996) Knee joint dynamics predict patellar tendinitis in elite volleyball players. Am J Sports Med 24: 676–683.
7. Lin HS, Huang TH, Wang HS, Mao SW, Tai YS, et al. (2013) Short-term free-fall landing causes reduced bone size and bending energy in femora of growing rats. J Sports Sci Med 12: 1–9.
8. Welch JM, Turner CH, Devareddy L, Arjmandi BH, Weaver CM (2008) High impact exercise is more beneficial than dietary calcium for building bone strength in the growing rat skeleton. Bone 42: 660–668.
9. Welch JM, Weaver CM, Turner CH (2004) Adaptations to free-fall impact are different in the shafts and bone ends of rat forelimbs. J Appl Physiol 97: 1859–1865.
10. Honda A, Umemura Y, Nagasawa S (2001) Effect of high-impact and low-repetition training on bones in ovariectomized rats. J Bone Miner Res 16: 1688–1693.
11. Ju YI, Sone T, Ohnaru K, Choi HJ, Choi KA, et al. (2013) Jump exercise during hindlimb unloading protect against the deterioration of trabecular bone microarchitecture in growing young rats. Springerplus 2: 35.
12. Ju YI, Sone T, Ohnaru K, Choi HJ, Fukunaga M (2012) Differential effects of jump versus running exercise on trabecular architecture during remobilization after suspension-induced osteopenia in growing rats. J Appl Physiol 112: 766–72.
13. Ju YI, Sone T, Okamoto T, Fukunaga M (2008) Jump exercise during remobilization restores integrity of the trabecular architecture after tail suspension in young rats. J Apple Physiol 104: 1594–1600.
14. Umemura Y, Ishiko T, Yamauchi T, Kurono M, Mashiko S (1997) Five jumps per day increase bone mass and breaking force in rats. J Bone Miner Res 12: 1480–1485.
15. Hildebrand T, Rüegsegger P (1997) A new method for the model-independent assessment of thickness in three-dimensional images. J Microsc 185: 67–75.
16. Chiba K, Nango N, Kubota S, Okazaki N, Taguchi K, et al. (2012) Relationship between microstructure and degree of mineralization in subchondral bone of osteoarthritis: a synchrotron radiation μCT study. J Bone Miner Res 27: 1511–1517.
17. Dempster DW, Compston JE, Drezner MK, Glorieus FH, Kanis JA, et al. (2013) Standardized nomenclature, symbols, and units for bone histomorphometry: a 2012 update of the report of the ASBMR Histomorphometry Nomenclature Committee. J Bone Miner Res 28: 1–16.
18. Forwood MR, Owan I, Takano Y, Turner CH (1996) Increased bone formation in rat tibiae after a single short period of dynamic loading in vivo. Am J Physiol 270: E419–23.
19. Judex S, Zernicke RF (2000) High-impact exercise and growing bone: relation between high strain rates and enhanced bone formation. J Appl Physiol 88: 2183–2191.
20. Fuchs RK, Bauer JJ, Snow CM (2001) Jumping improves hip and lumbar spine bone mass in prepubescent children: a randomized controlled trial. J Bone Miner Res 16: 148–156.
21. Kohrt WM, Bloomfield SA, Little KD, Nelson ME, Yingling VR (2004) American college of sports medicine. American college of sports medicine position stand: physical activity and bone health. Med Sci Sports Exerc 36: 1985–1996.
22. Yeow CH, Lee PV, Goh JC (2009) Regression relationships of landing height with ground reaction forces, knee flexion angles, angular velocities and joint powers during double-leg landing. Knee 16: 381–386.
23. Swift JM, Gasier HG, Swift SN, Wiggs MP, Hogan HA, et al. (2010) Increased training loads do not magnify cancellous bone gains with rodent jump resistance exercise. J Appl Physiol 109: 1600–1607.
24. Wu J, Ishizaki S, Kato Y, Kuroda Y, Fukashiro S (1998) The side-to-side differences of bone mass at proximal femur in female rhythmic sports gymnasts. J Bone Miner Res 13: 900–906.
25. Carroll AM, Lee DV, Biewener AA (2008) Differential muscle function between muscle synergists: long and lateral heads of the triceps in jumping and landing goats (Capra hircus). J Appl Physiol 105: 1262–1273.
26. Decker MJ, Torry MR, Wyland DJ, Sterett WI, Richard Steadman J (2003) Gender differences in lower extremity kinematics, kinetics and energy absorption during landing. Clin Biomech 18: 662–669.
27. Konow N, Azizi E, Roberts TJ (2012) Muscle power attenuation by tendon during energy dissipation. Proc Biol Sci 22: 1108–1113.
28. McGowan CP, Baudinette RV, Biewener AA (2005) Joint work and power associated with acceleration and deceleration in tammar wallabies (Macropus eugenii). J Exp Biol 208: 41–53.
29. Rittweger J (2008) Ten years muscle-bone hypothesis: what have we learned so far? - almost a festschrift-. J Musculoskelet Neuronal Interact 8: 174–178.
30. Lu TW, Taylor SJ, O'Connor JJ, Walker PS (1997) Influence of muscle activity on the forces in the femur: an in vivo study. J Biomech 30: 1101–1106.

31. Johannsen N, Binkly T, Englert V, Neiderauer G, Specker B (2003) Bone response to jumping is site-specific in children: a randomized trial. Bone 33: 533–539.

Physical Activity and Bone Mineral Accrual in Boys with Different Body Mass Parameters during Puberty: A Longitudinal Study

Donvina Vaitkeviciute[1], Evelin Lätt[1], Jarek Mäestu[1], Toivo Jürimäe[1], Meeli Saar[1], Priit Purge[1], Katre Maasalu[2], Jaak Jürimäe[1]*

1 Institute of Sport Pedagogy and Coaching Sciences, Faculty of Exercise and Sport Sciences, Centre of Behavioral, Social and Health Sciences, University of Tartu, Tartu, Estonia, **2** Department of Traumatology and Orthopedics, Faculty of Medicine, University of Tartu, Tartu, Estonia

Abstract

The aim of our longitudinal study was to investigate the relationships between physical activity and bone mass in boys with different body mass status during the years surrounding pubertal growth spurt. Two hundred and six boys entering puberty took part in this study. The subjects were divided into underweight ($BMI < 15.35$), normal weight ($BMI \geq 15.35 - 21.22$), overweight ($BMI \geq 21.22 - 26.02$) and obese ($BMI > 26.02$) groups at baseline according to age related categories. Whole-body DXA scans were performed at baseline, after 12 and 24 months to assess body composition (lean body mass, fat mass), and total body (TB), lumbar spine (LS) and femoral neck (FN) bone mineral density (BMD) parameters. Physical activity was measured by 7- day accelerometry. For longitudinal analysis, multilevel fixed effects regression models were constructed. Biological age, height and lean body mass had an effect for explanation of TB BMD, FN BMD and LS BMD. Moderate to vigorous physical activity (MVPA), vigorous physical activity (VPA) and sedentary time (SED) had the significant effect only on FN BMD. Being an underweight boy at the baseline indicated greater chance ($p<0.01$) to have lower TB BMD in the future (2 years at follow up) development, compared to normal weight (estimates = −0.038), overweight (estimates = −0.061) and obese boys (estimates = −0.106).

Editor: Yi-Hsiang Hsu, Harvard Medical School, United States of America

Funding: This study was supported by grant of Estonian Research Council IUT20-58 and SKKSP13188, http://www.etag.ee/en/, JJ. The funders had no role in study design, data collection and analysis, decision to publish, or preparation of the manuscript.

Competing Interests: The authors have declared that no competing interests exist.

* Email: jaak.jurimae@ut.ee

Introduction

Osteoporosis is the most common metabolic skeletal disease in humans and is a major public health problem. Optimising peak bone mass during puberty is an important key factor for the prevention of osteoporosis in later years [1]. Pubertal growth spurt is a period of rapid acceleration in the growth velocity of almost all skeletal tissue. Data from the longitudinal studies of bone mineral accrual reveal that the maximum bone growth velocity occurs during the 4-year period surrounding peak height velocity (PHV) with approximately 26% of adult total body bone mineral gained [2,3,4]. Peak height velocity (PHV) is an important somatic biological maturity parameter, widely used in growth studies and allows subjects to be compared by biological rather than by chronological age [5]. Underweight boys have been characterized by lower bone mineral density (BMD) compared to their normal weight peers and are at an increased risk of fractures [6]. Usually studies have examined differences in BMD between underweight boys attributed to diseases such as anorexia nervosa and their normal weight peers [7,8]. However, to our best of knowledge, there are no longitudinal studies performed that have investigated bone mineral accrual during puberty in healthy underweight boys.

There is a controversy in the literature as to whether obese boys have higher or lower bone mass compared with normal weights [9,10]. Studies in the literature are contradictory indicating that obese boys have increased [11,12], decreased [13,14], or similar [15,16] BMD values compared to normal weight peers. However, obese boys are also linked to an increased risk for bone fractures during rapid skeletal growth in pubertal period [17].

Physical activity (PA) is a major environmental factor that positively influences bone mineral accrual during puberty [18], however most studies have been carried out with exercise intervention programs [19–22]. Some studies have found positive cross-sectional data [23–26] and only one recent longitudinal study [27] investigating bone mineral parameters and PA relationships. However, it is relevant to continue investigating the amount and intensity of PA that could have valuable effect on bone mineral accrual during puberty in boys. The aim of the present study was to investigate the longitudinal relationships between physical activity and bone mineral parameters in boys with different body mass status during pubertal growth spurt.

Materials and Methods

Participants and Study Design

Study participants were recruited from different schools in Tartu city (Estonia) and its surrounding areas. At the baseline, the subjects were 12 years old and the measurements continued every year (in total 3 measurement sessions: at baseline, after 12 and 24 months). The present study sample consisted of 206 peripubertal boys. The inclusion criteria for current study were that a boy had to be healthy, took part in obligatory physical education (PE) lessons at school, and had the full set of PA data from all the measurement sessions.

Ethics statement

The subjects and their parents received information about the study and the procedures. The written signed informed consent was obtained from parents, while children gave the verbal assent. All procedures were reviewed and approved by the Medical Ethics Committee of the University of Tartu, Tartu, Estonia.

Anthropometry

Height (cm) was measured with a Martin metal anthropometer to the nearest 0.1 cm according to the standard technique (GPM anthropological instruments, Zurich, Switzerland). Body mass (kg) was measured using a medical electronic scale (A&D Instruments, Abingdon, UK) and recorded with 0.05 kg precision with the subject wearing light clothes. Body mass index (BMI; kg/m^2) was calculated as body mass (in kilograms) divided by height in square meters. The subjects were divided into underweight ($BMI < 15.35$), normal weight ($BMI \geq 15.35 - 21.22$), overweight ($BMI \geq 21.22 - 26.02$) and obese ($BMI > 26.02$) groups at baseline. The cut-off points for BMI were set according to Cole et al. [28].

Maturity Assessment

Pubertal development was assessed by self-report questionnaire of pubertal stages according to Tanner [29]. Each boy was given line drawings, pictures and descriptions representing genitalia and pubic hair development stages. The subject had to choose the one that most closely matched his own development. Age at peak height velocity (APHV) was assessed using gender specific anthropometric equations according to Mirwald et al. [30]. Biological age was calculated as the years from APHV.

Bone Densitometry and Body Composition

Bone mineral density (BMD; g/cm^2) of total body (TB), lumbar spine (LS) and femoral neck (FN), and body composition: fat mass (FM) and lean body mass (LBM) were measured using dual-energy x-ray absorptiometry (DXA; DPX-IQ densitometer, Lunar Corporation, Madison, USA) equipped with proprietary software (version 3.6). Boys were scanned in a supine position wearing light clothing. The medium scan mode and the standard subject positioning was used for total body measurements, which were analyzed using the extended analysis option. To reduce the impact of the operator variability factor, one qualified observer analyzed all scans over the 2-year period. The precision of measurement expressed as coefficient of variation (CV) was less than 2% for all bone mineral and body composition measurements. The ratio of LBM and height ($LBM/height$) was calculated.

Physical activity

A uniaxial accelerometer GT1M (ActiGraph, Pensacola, USA) was used to assess physical activity. GT1M accelerometer is a small ($3.8 \times 3.7 \times 1.8cm$) and lightweight (27 g) device that detects vertical accelerations ranging in magnitude from 0.05 to 2.00 G's with a frequency response of 0.25–2.50 Hz. The ActiGraph accelerometer has been previously validated in laboratory and free-living conditions in children and adolescents [31]. All participants wore the accelerometer on the right hip attached by an elastic belt and adjustable buckle for 7 consecutive days. Boys were instructed to remove the devices during showering, bathing, swimming and during sleep period. The used interval of time (epoch) was set at one minute. Data were uploaded to a computer after the measurements and were analyzed later. At least two workdays and one weekend day of recording with minimum 8 hours/day was set as an inclusion criterion and all sequences of 10 min or more of consecutive epoch with 0 counts were removed from the analyzes [32,33]. Total daily physical activity (TPA;$counts/\text{min}$) was calculated as the total number of counts divided by total daily registered time. The following PA thresholds were used: sedentary time (SED; $< 100counts/\text{min}$), light intensity PA (LPA; $100 - 1999counts/\text{min}$), moderate intensity PA (MPA; $2000 - 4000counts/\text{min}$) and vigorous intensity PA (VPA; $> 4000counts/\text{min}$) [34]. The time spent in moderate and vigorous intensity PA (MVPA; $\geq 2000counts/\text{min}$) was calculated as the sum of MPA and VPA.

Statistical Analysis

Statistical analysis was performed using SPSS software version 21.0 (SPSS Inc.) and SAS 9.2 (SAS Institute, Inc. Cary, NC, USA). Descriptive statistics were performed for all variables by BMI group at baseline and were presented as means and standard deviations (± SD). Normality of parameters was controlled by Shapiro-Wilks test and q-q plots. Analysis of variance (ANOVA) with Tukey *post hoc* was used to determine differences between underweight, normal weight, overweight and obese groups at baseline for anthropometric, body composition, maturity, bone mineral and physical activity parameters.

For longitudinal analyses, multilevel fixed effects regression models were constructed using PROC MIXED method (SAS version 9.2). Multilevel modeling allowed us to include participants who randomly missed some of the measurements. These models included time of measurements (0, 12, 24 months), biological age, height, LBM, SED, MVPA and group (underweight, normal weight, overweight and obese at baseline). To allow for the non-linearity biological age function was included into the linear models. The coefficients of fixed variables were used to predict TB BMD, FN BMD and LS BMD. A P-value less than 0.05 was considered significant for all analyses.

Results

Descriptive Characteristics

Data on participants' age, maturity, anthropometry, bone mineral parameters and physical activity levels at baseline are presented in Table 1. There was no difference in chronological age among all four groups with different body mass parameters (range, 11.7–12.1 yrs). However, biological age in underweight boys was significantly lower compared to other subgroups ($P < 0.05$). Underweight boys were significantly shorter compared to obese boys. All groups differed significantly from each other by body mass, FM and LBM ($P < 0.05$). In addition, TB BMD indicated significant differences in all four groups at baseline. LS BMD was significantly lower in underweight and normal weigh boys when compared to obese boys ($P < 0.05$), while FN BMD was significantly lower in underweight boys compared to normal weight and obese boys. No differences were found in SED time

Table 1. Mean (± SD) characteristics of the subjects at baseline measurement.

	Underweight	Normal weight	Overweight	Obese
	(n = 27)	(n = 133)	(n = 22)	(n = 24)
Age (years)	11.7±0.47	12.1±0.69	11.9±0.74	12.1±0.95
Biological age	−2.03±0.48[bcd]	−1.50±0.73[ad]	−1.39±0.54[ad]	−0.66±0.78[abc]
Tanner stage	2.29±0.47[b]	2.81±0.72[a]	2.41±0.67	2.79±0.78
I/II/III/IV/V	0/19/8/0/0	5/34/75/19/0	1/12/8/1/0	1/7/12/4/0
Height (cm)	152.0±6.86[d]	153.9±8.62[d]	154.6±7.06[d]	160.8±7.46[abc]
Body mass (kg)	35.2±3.98[bcd]	43.6±6.74[acd]	56.9±5.43[abd]	75.3±11.02[abc]
BMI (g/cm²)	15.1±0.59[bcd]	18.3±1.44[acd]	23.7±1.06[abd]	28.9±2.23[abc]
FM (kg)	4.4±1.17[bcd]	7.9±2.78[acd]	18.6±4.28[abd]	30.9±6.54[abc]
LBM (kg)	28.7±3.52[bcd]	33.3±5.97[ad]	34.5±5.08[ad]	40.8±6.36[abc]
LBM/height	0.18±0.143[bcd]	0.21±0.212[acd]	0.23±0.271[abd]	0.25±0.289[abc]
TB BMD (g/cm²)	0.932±0.053[bcd]	0.979±0.057[ad]	1.001±0.047[ad]	1.056±0.067[abc]
LS BMD (g/cm²)	0.796±0.088[d]	0.829±0.098[d]	0.849±0.094	0.898±0.084[ab]
FN BMD (g/cm²)	0.852±0.077[bd]	0.906±0.099[a]	0.913±0.092	0.938±0.088[a]
SED (min/day)	416.0±54.2	410.5±65.5	406.1±72.9	411.7±62.9
MVPA (min/day)	64.1±34.8[d]	60.6±25.8[d]	50.6±15.2	40.9±25.8[ab]
VPA (min/day)	15.3±16.1[d]	12.8±11.7[d]	7.2±4.6	5.1±7.7[ab]

[a]Significantly different from underweight boys;
[b]significantly different from normal weight boys;
[c]significantly different from overweight boys;
[d]significantly different from obese boys ($P<0.05$);
Biological age is years from APHV (age at peak height velocity); BMI, body mass index; TB BMD, total body bone mineral density; FN BMD, femoral neck bone mineral density; LS BMD, lumbar spine bone mineral density; SED, sedentary time; MVPA, moderate and vigorous physical activity.

among all groups of boys. However, underweight and normal weight boys showed higher MVPA and VPA levels compared to obese boys ($P<0.05$).

There was an increase in SED time for all the age groups during the 24-month study period (Table 2). Further, a significant decrease was seen in light PA at all measurement points. No change was seen in MPA, except for underweights where MPA had decreased at 24-month follow-up compared to baseline. Vigorous PA increased significantly for all weight groups (except for underweights) at 24 months follow-up compared to baseline.

Multilevel Regression Models for TB, FN and LS BMD

The variance of intercept for all models was significant, indicating that subjects varied significantly at each measurement occasion in their level of TB BMD ($P<0.001$), FN BMD ($P<0.001$) and LS BMD ($P<0.001$) (Tables 3 and 4). Multilevel models indicated that biological age, height and LBM had the significant effect for explanation of TB BMD, FN BMD and LS BMD in pubertal boys with different body mass values. However, the effect of LBM on TB BMD was not seen, but very close of being significant in the model if testing for the effect of SED time and VPA ($P=0.050$; Table 4). SED time and MVPA had a significant effect only in the explanation of FN BMD ($P=0.002$ and $P=0.006$, respectively; Table 3) as well as for SED and VPA ($P=0.001$; $P<0.001$, respectively; Table 4). However, time (testing at baseline, after 12 and after 24 months) had no effect on bone mineral parameters.

The group effect was significant only for TB BMD (estimates = 0.02520; $P<0.001$).

As four different BMI groups form group effect, we had to run further the mixed procedure (Table 5) to find which groups vary differently from each other. The further mixed procedure indicated that there was no significant difference for longitudinal model effect on TB BMD between normal weight and overweight groups ($P=0.084$), but the rest grouping had significant differences for longitudinal model effect on TB BMD.

The significant variance of biological age suggests that with the increasing biological age, boys varied by the changes in TB BMD, FN BMD and LS BMD. The tendency of variance could be seen in Figure 1, which presents changes of TB BMD during pubertal growth spurt, where 0 is APHV. We used the third year data to present this variance of changes and it indicated that all obese boys reached their APHV of being approximately 14 years old (variation range of biological age was 0–3 APHV for obese boys). While other groups had greater range of variation, their biological age varied from −2 to 3 APHV.

Discussion

In this study we aimed to investigate the relationships between PA and bone mass parameters in boys with different body mass values during the pubertal growth spurt. The current findings of multilevel regression models for longitudinal data indicated that MVPA, VPA and SED time had an effect on FN BMD over the 2-year period. However, no effect in the current study was found on TB BMD or LS BMD in boys during the puberty. Our findings confirm the results from the recent cross-sectional study of Kriemler et al. [24], who also found that VPA had significant effect on FN BMD in boys during pubertal growth spurt. Different authors have argued that FN is the site that is most responsive to PA, as loading forces have the most direct impact [35,36]. Our study results also indicated a decrease in overall physical activity in boys at the beginning of puberty and during further maturation

Table 2. The change of PA levels during the study period in four different groups of participants.

	At baseline	After 12 months	After 24 months
	Underweight		
	(n = 24)	**(n = 22)**	**(n = 22)**
SED (min/day)	416.0±54.2	463.7±72.2^{1}	565.7±111.3^{12}
LPA (min/day)	305.7±54.3	271.7±43.4^{1}	173.5±48.4^{12}
MPA (min/day)	48.8±21.9	42.2±16.3	34.7±16.9^{1}
VPA (min/day)	15.3±16.1	18.2±14.7	22.2±16.8
MVPA (min/day)	64.1±34.8	60.5±28.7	56.9±32.2
	Normal weight		
	(n = 110)	**(n = 92)**	**(n = 90)**
SED (min/day)	410.5±65.5	424.3±69.1	583±91.7^{12}
LPA (min/day)	308.2±59.3	278.2±53.9^{1}	174.3±43.1^{12}
MPA (min/day)	47.9±18.5	43.1±17.4	36.3±13.5^{1}
VPA (min/day)	12.8±11.7	15.9±13.6	20.6±16.2^{1}
MVPA (min/day)	60.6±25.8	59.0±26.9	56.9±25.3
	Overweight		
	(n = 21)	**(n = 17)**	**(n = 18)**
SED (min/day)	406.1±72.9	433.3±51.1	582.1±73.8^{12}
LPA (min/day)	315.6±54.5	270.0±65.3	182.5±43.8^{12}
MPA (min/day)	43.7±14.1	40.9±24.3	37.0±13.7
VPA (min/day)	7.2±4.6	12.0±7.9	15.2±10.1^{1}
MVPA (min/day)	50.6±15.2	52.9±27.4	52.2±18.4
	Obese		
	(n = 23)	**(n = 20)**	**(n = 17)**
SED (min/day)	411.7±62.9	431.4±66.3	565.7±74.7^{12}
LPA (min/day)	312.9±66.3	263.6±62.1	165.5±44.9^{12}
MPA (min/day)	35.5±19.9^{b}	34.7±17.6	38.9±14.8
VPA (min/day)	5.1±7.7^{ab}	9.5±7.9	14.3±10.2^{1}
MVPA (min/day)	40.9±25.8^{ab}	44.2±22.4	53.2±23.1

[a]Significantly different from underweight boys;
[b]significantly different from normal weight boys; ($P<0.05$);
[1]significantly different from baseline PA level;
[2]significantly different from PA level after 12 month;
SED, sedentary time; LPA, light physical activity; MPA, moderate physical activity; VPA, vigorous physical activity; MVPA, moderate to vigorous physical activity.

(see Table 2). Such decrease in habitual physical activity and increase in sedentary time with age is well known [37]. Differently from our results, Sherar et al. [38] found the faster decrease in VPA compared to MVPA in children aged 8 to 13 years old. However, in contrast, we found increase of VPA between the time points in every BMI group. This might be due to increase of participation in sports clubs or higher exercise intensities during the physical education lessons.

Underweight boys are less studied compared to underweight girls or overweight and obese boys. According to Misra et al. [8], one of the best predictors of BMD in underweights is LBM. In the current study, underweight boys had significantly lower absolute LBM values compared with normal weight, overweight and obese boys. LBM/height ratio showed that their low LBM is a result of true body composition difference rather than their shorter stature (Table 1). One of the factors for thinness in boys is due to malnutrition, but thin boys are not necessarily undernourished. The results of our longitudinal study confirm the findings that LBM had a major positive effect on bone mass parameters in boys as previously reported [9,39]. We indeed found the positive effect of LBM on FN BMD and LS BMD parameters in pubertal boys with different body mass status, however for underweights the effect of LBM was not seen if controlling for the effects of SED time and VPA (see Table 4). This might be explained by an additional loading of the LBM, as it has been found in cross-sectional design that for overweight boys even moderate PA may be significantly related to bone mineral parameters [18].

In the current study to assess PA levels we used accelerometry, which could measure the amount, but not the type of PA. Although the association of activity duration has found to be greater compared to the frequency of the activity [40], there is also indication that the high strain eliciting or weight-bearing PA has a greater effect on bone mineral parameters, compared to the amount of PA [41]. At baseline only underweight and normal

Table 3. Multilevel regression model for TB BMD, FN BMD and LS BMD controlling for biological age, height, lean body mass and testing for SED and MVPA.

Variables	TB BMD		FN BMD		LS BMD	
Fixed effect	**Estimates ± SE**	**P value**	**Estimates ± SE**	***p* value**	**Estimates ± SE**	***P* value**
Intercept	2.3717±0.2727	**<0.001**	1.8821±0.5465	**<0.001**	2.9526±0.4983	**<0.001**
Time	0.002705±0.0036	0.459	−0.00057±0.0066	0.931	0.000131±0.0064	0.983
Biological age	−0.01940±0.0034	**<0.001**	−0.01412±0.0068	**0.042**	−0.02969±0.0063	**<0.001**
Biological age^2	0.000065±0.00001	**<0.001**	0.000048±0.00002	**0.032**	0.000099±0.00002	**<0.001**
Height	0.02135±0.0057	**<0.001**	0.02826±0.0108	**0.010**	0.03115±0.01032	**0.003**
Lean body mass	0.001090±0.0005	**0.049**	0.002926±0.0010	**0.006**	0.004438±0.0010	**<0.001**
SED	−0.00001±0.00001	0.528	−0.00010±0.00003	**0.002**	−0.00001±0.00003	0.871
MVPA	0.000049±0.00006	0.421	0.000331±0.0001	**0.006**	0.000015±0.0001	0.892
Group	0.02520±0.0043	**<0.001**	0.007300±0.0073	0.321	0.001637±0.0071	0.818

SE is standard error. Biological age - years from age at peak height velocity (APHV). SED - sedentary time. MVPA - moderate to vigorous physical activity. Group effect is four different groups according to baseline BMI.

weight boys satisfied the recommendation of Physical Activity Guidelines for children and adolescents to spend at least 60 min in MVPA per day (see Table 1) [42]. Longitudinal multilevel model indicated that a boy with 60 min of MVPA had 0.00993 g/cm^2 higher FN BMD compared to a boy of the same biological age, height and LBM, but with 30 min of MVPA a day (0.000331×30; table 3). In comparison, after 24 months we had 35.4% of boys with $\leq 30\,min/day$ and only 5.4% of boys with $\geq 60\,\text{min}$ of MVPA in average (Table 2). In contrast, Gracia-Marco et al. [25] reported that more than 78 min/day of MVPA (>3 METs) or 32 min/day of VPA (>6 METs) was associated with increased FN BMD in adolescents, however, the study of Gracia-Marco et al [25] used epoch of 15 sec in accelerometry, while it was 60 sec in the current study, which might estimate differently, for example, the amount of vigorous PA. Our longitudinal analysis indicated that a boy with $\geq 32\,\text{min}$ of VPA had 0.02273 g/cm^2 higher FN BMD compared to a boy of the same biological age, height and LBM, but with less than 10 min VPA a day $(0.001033 \times 32) - (0.001033 \times 10)$(Table 4). Furthermore, our data confirms the findings of Cardareiro et al. [43] who found that 10 min/day of VPA would be expected to result in a ~1% higher FN BMD in boys. Results from our study show ~1.2% higher FN BMD in boys with every 10 min/day of VPA and ~3.7% higher FN BMD in boys with 32 min/day of VPA.

Sedentary behavior is becoming more important and interesting topic in relation to bone mineralization, as it could result a higher bone resorption leading to reduced BMC (bone mineral content) [44]. Results from our study showed the significant increase in sedentary time over the 3-year period in all four groups of the boys (Table 2). Pate et al. (2008) reported that subject has to stay in low energy expenditure zone (<1.5 MET) for at least several hours to call it sedentary behavior [45]. The last year of the present study boys accumulated more than 9 hours of SED time (studying, watching television or surfing the internet) (Table 2). The study of Vicente-Rodriguez (2009) indicated that watching television for 3 or more hours a day is increasing risk for low BMC in male adolescents, however it is important to emphasize that this association is mediated by participation in PA and authors suggest that negative consequences of sedentary behavior on adolescent bone health could be counteracted by sport participation [46].

Table 4. Multilevel regression model for TB BMD, FN BMD and LS BMD values when controlling for biological age, height, lean mass and testing for SED and VPA.

Variables	TB BMD		FN BMD		LS BMD	
Fixed effect	**Estimates ± SE**	***P* value**	**Estimates ± SE**	***P* value**	**Estimates ± SE**	**P value**
Intercept	2.3514±0.2715	**<0.001**	1.8034±0.5430	**<0.001**	2.9229±0.4971	**<0.001**
Time	0.002310±0.0036	0.528	−0.00285±0.0066	0.666	−0.00036±0.0064	0.956
Biological age	−0.01912±0.0034	**<0.001**	−0.01289±0.0068	**0.061**	−0.02939±0.0063	**<0.001**
Biological age^2	0.000064±0.00001	**<0.001**	0.000043±0.00002	**0.049**	0.000098±0.00002	**<0.001**
Height	0.02115±0.0057	**<0.001**	0.02823±0.0107	**0.009**	0.03055±0.01029	**0.003**
Lean body mass	0.001078±0.0005	0.050	0.002920±0.0010	**0.005**	0.004354±0.0010	**<0.001**
SED	−0.00001±0.00002	0.519	−0.00010±0.00003	**<0.001**	−0.00001±0.00003	0.936
VPA	0.000214±0.00013	0.108	0.001033±0.00025	**<0.001**	0.000265±0.0002	0.284
Group	0.02574±0.0043	**<0.001**	0.009473±0.0073	0.196	0.002946±0.0071	0.679

SE is standard error. Biological age - years from age at peak height velocity (APHV). SED - sedentary time. VPA - vigorous physical activity. Group effect is four different groups according to baseline BMI.

Table 5. Differences between groups on the effect of model to TB BMD.

Effect	Group	Group	Estimates	*P* value
Group	Underweight	Normal weight	−0.03831±0.01187	**<0.001**
Group	Underweight	Overweight	−0.06080±0.01615	**<0.001**
Group	Underweight	Obese	−0.1056±0.01577	**<0.001**
Group	Normal weight	Overweight	−0.02250±0.01294	0.084
Group	Normal weight	Obese	−0.06726±0.01247	**<0.001**
Group	Overweight	Obese	−0.04476±0.01660	**0.008**

Similarly, Gracia-Marco (2012) found that use of the internet for non-study purposes was negatively associated with TB BMC and FN BMC in adolescent boys even after controlling for LBM and MVPA, also it was reported that total SED time was negatively associated with TB BMC in boys, but after controlling for LBM the association disappeared [47]. Our longitudinal models showed that SED time has a significant effect only on FN BMD (see Tables 3 and 4) and supports the main findings of the Gracia-Marco et al. (2012) study where they found negative association between total SED time and FN BMC after controlling for LBM and MVPA [47]. Our previous study regarding one year observation period indicated that SED time has an impact on bone mineral parameters, however using a longitudinal model the effect was stronger, which further indicates the need for longer observation periods in order to study the effect of sedentary time to bone mineral parameters [36]. Current and previously reported studies [36,46,47] provides important evidence of negative effect of SED time on bone mineralization in adolescents. However it is needed to carry out more longitudinal studies' to study the interaction between SED time and bone mass parameters.

Our presented models indicated that the group effect is not significantly important for FN BMD and LS BMD in boys, and that does not show differences between the groups when looking for effect of MVPA, VPA and SED time on FN BMD or LS BMD (see Tables 3 and 4). This indicates that being underweight, normal weight, overweight or obese boy at baseline (12 years old in our case) has no effect on future (2 years of follow up) FN BMD or LS BMD. However, there was a significant group effect of SED time, MVPA and VPA on TB BMD ($P<0.001$, see Tables 3 and 4). Further mixed procedure showed that being an underweight boy at baseline is related to higher chance to have lower TB BMD in the future (2 years at follow up) development compared to normal weight, overweight and obese boys (see Table 5). We have recently found that the cut-offs for PA, taking into account its effect on fitness and fatness parameters should be at least 59 min MVPA including 14 min VPA [43]. As the underweight boys fulfilled the criteria for healthy PA ($64.1 \pm 34.8\ \text{min}/day$), that even included $15.3 \pm 16.1\ \text{min}/day$ for VPA), it can be considered that the PA guidelines [25] for healthy bone development may not be sufficient for underweights. This result is very relevant, taking into account that femoral neck is very important for its clinical relevance to osteoporosis. Unfortunately, due to too small sample size in underweight, overweight and obese groups we could not run multilevel model for sufficient power for each group separately to check the effects of MVPA, VPA and SED time on TB BMD. However, there was a tendency that MVPA and VPA had a significant effect on TB BMD in overweight boys (data not shown). In underweight and normal weight boys, only LBM had a strong positive effect on TB BMD and in obese boys nor LBM, MVPA or SED had an effect on TB BMD (data not shown).

Our research has some limitations. Our major limitation is a relatively small number of subjects in underweight, overweight and obese groups. Because of that we could not run group-based longitudinal multilevel models for sufficient power. Further, the use of 1-min epoch in accelerometry might have some effect on short bouts of VPA and therefore, might probably underestimate the amount of VPA [48]. However, the strengths of the current study is the relatively long investigation period that covers two years during the puberty ending with PHV with objective measures of PA and bone mineral density.

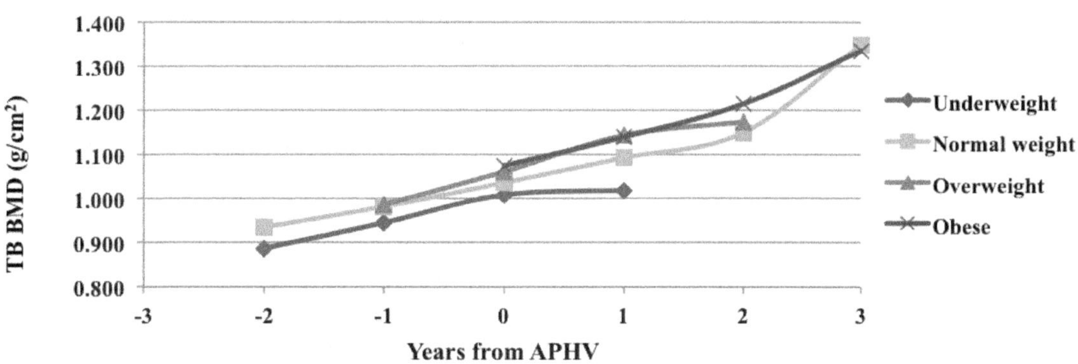

Figure 1. TB BMD changes during pubertal growth spurt. Comparing four different groups – underweight, normal weight, overweight and obese pubertal boys. APHV - age of peak height velocity.

Conclusions

This study is unique in examining longitudinally the influence of PA and body composition on BMD parameters in boys during pubertal growth spurt. Our longitudinal multilevel models indicated that the LBM had a positive significant effect on TB BMD, FN BMD and LS BMD in boys during pubertal growth spurt. MVPA, VPA and SED time had significant effect only on FN BMD. Being an underweight boy at the baseline indicated greater chance ($p<0.01$) to have lower TB BMD in the future (2 years at follow up) development, compared to normal weight (estimates = −0.038), overweight (estimates = −0.061) and obese boys (estimates = −0.106).

Acknowledgments

We gratefully acknowledge children and their parents for the contribution to this project.

Author Contributions

Conceived and designed the experiments: TJ JJ. Performed the experiments: EL PP MS. Analyzed the data: DV JM. Contributed reagents/materials/analysis tools: KM. Wrote the paper: DV JM JJ.

References

1. Rizzoli R, Bianchi ML, Garabedian M, McKay HA, Moreno LA (2010) Maximizing bone mineral mass gain during growth for the prevention of fractures in the adolescents and the elderly. Bone 46: 294–305.
2. Bailey DA (1997) The Saskatchewan Pediatric Bone Mineral Accrual Study: bone mineral acquisition during the growing years. Int J Sports Med 18: 191–194.
3. Bailey DA, McKay HA, Mirwald RL, Crocker PR, Faulkner RA (1999) A six-year longitudinal study of the relationship of physical activity to bone mineral accrual in growing children: The University of Saskatchewan Bone Mineral Accrual Study. J Bone Miner Res 14: 1672–1679.
4. Bailey DA, Martin AD, McKay HA, Whiting S, Mirwald R (2000) Calcium accretion in girls and boys during puberty: a longitudinal analysis. J Bone Miner Res 15: 2245–2250.
5. Baxter-Jones AD, Mirwald RL, McKay HA, Bailey DA (2003) A longitudinal analysis of sex differences in bone mineral accrual in healthy 8–19-year-old boys and girls. Ann Hum Biol 30: 160–175.
6. Galusca B, Zouch M, Germain N, Bossu C, Frere D, et al. (2008) Constitutional thinness: unusual human phenotype of low bone quality. J Clin Endocrinol Metab 93: 110–117.
7. Castro J, Toro J, Lazaro L, Pons F, Halperin I (2002) Bone mineral density in male adolescents with anorexia nervosa. J Am Acad Child Adolesc Psychiatry 41: 613–618.
8. Misra M, Katzman DK, Cord J, Manning SJ, Mendes N, et al. (2008) Bone metabolism in adolescent boys with anorexia nervosa. J Clin Endocrinol Metab 93: 3029–3036.
9. Gracia-Marco LA, Ortega FB, Jimenez-Pavon D, Rodriguez G, Castillo MJ, et al. (2012) Adiposity and bone health in Spanish adolescents. The HELENA Study. Osteoporos Int, 23: 937–947.
10. Ivuskans A, Lätt E, Mäestu J, Saar M, Purge P, et al. (2013) Bone mineral density in 11–13-year-old boys: relative importance of the weight status and body composition factors. Rheum Int 33: 1681–1687.
11. Vandewalle S, Taes Y, Van Helvoirt M, Debode P, Herregods N, et al. (2013) Bone size and bone strength are increased in obese male adolescents. J Clin Endocrinol Metab 98: 3019–3028.
12. Leonard MB, Shults J, Wilson BA, Tershakovec AM, Zemel BS (2004) Obesity during childhood and adolescence augments bone mass and bone dimensions. Am J Clin Nutr 80: 514–523.
13. Dimitri P, Wales JK, Bishop N (2010) Fat and bone in children: differential effects of obesity on bone size and mass according to fracture history. J Bone Miner Res 25: 527–536.
14. Rocher E, Chappard C, Jaffre C, Benhamou CL, Courteix D (2008) Bone mineral density in prepubertal obese and control children: relation to body weight, lean mass, and fat mass. J Bone Miner Metab 26: 73–78.
15. Fintini D, Brufani C, Grossi A, Ubertini G, Fiori R, et al. (2011) Gender differences in bone mineral density in obese children during pubertal development. J Endocrinol Invest 34: 86–91.
16. Hasanoglu A, Bideci A, Cinaz P, Tumer L, Unal S (2000) Bone mineral density in childhood obesity. J Pediatr Endocrinol Metab 13: 307–311.
17. Dimitri P, Bishop N, Walsh JS, Eastell R (2012) Obesity is a risk factor for fracture in children but is protective against fracture in adults: a paradox. Bone 50: 457–466.
18. MacKelvie KJ, Petit MA, Khan KM, Beck TJ, McKay HA (2004) Bone mass and structure are enhanced following a 2-year randomised controlled trial of exercise in prepubertal boys. Bone 34: 755–764.
19. Ivuskans A, Mäestu J, Jürimäe T, Lätt E, Purge P, et al. The role of physical activity in bone health in peripubertal boys. Pediatr Int In press.
20. McKay HA, Petit MA, Schutz RW, Prior JC, Barr SI, et al. (2000) Augmented trochanteric bone mineral density after modified physical education classes: a randomized school-based exercise intervention study in prepubescent and early pubescent children. J Pediatr 136: 156–162.
21. Fuchs RK, Bauer JJ, Snow CM (2001) Jumping improves hip and lumbar spine bone mass in prepubescent children: a randomized controlled trial. J Bone Miner Res 16: 148–156.
22. Weeks BK, Young CM, Beck BR (2008) Eight months of regular in- school jumping improves indices of bone strength in adolescent boys and girls: the POWER PE study. J Bone Miner Res 23: 1002–1011.
23. Tobias JH, Steer CD, Mattocks CG, Riddoch C, Ness AR (2007) Habitual levels of physical activity influence bone mass in 11-year-old children from the United Kingdom: findings from a large population-based cohort. J Bone Miner Res 22: 101–109.
24. Kriemler S, Zahner L, Puder JJ, Braun-Fahrlander C, Schindler C, et al. (2008) Weight-bearing bones are more sensitive to physical exercise in boys than in girls during pre- and early puberty: a cross-sectional study. Osteoporos Int 19: 1749–1758.
25. Gracia-Marco L, Moreno LA, Ortega FB, Leon F, Sioen I, et al. (2011) Levels of physical activity that predicts optimal bone mass in adolescents: The HELENA Study. Am J Prev Med 40: 599–607.
26. Sayers A, Mattocks C, Deere K, Ness A, Riddoch C, et al. (2011) Habitual levels of vigorous, but not moderate or light, physical activity is positively related to cortical bone mass in adolescents. J Clin Endocrinol Metab 96: 793–802.
27. Heidemann M, Molgaard C, Husby S, Schou AJ, Klakk H, et al. (2013) The intensity of physical activity influences bone mineral accrual in childhood: the childhood health, activity and motor performance school (the CHAMPS) study, Denmark. BMC Pediatr 13:32.
28. Cole TJ, Flegal KM, Nicholls D, Jackson AA (2007) Body mass index cut offs to define thinness in children and adolescents: international survey. Br Med J 335: 194–201.
29. Tanner J (1962) Growth at Adolescence, 2nd ed. Oxford: Blackwell Scientific Publications.
30. Mirwald RL, Baxter-Jones AD, Bailey DA, Beunen GP (2002) An assessment of maturity from anthropometric measurements. Med Sci Sports Exerc 34: 689–694.
31. Freedson P, Pober D, Janz KF (2005) Calibration of accelerometer output for children. Med Sci Sports Exerc 37: 523–530.
32. Rizzo NS, Ruiz JR, Oja L, Veidebaum T, Sjöström M (2008) Associations between physical activity, body fat, and insulin resistance (homeostasis model assessment) in adolescents: the European Youth Heart Study. Am J Clin Nutr 87: 586–592.
33. Martinez-Gomez D, Ruiz JR, Ortega FB, Casajús JA, Veiga OL, et al. (2010) Recommended levels and intensities of physical activity to avoid low cardiorespiratory fitness in European adolescents. The HELENA Study. Am J Hum Biol 22: 750–756.
34. Ekelund U, Anderssen SA, Froberg K, Sardinha LB, Andersen LB, et al. (2007) Independent associations of physical activity and cardiorespiratory fitness with metabolic risk factors in children: the European Youth Heart Study. Diabetologia 50: 1832–1840.
35. Baptista F, Barrigas C, Vieira F, Santa-Clara H, Homens PM, et al. (2012) The role of lean body mass and physical activity in bone health in children. J Bone Miner Metab 30: 100–108.
36. Ivuskans A, Mäestu J, Jürimäe T, Lätt E, Purge P, et al. Sedentary time has a negative influence on bone mineral parameters: a 1-year prospective study. J Bone Mineral Metab. In press.
37. Knuth AG, Hallal PC (2009) Temporal trends in physical activity: a systematic review. J Phys Act Health 6: 548–559.
38. Sherar LB, Esliger DW, Baxter-Jones AD, Tremblay MS (2007) Age and gender differences in youth physical activity: does physical maturity matter? Med Sci Sports Exerc 39: 830–835.
39. Pietrobelli A, Faith MS, Wang J, Brambilla P, Chiumello G, et al. (2002) Association of lean tissue and fat mass with bone mineral content in children and adolescents. Obes Res 10: 56–60.
40. Farr JN, Blew RM, Lee VR, Lohman TG, Going SB (2011) Associations of physical activity duration, frequency, and load with volumetric BMD, geometry, and bone strength in young girls. Osteoporos Int 22: 1419–1430.
41. Vicente-Rodriguez G (2006) How does exercise affect bone development during growth? Sports Med 36: 561–569.
42. DHHS. Key guidelines for children and adolescents. Available: http://www.health.gov/PAGuidelines/. Accessed 16 August 2013.

43. Cardadeiro G, Baptista F, Ornelas R, Janz KF, Sardinha LB (2012) Sex Specific Association of Physical Activity on Proximal Femur BMD in 9 to 10 Year-Old Children. PLoS ONE 7(11): e50657. doi:10.1371/journal.pone.0050657
44. Tremblay MS, Colley RC, Saunders TJ, Healy GN, Owen N (2008) Physiological and health implications of a sedentary lifestyle. Appl Physiol Nutr Metab 35: 725–740.
45. Pate RR, O'Neill JR, Lobelo F (2008) The evolving definition of "sedentary". Exerc Sport Sci Rev 36: 173–178.
46. Vicente-Rodriguez G, Ortega FB, Rey-Lopez JP, Espana-Romero V, Blay VA, et al. (2009) Extracurricular physical activity participation modifies the association between high TV watching and low bone mass. Bone 45: 925–930.
47. Gracia-Marco L, Rey-Lopez JP, Santaliestra-Pasias AM, Jimenez-Pavon D, Diaz LE, et al. (2012) Sedentary behaviors and its association with bone mass in adolescents: the HELENA cross-sectional study. BMC Public Health 4: 628–635.
48. Welk GJ (2002) Use of accelerometer-based activity monitors to assess physical activity. In: Welk GJ, editor. Physical Activity Assessments for Health-Related Research. Human Kinetics 125–142.

7

Physical Activity and Cardiorespiratory Fitness Are Beneficial for White Matter in Low-Fit Older Adults

Agnieszka Zofia Burzynska[1]*, Laura Chaddock-Heyman[1], Michelle W. Voss[2], Chelsea N. Wong[1], Neha P. Gothe[3], Erin A. Olson[3], Anya Knecht[1], Andrew Lewis[1], Jim M. Monti[1], Gillian E. Cooke[1], Thomas R. Wojcicki[3], Jason Fanning[3], Hyondo David Chung[3], Elisabeth Awick[3], Edward McAuley[1,3], Arthur F. Kramer[1]

1 The Beckman Institute for Advanced Science and Technology, University of Illinois, Urbana, Illinois, United States of America, **2** Department of Psychology, University of Iowa, Iowa City, Iowa, United States of America, **3** Department of Kinesiology and Community Health, University of Illinois, Urbana, Illinois, United States of America

Abstract

Physical activity (PA) and cardiorespiratory fitness (CRF) are associated with better cognitive function in late life, but the neural correlates for these relationships are unclear. To study these correlates, we examined the association of both PA and CRF with measures of white matter (WM) integrity in 88 healthy low-fit adults (age 60–78). Using accelerometry, we objectively measured sedentary behavior, light PA, and moderate to vigorous PA (MV-PA) over a week. We showed that greater MV-PA was related to lower volume of WM lesions. The association between PA and WM microstructural integrity (measured with diffusion tensor imaging) was region-specific: light PA was related to temporal WM, while sedentary behavior was associated with lower integrity in the parahippocampal WM. Our findings highlight that engaging in PA of various intensity in parallel with avoiding sedentariness are important in maintaining WM health in older age, supporting public health recommendations that emphasize the importance of active lifestyle.

Editor: Daniel Margulies, Max Planck Institute for Human Cognitive and Brain Sciences, Germany

Funding: This work was supported by the National Institute on Aging (NIA) grant (R37-AG025667) and a grant from Abbott Nutrition through the Center of Nutrition, Learning and Memory at the University of Illinois. A.Z.B was supported by the "Changing Viewpoints" grant from the Robert Bosch Foundation (http://www.bosch-stiftung.de/content/language2/html/39607.asp). The funders had no role in study design, data collection and analysis, decision to publish, or preparation of the manuscript.

Competing Interests: The authors have declared that no competing interests exist.

* Email: agaburza@illinois.edu

Introduction

Participation in physical activity and high levels of cardiorespiratory fitness (CRF) have protective effects on brain structure and function and are associated with later onset or lower degree of age-related cognitive decline [1,2]. Disruption of axons and myelin in white matter (WM) is considered one of the primary mechanisms underlying age-related cognitive decline [3,4]. Therefore, maintaining WM structural connectivity may be one of the key factors for preserving brain function and high cognitive performance necessary for independent living in old age. However, little is known about the associations of different levels of physical activity (PA), sedentary behavior, and CRF with the integrity of aging WM.

Much of the research examining PA and brain health has relied on subjective assessments of PA. Such self-reports, in contrast to quantitative measures such as accelerometry, fail to provide objective and accurate estimates of non-exercise lifestyle activities such as moderate PA (climbing stairs), light PA (housework, gardening) and sedentary behavior (prolonged periods of sitting with little movement, such as watching TV [5]). Importantly, different levels of PA are associated with different physiological mechanisms and benefits; for example, general sedentariness may even negate the benefits of sporadic MV-PA [6,7]. Surprisingly, objective measures of PA using accelerometry have never been examined in association with brain health in older adults. Thus, the independent effects of sedentariness, PA, and CRF are on brain health remain unclear. Epidemiological studies using objective measures of energy expenditure have shown that greater overall PA is related to lower incident of dementia [8]. In adults who do not exercise, which is true for most older adults, it is low intensity PA, not MV-PA, that accounts for most energy expenditure [9]. In addition, more time spent on light PA means less sedentary behavior, which has strong adverse effects on the cardiovascular system, metabolism, and is related to higher mortality [10]. These findings highlight the necessity of objectively measuring PA to tease apart physiological mechanisms associated with PA of different intensity levels, which may differentially relate to the brain health. Finally, although MV-PA is more efficient for increasing CRF than light PA [11], studies using objective measures of PA revealed that middle and older age women who meet the guidelines for engagement in limited MV-PA do not spend less time in sedentary behavior than their low-active peers [6]. Therefore, adults engaging in MV-PA may still experience some negative physiological effects of sedentary behavior [7], which may obscure the associations between CRF and brain health measures. Clearly, some aspects of lifestyle behaviors that influence brain aging cannot be captured by the CRF measure alone. CRF typically measured objectively as maximum oxygen consumption is a sum of oxygen "supply factors" (pulmonary diffusion capacity, cardiac output, erythrocyte levels, and capillary density in muscles) and muscle mitochondrial respiration rate [12–14]. Although CRF can be increased by PA, genetic factors also contribute to CRF that can boost or limit activity-induced gains [15]. Thus, in order to understand the independent effects of physical activity (sedentariness, light PA, MV-PA) and CRF on WM integrity in aging, different intensities of PA need to be objectively assessed, in addition to CRF.

Magnetic resonance imaging enables the non-invasive assessment of integrity of aging WM. Age is the primary predictor of the appearance of lesions called WM hyperintensities (WMH) on T2-weighted images [16]. The pathogenesis of WMH is complex and includes occlusion of small cerebral vessels, local ischemic changes, and damage to the blood-brain barrier with chronic leakage of ventricular and blood plasma fluid into the WM [17,18]. Second, age-related degeneration of WM microstructure can be captured as decreased fractional anisotropy (FA) measured with diffusion tensor imaging (DTI). FA is a measure of the directional dependence of diffusion [19], and reflects fiber density, integrity, and coherence within a voxel [20]. Reduced FA in aging has been linked to loss of axon and myelin integrity [21,22]. Thus far, only four studies have investigated the relation between CRF and WM structure in healthy older adults. Three relatively small cross-sectional studies including a large fraction of very high fit older adults showed a positive relationship between CRF and FA in the anterior body corpus callosum ([23]; n = 26), anterior cingulum ([24]; n = 15), and single clusters in the inferior and superior longitudinal fasciculi ([25]; n = 20). A one-year aerobic exercise intervention study showed that increases in CRF were positively related to increases in general frontal and temporal lobe FA ([26]; n = 70). In addition, [25] showed that life-long engagement in MV-PA was linked to 83% reduction in deep WMH volume in Master's athletes compared to low-active controls. Although not representative of a typical low-active aging population, these preliminary studies on samples with very fit older adults are important by showing there may be a positive relationship between CRF and WM microstructure in anterior corpus callosum, cingulum, fronto-parietal connections and temporal WM, as well as associations between life-long history of MV-PA and WMH volume in healthy older individuals.

Our study goes beyond the above studies by combining objective measures of PA and CRF with two MRI measures of WM health (FA and WMH volume) in a large group of typically low–fit healthy adults (n = 88, age 60–78, 33 males). PA was objectively measured with an accelerometer worn on the hip for at least 10 waking hours for 7 days and was classified into sedentary behavior, light PA, and MV-PA [5]. We assessed CRF as the maximum oxygen consumption during a graded maximal exercise test. Unlike previous studies (e.g. [23]), we did not exclude participants with WMH but instead quantified the lesion volume on T2-weighted images as a marker of age-related WM damage. This made our sample more generalizable to a normal aging population and allowed inclusion of participants older than 70, given that only 4% of adults above age of 65 do not present WMH [27].

Our study had two main aims. First, we aimed to test whether in healthy low-active and low-fit older adults CRF conjointly with and PA is related to WM health, measured by combining FA with WMH volume. We predicted that, in general, greater CRF and PA would be related to higher WM integrity. The second aim, given that our first hypothesis is true, was to investigate in more detail the multiple interacting pathways linking PA to WM health. Here, our main goal was to identify in post-hoc exploratory analyses the relationships between different levels of PA intensity and WM health in older adults, and to test the role of CRF in these relationships. We predicted that greater PA would be related to lower WMH volume [25] and higher FA in five regions. These included two regions within the temporal lobe: parahippocampal WM and core temporal WM containing the inferior longitudinal fasciculus, given that exercise interventions and higher CRF showed beneficial effects on temporal regions and the hippocampus [28–33]. In addition, we revisited previous findings by measuring FA in three frontal regions that related to greater CRF: anterior corpus callosum, dorsal anterior cingulum, and superior longitudinal fasciculi [23–25]. With regard to PA intensity, we considered two alternative hypotheses. Better WM health could be related to greater MV-PA, as MV-PA is most efficient in increasing CRF and inducing CRF-related protective effects on the brain. Alternatively, in older population, higher levels of light PA or less sedentary behavior could act on WM via higher overall energy expenditure and reducing risks related to sedentariness. In addition, although FA and WMH are often related in the posterior periventricular regions, in other regions they probe different aspects of WM health and are not redundant [22,34]. As outlined above, the same holds for PA and CRF. Thus, we hypothesized there may be a dissociation of the effects of CRF and PA on WMH and FA in healthy aging.

Our findings confirmed our expectations that better physical health was related to WM health. In particular, greater PA and lower sedentariness were associated with lower WMH volume and higher FA, especially in the temporal WM regions, but our data did not support a significant relationship between CRF and WM health in the frontal regions.

Methods

Participants

We recruited 103 community-dwelling healthy, older adults (33 males). The sample contained more females because less older males met the inclusion criteria or showed willingness to participate in the study. Eligible participants met the following criteria: (1) were between the ages of 60 and 79 years old, (2) were free from psychiatric and neurological illness and had no history of stroke or transient ischemic attack, (3) scored ≥23 on the Mini-Mental State Exam (MMSE) and >21 on a Telephone Interview of Cognitive Status (TICS-M) questionnaire, (4) scored <10 on the geriatric depression scale (GDS-15), (5) scored ≥75% right-handedness on the Edinburgh Handedness Questionnaire, (6) demonstrated normal or corrected-to-normal vision of at least 20/40 and no color blindness, (7) cleared for suitability in the MRI environment; that is, no metallic implants that could interfere with the magnetic field or cause injury, no claustrophobia, and no history of head trauma. The participants were a pre-intervention cross-sectional subsample from an on-going randomized controlled exercise trial ("Influence of Fitness on Brain and Cognition II" at ClinicalTrials.gov, clinical study identifier NCT01472744), from whom good quality DTI and T2 data (as described in the following sections), as well as CRF and PA data were available. We furthermore excluded participants who had MMSE score <27, in order to limit the analyses to cognitively healthy older adults and exclude those with possible mild cognitive impairment. Seventy-two participants (83%) of the sample reported no participation in regular PA (maximum of two moderate bouts of PA/week) in the past six months. The remaining 17% reported engaging in some exercise upon recruitment; however, the subsequent accelerometer data analysis revealed that as many as 40% of them did not met the minimum recommendations for PA (>150 min of moderate PA per week). Similarly, fourteen (19%) of the self-reported "low-active" adults met the criteria of >150 min of moderate PA per week. This highlights the necessity of objective assessment of PA for accurate sample description, in addition to self-reports. In total, based on the accelerometer data, only 26% (n = 23, 9 women) of the 88 participants met the minimum criteria for PA for older adults and only 3 of them met the recommended criteria based on vigorous activity (>60 min/week; [35]; one was subsequently excluded due to high CRF, see Section 2.3). In sum, we define our sample as low-fit and low-active although capable of performing exercise (i.e. no physical disability that prohibits mobility).

The 88 participants had mean body mass index (BMI) $M_{BMI} = 30 \pm 6$ kg/m^2, systolic blood pressure $M_{sysBP} = 131 \pm 13$ mm Hg and diastolic blood pressure $M_{diasBP} = 81 \pm 7$ mm Hg. Out of 88 participants, 69 (78%) were normotensive, while 18 (22%) were hypertensive, defined as either systolic BP >140 mmHg or diastolic BP >90 mm Hg. Twenty participants (23%) had normal BMI, while 68 (77%) were overweight (BMI >25). If stratified based on BMI or BP, the groups did not differ on any of the WM or fitness variables of interest, and therefore BMI and BP were not included as in the following analyses.

Physical activity assessment

Participants were instructed to wear the GT3× ActiGraph accelerometer (ActiGraph; Pensacola, Florida) for seven consecutive days on an elastic belt on the left hip during all waking hours, except for when bathing or swimming. The participants completed a daily log to record the time that the accelerometer was worn, and this log was used to verify the accelerometer data for processing with the ActiLife v5.6.0 software. For the purposes of this study, a valid day of data consisted of at least 10 hours of valid wear-time, with a valid hour defined as no more than 30 consecutive minutes of zero counts with one minute sampling epochs (Table 1). Only data for individuals with a minimum of three valid days of wear time were included in analyses [36]. Based on this criterion, two females were excluded from analyses. The remaining 86 participants (28 males) had on average 6.8±0.8 valid days of measurement (range 3–8), resulting in 90.7% of the sample having 6 or more valid days required to reliably measure sedentary behavior [36].

Each valid measurement epoch was classified into sedentary, light, moderate, and vigorous physical activity based on displacement magnitude and frequency. We used activity intensity cut-off ranges appropriate for older adults [5] using MeterPlus v4.2 software (Santech, Inc.; San Diego, CA). Sedentary behavior was defined as <100, light activity as 100–1951, moderate activity as 1952–5723, and vigorous activity as >5724 counts/epoch. The total epochs (i.e. minutes) of each intensity, divided by total valid days, yielded average time spent daily in a specific physical activity intensity (note that in Table 1 we further divided these variables by 60 to express the time in hours). Only nine participants showed any vigorous activity during the measurement week. We therefore summed moderate and vigorous activity to obtain a "moderate-to-vigorous activity" (MV-PA) variable [37]. Observed MV-PA was positively skewed and we performed a natural log-transformation of this variable for further analyses. The daily valid hours of two participants were >2.5SD and were winsorized with respect to the distribution of the whole sample before being entered into correlations and regressions.

Cardiorespiratory fitness assessment

All participants obtained physician's approval to engage in cardiorespiratory fitness (CRF) testing. CRF was defined as peak oxygen consumption [ml/kg/min], measured with indirect calorimetry during a modified Balke graded maximal exercise test on a motor-driven treadmill test. Oxygen consumption (VO_2) was calculated from expired air sampled at 30-s intervals until peak VO_2 was reached or the test was terminated due to volitional exhaustion and/or symptom limitation. CRF was defined as the highest recorded VO_2 value (VO_2max) after two of three criteria were met: (1) a plateau in VO_2 after increase in workload; (2) a respiratory exchange ratio >1.10, and (3) a maximal heart rate within 10 bpm of their age-predicted maximum. Our subjects represented a broad range of CRF values, with extremely high values for 2 female participants (>±2.5 SD and beyond the 90% peak VO_2max percentile (superiorly/excellent fit) according to gender- and age-specific norms; ACSM's Guidelines for Exercise Testing and Prescription, www.acsm.org. Accessed 2014 June 12). They were therefore considered outliers in our largely low-fit sample and their values were removed from further analyses. As one female participant did not complete the treadmill test, the final sample for CRF assessment was 83 (28 males).

MRI acquisition

Diffusion-weighted and high in-plane resolution T2-weighted images (for WMH volume estimation) were acquired on a 3T Siemens Trio Tim system with 45 mT/m gradients and 200 T/m/sec slew rates (Siemens, Erlangen, Germany). All images were obtained parallel to the anterior-posterior commissure plane with no interslice gap. T2-weighted images consisted of 35 4-mm-thick slices with an in-plane resolution of 0.86×0.86 (256×256 matrix, TR/TE = 2400/63 ms, FA = 120). DTI images were acquired with a twice-refocused spin echo single-shot Echo Planar Imaging sequence [38] to minimize eddy current-induced image distortions. The protocol consisted of a set of 30 non-collinear diffusion-weighted acquisitions with b-value = 1000 s/mm^2 and two T2-weighted b-value = 0 s/mm^2 acquisitions, repeated two times (TR/TE = 5500/98 ms, 128×128 matrix, 1.7×1.7 mm^2 in-plane resolution, FA = 90, GRAPPA acceleration factor 2, and bandwidth of 1698 Hz/Px, comprising 40 3-mm-thick slices).

Assessment of White Matter Hyperintensity (WMH) volume

We estimated WMH volume on T2-weighted images using a semi-automated procedure based on FMRIB's Automated Segmentation Tool (FAST in FSL v.5.0.1, [39]. The procedure included: a) removal of the skull and non-brain tissue using the Brain Extraction Tool (BET) [40], b) segmentation of the image into three tissue types (grey and white matter, cerebrospinal fluid). All segmentation results were visually checked by AZB, c) manual masking of WMH regions within the cerebrospinal fluid segmentation (done by AZB, Figure 1-A). WMH volume was reported in voxel number classified in the above procedure as hyperintense, where voxel size was 0.86×0.86×4 mm^3. The WMH volume was positively skewed (Kolmogorov-Smirnov test $D(60) = 0.28$, $p < 0.05$) and we performed a natural log-transformation of this variable for further analyses.

DTI analysis

DTI allows inferences about WM microstructure in vivo by quantifying the magnitude and directionality of diffusion of water within a tissue [20]. Visual checks were performed on every volume of the raw data of every participant by AZB. In one

Table 1. Variables of interest: descriptive statistics and correlations with age.

Variable	n	Mean±SD*	Range*	r with age**	p-value
Age (years)	88	65±4	60–78	–	–
Education (years)	86	16±3	11–26	−0.21	0.059
CRF (mL/kg/min) ***					
Males	28	26±7	12–43	**−0.47**	0.012
Females	55	20±4	12–31	−0.06	0.661
Physical activity (hours/day)					
Sedentary	86	8.9±1.3	5.8–11.6	0.08	0.489
Light	86	4.6±1.2	2.3–7.6	0.01	0.938
MV-PA	86	0.27±0.25	0.01–1.22	**−0.26**	0.016
Aceelerometer valid hours/day	86	13.7±1.3	11.4–19.4	0.05	0.652
WMH volume (voxels)	86	813±1233	1–7290	**0.25**	0.021
Fractional anisotropy (FA)					
Anterior cc	86	.67±.03	.59–.75	**−0.22**	0.046
Anterior cingulum	86	.47±.03	.40–.54	**−0.27**	0.012
Superior longitud. fasci.	86	.46±.03	.41–.52	**−0.24**	0.025
Parahippocampal WM	81	.55±.03	.49–.62	**−0.39**	<.001
Temporal lobe WM	81	34±.03	.27–.42	−0.15	0.172

*Raw data.
** WMH and MV-PA were ln-transformed for correlations with age and valid hours were winsorized.
*** The values are after excluding two outliers >2.5 SD.

dataset, one volume with the corresponding b-vectors and b-values was deleted from the dataset before processing due to artifact. Next, DTI data were processed using the FSL Diffusion Toolbox v.3.0 in a standard multistep procedure, including: a) motion and eddy current correction of the images and corresponding b-vectors, b) removal of the skull and non-brain tissue using the Brain Extraction Tool [40], and c) voxel-by-voxel calculation of the diffusion tensors. Using the diffusion tensor information, FA maps were computed using DTIFit within the FDT. All motion- and eddy-current outputs, as well as FA images were visually inspected.

We used tract-based spatial statistics (TBSS; 41,42], a toolbox within FSL v5.0.1 [43], to create a representation of main WM tracts common to all subjects (WM "skeleton"). This included: (1) nonlinear alignment of each participant's FA volume to the $1\times1\times1$ mm^3 standard Montreal Neurological Institute (MNI152) space via the FMRIB58_FA template using the FMRIB's Nonlinear Registration Tool (FNIRT, [44]), (2) calculation of the mean of all aligned FA images, (3) creation of the WM "skeleton" by perpendicular non-maximum-suppression of the mean FA image and setting the FA threshold to 0.25, and (4) perpendicular projection of the highest FA value (local center of the tract) onto the skeleton, separately for each subject. The outputs of all the above processing steps were carefully inspected by AZB.

To verify how the tracts of interest were related to CRF and PA, we extracted FA values from five regions: anterior corpus callosum (antCC; two most anterior sections of the corpus callosum as segmented after [45], anterior cingulum (antCING), superior longitudinal fasciculi (SLF), temporal lobe WM (TEMP), and WM of the medial temporal lobe (parahippocampal WM, paraHIPP; Figure 1-B; [46]. The regions were identified on the TBSS skeleton with the use of the DTI WM atlas to probe FA in the core parts of the selected tracts [47]. DTI data of five participants did not entirely cover the temporal lobes. Therefore, the above analyzes were done twice: once with all participants and once without the five participants (n = 78). The full sample analysis resulted in common mask not covering the temporal lobes and therefore those five subjects had missing data in those tracts.

It is important to note that the TBSS analysis used here inherently focuses on normal appearing WM, as the highest FA values perpendicular to the tract are being projected to the WM skeleton for further analysis. This means that there may be some bias for excluding voxels affected by WMH from FA analyses. We thus consider TBSS approach most suitable for the current study as it maximizes the independence of FA measures from WMH, in addition to circumventing the inter-subject anatomical variability in older populations.

An exploratory analysis relating CRF with FA across the whole WM skeleton was carried out in randomize, a voxel-wise permutation-based (5000 permutations) inference (Nichols and Holmes, 2002), with the threshold-free cluster enhancement option, and controlling for age and gender.

Statistical analyses

To test the first study hypothesis, we performed a dimensionality reduction by running two separate principal component analyses (PCA) with varimax rotation. The first model included the four variables: CRF, sedentary time, light PA, and MV-PA. The second model included the WM health indices: five FA values and WMH volume. Both analyses yielded a one-component model and therefore represented "CRF and PA" and "WM health", respectively. Importantly, a PCA analysis replacing the five FA

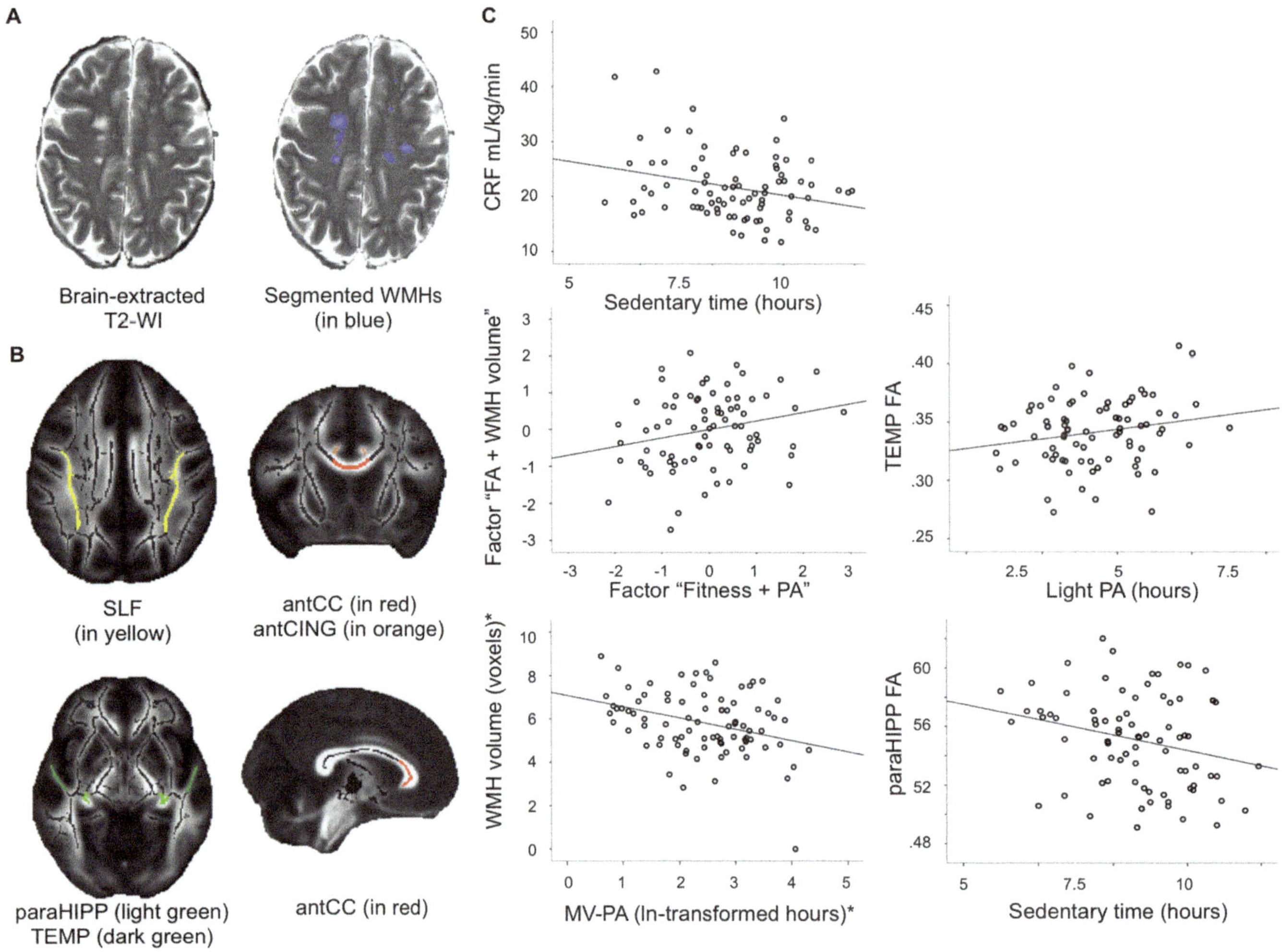

Figure 1. Illustration of WMH volume and FA analyses. A: An example of segmentation of WMHs on a T2-weighted image. B: Regions of interest for DTI analysis. Mean WM skeleton overlaid on FMRIB58_FA mean FA image. Anterior corpus callosum (antCC), anterior cingulum (antCING), superior longitudinal fasciculus (SLF), temporal lobe WM (TEMP), and parahippocampal WM (paraHIPP). C: Scatterplots showing the representative relationships between PA, CRF, and WM integrity. *Indicates that the variable was ln-transformed.

values with global FA measure (mean FA over the entire WM skeleton) yielded the same outcome, confirming that the FA in the five WM regions are representative for the overall WM health.

All statistical analyses were performed using SPSS (v.16, SPSS Inc., Chicago, IL, USA). We used partial 2-tailed correlations (controlling for chronological age and gender) and multiple step-wise linear regressions to investigate the relationships among CRF, PA, WMH volume, and FA. The p values in these post-hoc analyses were not corrected for multiple comparisons.

The raw CRF, PA, WMH volume, and FA values is made available in Data S1.

Ethics statement

A University of Illinois Institutional Review Board approved the study, and written informed consent was obtained from all participants and the study was performed in accordance with the 1964 Declaration of Helsinki. Participants received financial reimbursement.

Results

PA, CRF, and WM integrity: age- and gender-related trends

We summarized the descriptive statistics of main variables in our study and their correlations with chronological age in Table 1. There were no gender differences except for CRF (higher in males, $p = .001$). CRF in males, MV-PA, and FA (except for temporal lobe WM) decreased with age, while WMH volume increased with age. The WMH volume and FA values are comparable with previous reports for healthy adults in this age range [22], [48]. Given age and gender differences in key variables, we included age and gender as covariates in further analyses.

CRF was positively related to light and MV-PA, and negatively related to sedentary behavior (all controlled for age and gender, Table 2; Figure 1-C). These results are important in showing that, in this sample of older low-active adults, all levels of PA as well as sedentary behavior were moderately related to CRF. We also investigated how daily wear time (valid hours), to a large extent reflecting waking hours, was related to different PA levels. As expected, we found that all levels of PA were positively related to valid hours, but not CRF (Table 2). In particular, sedentary hours

Table 2. Partial correlations between CRF and levels of PA.

	1. Valid hours	2. Sedentary	3. Light PA	4. MV-PA	5. CRF
1. Valid hours	1	**pr = .53**	**pr = .45**	**pr = .22**	pr = .18
		p< .001	p< .001	p= .041	p= .106
		df =82	df =82	df =82	df =79
2. Sedentary		1	**pr =−.48**	**pr =−.27**	**pr =−.36**
			p< .001	p= .013	p= .001
			df =82	df =82	df =79
3. Light PA		-	1	**pr = .35**	**pr = .43**
				p= .001	p< .001
				df =82	df =79
4. MV-PA		-	-	1	**pr = .55**
					p< .001
					df =79
5. CRF		-	-	-	1

All correlations controlled for age and gender. pr denotes partial correlation. CRF data is in units of mL/kg/min, Sedentary, Light, and MV-PA are expressed in hours (ln-transformed for MV-PA, winsorized for valid hours).

accounted for most of the variability in the wearing time among our participants.

Finally, we examined the relationships between WMH volume and FA in the five WM regions. We found no significant relationship between WMH volume and FA (controlled for age and gender). This confirmatory analysis showed that in the five regions, WMH and DTI are not redundant measures of WM health.

Greater CRF and PA are associated with better WM health

Dimensionality reduction using PCA separately on WM and CRF and PA measures yielded single factors for "CRF and PA" and "FA and WMH volume". In other words, participants with greater "CRF and PA" factor scores had higher CRF, showed more light and MV-PA, and less sedentary behavior. Participants with higher WM health factor score had higher FA in all five regions and lower WMH volume. As predicted, we found a positive association between "CRF and PA" and "FA and WMH volume" ($r = .24$, $p = .037$, $n = 77$), which was a prerequisite for the following post-hoc analyses (Figure 1-C).

Relationships of PA with WM health (FA and WMH volume)

MV-PA ($pr = -.31$ $p = .004$, $df = 82$), but not sedentary or light daily PA was related to WMH volume (all controlled for age and gender; Figure 1-C). A multiple hierarchical regression showed that MV-PA was associated with WMH volume in addition to variance explained by age, gender, and CRF (Model 1 in Table 3).

Greater light PA ($pr = .25$, $p = .026$, $df = 77$) was associated with higher FA in the temporal lobe WM (Figure 1-C). A multiple hierarchical regression showed that light PA was not associated with temporal lobe FA in addition to variance explained by age, gender, and CRF (Model 2 in Table 3).

Sedentary behavior was inversely related to FA in the parahippocampal WM. That is, participants who spent more time on sedentary behavior had lower FA adjacent to the hippocampus ($pr = -.24$, $p = .035$, $df = 77$; controlled for age and gender; Figure 1-C). The negative relationship between sedentary behavior and temporal lobe FA ($pr = -.21$, $p = .066$, $df = 77$) was at trend level. Again, as sedentary behavior was negatively associated with CRF, we examined whether the effect of sedentariness on parahippocampal FA was independent of CRF in a hierarchical multiple regression. We found that sedentary behavior explained a significant amount of variance in parahippocampal FA, independently of variance explained by age, gender, and CRF (Model 3 in Table 3). The results of all of the above analyses were unchanged if valid hours were included as covariates in addition to age, gender, and CRF. Only the partial correlation between sedentary time and the parahippocampal WM FA was at a trend level after controlling for valid hours in addition to age and gender ($pr = -.20$, $p = .076$, $df = 76$). This was expected, given that the variance in valid hours was mainly associated with variance in sedentary time and, to a lesser extent, to light and MV-PA. Together, these results suggest that daily valid PA measurement hours, likely reflecting waking hours, are to some extent related to the PA counts, but do not account for the relationships between PA and WM health.

Finally, the mechanisms linking sedentary behavior to brain integrity may differ from those related to MV-PA [7]. Indeed, a hierarchical multiple regression showed that sedentary behavior explained a significant amount of variance in parahippocampal FA, independently of variance explained by age, gender, and MV-PA (Model 4 in Table 3).

Figure 1-C shows scatterplots of the representative relationships between CRF, PA, and WM integrity.

Relationships of CRF with WM health (FA and WMH volume)

To revisit the findings from previous studies [23–25] we tested the relationship between CRF and FA three prefrontal WM regions in our low-active and low-fit sample. We found no significant associations in the ROI-based analysis as well as whole-brain exploratory TBSS analysis. There was no significant relationship between CRF and WMH volume ($pr = -.16$, $p = .143$, $df = 79$).

We found a positive association only between temporal lobe FA and CRF; however, after controlling for age and gender it remained at trend level ($pr = .20$, $p = .078$, $df = 74$).

Table 3. Regression models predicting WM integrity.

Dependent variables	Predictors	R^2 change	F change	df	p-value F change
1. WMH volume (voxels)	Age, gender	.15	7.13	80/2	**.001**
	CRF	.02	2.19	79/1	.143
	MV-PA	.50	5.06	78/1	**.027**
2. Temporal WM	Age, gender	.08	3.10	75/2	**.051**
	CRF	.04	3.20	74/1	**.078**
	Light PA	.02	2.07	73/1	**.155**
3. Parahippocampal FA	Age, gender	.14	6.10	75/2	**.004**
	CRF	.002	0.16	74/1	.689
	Sedentary time	.08	7.03	73/1	**.010**
4. Parahippocampal FA	Age, gender	.15	7.08	78/2	**.001**
	MV-PA	.001	.09	77/1	.764
	Sedentary time	.05	4.55	76/1	**.036**

CRF data is in units of mL/kg/min, Sedentary and MV-PA are expressed in hours (ln-transformed for MV-PA).

Discussion

We studied the relationships among CRF, PA, and WM health in a sample of 88 healthy low-active older adults. We found that "CRF and PA", measured as a factor combining CRF and three levels of PA, was positively associated with WM health, represented by a factor "FA and WMH volume". Post hoc analyses showed that this general result was driven by several WM-PA relationships. Specifically, higher MV-PA was associated with lower WMH volume, independent of age, gender, and CRF. Additionally, less time spent in sedentariness was linked with higher FA in the parahippocampal WM, and this association was independent of age, gender, and MV-PA. Our findings suggest that different levels of PA, although related, are associated with different aspects of WM integrity in a region-specific way. Here we focus on the specific post-hoc results and discuss how different mechanisms related to physical activity and sedentariness, such as cerebrovascular health, neurotrophic factors, or glucose and lipid metabolism, could underlie the observed relationships in specific brain regions.

PA is related to WMH volume

We found that higher MV-PA was related to lower volume of WMH. We propose that the mechanism underlying this association is the beneficial effect of the MV-PA on the cerebrovascular system.

Aging is associated with stiffening and dilation of aorta and proximal elastic arteries due to accumulating "wear and tear" of their elastic and muscular components. This results in hypertension and impaired cushioning function of the arterial system, i.e. the ability to change the pulsatile flow in arteries to steady flow in the capillaries. This impaired cushioning increases vascular wall tension in arterioles and capillaries, particularly those of the brain [49]. This causes mechanical damage to blood vessel, arteriosclerotic changes, inflammation, as well as alterations in mechanosensitive gene expression, leading to vascular remodeling and oxidative stress [49,50].

These age-related vascular changes are said to be counteracted by mainly moderate PA, captured as MV-PA by accelerometry. The effects of MV-PA include reduction in arterial stiffness and blood pressure [51], preserved arterial elasticity, blood flow, and reduced formation of arteriosclerotic lesions [52]. Clearly, these age-related vascular changes, which are modifiable by PA, overlap with the factors involved in the pathogenesis of WMH (permanent vessel dilation, damage to the vascular wall, disruption of the blood-brain-barrier, leakage of fluid from the blood vessel lumen to the surrounding tissue [17,53]. Indeed, the association between hypertension and higher risk of WMH is well documented in large samples of older adults [54,55]. However, the current study is first to report that link between lifestyle behavior relevant for cardiovascular health and WMH burden. To directly investigate how cerebrovascular factors relate to WM health, we are currently analyzing the relationships between cerebral arterial elasticity and WMH volume in another aging sample. We also speculate that in our relatively low-active and low-fit but healthy sample MV-PA may be a more sensitive correlate of WMH and FA than CRF, as VO_2max reflects not only cardiovascular health, but also reflects body composition, genetic factors, and muscle metabolic rate. An ongoing exercise intervention study will shed more light on the discrepancy between CRF and MV-PA measures in relation to WM health.

Time spent on light PA is related to temporal lobe WM integrity

Light PA was positively related to FA in the temporal lobe WM. Our results are novel in showing that not only exercise aimed to increase CRF, but also light PA may be beneficial for the temporal lobe during aging. It is worth noting, however, that in our low-fit sample, greater daily light PA (and not only MV-PA) was also associated with greater CRF, and light PA no longer significantly predicted temporal FA after accounting for CRF. Therefore, we speculate that the effect of PA on temporal WM may be related to mechanisms related to CRF.

The beneficial effects of CRF and exercise on temporal lobe structures are well known in both animals and humans [56]. Specifically, in older adults, aerobic exercise interventions aimed to increase CRF are related to increased gray matter density in the lateral temporal cortex [57]. A recent study showed that improvement in CRF due to aerobic exercise training correlated with an increase in FA of temporal and frontal lobes in older adults [58].

Aerobic exercise upregulates the expression and release of important neuronal growth factors such as brain-derived neurotrophic factor (BDNF) [31,58–60] and insulin-like growth factor I (IGF-1; a potent survival factor for neurons and oligodendrocytes) [61]. Therefore, structural and functional brain changes related to improved oxidative capacity have been largely attributed to the action of neurotrophins. For example, an aerobic walking intervention in older adults resulted in increased temporal lobe functional connectivity, associated with increased BDNF, IGF-1, and vascular endothelial growth factor serum levels [58].

BDNF supports survival and growth of many neuronal subtypes and is a mediator of synaptic efficacy and use-dependent plasticity [62]. Still, the effects of BDNF on WM are poorly understood. Therefore the link between CRF, neurotrophin upregulation, and temporal WM integrity in healthy humans is less straightforward. Healthy adult Val/Val homozygotes of the BDNF $Val^{66}Met$ polymorphism (increased levels of activity-dependent release) had decreased FA compared to Met-allele carriers [63,64], and lower structural brain connectivity [65]. Therefore, while for grey matter the met66 allele is almost invariably protective, BDNF seems to be a "punitive" signal in axonal pruning, i.e. higher BDNF secretion from stimulated axons results in its higher binding to p75 neurotrophin receptor on less active axons, which leads to neurite elimination [66] BDNF has neuroprotective role of on WM in clinical studies [67,68] and plays a role in normal axonal pruning and maintenance observed in animals [66,69]. Therefore, further research combining various MRI modalities to serum levels of neurotrophins is necessary to understand their role in mature as well as aging WM, and the link between light PA and temporal lobe WM.

It is also possible that the positive effects of light PA on temporal lobe WM integrity are mediated by changes in cerebrovascular supply factors related to CRF, reducing the oxygenative stress in the tissue [12]. Aerobic training correlates with increased capillary density in brain parenchyma [70] and higher number and integrity of small blood vessels as measured by MRI angiography [71]. Together, these changes may lead to increased ratio of blood vessels to brain volume [72] and more efficient oxygen delivery.

An alternative, although not mutually exclusive, explanation for the observed association between PA and WM integrity (both FA and WMH) is that individuals with higher WMH burden or decreases in FA are at more risk of impaired mobility [73], gait and balance dysfunction [74–79], and physical disability [80–82]. This could lead to their lower mobility and engagement in PA. Still, a study comparing athletes with non-exercising controls indicated that life-long exercise is associated with reduced WMH and age-related decline in FA [25]. We will test these alternative hypotheses in an ongoing randomized control study with exercise intervention.

In sum, our results suggest that not only structured exercise, but also light PA may be associated with greater WM microstructural integrity in temporal regions, known to be prone to age-related changes and sensitive to CRF-related benefits. Future analyses linking temporal WM FA to cognitive measures, local structure, and neural activity will allow assessing the functional relevance of the reported associations.

Sedentary behavior may relate to WM via different mechanisms than PA

We found that older adults who spent more time in sedentary behavior had lower FA in the parahippocampal WM. Importantly, more sedentary behavior was related not only to less light PA, but also to less MV-PA, and lower CRF. Therefore, more sedentary older individuals were less exposed to beneficial effects of light and MV-PA, but also more prone to deleterious effects of sedentariness, such as increased metabolic risk [83,84]. The association between sedentariness and parahippocampal WM, however, was independent from MV-PA. This is in line with recent hypotheses that sedentariness may act via different mechanisms than MV-PA, and may even offset the benefits of MV-PA [7,85]. Specifically, both acute and chronic sedentariness is related to reduced activity of lipoprotein lipase activity [86], which facilitates uptake of fatty acids into muscle and adipose tissue. This causes increased plasma levels of triglycerides, total cholesterol, and decreased levels of high-density lipoprotein cholesterol [84,87]. In addition, sedentary behavior is related to insulin resistance and increased glucose plasma levels [84].

Physiological differences between sedentary behavior and lack of MV-PA [7,85] may partly explain the specificity of sedentary behavior for parahippocampal WM integrity. For instance, insulin receptors are highly expressed in the hippocampus and play a modulatory role in learning and memory processing [88]. Both insulin deficiency and resistance impairs hippocampus-dependent memory, long-term potentiation along the perforant pathway, and adult neurogenesis in rats [89]. Insulin resistance in humans is associated with similar cognitive deficits as in rodents [90]. Similarly, elevation in serum cholesterol change hippocampus lipid metabolism and induce oxygenative stress in rats [91]. As hyperlipidemia often presages insulin resistance, we speculate that sedentariness-induced changes in plasma lipids and glucose may have negative effect on hippocampus in low-active older adults, even in the absence of diagnosed diabetes. Deleterious changes in medial temporal lobe structures should be tightly linked to WM tracts connecting these regions. Little is known, however, about mechanisms linking plasma lipids and glucose levels to WM integrity, i.e. myelin turnover and repair, oligodendrocyte viability, axonal transport and integrity. Clearly, more research is needed to understand how sedentary behavior physiology interacts with the integrity of WM. Ideally, future studies will combine PA measures, structural and functional MRI with blood metabolite assays.

Finally, we observed no relationships between CRF with WMH volume or FA in the corpus callosum, the cingulum bundle, or superior longitudinal fasciculi, as reported previously by [23–25]. The earlier studies may have limited generalizability due to size ($n \leq 26$) and characteristics of the sample: [23] sample consisted of 26% superiorly fit individuals according to ACSM's Guidelines for Exercise Testing and Prescription ($V0_2max > 42.7$ for men in 7th decade of life), 53% participants in [24] had a history of minimum 10 years of exercise 3 hours/week and mean $V0_2max = 38$, while half of [25] sample included Masters athletes. These effects observed in small samples including superiorly fit older individuals might not be reproducible in larger, low-active aging samples with narrower range of CRF, like ours. The causality of the relationships is also speculative, as some genetic or environmental factors, unrelated to PA, may have predisposed Masters athletes for high performance in aerobic sports and may be also linked to WM properties.

Conclusions

We explored the associations of objective measures of CRF and PA with measures of WM health in older low-fit and low-active adults. We showed that higher levels of MV-PA were linked to lower WMH volume. We propose that MV-PA allows keeping WMHs in check via cerebrovascular mechanisms, such as preserving higher blood vessel elasticity and wall integrity. We found an association between light PA and WM integrity in the temporal lobe while sedentary behavior was related to lower FA in the parahippocampal WM. We speculate that these associations are related to neurotrophic, cerebrovascular, lipid and insulin metabolic mechanisms related to PA or lack thereof. Together, our findings suggest that PA is associated with WM health in aging in an intensity- and region-specific manner. Our results are optimistic in showing that modifiable lifestyle factors such as increasing PA and reducing sedentariness may be beneficial for brain health. We are currently assessing in a randomized exercise intervention trial whether increases in CRF and changes in PA behavior may induce changes in WM health over shorter periods of time.

We conclude that PA and CRF are related but not equivalent in their relationships with WM health in aging. Specifically, the effects are WM measure- and region-specific, showing the importance of using multiple, objective, and independent measures to assess fitness, physical activity and sedentariness, and brain integrity. Our findings pave the way for testing more targeted hypotheses linking bodily fitness and WM integrity in longitudinal designs, with improved public health recommendations on PA being the longer-term outcome of such studies.

Acknowledgments

The authors thank Chanheng He, Meera Zukosky, Kishan Patel for help with data management, Holly Tracy and Nancy Dodge for MRI data collection, Sarah Banducci for help in data analyses, and Susan H. Herrel for project coordination.

Author Contributions

Conceived and designed the experiments: MWV AFK EM. Performed the experiments: AZB GEC JM CNW NPG EAO AK AL TRW JF HDC EA. Analyzed the data: AZB. Contributed reagents/materials/analysis tools: AZB CNW. Wrote the paper: AZB LCH MWV AFK.

References

1. Kramer AF, Hahn S, Cohen NJ, Banich MT, McAuley E, et al. (1999) Ageing, fitness and neurocognitive function.
2. Hillman CH, Erickson KI, Kramer AF (2008) Be smart, exercise your heart: exercise effects on brain and cognition. Nat Rev Neurosci 9: 58–65.
3. Madden DJ, Bennett IJ, Burzynska A, Potter GG, Chen N-K, et al. (2012) Diffusion tensor imaging of cerebral white matter integrity in cognitive aging. Biochim Biophys Acta 1822: 386–400.
4. Raz N, Rodrigue KM (2006) Differential aging of the brain: patterns, cognitive correlates and modifiers. Neurosci Biobehav Rev 30: 730–748.
5. Freedson PS, Melanson E, Sirard J (1998) Calibration of the Computer Science and Applications, Inc. accelerometer. Med Sci Sports Exerc 30: 777–781.
6. Craft LL, Zderic TW, Gapstur SM, Vaniterson EH, Thomas DM, et al. (2012) Evidence that women meeting physical activity guidelines do not sit less: an observational inclinometry study. Int J Behav Nutr Phys Act 9: 122.
7. Voss MW, Carr LJ, Clark R, Weng T (2014) Revenge of the "sit" II: Does lifestyle impact neuronal and cognitive health through distinct mechanisms associated with sedentary behavior and physical activity? Ment Health Phys Act.
8. Middleton LE, Manini TM, Simonsick EM, Harris TB, Barnes DE, et al. (2011) Activity energy expenditure and incident cognitive impairment in older adults. Arch Intern Med 171: 1251–1257.
9. Donahoo WT, Levine JA, Melanson EL (2004) Variability in energy expenditure and its components. Curr Opin Clin Nutr Metab Care 7: 599–605.
10. Dunstan DW, Howard B, Healy GN, Owen N (2012) Too much sitting–a health hazard. Diabetes Res Clin Pract 97: 368–376.
11. Helgerud J, Høydal K, Wang E, Karlsen T, Berg P, et al. (2007) Aerobic high-intensity intervals improve VO2max more than moderate training. Med Sci Sports Exerc 39: 665–671.
12. Bassett DR, Howley ET (2000) Limiting factors for maximum oxygen uptake and determinants of endurance performance. Med Sci Sports Exerc 32: 70–84.
13. Spina RJ, Ogawa T, Kohrt WM, Martin WH, Holloszy JO, et al. (1993) Differences in cardiovascular adaptations to endurance exercise training between older men and women. J Appl Physiol 75: 849–855.
14. Hoppeler H, Howald H, Conley K, Lindstedt SL, Claassen H, et al. (1985) Endurance training in humans: aerobic capacity and structure of skeletal muscle. J Appl Physiol 59: 320–327.
15. Peter I, Papandonatos GD, Belalcazar LM, Yang Y, Erar B, et al. (2014) Genetic modifiers of cardiorespiratory fitness response to lifestyle intervention. Med Sci Sports Exerc 46: 302–311.
16. Baloh RW, Vinters HV (1995) White matter lesions and disequilibrium in older people. II. Clinicopathologic correlation. Arch Neurol 52: 975–981.
17. Pantoni L (2002) Pathophysiology of age-related cerebral white matter changes. Cerebrovasc Dis 13 Suppl 2: 7–10.
18. Schmidt R, Enzinger C, Ropele S, Schmidt H, Fazekas F (2003) Progression of cerebral white matter lesions: 6-year results of the Austrian Stroke Prevention Study. Lancet 361: 2046–2048.
19. Basser PJ (n.d.) Inferring microstructural features and the physiological state of tissues from diffusion-weighted images. NMR Biomed 8: 333–344.
20. Beaulieu C (n.d.) The basis of anisotropic water diffusion in the nervous system - a technical review. NMR Biomed 15: 435–455.
21. Bennett IJ, Madden DJ, Vaidya CJ, Howard DV, Howard JH (2010) Age-related differences in multiple measures of white matter integrity: A diffusion tensor imaging study of healthy aging. Hum Brain Mapp31: 378–390.
22. Burzynska AZ, Preuschhof C, Bäckman L, Nyberg L, Li S-C, et al. (2010) Age-related differences in white matter microstructure: region-specific patterns of diffusivity. Neuroimage 49: 2104–2112.
23. Johnson NF, Kim C, Clasey JL, Bailey A, Gold BT (2012) Cardiorespiratory fitness is positively correlated with cerebral white matter integrity in healthy seniors. Neuroimage 59: 1514–1523.
24. Marks BL, Katz LM, Styner M, Smith JK (2011) Aerobic fitness and obesity: relationship to cerebral white matter integrity in the brain of active and sedentary older adults. Br J Sports Med 45: 1208–1215.
25. Tseng BY, Gundapuneedi T, Khan MA, Diaz-Arrastia R, Levine BD, et al. (2013) White matter integrity in physically fit older adults. Neuroimage 82: 510–516.
26. Voss MW, Heo S, Prakash RS, Erickson KI, Alves H, et al. (2012) The influence of aerobic fitness on cerebral white matter integrity and cognitive function in older adults: Results of a one-year exercise intervention. Hum Brain Mapp.
27. De Leeuw FE, de Groot JC, Achten E, Oudkerk M, Ramos LM, et al. (2001) Prevalence of cerebral white matter lesions in elderly people: a population based magnetic resonance imaging study. The Rotterdam Scan Study. J Neurol Neurosurg Psychiatry 70: 9–14.
28. McAuley E, Szabo AN, Mailey EL, Erickson KI, Voss M, et al. (2011) Non-Exercise Estimated Cardiorespiratory Fitness: Associations with Brain Structure, Cognition, and Memory Complaints in Older Adults. Ment Health Phys Act 4: 5–11.
29. Szabo AN, McAuley E, Erickson KI, Voss M, Prakash RS, et al. (2011) Cardiorespiratory fitness, hippocampal volume, and frequency of forgetting in older adults. Neuropsychology 25: 545–553.
30. Voss MW, Erickson KI, Prakash RS, Chaddock L, Malkowski E, et al. (2010) Functional connectivity: a source of variance in the association between cardiorespiratory fitness and cognition? Neuropsychologia 48: 1394–1406.
31. Erickson KI, Voss MW, Prakash RS, Basak C, Szabo A, et al. (2011) Exercise training increases size of hippocampus and improves memory. Proc Natl Acad Sci U S A 108: 3017–3022.
32. Erickson KI, Prakash RS, Voss MW, Chaddock L, Hu L, et al. (2009) Aerobic fitness is associated with hippocampal volume in elderly humans. Hippocampus 19: 1030–1039.
33. Voss MW, Heo S, Prakash RS, Erickson KI, Alves H, et al. (2013) The influence of aerobic fitness on cerebral white matter integrity and cognitive function in older adults: results of a one-year exercise intervention. Hum Brain Mapp34: 2972–2985.
34. Vernooij MW, de Groot M, van der Lugt A, Ikram MA, Krestin GP, et al. (2008) White matter atrophy and lesion formation explain the loss of structural integrity of white matter in aging. Neuroimage 43: 470–477.
35. Haskell W, Lee I-M, Pate R, Powell K, Blair S, et al. (2007) Physical Activity and Public Health: Updated Recommendation for Adults From the American College of Sports Medicine and the American Heart Association. Circulation 116: 1081–1093.
36. Hart TL, McClain JJ, Tudor-Locke C (2011) Controlled and free-living evaluation of objective measures of sedentary and active behaviors. J Phys Act Health 8: 848–857.
37. Troiano RP, Berrigan D, Dodd KW, Mâsse LC, Tilert T, et al. (2008) Physical activity in the United States measured by accelerometer. Med Sci Sports Exerc 40: 181–188.
38. Reese TG, Heid O, Weisskoff RM, Wedeen VJ (2003) Reduction of eddy-current-induced distortion in diffusion MRI using a twice-refocused spin echo. Magn Reson Med 49: 177–182.
39. Zhang Y, Brady M, Smith S (2001) Segmentation of brain MR images through a hidden Markov random field model and the expectation-maximization algorithm. IEEE Trans Med Imaging 20: 45–57.
40. Smith SM (2002) Fast robust automated brain extraction. Hum Brain Mapp17: 143–155.
41. Smith SM, Jenkinson M, Johansen-Berg H, Rueckert D, Nichols TE, et al. (2006) Tract-based spatial statistics: voxelwise analysis of multi-subject diffusion data. Neuroimage 31: 1487–1505.

42. Smith SM, Johansen-Berg H, Jenkinson M, Rueckert D, Nichols TE, et al. (2007) Acquisition and voxelwise analysis of multi-subject diffusion data with tract-based spatial statistics. Nat Protoc 2: 499–503.
43. Smith SM, Jenkinson M, Woolrich MW, Beckmann CF, Behrens TEJ, et al. (2004) Advances in functional and structural MR image analysis and implementation as FSL. Neuroimage 23 Suppl 1: S208–19.
44. Rueckert D, Sonoda LI, Hayes C, Hill DL, Leach MO, et al. (1999) Nonrigid registration using free-form deformations: application to breast MR images. IEEE Trans Med Imaging 18: 712–721.
45. Hofer S, Frahm J (2006) Topography of the human corpus callosum revisited–comprehensive fiber tractography using diffusion tensor magnetic resonance imaging. Neuroimage 32: 989–994.
46. Burzynska AZ, Garrett DD, Preuschhof C, Nagel IE, Li S-C, et al. (2013) A scaffold for efficiency in the human brain. J Neurosci 33: 17150–17159.
47. Mori S, Wakana S, Nagae-Poetscher LM, Van Zijl PCM (2005) MRI Atlas of Human White Matter. Elsevier, editor Elsevier.
48. Bhagat YA, Beaulieu C (2004) Diffusion anisotropy in subcortical white matter and cortical gray matter: changes with aging and the role of CSF-suppression. J Magn Reson Imaging 20: 216–227.
49. O'Rourke MF, Hashimoto J (2007) Mechanical factors in arterial aging: a clinical perspective. J Am Coll Cardiol 50: 1–13.
50. Ungvari Z, Kaley G, de Cabo R, Sonntag WE, Csiszar A (2010) Mechanisms of vascular aging: new perspectives. J Gerontol A Biol Sci Med Sci 65: 1028–1041.
51. McDonnell BJ, Maki-Petaja KM, Munnery M, Yasmin, Wilkinson IB, et al. (2013) Habitual exercise and blood pressure: age dependency and underlying mechanisms. Am J Hypertens 26: 334–341.
52. Vaitkevicius PV, Fleg JL, Engel JH, O'Connor FC, Wright JG, et al. (1993) Effects of age and aerobic capacity on arterial stiffness in healthy adults. Circulation 88: 1456–1462.
53. Schmidt R, Petrovic K, Ropele S, Enzinger C, Fazekas F (2007) Progression of leukoaraiosis and cognition. Stroke 38: 2619–2625.
54. Longstreth WT, Manolio TA, Arnold A, Burke GL, Bryan N, et al. (1996) Clinical correlates of white matter findings on cranial magnetic resonance imaging of 3301 elderly people. The Cardiovascular Health Study. Stroke 27: 1274–1282.
55. Van Dijk EJ, Breteler MMB, Schmidt R, Berger K, Nilsson L-G, et al. (2004) The association between blood pressure, hypertension, and cerebral white matter lesions: cardiovascular determinants of dementia study. Hypertension 44: 625–630.
56. Voss MW, Vivar C, Kramer AF, van Praag H (2013) Bridging animal and human models of exercise-induced brain plasticity. Trends Cogn Sci 17: 525–544.
57. Colcombe SJ, Erickson KI, Scalf PE, Kim JS, Prakash R, et al. (2006) Aerobic exercise training increases brain volume in aging humans. J Gerontol A Biol Sci Med Sci 61: 1166–1170.
58. Voss MW, Erickson KI, Prakash RS, Chaddock L, Kim JS, et al. (2013) Neurobiological markers of exercise-related brain plasticity in older adults. Brain Behav Immun 28: 90–99.
59. Rasmussen P, Brassard P, Adser H, Pedersen M V, Leick L, et al. (2009) Evidence for a release of brain-derived neurotrophic factor from the brain during exercise. Exp Physiol 94: 1062–1069.
60. Zoladz JA, Pilc A, Majerczak J, Grandys M, Zapart-Bukowska J, et al. (2008) Endurance training increases plasma brain-derived neurotrophic factor concentration in young healthy men. J Physiol Pharmacol 59 Suppl 7: 119–132.
61. Carro E, Nuñez A, Busiguina S, Torres-Aleman I (2000) Circulating insulin-like growth factor I mediates effects of exercise on the brain. J Neurosci 20: 2926–2933.
62. Cotman CW, Berchtold NC (2002) Exercise: A behavioral intervention to enhance brain health and plasticity. Trends Neurosci 25: 295–301.
63. Chiang M-C, Barysheva M, Toga AW, Medland SE, Hansell NK, et al. (2011) BDNF gene effects on brain circuitry replicated in 455 twins. Neuroimage 55: 448–454.
64. Tost H, Alam T, Geramita M, Rebsch C, Kolachana B, et al. (2013) Effects of the BDNF Val66Met polymorphism on white matter microstructure in healthy adults. Neuropsychopharmacology 38: 525–532.
65. Ziegler E, Foret A, Mascetti L, Muto V, Le Bourdiec-Shaffii A, et al. (2013) Altered white matter architecture in BDNF met carriers. PLoS One 8: e69290.
66. Cao L, Dhilla A, Mukai J, Blazeski R, Lodovichi C, et al. (2007) Genetic modulation of BDNF signaling affects the outcome of axonal competition in vivo. Curr Biol 17: 911–921.
67. Husson I, Rangon C-M, Lelièvre V, Bemelmans A-P, Sachs P, et al. (2005) BDNF-induced white matter neuroprotection and stage-dependent neuronal survival following a neonatal excitotoxic challenge. Cereb Cortex 15: 250–261.
68. Weinstock-Guttman B, Zivadinov R, Tamaño-Blanco M, Abdelrahman N, Badgett D, et al. (2007) Immune cell BDNF secretion is associated with white matter volume in multiple sclerosis. J Neuroimmunol 188: 167–174.
69. Singh KK, Park KJ, Hong EJ, Kramer BM, Greenberg ME, et al. (2008) Developmental axon pruning mediated by BDNF-p75NTR-dependent axon degeneration. Nat Neurosci 11: 649–658.
70. Black JE, Isaacs KR, Anderson BJ, Alcantara AA, Greenough WT (1990) Learning causes synaptogenesis, whereas motor activity causes angiogenesis, in cerebellar cortex of adult rats. Proc Natl Acad Sci U S A 87: 5568–5572.
71. Bullitt E, Rahman FN, Smith JK, Kim E, Zeng D, et al. (2009) The effect of exercise on the cerebral vasculature of healthy aged subjects as visualized by MR angiography. AJNR Am J Neuroradiol 30: 1857–1863.
72. Thomas C, Baker CI (2013) Teaching an adult brain new tricks: a critical review of evidence for training-dependent structural plasticity in humans. Neuroimage 73: 225–236.
73. Wakefield DB, Moscufo N, Guttmann CR, Kuchel GA, Kaplan RF, et al. (2010) White matter hyperintensities predict functional decline in voiding, mobility, and cognition in older adults. J Am Geriatr Soc 58: 275–281.
74. Whitman GT, Tang Y, Lin A, Baloh RW, Tang T (2001) A prospective study of cerebral white matter abnormalities in older people with gait dysfunction. Neurology 57: 990–994.
75. Starr JM, Leaper SA, Murray AD, Lemmon HA, Staff RT, et al. (2003) Brain white matter lesions detected by magnetic resonance [correction of resosnance] imaging are associated with balance and gait speed. J Neurol Neurosurg Psychiatry 74: 94–98.
76. Srikanth V, Beare R, Blizzard L, Phan T, Stapleton J, et al. (2009) Cerebral white matter lesions, gait, and the risk of incident falls: a prospective population-based study. Stroke 40: 175–180.
77. Srikanth V, Phan TG, Chen J, Beare R, Stapleton JM, et al. (2010) The location of white matter lesions and gait—a voxel-based study. Ann Neurol 67: 265–269.
78. Bhadelia RA, Price LL, Tedesco KL, Scott T, Qiu WQ, et al. (2009) Diffusion tensor imaging, white matter lesions, the corpus callosum, and gait in the elderly. Stroke 40: 3816–3820.
79. Van Impe A, Coxon JP, Goble DJ, Doumas M, Swinnen SP (2012) White matter fractional anisotropy predicts balance performance in older adults. Neurobiol Aging 33: 1900–1912.
80. Sachdev PS, Wen W, Christensen H, Jorm AF (2005) White matter hyperintensities are related to physical disability and poor motor function. J Neurol Neurosurg Psychiatry 76: 362–367.
81. Gouw AA, Van der Flier WM, van Straaten ECW, Barkhof F, Ferro JM, et al. (2006) Simple versus complex assessment of white matter hyperintensities in relation to physical performance and cognition: the LADIS study. J Neurol 253: 1189–1196.
82. Zheng JJJ, Delbaere K, Close JCT, Sachdev P, Wen W, et al. (2012) White matter hyperintensities are an independent predictor of physical decline in community-dwelling older people. Gerontology 58: 398–406.
83. Demiot C, Dignat-George F, Fortrat J-O, Sabatier F, Gharib C, et al. (2007) WISE 2005: chronic bed rest impairs microcirculatory endothelium in women. Am J Physiol Heart Circ Physiol 293: H3159–64.
84. Hamburg NM, McMackin CJ, Huang AL, Shenouda SM, Widlansky ME, et al. (2007) Physical inactivity rapidly induces insulin resistance and microvascular dysfunction in healthy volunteers. Arterioscler Thromb Vasc Biol 27: 2650–2656.
85. Tremblay MS, Colley RC, Saunders TJ, Healy GN, Owen N (2010) Physiological and health implications of a sedentary lifestyle. Appl Physiol Nutr Metab 35: 725–740.
86. Hamilton MT, Hamilton DG, Zderic TW (2004) Exercise physiology versus inactivity physiology: an essential concept for understanding lipoprotein lipase regulation. Exerc Sport Sci Rev 32: 161–166.
87. Yanagibori R, Kondo K, Suzuki Y, Kawakubo K, Iwamoto T, et al. (1998) Effect of 20 days' bed rest on the reverse cholesterol transport system in healthy young subjects. J Intern Med 243: 307–312.
88. Wickelgren I (1998) Tracking insulin to the mind. Science 280: 517–519.
89. Stranahan AM, Arumugam TV, Cutler RG, Lee K, Egan JM, et al. (2008) Diabetes impairs hippocampal function through glucocorticoid-mediated effects on new and mature neurons. Nat Neurosci 11: 309–317.
90. Greenwood CE, Winocur G (2005) High-fat diets, insulin resistance and declining cognitive function. Neurobiol Aging 26 Suppl 1: 42–45.
91. Stranahan AM, Cutler RG, Button C, Telljohann R, Mattson MP (2011) Diet-induced elevations in serum cholesterol are associated with alterations in hippocampal lipid metabolism and increased oxidative stress. J Neurochem 118: 611–615.

8

Reliability and Validity of the Transport and Physical Activity Questionnaire (TPAQ) for Assessing Physical Activity Behaviour

Emma J. Adams[1]*, Mary Goad[1], Shannon Sahlqvist[2], Fiona C. Bull[3], Ashley R. Cooper[4], David Ogilvie[5] on behalf of the iConnect Consortium

1 British Heart Foundation National Centre for Physical Activity and Health, School of Sport, Exercise and Health Sciences, Loughborough University, Loughborough, United Kingdom, **2** Centre for Physical Activity and Nutrition Research (C-PAN), School of Exercise and Nutrition Sciences, Deakin University, Geelong, Australia, **3** Centre for the Built Environment and Health, School of Population Health, University of Western Australia, Perth, Australia, **4** Centre for Exercise, Nutrition and Health Sciences, School for Policy Studies, University of Bristol, Bristol, United Kingdom, **5** Medical Research Council Epidemiology Unit and UKCRC Centre for Diet and Activity Research (CEDAR), University of Cambridge, Cambridge, United Kingdom

Abstract

Background: No current validated survey instrument allows a comprehensive assessment of both physical activity and travel behaviours for use in interdisciplinary research on walking and cycling. This study reports on the test-retest reliability and validity of physical activity measures in the transport and physical activity questionnaire (TPAQ).

Methods: The TPAQ assesses time spent in different domains of physical activity and using different modes of transport for five journey purposes. Test-retest reliability of eight physical activity summary variables was assessed using intra-class correlation coefficients (ICC) and Kappa scores for continuous and categorical variables respectively. In a separate study, the validity of three survey-reported physical activity summary variables was assessed by computing Spearman correlation coefficients using accelerometer-derived reference measures. The Bland-Altman technique was used to determine the absolute validity of survey-reported time spent in moderate-to-vigorous physical activity (MVPA).

Results: In the reliability study, ICC for time spent in different domains of physical activity ranged from fair to substantial for walking for transport (ICC = 0.59), cycling for transport (ICC = 0.61), walking for recreation (ICC = 0.48), cycling for recreation (ICC = 0.35), moderate leisure-time physical activity (ICC = 0.47), vigorous leisure-time physical activity (ICC = 0.63), and total physical activity (ICC = 0.56). The proportion of participants estimated to meet physical activity guidelines showed acceptable reliability (k = 0.60). In the validity study, comparison of survey-reported and accelerometer-derived time spent in physical activity showed strong agreement for vigorous physical activity ($r = 0.72$, $p < 0.001$), fair but non-significant agreement for moderate physical activity ($r = 0.24$, $p = 0.09$) and fair agreement for MVPA ($r = 0.27$, $p = 0.05$). Bland-Altman analysis showed a mean overestimation of MVPA of 87.6 min/week ($p = 0.02$) (95% limits of agreement −447.1 to +622.3 min/week).

Conclusion: The TPAQ provides a more comprehensive assessment of physical activity and travel behaviours and may be suitable for wider use. Its physical activity summary measures have comparable reliability and validity to those of similar existing questionnaires.

Editor: Conrad P. Earnest, Texas A&M University, United States of America

Funding: The iConnect consortium is funded by the Engineering and Physical Sciences Research Council (grant reference EP/G00059X/1). The funders had no role in study design, data collection and analysis, decision to publish, or preparation of the manuscript. DO is also supported by the Medical Research Council [Unit Programme number MC_UU_12015/6] and the Centre for Diet and Activity Research (CEDAR), a UKCRC Public Health Research Centre of Excellence that is funded by the British Heart Foundation, Economic and Social Research Council, Medical Research Council, National Institute for Health Research and the Wellcome Trust. The views expressed in this paper are those of the authors and do not necessarily reflect those of the study funders, the NIHR, or the Department of Health.

Competing Interests: The authors have declared that no competing interests exist.

* Email: e.j.adams@lboro.ac.uk

Introduction

Current approaches for increasing population levels of physical activity include promoting walking and cycling for transport and recreation. This has the potential to support policy goals in a number of sectors including public health (increasing physical activity levels), transport (increasing the use of sustainable travel modes) and environment (reducing carbon emissions) [1–3]. Increasingly, interdisciplinary research teams are working together to advance research in this area and require comprehensive measures of physical activity and travel behaviours to meet their different needs [3–5]. These measures need to enable assessment of the frequency and duration of participation in specific domains of physical activity, the total amount of physical activity undertaken, and the time spent and distance travelled using different modes of motorised and non-motorised transport for specific journey purposes. To date, no such comprehensive instruments have been developed and tested for their reliability and validity. A few instruments do cover some of these items, but these generally omit certain domains of activity (such as recreational activity), journeys made for certain purposes or the use of modes of transport other than walking and cycling [6,7]. In some cases the use of modes of transport other than walking and cycling is measured but the modes are grouped collectively under the term 'motorised vehicles', as in the long version of the International Physical Activity Questionnaire (IPAQ) [8]. This means it is not possible to assess the use of individual modes of motorised travel, such as car, train or bus, separately.

The development of a comprehensive instrument presents a challenge because of differences in the measures and approaches used by each discipline for assessing the different behaviours of interest. Physical activity research in adults typically uses self-report questionnaires or telephone surveys which ask about physical activity participation in different domains in the previous week or month [9]. The reliability and validity of instruments of this kind, such as the IPAQ [8], Global Physical Activity Questionnaire (GPAQ) [10] and Neighbourhood Physical Activity Questionnaire (NPAQ) [11], are usually tested and reported. However, in the transport sector, trip diaries and intercept surveys are more commonly used and the measurement properties of these instruments are often not tested or reported [12].

Although many physical activity questionnaires already exist and have been tested for reliability and validity, these instruments are often amended by researchers, who have slightly differing needs for their specific research project, without further reliability and validity testing. The effect of making these small changes on reliability and validity is largely unknown which raises a question as to whether further reliability and validity studies are needed each time an existing survey is adapted or whether it is safe to assume that the measurement properties are likely to remain similar.

The current study was conducted within the iConnect (Impact of COnstructing Non-motorised Networks and Evaluating Changes in Travel) project, a five year natural experimental study to assess the impact of improving walking and cycling infrastructure on travel, physical activity and carbon emissions [13]. In view of the lack of suitable existing instruments for assessing physical activity, walking and cycling for recreation, walking and cycling for transport and detailed measures of travel behaviour using other modes, a new transport and physical activity questionnaire (TPAQ) was developed. This paper reports on the development of the TPAQ, the test-retest reliability and validity of the physical activity items in the TPAQ and the impact of modifying an existing instrument, the IPAQ [8].

Methods

Development and content of the TPAQ. The TPAQ was developed by an interdisciplinary consortium as part of the iConnect study in the UK. Full details of the study, including a freely downloadable copy of the survey which incorporates the TPAQ, are provided elsewhere [14]. The development phase included a feasibility study [15] and pilot reliability and validity studies (not reported). The TPAQ was designed to enable a detailed assessment of time spent and distance travelled using different modes of transport overall and for different journey purposes, as well as time spent in different domains of recreational physical activity. First, travel behaviour in the last seven days was assessed across five categories of trip purpose: 1. to and from work, 2. for business purposes, 3. to and from a place of study, 4. for shopping and personal business, and 5. to visit friends or family or for other social activities. For each journey purpose participants were asked to report the number of trips, the total time spent (in hours and minutes) and the total distance (in miles) travelled in the last seven days for each of six specified modes of transport (walking, cycling, bus, train, car as a driver and car as a passenger) or any 'other' mode (which captured modes such as taxi and van). Four domains of activity (walking for recreation, cycling for recreation, moderate leisure-time activity and vigorous leisure-time activity) were assessed using items adapted from the short form of the IPAQ [8]. The questions asked participants to report the number of sessions and the total duration of participation (in hours and minutes) in each of the four domains of activity in the last seven days excluding any activity they had previously reported. The items were then used to create a number of key physical activity summary variables (Table 1). In addition the survey asked respondents to report their sex, age, ethnic group, educational qualifications, housing tenure, and the number of cars and bicycles in the household. This paper reports on the reliability and validity of the physical activity summary variables measured using the TPAQ. The reliability and validity of the travel behaviour measures will be reported separately.

Ethics statement

The reliability and validity studies received ethical approval from the University of Southampton Ethics Committee (CEE 200809-15).

Reliability study

Participants and procedures. In October 2010, 3000 adults were randomly selected from the edited electoral register for six wards in the town of Loughborough, UK and invited to complete the iConnect survey on two separate occasions, approximately seven days apart. The initial mailing contained a letter of invitation, a copy of the survey, a consent form and a freepost return envelope. Individuals who completed and returned the first survey (n = 216) were then posted the second survey and asked to complete and return it as soon as possible. Participants who did not return the second survey within seven days received a reminder phone call or letter. A prize draw to win one of twenty £25 gift vouchers was offered for those who completed both surveys as an incentive for participation.

Physical activity summary variables. Seven continuous physical activity summary variables (number of minutes spent in the past week in walking for transport, cycling for transport, walking for recreation, cycling for recreation, moderate leisure-time physical activity, vigorous leisure-time physical activity and total physical activity) and one categorical variable (proportion meeting current UK physical activity guidelines) were computed. Time spent walking for transport for each of the five journey purposes was summed to give the total time spent walking for transport. A similar process was followed for total time spent cycling for transport. A measure of total physical activity was computed by summing time spent walking and cycling for transport, time spent walking and cycling for recreation and time spent in moderate and vigorous leisure-time physical activity. This measure was also used to derive a categorical variable indicating whether respondents met the level of physical activity for adults recommended in the 2011 UK guidelines of at least 150 minutes of moderate intensity activity per week [16].

Analyses. The test-retest reliability of the seven continuous physical activity summary variables and the categorical variable was assessed. In secondary analyses, the reliability of the frequency

Table 1. Questionnaire items and physical activity summary variables in TPAQ.

Questionnaire item	Response	Items included in physical activity summary variables									
		Reliability study							Validity study		
TRAVEL BEHAVIOUR		Wt^r	Ct^r	Wr^r	Cr^r	MPA^r	VPA^r	TPA^r	MPA^v	VPA^v	MVPA^v
For each of five journey purposes†:											
How often did you make such a journey over the last 7 days?	Number of times										
How much time in total over the last 7 days did you spend travelling to and from work by:	Hours/minutes spent:										
	Walking	✓♦						✓♦	✓♦		✓♦
	Cycle		✓♦					✓♦			
	Bus										
	Train										
	Car, as a driver										
	Car, as a passenger										
	Other (specify)										
PHYSICAL ACTIVITY											
In the last 7 days, how many times did you **walk** for recreation, health or fitness (including walking your dog)?	Number of times			✓^{f}							
Please estimate the total time you spent **walking** for recreation, health or fitness in the last 7 days.	Hours Minutes			✓				✓	✓		✓
In the last 7 days, how many times did you **cycle** for recreation, health or fitness?	Number of times				✓^{f}						
Please estimate the total time you spent **cycling** for recreation, health or fitness in the last 7 days.	Hours Minutes				✓			✓			
During the last 7 days, how many times did you do **moderate intensity leisure time** physical activities which make you breathe somewhat harder than normal?	Number of times					✓^{f}					
What do you estimate is the total time you spent doing **moderate intensity leisure time** physical activities in the last 7 days?	Hours Minutes					✓		✓	✓		✓
During the last 7 days, how many times did you do **vigorous intensity leisure time** physical activities which makes you breathe harder or puff and pant?	Number of times						✓^{f}				
What do you estimate is the total time you spent doing **vigorous intensity leisure time** physical activities in the last 7 days?	Hours Minutes						✓	✓		✓	✓

†Journey purposes: to and from work; business journeys; to and from a place of study or to and from school; for shopping and personal business; to visit friends and relatives and for other social activities. Wt = walking for transport; Ct = cycling for transport; Wr = Walking for recreation; Cr = cycling for recreation; VPA = vigorous physical activity; MPA = moderate physical activity; TPA = Total physical activity; MPA = moderate physical activity; TPA = Total physical activity; MVPA = moderate-to-vigorous physical activity.

^{r} = reliability study;

^{v} = validity study;

^{f} = frequency of participation assessed in reliability study as separate variable;

♦ summed across all journey purposes. The full survey is available at http://bmjopen.bmj.com/content/suppl/2012/02/04/bmjopen-2011-000694.DC1/bmjopen-2011-000694-s1.pdf

of participation (number of sessions per week) was assessed for walking for recreation, cycling for recreation, moderate leisure-time physical activity and vigorous leisure-time physical activity.

Descriptive results are reported as mean ± standard deviation (SD). Intra-class correlation coefficients (ICC) were used to assess the reliability of each of the continuous variables and Kappa scores were used to assess the reliability of the categorical variable. For the purposes of this study, coefficient values of ≤0.20 were taken to indicate poor agreement; 0.21–0.40 represented fair agreement; 0.41–0.60 represented moderate or acceptable agreement; 0.61–0.80 represented substantial agreement; and 0.81–1.0 represented almost perfect agreement [17].

Validity study

Participants and procedures. The validity study was conducted between June and October 2011. Participants who took part in the reliability study and who had agreed to take part in future studies (n = 136) were sent a letter inviting them to take part in the validity study. In addition, employees from Loughborough University and three local small-to-medium-sized businesses were invited to take part in the project via email and word of mouth.

Individuals who registered their interest in participating in the study were invited to attend a group meeting where they were provided with an accelerometer (Actigraph GT3X, Actigraph, Pensacola, Florida, USA), a global positioning system (GPS) data logger (QSTARZ BT-Q1000) and a copy of the iConnect survey. A researcher explained the study to participants, including how to use the accelerometer and GPS device and when to complete the survey, and obtained written consent from each participant. Participants were instructed to wear the accelerometer and GPS device around their waist on the right hip for seven consecutive days from getting out of bed in the morning until going to bed at night, except when participating in water-based activities. Participants were asked to complete the survey on the eighth day. To maximise adherence to the study protocol, on the third day of monitoring participants received a follow-up telephone call or email to resolve any issues or concerns about the study. Participants were also contacted on day seven to remind them to complete the survey the following day and to arrange a time and place for the researcher to collect the study materials. Each participant in the validity study received a £5 gift voucher.

This study reports on the validity of the survey-derived physical activity summary variables using accelerometer data. GPS data were used only for the validation of the travel behaviour measures, which will be reported separately.

Data processing and accelerometer-derived physical activity summary variables. Accelerometers were programmed to record data at ten second epochs. Raw accelerometer data were processed using MAHUffe (MRC Epidemiology Unit, Cambridge, http://www.mrc-epid.cam.ac.uk). The last day of recording (the day on which the accelerometer was collected from the participant) and continuous periods where 60 or more minutes of zero values were recorded were considered to be non-wear time and were excluded. To maximise study quality we applied a strict inclusion criterion whereby participants were only included in analyses if they had worn the accelerometer for six or more days for at least 10 hours per day and had completed the survey within 2 days of their last day of accelerometry (n = 54). For participants with only six days of objectively measured physical activity (n = 9), the mean values for time spent in physical activity across the six recorded days were calculated and added to the six day total to estimate a value for seven days, the time period required for comparison with the survey data. Data were aggregated into 60 second epochs and cut points were used to classify data into different intensity activities: sedentary (0–199 counts per minute (cpm)), light intensity activity (200–2019 cpm), moderate intensity activity (2020–5998 cpm), or vigorous/very vigorous intensity activity (>5998 cpm) [18,19]. Summary variables were then computed representing time spent in moderate physical activity; time spent in vigorous physical activity (includes vigorous/very vigorous intensity activity) and time spent in moderate-to-vigorous physical activity (MVPA) (sum of time spent in moderate and vigorous physical activity).

Survey-derived physical activity summary variables. Three physical activity summary variables (moderate physical activity, vigorous physical activity and MVPA) were computed using survey data for comparison with accelerometer data. Times spent walking for transport, walking for recreation and in moderate leisure-time physical activity were summed to give time spent in moderate physical activity. Self-reported time spent in vigorous leisure-time physical activity was used for comparison with accelerometer-derived time spent in vigorous activity. A measure of total MVPA was computed by summing time spent walking for transport, time spent walking for recreation and time spent in moderate and vigorous leisure-time physical activity. Cycling was excluded from the survey-derived physical activity summary variables used in the validity study because hip-worn accelerometers have limited capacity to detect cycling [20] and time spent cycling has been shown to be a significant contributor to the disagreement between self-reported and objectively measured estimates of activity [21]. A sensitivity analysis was, however, conducted to determine whether this had any impact on the results (see below).

Analyses. Descriptive statistics are reported as mean ± standard deviation (SD). Correlation coefficients were calculated for survey-reported and accelerometer-derived summary physical activity variables using Spearman's rho because the data were not normally distributed.

Absolute validity was assessed by determining the agreement between self-reported total time spent in MVPA and accelerometer-derived total time spent in MVPA using the Bland-Altman technique [22]. A mean bias was defined as a significant mean difference obtained by subtracting objectively measured time spent in physical activity from self-reported time spent in physical activity. The error was defined as 2 SD of the mean bias.

Analyses for the reliability and validity studies were conducted using Statistical Package of Social Sciences, version 19.0.0 for Windows (IBM SPSS Inc, Chicago, Illinois, USA). Bland-Altman analyses were conducted using STATA 13 (StataCorp LP, College Station, Texas, USA).

Sensitivity analysis. A sensitivity analysis was conducted to determine the impact of including cycling in the survey-derived data for the analyses. Additionally, because participants may have reported transport or recreational walking undertaken at light intensity (<3 METs) [23] we conducted a second sensitivity analysis in which time spent in objectively-measured light intensity activity was included in the accelerometer-derived summary variables for total physical activity and moderate intensity physical activity. For both analyses, correlation co-efficients were calculated and absolute validity was assessed.

Results

Reliability study

Of the 3000 adults invited to take part in the reliability study, 166 completed and returned both surveys (a response rate of 6%) and were included in the analysis (Table 2).

Table 2. Sample characteristics.

Characteristic		Reliability study		Validity study	
		n = 166		n = 54[a]	
		n[b]	%	n[b]	%
Sex	Male	77	46.7	19	35.2
Age (years)	<30	19	11.7	12	22.2
	30–44	40	24.5	13	24.1
	45–64	59	36.2	25	46.3
	≥65	45	27.6	4	7.4
Ethnicity	White	147	90.7	53	98.1
	Other	15	9.3	1	1.9
Education	Degree	51	31.7	35	64.8
	GCE 'A' Level	28	17.4	10	18.5
	GCSE Grades A to C	39	24.2	5	9.3
	No formal qualification	43	26.7	4	7.4
Housing tenure	Owned	133	81.1	44	81.5
	Rented from private landlord	10	6.1	9	16.7
	Rented from local authority	19	11.6	1	1.9
	Other	2	1.2	0	0.0
Household cars	0	20	12.3	6	11.1
	1	71	43.8	18	33.3
	2 or more	71	43.8	30	55.6
Household bicycles	0	57	34.3	7	13.0
	1 more	109	65.7	47	87.0

[a] Included in analysis.
[b] Numbers do not sum to totals due to missing responses.

For each of the physical activity summary variables the mean weekly duration of physical activity was lower at the second survey administration (T2), which took place on average 12.4±6.6 days after the first survey administration (T1) (Table 3). The reliability of the survey-based time measures differed according to the specific activities being assessed. For transport-related activity, the intra-class correlation (ICC) of items was substantial for time spent cycling for transport (ICC = 0.61) and acceptable for time spent walking for transport (ICC = 0.59). For recreational activities, there was acceptable agreement for time spent walking for recreation (ICC = 0.48) but only fair agreement for time spent cycling for recreation (ICC = 0.35). Agreement was substantial for time spent in vigorous leisure-time physical activity (ICC = 0.63) and acceptable for time spent in moderate leisure-time intensity physical activity (ICC = 0.47) (Table 3). There was acceptable agreement between the two survey administrations for total duration of physical activity (ICC = 0.56) (Table 3) and for the proportion of respondents meeting physical activity recommendations (Kappa = 0.60) (data not shown).

For frequency of participation, there was substantial agreement for the number of sessions of walking (ICC = 0.80) and cycling (ICC = 0.63) for recreation, acceptable agreement for the number of sessions of vigorous intensity leisure-time physical activity (ICC = 0.52) and poor agreement for the number of sessions of moderate intensity leisure-time physical activity (ICC = 0.13) (Table 4).

Validity study

A total of 72 participants took part in the validity study. These were recruited from among those who took part in the reliability study (n = 25; a response rate of 18%) and from the convenience samples of staff and students of Loughborough University (n = 27) and local small-to-medium-sized businesses (n = 20). Of those who took part in the validity study 54 participants were eligible for inclusion in the analysis (Table 2).

In comparison to objectively-measured data, participants tended to over-report moderate and vigorous physical activity which resulted in an over-reporting of total physical activity in the survey (Table 5). Survey-reported moderate physical activity (including moderate leisure-time physical activity, walking for transport and walking for recreation, but excluding any cycling) showed fair agreement with objectively measured time spent in moderate physical activity ($r = 0.24$, $p = 0.085$). In contrast, survey-reported vigorous physical activity showed strong agreement with objectively-measured vigorous physical activity ($r = 0.72$, $p < 0.001$), although this relatively high correlation concealed large differences in the absolute estimates in that the mean duration of survey-reported vigorous physical activity (99.2 min/week) was more than three times higher than that of objectively-measured vigorous physical activity (30.2 min/week). Agreement between survey-reported MVPA and objectively-measured MVPA was fair and of borderline statistical significance ($r = 0.27$, $p = 0.051$) (Table 5).

In sensitivity analysis, including light intensity activity in the accelerometer-derived summary variables reduced the agreement

Table 3. Intra-class correlations for time spent in transport-related and recreational physical activity overall and by domain.

Physical activity domain		T1	T2	
	n	Mean minutes in last week ±SD	Mean minutes in last week ±SD	ICC (95% CI)
Walking for transport	164	142.0±256.6	129.6±194.4	0.59 (0.48, 0.68)
Cycling for transport	164	25.7±92.6	21.5±92.6	0.61 (0.50, 0.70)
Walking for recreation	165	117.1±192.2	116.6±207.4	0.48 (0.35, 0.59)
Cycling for recreation	165	27.4±104.6	20.4±105.8	0.35 (0.20, 0.47)
Moderate intensity leisure-time physical activity	165	80.7±168.4	63.2±131.8	0.47 (0.34, 0.58)
Vigorous intensity leisure-time physical activity	163	60.6±134.2	49.8±97.1	0.63 (0.53, 0.71)
Total physical activity†	161	441.2±455.3	387.4±374.0	0.56 (0.45, 0.66)

T1 = Survey time point 1;
T2 = Survey time point 2;
†Total physical activity includes vigorous and moderate leisure-time activity and walking and cycling for transport and recreation.

between self-reported and objectively-measured moderate physical activity ($r = 0.17$, $p = 0.226$) whereas the agreement for MVPA improved slightly and became significant ($r = 0.29$, $p = 0.037$). Including cycling in the survey-derived summary variables reduced the agreement between survey-reported and objectively-measured moderate physical activity ($r = 0.10$, $p = 0.495$) and between survey-reported and objectively-measured MVPA ($r = 0.09$, $p = 0.518$) (data not shown).

A Bland-Altman plot for the main analysis is shown in Figure 1. The difference between self-reported and accelerometer-derived MVPA for each participant is plotted on the *y* axis against their accelerometer-derived MVPA on the *x* axis. A mean overestimation of self-reported MVPA of 87.6 min/week ($p = 0.02$) was observed and the 95% limits of agreement were wide (−447.1 to +622.3 min/week).

In sensitivity analysis including light intensity accelerometer activity, the mean difference was greater at −1407.5 min/week ($p<0.001$) with commensurately wider 95% limits of agreement (−2314.4 to −500.6 min/week). In sensitivity analysis including cycling for transport and recreation in survey-reported total physical activity, the mean difference was 202.4 min/week ($p<0.001$) with 95% limits of agreement of −473.6 to +878.3 min/week (data not shown).

Discussion

A new instrument (the TPAQ) was developed for use in interdisciplinary research on physical activity and travel behaviours. The instrument allows specific target behaviours (walking and cycling separately and for different purposes) to be measured as well as providing an estimate of total physical activity. Developing such instruments is challenging given the different approaches typically used by different disciplines to assess the behaviours of interest and differences in terminology applied to similar constructs.

Reliability and validity of physical activity summary variables derived from TPAQ

TPAQ, which combines new items on travel behaviour with an adapted version of the short form of IPAQ, appears to be an acceptably reliable measure of time spent in different domains of physical activity as well as total physical activity. In most respects its reliability was comparable to that of other similar instruments used for measuring physical activity [8,10,11,24,25]. We used the last seven days as the reference period, which may have resulted in lower stability in our measures of behaviours such as walking and cycling for transport and recreation than would have been observed using an instrument framed in terms of a 'usual' week.

The reported frequency of participation in most types of leisure-time physical activity (walking for recreation, cycling for recreation and vigorous intensity physical activity) showed greater reliability than that for the reported duration of activity. Similar findings have been reported elsewhere [11], raising the question of whether it may be more appropriate to assess frequency of participation than to assess duration. However, the test-retest reliability of reported frequency of moderate intensity physical activity was poor, and it is more difficult to impute health benefits to a measure of frequency of participation than to an estimate of total volume (e.g. duration) of activity.

Table 4. Intra-class correlations for frequency of participation in recreational physical activity.

Physical activity domain		T1	T2	
	n	Mean times in last week (±SD)	Mean times in last week (±SD)	ICC (95% CI)
Walking for recreation	165	2.6±4.2	2.4±4.1	0.80 (0.73, 0.85)
Cycling for recreation	165	0.4±1.3	0.4±1.2	0.63 (0.53, 0.71)
Moderate intensity leisure-time physical activity	166	1.0±1.7	0.8±2.4	0.13 (−0.02, 0.28)
Vigorous intensity leisure-time physical activity	166	1.1±1.9	0.9±1.8	0.52 (0.40, 0.62)

T1 = Survey time point 1;
T2 = Survey time point 2.

Table 5. Validity of physical activity measures overall and by domain.

Physical activity domain	n	Survey items included in summary variable	Accelerometer-derived data included in summary variable	Survey data Mean minutes (±SD)	Accelerometer data Mean minutes (±SD)	r	p
Moderate physical activity	53	Moderate intensity leisure-time physical activity	Moderate intensity physical activity	307.9±227.2	294.5±133.5		
		Walking for transport					
		Walking for recreation					
Vigorous physical activity	46	Vigorous intensity leisure-time physical activity	Vigorous intensity physical activity	99.1±141.6	30.2±67.5	0.72	<.001
Moderate-to-vigorous physical activity	52	Vigorous intensity leisure-time physical activity	Vigorous intensity physical activity	431.1±256.7	343.5±164.4	0.27	.051
		Moderate intensity leisure-time physical activity	Moderate intensity physical activity				
		Walking for transport					
		Walking for recreation					

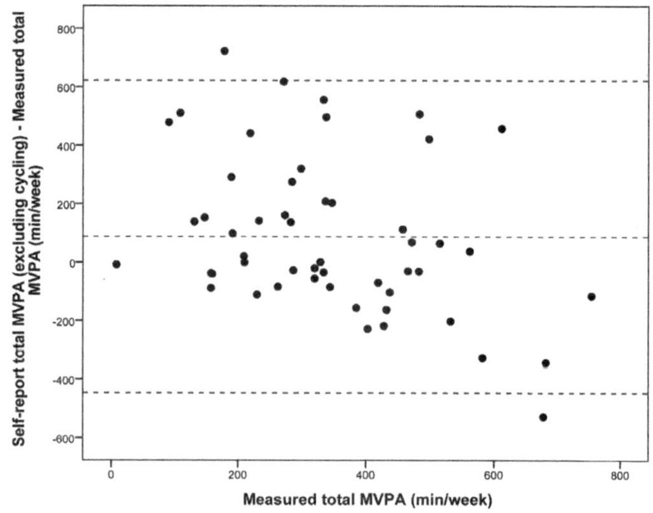

Figure 1. Bland-Altman plot for time spent in moderate-to-vigorous physical activity. The difference between objectively measured time spent in total MVPA (min/week) and self-reported time spent in MVPA excluding cycling (min/week) plotted against objectively measured time spent in MVPA (min/week). Mean difference: 87.6 min/week (p = 0.02); limits of agreement: −447.1 min/week, +622.3 min/week.

Compared to an accelerometer-derived criterion, TPAQ produced an estimate of total time spent in physical activity of comparable validity to that of the short IPAQ [8,25] and most other off-the-shelf questionnaires of similar length currently in use. In Bland-Altman analysis, TPAQ significantly overestimated MVPA in comparison to accelerometer-derived estimates by 88 minutes per week, with no clear pattern of any change in bias with higher levels of self-reported physical activity. Other studies have also reported an overestimation of self-reported MVPA in comparison to accelerometer-measured MVPA, although these differences have been much larger than those observed in our study. For example, one recent study found an overestimation of 46 minutes per day between GPAQ and objectively-measured MVPA, and 76 minutes per day between short IPAQ and objectively-measured MVPA [26]. The observed limits of agreement in our study were very wide (over 10 hours per week) however other studies comparing self-reported MVPA with objectively-measured MVPA have reported even larger limits of agreement, for example up to 17 hours per week using long IPAQ [27] or two hours per day using short IPAQ [28]. We therefore conclude that TPAQ is as acceptable as other similar instruments for use in measuring MVPA, notwithstanding the widely recognised limitations of all self-reported estimates of physical activity.

The substantial agreement observed for vigorous physical activity estimated using the TPAQ is higher than that reported elsewhere [25]. However it appears that the TPAQ may overestimate the time spent in this domain of activity and thus overall physical activity. The poor agreement between survey-reported and accelerometer-measured moderate physical activity has also been observed in a number of other studies [25]. This may reflect participants having reported light intensity activities in the survey, as TPAQ does not specify the intensity of walking and cycling for transport or recreation that should be reported. Participants may therefore have reported walking or cycling of any intensity. Including light intensity accelerometer-derived activity in a sensitivity analysis did improve the agreement slightly for total physical activity. These findings suggest that the performance of TPAQ as a measure of moderate and vigorous physical activity could be improved by specifying the intensity of walking and cycling that should be reported and more clearly defining which activities should be reported as being of vigorous intensity. The inclusion of cycling in survey-reported measures reduced the agreement with accelerometer-derived variables, supporting previous findings that time spent cycling may contribute to the disagreement between self-reported and objectively measured estimates of activity [21].

TPAQ asks about participation in a number of different domains of physical activity in order to provide more specific outcome measures for particular interventions that might target, for example, walking or cycling for transport or recreation. In the validity study, this appeared to lead to an over-reporting of physical activity compared to accelerometer-derived estimates. It is not yet clear whether disaggregating physical activity behaviours in this way leads to over-reporting, or whether it increases accuracy because participants can recall the time they have spent in more specific activities more precisely than they can provide a more global estimate of time spent in overall physical activity. Other possible reasons for the higher estimates from self-report data include social desirability bias which may have led to participants over-reporting their activity; difficulties in recalling activities over the past week; inclusion of short (<10 minute) bouts of activity; or the need for participants to sum time spent in different activities over the previous week. High estimates may also be due to participants reporting walking or cycling under both 'transport' and 'recreation, health or fitness' headings, because it is sometimes difficult to distinguish these purposes.

Adaptation of physical activity items from existing instruments

Instruments used to assess physical activity behaviour are often adapted by investigators for use in their research projects without further reliability and validity testing. In developing the TPAQ, recreational and leisure-time physical activity items were adapted from an existing instrument, the short IPAQ. We found the physical activity summary variables derived from TPAQ to have broadly comparable reliability and validity to those of the original IPAQ [8], suggesting that minor modifications to survey instruments may not necessarily alter their reliability and validity to the extent that their measurement properties would always need to be reassessed. However, IPAQ itself has been tested in a large number of different populations from different countries [8,9,25] with varying findings, suggesting that it is not only the wording of the surveys but also the target group and context in which they are used that may affect reliability and validity.

Strengths and limitations

We successfully developed an instrument to meet the needs of interdisciplinary research on physical activity and travel behaviour. We tested its reliability and validity predominantly using a community sample rather than a convenience sample, which helps to improve the generalisability of our findings. Although the response rate to the reliability study was low, our sample had a similar gender and ethnic composition to that of the 2011 Census findings [29] for the local borough of Charnwood from which our sample was recruited. There was a small difference in age distribution, with a lower proportion of those aged under 30 and a higher proportion of those aged over 45 represented in our sample. In the validity study additional strategies were necessary to recruit sufficient participants, resulting in the inclusion of staff and students from within the University and local workplaces that may have reduced the overall representativeness of the study population.

Adherence with the validity study protocol was generally very high, although a small number of participants did not wear the accelerometer for sufficient time on all seven days of the measurement period. We were able to adjust for this in the analysis using standard procedures. Some participants were excluded from the analysis because they did not meet the strict accelerometer wear time criteria or did not complete the survey with two days of their final day of wearing the accelerometer. There were no significant differences in key characteristics between participants included and excluded for these reasons, except that a higher proportion of those excluded were aged 30–44 (data not shown). Given the low number of participants in the validity study, and the inclusion of only a small number of adults aged 65 and over, further investigation may be required to assess the measurement properties of the TPAQ in different age groups and in different contexts.

Finally, it is difficult to distinguish between different forms of activity using conventional methods of processing accelerometer data, and it was therefore not possible to assess the validity of self-reported estimates of time spent in the specific behaviours of walking and cycling in this study. To derive objective measures of mode-specific travel times in this sample requires a combination of accelerometer and GPS data that will be pursued in subsequent analyses.

Conclusions

This study reports on the development and selected measurement properties of a new comprehensive instrument (the TPAQ) for use in the assessment of physical activity and travel behaviours. Overall, the reliability and validity of the TPAQ for measuring total physical activity, and specific domains of physical activity including walking and cycling for different purposes, are comparable to those of existing physical activity questionnaires of similar length currently being used. The TPAQ may therefore provide an alternative instrument suitable for wider use.

Acknowledgments

This paper was written on behalf of the iConnect consortium (www.iconnect.ac.uk: Christian Brand, Fiona Bull, Ashley Cooper, Andy Day, Nanette Mutrie, David Ogilvie, Jane Powell, John Preston and Harry Rutter). We thank the study participants for their cooperation and Aron Sherry for co-ordinating the reliability study.

Author Contributions

Conceived and designed the experiments: EA SS FB AC DO. Performed the experiments: EA MG. Analyzed the data: EA MG SS AC DO. Wrote the paper: EA MG SS FB AC DO.

References

1. Department of Health and Department for Transport (2010) Active Travel Strategy. London, UK. Available: http://webarchive.nationalarchives.gov.uk/20130107105354/http:/www.dh.gov.uk/en/Publicationsandstatistics/Publications/PublicationsPolicyAndGuidance/DH_113102. Accessed 2014 Aug 25.
2. de Nazelle A, Nieuwenhuijsen MJ, Anto JM, Brauer M, Briggs D, et al. (2011) Improving health through policies that promote active travel: A review of evidence to support integrated health impact assessment. Environ Int 37: 766–777.

3. National Institute for Health and Care Excellence (2012) Walking and cycling: Local measures to promote walking and cycling as forms of travel or recreation. NICE Public Health Guidance 41.
4. Handy SL, Boarnet MG, Ewing R, Killingsworth RE (2002) How the built environment affects physical activity - views from urban planning. Am J Prev Med 23: 64–73.
5. Krizek KJ, Handy SL, Forsyth A (2009) Explaining changes in walking and bicycling behaviour: Challenges for transportation research. Environ Plann B 36: 725–740.
6. Badland H, Schofield G (2006) Test-retest reliability of a survey to measure transport-related physical activity in adults. Res Q Exerc Sport 77: 386–390.
7. Forsyth A, Agrawal AW, Krizek KJ (2012) Simple, inexpensive approach to sampling for pedestrian and bicycle surveys approach developed in pedestrian and bicycling survey. Transp Res Rec 2299: 22–30.
8. Craig CL, Marshall AL, Sjostrom M, Bauman AE, Booth ML, et al. (2003) International Physical Activity Questionnaire: 12-country reliability and validity. Med Sci Sports Exerc 35: 1381–1395.
9. van Poppel MNM, Chinapaw MJM, Mokkink LB, van Mechelen W, Terwee CB (2010) Physical activity questionnaires for adults A systematic review of measurement properties. Sports Med 40: 565–600.
10. Bull FC, Maslin TS, Armstrong T (2009) Global Physical Activity Questionnaire (GPAQ): Nine country reliability and validity study. J Phys Act Health 6: 790–804.
11. Giles-Corti B, Timperio A, Cutt H, Pikora TJ, Bull FCL, et al. (2006) Development of a reliable measure of walking within and outside the local neighborhood: RESIDE's neighborhood physical activity questionnaire. Prev Med 42: 455–459.
12. Forsyth A, Krizek KJ, Agrawal AW (2010) Measuring walking and cycling using the PABS (pedestrian and bicycling survey) approach: A low-cost survey method for local communities. CA-MTI-10-2907.
13. Ogilvie D, Bull F, Powell J, Cooper AR, Brand C, et al. (2011) An applied ecological framework for evaluating infrastructure to promote walking and cycling: The iConnect study. Am J Public Health 101: 473–481.
14. Ogilvie D, Bull F, Cooper A, Rutter H, Adams E, et al. (2012) Evaluating the travel, physical activity and carbon impacts of a 'natural experiment' in the provision of new walking and cycling infrastructure: Methods for the core module of the iConnect study. BMJ Open 2: e000694.
15. Sahlqvist S, Song Y, Bull F, Adams E, Preston J, et al. (2011) Effect of questionnaire length, personalisation and reminder type on response rate to a complex postal survey: Randomised controlled trial. BMC Med Res Methodol 11: 62–62.
16. Department of Health (2011) Start Active, Stay Active: A report on physical activity from the four home countries' Chief Medical Officers. London, UK. Available: https://www.gov.uk/government/publications/start-active-stay-active-a-report-on-physical-activity-from-the-four-home-countries-chief-medical-officers. Accessed 2014 Aug 25.
17. Landis JR, Koch GG (1977) Measurement of observer agreement for categorical data. Biometrics 33: 159–174.
18. Craig R, Mindell J, Hirani V (2009) Health Survey for England 2008 Volume 1. Physical activity and fitness. NHS Information Centre for Health and Social Care. London, UK.
19. Troiano RP, Berrigan D, Dodd KW, Masse LC, Tilert T, et al. (2008) Physical activity in the United States measured by accelerometer. Med Sci Sports Exerc 40: 181–188.
20. De Vries SI, Engels M, Garre FG (2011) Identification of children's activity type with accelerometer-based neural networks. Med Sci Sports Exerc 43: 1994–1999.
21. Slootmaker SM, Schuit AJ, Chinapaw MJM, Seidell JC, van Mechelen W (2009) Disagreement in physical activity assessed by accelerometer and self-report in subgroups of age, gender, education and weight status. Int J Behav Nutr Phys Act 6: 17.
22. Bland JM, Altman DG (2010) Statistical methods for assessing agreement between two methods of clinical measurement. Int J Nurs Stud 47: 931–936.
23. Ainsworth BE, Haskell WL, Herrmann SD, Meckes N, Bassett DR Jr, et al. (2011) 2011 compendium of physical activities: A second update of codes and MET values. Med Sci Sports Exerc 43: 1575–1581.
24. Helmerhorst HJF, Brage S, Warren J, Besson H, Ekelund U (2012) A systematic review of reliability and objective criterion-related validity of physical activity questionnaires. Int J Behav Nutr Phys Act 9: 103.
25. Lee PH, Macfarlane DJ, Lam TH, Stewart SM (2011) Validity of the International Physical Activity Questionnaire short form (IPAQ-SF): A systematic review. Int J Behav Nutr Phys Act 8: 115.
26. Herrmann SD, Heumann KJ, Der Ananian CA, Ainsworth BE (2013) Validity and reliability of the Global Physical Activity Questionnaire (GPAQ). Meas Phys Educ Exerc Sci 17: 221–235.
27. Hagstromer M, Oja P, Sjostrom M (2006) The International Physical Activity Questionnaire (IPAQ): A study of concurrent and construct validity. Public Health Nutr 9: 755–762.
28. Ekelund U, Sepp H, Brage S, Becker W, Jakes R, et al. (2006) Criterion-related validity of the last 7-day, short form of the International Physical Activity Questionnaire in Swedish adults. Public Health Nutr 9: 258–265.
29. Office for National Statistics (2011) 2011 Census for England and Wales. Available: http://www.ons.gov.uk/ons/guide-method/census/2011/index.html?utm_source=twitterfeed&utm_medium=twitter. Accessed 2014 Aug 25.

9

Attitudes and Barriers to Exercise in Adults with Type 1 Diabetes (T1DM) and How Best to Address Them

Nadia Lascar[1,2], Amy Kennedy[1,2], Beverley Hancock[3], David Jenkins[2], Robert C. Andrews[3], Sheila Greenfield[4], Parth Narendran[1,2*]

1 School of Clinical and Experimental Medicine, University of Birmingham, Edgbaston, Birmingham, United Kingdom, 2 Department of Diabetes, Nuffield House, The Queen Elizabeth Hospital, Edgbaston, Birmingham, United Kingdom, 3 School of Clinical Sciences, University of Bristol, Bristol, United Kingdom, 4 Primary Care Clinical Sciences, University of Birmingham, Edgbaston, Birmingham, United Kingdom

Abstract

Background: Regular physical activity has recognised health benefits for people with T1DM. However a significant proportion of them do not undertake the recommended levels of activity. Whilst questionnaire-based studies have examined barriers to exercise in people with T1DM, a formal qualitative analysis of these barriers has not been undertaken. Our aims were to explore attitudes, barriers and facilitators to exercise in patients with T1DM.

Methodology: A purposeful sample of long standing T1DM patients were invited to participate in this qualitative study. Twenty-six adults were interviewed using a semi-structured interview schedule to determine their level of exercise and barriers to initiation and maintenance of an exercise programme.

Principal findings: Six main barriers to exercise were identified: lack of time and work related factors; access to facilities; lack of motivation; embarrassment and body image; weather; and diabetes specific barriers (low levels of knowledge about managing diabetes and its complications around exercise). Four motivators to exercise were identified: physical benefits from exercise; improvements in body image; enjoyment and the social interaction of exercising at gym or in groups. Three facilitators to exercise were identified: free or reduced admission to gyms and pools, help with time management, and advice and encouragement around managing diabetes for exercise.

Significance: Many of the barriers to exercise in people with T1DM are shared with the non-diabetic population. The primary difference is the requirement for education about the effect of exercise on diabetes control and its complications. There was a preference for support to be given on a one to one basis rather than in a group environment. This suggests that with the addition of the above educational requirements, one to one techniques that have been successful in increasing activity in patients with other chronic disease and the general public should be successful in increasing activity in patients with T1DM.

Editor: Irene Petersen, UCL, United Kingdom

Funding: The study was funded by the Insulin Dependent Diabetes Trust (http://iddt.org/). PN received the funding. The study was funded for £9,600. The study was sponsored by The University of Birmingham, United Kingdom. The funders had no role in study design, data collection and analysis, decision to publish, or preparation of the manuscript.

Competing Interests: The authors have declared that no competing interests exist.

* Email: p.narendran@bham.ac.uk

These authors contributed equally to this work.

Introduction

Type 1 diabetes is a chronic autoimmune disease characterized by the loss of insulin producing cells in the pancreas. It is treated by strict management of lipids, blood pressure and glucose levels, the latter through the injection of insulin [1]. Regular physical activity is also recognized to play a key role in the management of patients with T1DM. It improves insulin sensitivity, reduces cardiovascular risk factors, improves quality of life and reduces mortality [2]. Guidelines for patients with T1DM currently recommend they undertake at least 150 minutes (mins) per week of moderate to vigorous aerobic exercise, spread out during at least 3 days during the week, with no more than two consecutive days between bouts of aerobic activity. They should also be encouraged to perform resistance exercise 'at least twice weekly on non-consecutive days' [3,4].

A large percentage of patients with T1DM do not reach these guidelines [5]. In the Finnish Diabetic Neuropathy Study, 23% of patients with T1DM were classed as sedentary and a further 21% were doing less than 1 session of exercise per week [6].

In a retrospective analysis of the Diabetes and Complications Trial, Makura and colleagues showed that 271 (19%) of the 1441 participants were not achieving the ADA recommendation for activity levels [7]. In a prospective cohort study of 2185 patients with T1DM from 16 European countries (The EURODIAB Prospective Complications Study), Tielemans and colleagues demonstrated that 786 (36%) of patients were doing none or only mild physical activity [8]. To date, there has only been one study that examines barriers to exercise in T1DM. Based in North America and using a questionnaire, this study found that fear of hypoglycaemia, work schedule and loss of control over their diabetes were the main barriers to exercise [9]. They also identified that knowledge of insulin pharmacokinetics, awareness of strategies to reduce hypoglycaemia, and increased social support (including having someone to exercise with) was associated with fewer barriers. Culture, diet and diabetes education vary significantly between countries [10] and therefore these findings in the North American population urgently need to be validated in other populations. By interviewing adults with T1DM this study aimed to qualitatively explore attitudes and barriers to the uptake and maintenance of exercise. This should provide a more in-depth understanding than that provided by questionnaires, and should allow the development of strategies to increase exercise to the recommended levels in patients with T1DM.

Methods

Sampling and recruitment

Purposeful sampling to include both genders and across all adult age groups was used to recruit adults with a clinical diagnosis of T1DM to participate in individual face to face interviews.

Patients aged between 18 to 80 years were recruited from the Diabetes Unit of Selly Oak Hospital, University Hospitals Birmingham NHS Foundation Trust, Birmingham, UK. Patients were approached to participate in the study whilst waiting for their diabetes appointment, and/or directly by their clinician at the end of their diabetes appointment. If patients were interested in taking part in the study, their details were taken and information sheets were sent to them. They were then contacted to confirm they remained interested in taking part in the interview, and a date scheduled for interview.

Ethics statement

Ethical approval was granted by Birmingham East North and Solihull Research Ethics Committee. The study was sponsored by The University of Birmingham, UK. Informed written consent was obtained from all the participants. All participants were adults older than 18 years.

Interviews

Each interview lasted an average of 30 minutes and was undertaken in the Diabetes Unit of Selly Oak Hospital. We ensured that the clinicians and allied health care professionals who were involved in managing the patient were not involved in any way in the interview so that the patient responses would not be influenced by their presence.

All interviews were carried out by one experienced qualitative researcher using a topic guide (see Table 1) which asked about patients' level of exercise, reasons why they do not exercise, and barriers to initiation and maintenance of an exercise programme. Resistance to change, individual needs and preferences, use of exercise diaries, approaches to monitoring levels of exercise and acceptability of different types of intervention delivery were also explored. At the beginning of the interview patients were asked about their diagnosis, family history of T1DM, treatment regime and control, to provide the context to explore each individual's relationship with diabetes and how this might impact on their activity and exercise behaviour. All patients were made aware that the interview would be recorded, transcribed and analysed anonymously.

Data handling and analysis

The interviews were recorded and transcribed. Data were analysed using a framework approach [11] which involved reading through the transcripts and developing a matrix of overarching and supporting themes.

Results

Patients

Over a four month period (April to July 2010), 48 patients expressed interest in the study. Six did not respond to repeated telephone messages and five were unavailable for interview because of their work or living away. Interviews were arranged with 32/48 patients and six subsequently failed to attend or cancelled at very late notice.

A further five, recruited towards the end of the study, were not interviewed because they belonged to subgroups already well represented in the sample and also because data saturation had been achieved. In total 26 interviews were undertaken.

Characteristics of the sample

12 females and 14 males were interviewed (Table 2). The females were aged between 21 and 62 years (mean 40.7±13.9 years) and the males were aged between 21 and 65 (mean 42.6±13.3). Time since diagnosis ranged from two weeks to 50 years (mean 17.6±15.7 years), and age at diagnosis ranged from nine months to 57 years (mean 25.3±14.1 years). The treatment regime was insulin injections for 19 patients. Five patients used an insulin pump. The treatment regime was not recorded for two patients.

Framework analysis of the data revealed three major themes and supporting themes around exercise: physical activity and exercise behaviour; barriers to exercise; facilitating and encouraging exercise (see Table 3).

Theme 1: Physical activity and Exercise Behaviour

Activity levels. Patients were asked to describe how active they were in terms of lifestyle and work.

A recurring theme was interviewees confusing an *active* lifestyle with a *busy* lifestyle.

Many cited walking when describing activity levels but the amount of walking varied and few walked a total of thirty minutes or more on a daily basis. Having a dog to walk or not having a car was associated with regular walking but people with cars were more likely to drive than walk, often citing the distances they had to cover between home and work as being the main reason although bad weather and not having time to walk were additional reasons. A number of participants described walking for pleasure but probing revealed that this usually meant when they were on holiday and not as a regular activity. Similarly, six people (all men) said they either cycled occasionally or that they had been cyclists when they were younger, though they were not currently regular cyclists.

Exercise behaviour. Over half of the group (16) claimed to do some form of exercise but probing revealed that more than half

Table 1. Interview schedule.

1	Can you tell me a little bit about your diabetic history: when were you first diagnosed, has anyone else in your family had diabetes, how your diabetes is managed, that sort of thing?
2	How does the diabetes affect your lifestyle?
3	As you know, the research is about physical activity. What kinds of physical activity do you do?
4	Do you do any exercise or take part in any sports?
5	Would you like to be more physically active?/Would you like to do more exercise?
6	What do you think prevents you from taking exercise?
7	What would help or encourage you to do more exercise?
8	Some things have been suggested that might help people to take up, and keep doing, more exercise. Would any of these be of interest to you? - one to one advice from a health and fitness advisor - attending an exercise group organised by the hospital or your GP - motivational support – someone who keeps in touch to see how you are doing with your exercise programme
9	The latest health recommendation is that we all undertake a minimum of 150 minutes of exercise a week – half an hour, five times a week. What do you think about that? Do you think you could achieve that target?
10	Follow up: what is the one thing that would most help you to increase your level of exercise?

of them only exercised an average of once or twice a week and sometimes not at all; some described "going through phases".

Swimming and going to the gym were the most frequent forms of exercise. Individuals participated in a range of other exercise activities and sports including fencing, badminton, tennis, yoga and skiing but not on a regular (weekly) basis. Although some of the men had previously played football when they were younger, none of the participants took part in team sports currently.

Table 2. Interviewee Characteristics.

Interview order	Gender	Age	Age diagnosed	Time since diagnosis	Treatment
1	M	57	49 years	7 years	Injection
2	M	21	20 years	10 months	Injection
3	F	23	18 years	5 years	Injection
4	M	31	29 years	Less than 2 years	Injection
5	F	54	27 years	27 years	Pump
6	F	21	9 years	12 years	Pump
7	M	34	32 years	18 months	Injection
8	F	38	31 years	7 years	Injection
9	M	33	33 years	2 weeks	Injection
10	M	55	43 years	12 years	Injection
11	F	24	9 years	15 years	Pump
12	M	53	27 years	26 years	Injection
13	M	64	14 years	50 years	Injection
14	F	40	25 years	15 years	Pump
15	F	39	21 years	18 years	Injection
16	F	33	21 years	12 years	Injection
17	F	50	10 years	40 years	Injection
18	M	35	30 years	5 years	Injection
19	M	50	45 years	5 years	Injection
20	M	50	9 months	50 years	Injections
21	F	62	19 years	43 years	Pump
22	M	44	28 years	16 years	Injection
23	M	22	13 years	9 years	Not recorded
24	M	47	4 years	43 years	Not recorded
25	F	59	57 years	Nearly 3 years	Injection
26	F	45	42 years	3 years	Injection

Table 3. Interview Themes.

Overarching themes	Supporting themes	
Activity and exercise behaviour	Physical activity	
	Exercise behaviour	
	Perceptions of activity and exercise levels	
	Present and desired activity levels	
	Achieving targets	
Barriers to exercise	Time, work and lifestyle	
	Health and medical	
	Social and personal	
	Environmental	
Facilitating, motivating and encouraging exercise	**Facilitators and Motivators**	**Interventions to encourage exercise**
	Enjoyment	One to one advice from a health and fitness advisor
	Rewards	Attending an exercise group organised by the hospital or GP
	Support and encouragement	Motivational support
	Access	
	Knowledge and advice	
	Time management	

Whilst swimming was given as an example of preferred exercise by half of the people (13), it emerged that half of them (7) only swam occasionally such as when they were on holiday. Three people explained that although they enjoyed swimming they were worried about doing so because they felt less in tune with their bodies when they were in the water and at greater risk of a hypoglycaemic attack. Two people did not swim because they were embarrassed at being seen in swimwear.

One third of participants (9) stated that they exercised at a gym and three of these went to a gym once a week or less. Although a couple of the regular gym users identified social as well as health reasons for going, most gave the impression that they had to make an effort to go but did so for the health benefits they derived.

Some of those who did not use a gym volunteered why: they believed they could exercise equally well elsewhere, they preferred to take part in a sport or activity outside or they felt they weren't "gym people".

Increasing activity levels. Participants were informed of the health recommendation that they take a minimum of 150 mins of moderate intensity exercise every week. A third (9) claimed that they were achieving that target (when they included walking as part of their regime). Many of these people did not exercise for 30 mins a day on five days a week, but rather longer bouts of exercise on fewer than five times a week.

Of those 17 people that said they were not achieving the target, five thought it was possible for them to increase their exercise levels to achieve the target. Seven people did not believe they could achieve the target, and some suggested that the target was unrealistic.

Well over half (18) said they would like to be more active. The reasons why they did not exercise and the things that might help them to be more active are discussed in the next two themes.

Theme 2: Barriers to Exercise

Participants identified four main barriers 'health and medical', 'time', 'work and lifestyle', 'social and personal' and 'environmental', to exercise.

Health and Medical. Four people cited non-diabetes related health problems as reasons for not exercising: asthma, arthritis and sports related injury. More people (nine) attributed their under active lifestyle to diabetes, although it was not necessarily a barrier for them. Many more than this talked about exercise and diabetes in ways that illustrated that they recognised a link between exercise and management of diabetes but many did not fully understand the relationship and how blood sugar could be affected by activity.

> *"I'm never sure why my sugar levels do actually shoot after I've exercised. They can go up really high and sometimes that is not a worry but it's just like why can't I suss this? I still don't understand what the logic is behind that."*
>
> (Int 15, F, 39)

Many participants talked about the risk of hypoglycaemia when exercising but very few cited fear of a hypoglycaemic attack as a specific reason for not exercising.

Similarly, complications due to diabetes were another potential condition-related barrier to exercise but it tended to influence the type of exercise or limit the amount of exercise people could do rather than stop them completely.

Time, work and lifestyle. People's lifestyles, their work and demands on their time was a far greater barrier than diabetes for most people. Half (12) cited lack of time as a barrier. Working full time, the type of work people did and shift work were all described as restricting people's ability to exercise. Added to this were demands in the home or caring for children or relatives.

However, several interviewees admitted that the problem was not so much lack of time but more a problem of time management or prioritisation. However, when combined with other factors – such as low motivation to exercise, bad weather, erratic lifestyle – a perceived lack of time became the excuse for not exercising.

Social and personal. A wide range of additional factors contributed to individual reluctance to exercise. None of them were major factors for the group but they influenced individual behaviour.

Lack of motivation to exercise was described by four people, another three more bluntly stated that they were lazy and among those who described time as a barrier it emerged that not prioritising exercise was at least partly due to a lack of interest in being more active.

"I don't know that if I'd not been a diabetic I'd be doing any more exercise than in fact I am. My interests tend to be more mental, cerebral than physical anyway and I don't think the fact I was diagnosed diabetic has really had much impact on that. Not to my knowledge. That's how I feel about it, anyway."
(Int 24, M, 47)

Six participants felt inhibited to exercise because of embarrassment or fear of failure. This was not restricted to a specific gender or age group. Three participants related embarrassment to body image but it was also related to fears of not being as good as other people.

Environmental. Access to a gym or swimming pool was raised as a problem by a few people, usually in relation to finance although several interviewees pointed out that there were a number of local authority initiatives in the area that provided free or reduced cost access to facilities. However, the concession often applied during the day, not at evenings or weekends when some of the employed people or students would prefer to use the facility.

Another issue was weather. Four people specifically stated that bad weather – or even good weather if the temperature was too high – stopped them from cycling or walking.

Theme 3: Facilitating and encouraging exercise

Participants were asked about what would help or encourage them to take more exercise and we called these Facilitators (free or reduced admission to gyms and pools) and Motivators (health benefits, body image, enjoyment, support and encouragement, advice and information, time management).

Although only a small number of people cited cost as a barrier to exercise, more thought that free passes or reduced membership of gyms and swimming pools would be a facilitator. Interestingly some of them were aware of council schemes providing this, yet they did not take advantage of the schemes. The social aspect of exercise was seen as helping with motivation. Several interviewees, especially older people (over 50) with partners, explained that they liked to exercise with someone else. Those with children also expressed a preference for physical activities that they could do as a family. These groups usually referred doing more walking or swimming to increase their activity levels.

The Social Facilitator also included a practical, security element, e.g. when applied to swimming or going to a gym so that someone could spot if they were having a hypo.

Some interviewees felt that the health benefits were an important motivator to exercise:

"I'd do anything to help my body now if it means that the diabetes is going to live healthier if that makes sense, if I've going to manage it better, then I'll do anything."
(Int 9, M, 33)

Investing in their health avoiding complications in the future and improving body image were all quoted as motivators.

Enjoyment seemed to be an important element of exercise: the interviews contained many examples of how people enjoyed a wide range of activities. Meeting the target of 150 mins of exercise each week was more common among those who described the pleasure they derived from exercise. Consequently, finding an exercise or a sport that people enjoyed emerged as an important factor in motivating people to exercise.

Among the barriers to exercise were lack of motivation and a perceived lack of time so providing external motivators was important for some people. This took various forms but convenience and access to people who could help them were important elements.

A quarter of interviewees said that advice or information about what exercises and why would encourage them to exercise more. This would help them to understand the relationship between exercise and blood sugar levels.

Allied to this was the power of medical advice to influence behaviour:

"If they said to me, 'Look, you'll extend your life if you do more exercise,' obviously you would. Or, 'You'd feel better in yourself.' Obviously you'd try your damned hardest to do more exercise...If he said it genuinely. If he said, 'Look, I'm serious.'
(Int 1, M, 57)

Time has already been identified as a perceived barrier to exercise and consequently, having more time was posed as the solution.

While creating more time is clearly not possible, time management can release time and opportunity for exercise, a conclusion that some participants came to as the interview progressed.

Encouraging exercise

Interviewees were presented with three interventions aimed at encouraging exercise and asked for their views on each.

Option 1: one to one advice from a health and fitness advisor. This was the intervention that appealed to the greatest number of people (20 people). There were three main reasons given for supporting this intervention. The first was the perception that one to one advice would be tailored to individual needs and provided the opportunity to learn how specific exercises or gym equipment could be used to work to personal goals such as improving fitness or losing weight.

Seven participants stressed that the personal trainer should be someone who understood diabetes and was considered helpful because it provided an external motivator.

Option 2: attending an exercise group organised by the hospital or General Practitioner (GP). Half of the participants (13) supported the idea of an exercise group organised by the hospital or GP. The main attraction was the social aspect of being in a group and having peer support that comes with being part of a group.

The composition of the group was raised as an important factor, reinforcing the desirability of being with "likeminded people" (Int 20, M, 50) although this meant different things for different people: age, similar level of fitness, other diabetics or a mixed group including non diabetics.

"I'd like it to be people my age"
(Int 14, F, 40)

> *"That would be a brilliant idea. Brilliant, yeah. I would go to it if I knew that it was run by someone that understands it and that there'd be other diabetics there. I would go, definitely."*
> (Int 26, F, 45)

The main objections to the group intervention were almost the opposite of the reasons for supporting the idea: a dislike of group situations and preconceived ideas of who would be in the group and not wanting to identify with them.

> *"I don't really like group activities. I'd much rather, when I exercise, do things by myself or I go with a member of the family to play a sport. I'm not so keen on the group activities."*
> (Int 6, F, 21)

There were further reasons for not supporting this type of intervention. There was a degree of embarrassment among some of those who said they disliked group exercise. Several interviewees did not think they could commit to a regular group and others felt they did not need the intervention because they didn't need to increase their activity levels.

Option 3: motivational support. Eleven people supported the third intervention, motivational support, but it was the least popular of the three options and 12 actively expressed a dislike. A third of interviewees (8) thought it might help to motivate them and encourage them to meet their goals.

The main reasons for rejecting option 3 were that it would be easy to deceive the person providing support and the perception that this approach would be "childish" or "nagging".

> *"That would be a no no. I wouldn't mind going to like your Weightwatchers, things like that because you're choosing to go there. And again that guilt thing, I've got a terrible guilt thing where food and exercise are concerned. And knowing that someone was going to phone me to check up, no, I wouldn't like that."*
> (Int 8, F, 38)

One interviewee aptly summarised the potential benefit of support from a mentor but not by telephone:

> *"It would be great if it was over the phone because you could lie madly. 'Oh yes, I've lost two stone and I'm really trim. 'I'm a great believer in mentors; I really am. But I think the mentor has to be tangible. You have to be able to go and see them and you have to care about whether they approve or encourage you or not. But no, not a voice over the phone."*
> (Int 25, F, 59)

Discussion

Statement of, and reflection on the principal findings

Six main barriers to exercise were identified in this study (see Table 4). These were: lack of time; work related factors; difficulties with access to facilities (distance and cost); lack of motivation; low confidence (embarrassment about body image and fear of failing); weather; and health specific barriers (low levels of knowledge about managing diabetes around exercise and diabetes complications).

The first five of these barriers have been reported in many studies of barriers to exercise: individuals at high risk [12] or already affected by type 2 diabetes [13–17]; people with disabilities and chronic health conditions [18–20]; people with cancer [21]; and the general population [22,23] have identified these factors as barriers to exercise.

Only one study has looked at barriers to exercise in patients with T1DM. Using a questionnaire, Brazeau et al, identified four main barriers to exercise in 100 patients with T1DM: fear of hypoglycaemia; work schedule; loss of control over diabetes; and low fitness level.

Our study identified similar barriers to exercise. Many patients stated that work schedules were a barrier to exercise. Whilst many patients were aware of the risks of hypoglycaemia with exercise, the fear of hypoglycaemia was not specifically stated as a reason for not exercising. However a few patients did allude to this fear, mentioning that one advantages for going to the gym or swimming pool was that they would be around people who would notice if they went hypo. Again although patients did not explicitly say that loss of diabetes control was a barrier to exercise, many patients expressed frustration at not understanding why in certain situations their blood sugars rose with exercise, and felt that having more information around how exercise can affect glucose levels in diabetes would encourage them to exercise. In addition we found that the presence of diabetes related complications and other co-morbidities was not a major barrier to exercise in this study, though it did influence the type of exercise that patients chose to undertake.

Our interviews identified 4 main factors that motivated patients to exercise: physical benefits from exercise; improvements in body image; enjoyment of the exercise and the social interaction of exercising at gym or in groups.

These factors have also been found to be important in individuals at high risk [12] or already affected by type 2 diabetes [13–17]; people with disabilities and chronic health conditions [18–20]; people with cancer [21]; and the general population [22,23]. Weight control, which was cited as an incentive to exercise by people with pre-diabetes, type 2 diabetes [14,17] and cancer [21], and positive emotions and improvements in mental well-being, cited by cancer patients [21], were not cited as motivators to exercise in our patients.

Three factors were identified by our patients that would encourage them to increase their exercise levels. These were free or reduced admission to gyms and pools, help with time management, and better advice about what exercise they should do, why and how this would affect their blood sugars. Similar findings have been found in other populations [24].

In order to overcome exercise barriers, other studies have found community-based exercise programmes [23,25] and group activities [20] to be the most useful programmes with people with disabilities or chronic health conditions stating that these programmes were helpful as they could exercise with patients of similar abilities and share their experiences of their illnesses [21]. In contrast our T1DM patients preferred individually tailored exercise support, designed with consideration of their preferences, circumstances and fitness levels. They also were not keen on motivational interviewing, particularly if telephone based, a well accepted approach to promote exercise among people with other health problems [20,26,27].

Strengths and weaknesses of the study

The strengths of this study are that it is the first qualitative study of barriers and facilitators of exercise for patients with T1DM. It includes male and females with a broad age range (21–64) and diabetes duration, and on both insulin injection and pump therapy. The weaknesses are that patients were only recruited

Table 4. Barriers, Facilitators and Motivators.

BARRIERS TO EXERCISE	
Lack of knowledge on the management diabetes for exercise	
Time and work	
Access to facilities (distance and cost)	
Embarrassment, body image, fear of failure	
Lack of motivation	
Weather	
MOTIVATORS	**FACILITATORS**
Health benefits	Free or reduced admission gyms/pools
Body image	Better time management
Enjoyment	Support and encouragement
Social Aspects	Advice and information

from one clinical centre, ethnic diversity was low and the majority were inactive.

Conclusions and recommendations

In this study we have shown that many of the barriers, motivators and facilitators of exercise in patients with T1DM are similar to patients with other chronic diseases and the general public. The only difference are that patients with T1DM require education about the effect of exercise on diabetes control and they prefer support to be given on a one to one basis rather than in a group environment. This suggests that with the addition of the above educational requirements, one to one techniques that have been successful in increasing activity in patients with other chronic diseases and the general public should be successful in increasing activity in patients with T1DM.

Acknowledgments

We would like to thank all the patients who gave up their time to participate in these interviews and to share their views for research purposes.

Author Contributions

Conceived and designed the experiments: PN SG. Performed the experiments: BH. Analyzed the data: BH AK NL SG RA PN DJ. Contributed to the writing of the manuscript: BH AK NL SG RA PN. Undertook the questionnaire audit of exercise in T1D patients: DJ.

References

1. Atkinson MA, Eisenbarth GS, Michels AW (2014) Type 1 Diabetes. The Lancet 383(9911): 69–82.
2. Chimen M, Kennedy A, Nirantharakumar K, Pang TT, Andrews R, et al. (2012) What are the health benefits of physical activity in type 1 diabetes mellitus? A literature review. Diabetologia ;55(3): 542–51.
3. Colberg SR, Sigal RJ, Fernhall B, Regensteiner JG, Blissmer BJ, et al. (2010) Exercise and type 2 diabetes: the American College of SportsMedicine and theAmerican Diabetes Association: joint position statement. Diabetes Care 33: e147–e167.
4. Ryden L, Standl E, Bartnik M, Van den Berghe G, Betteridge J, et al. (2007) Guidelines on diabetes, pre-diabetes, and cardiovascular diseases: executive summary. The Task Force on Diabetes and Cardiovascular Diseases of the European Society of Cardiology (ESC) and of the European Association for the Study of Diabetes (EASD). Eur Hear J 28: 88–136.
5. WHO (2003) Adherence to long-term therapies:Evidence for Action. ISBN 92 4 154599 2. Available: http://www.who.int/chp/knowledge/publications/adherence_report/en/ Accessed 2014 Jul 2.
6. Wadén J, Forsblom C, Thorn LM, Saraheimo M, Rosengård-Bärlund M, et al. (2008) Physical activity and diabetes complications in patients with type 1 diabetes: the Finnish Diabetic Nephropathy (FinnDiane) Study. Diabetes Care 31(2): 230–2.
7. Makura CB, Ninantharakumar K, Girling AJ, Saravanan P, Narendran P (2013) Effects of physical activity on the development and progression of microvascular complications in type 1 diabetes: retrospective analysis of the DCCT study.BMC Endocr Disord.13(1): 37.
8. Tielemans SM, Soedamah-Muthu SS, De Neve M, Toeller M, Chaturvedi N, et al. (2013) Association of physical activity with all-cause mortality and incident and prevalent cardiovascular disease among patients with type 1 diabetes: the EURODIAB Prospective Complications Study.Diabetologia 56(1): 82–91.
9. Brazeau AS, Rabasa-Lhoret R, Strychar I, Mircescu H (2008) Barriers to physical activity among patients with type 1 diabetes. Diabetes Care 31(11): 2108–9.
10. Peyrot M, Rubin RR, Lauritzen T, Skovlund SE, Snoek FJ, et al. (2006) Patient and provider perceptions of care for diabetes: results of the cross-national DAWN Study. Diabetologia 49(2): 279–88.
11. Ritchie J, Spencer L (1994) Qualitative data analysis for applied policy research. In: Bryman A, Burgess RG (Eds) *Analysing Qualitative Data,* London: Routledge.
12. Korkiakangas EE, Alahuhta MA, Husman PM, Keinänen-Kiukaanniemi S, Taanila AM, et al. (2011) Motivators and barriers to exercise among adults with a high risk of type 2 diabetes: a qualitative study. Scand J Caring Sci. 25(1): 62–9.
13. Dubé MC, Valois P, Prud'homme D, Weisnagel SJ, Lavoie C (2006) Physical activity barriers in diabetes: development and validation of a new scale. Diabetes Res Clin Pract. 72(1): 20–7.
14. Casey D, De Civita M, Dasgupta K (2010) Understanding physical activity facilitators and barriers during and following a supervised exercise programme in Type 2 diabetes: a qualitative study. Diabet. Med. 27, 79–84.
15. Egan AM, Mahmood WA, Fenton R, Redziniak N, Kyaw Tun T, et al. (2013) Barriers to exercise in obese patients with type 2 diabetes. QJM. 106(7): 635–8.
16. Thomas N, Alder E, Leese GP (2004) Barriers to physical activity in patients with diabetes. Postgrad Med J 80: 287–291.
17. Booth AO, Lowis C, Dean M, Hunter SJ, McKinley MC (2013) Diet and physical activity in the self-management of type 2 diabetes: barriers and facilitators identified by patients and health professionals. Prim Health Care Res Dev.14(3): 293–306.
18. Malone LA, Barfield JP, Brasher JD (2012) Perceived benefits and barriers to exercise among persons with physical disabilities or chronic health conditions within action or maintenance stages of exercise. Disability and Health Journal 5; 254e260.
19. Slade SC, Patel S, Underwood M, Keating JL (2013) What are Patient Beliefs and Perceptions about Exercise for Non-specific Chronic Low Back Pain? A Systematic Review of Qualitative Studies. Clin J Pain. Epub ahead of print.
20. Roberts SH, Bailey JE (2011) Incentives and barriers to lifestyle interventions for people with severe mental illness: a narrative synthesis of quantitative, qualitative and mixed methods studies. J Adv Nurs ;67(4): 690–708.
21. Brunet J, Taran S, Burke S, Sabiston CM (2013) A qualitative exploration of barriers and motivators to physical activity participation in women treated for breast cancer. Disabil Rehabil ;35(24): 2038–45.

22. Biedenweg K, Meischke H, Bohl A, Hammerback K, Williams B, et al. (2014) Understanding older adults' motivators and barriers to participating in organized programs supporting exercise behaviors. J Prim Prev;35(1): 1–11.
23. Justine M, Azizan A, Hassan V, Salleh Z, Manaf H (2013) Barriers to participation in physical activity and exercise among middle-aged and elderly individuals. Singapore Med J 2013; 54(10): 581–586.
24. Donahue KE, Mielenz TJ, Sloane PD, Callahan LF, Devellis RF (2006) Identifying Supports and Barriers to Physical Activity in Patients at Risk for Diabetes. Prev Chronic Dis. 3(4): A119.
25. Mulligan H, Treharne GJ, Hale LA, Smith C (2013) Combining self-help and professional help to minimize barriers to physical activity in persons with multiple sclerosis: a trial of the "Blue Prescription" approach in New Zealand. J Neurol Phys Ther. ;37(2): 51–7.
26. Tse MM, Vong SK, Tang SK (2013) Motivational interviewing and exercise programme for community-dwelling older persons with chronic pain: a randomised controlled study. J Clin Nurs. ;22(13–14): 1843–56.
27. Lilienthal KR, Pignol AE, Holm JE, Vogeltanz-Holm N (2013) Telephone-Based Motivational Interviewing to Promote Physical Activity and Stage of Change Progression in Older Adults. J Aging Phys Act.

10

Peak Oxygen Uptake after Cardiac Rehabilitation: A Randomized Controlled Trial of a 12-Month Maintenance Program versus Usual Care

Erik Madssen[1,2], Ingerid Arbo[1], Ingrid Granøien[3], Liv Walderhaug[3], Trine Moholdt[1,4]*

1 K.G. Jebsen Center of Exercise in Medicine, Department of Circulation and Medical Imaging, Faculty of Medicine, Norwegian University of Science and Technology, Trondheim, Norway, **2** Department of Pulmonary Medicine, St. Olavs Hospital, Trondheim, Norway, **3** Ålesund Hospital, Ålesund, Norway, **4** Women's Clinic, St. Olavs Hospital, Trondheim, Norway

Abstract

Background: Exercise capacity is a strong predictor of survival in patients with coronary artery disease (CAD). Exercise capacity improves after cardiac rehabilitation exercise training, but previous studies have demonstrated a decline in peak oxygen uptake after ending a formal rehabilitation program. There is a lack of knowledge on how long-term exercise adherence can be achieved in CAD patients. We therefore assessed if a 12-month maintenance program following cardiac rehabilitation would lead to increased adherence to exercise and increased exercise capacity compared to usual care.

Materials and Methods: Two-centre, open, parallel randomized controlled trial with 12 months follow-up comparing usual care to a maintenance program. The maintenance program consisted of one monthly supervised high intensity interval training session, a written exercise program and exercise diary, and a maximum exercise test every third month during follow-up. Forty-nine patients (15 women) on optimal medical treatment were included following discharge from cardiac rehabilitation. The primary endpoint was change in peak oxygen uptake at follow-up; secondary endpoints were physical activity level, quality of life and blood markers of cardiovascular risk.

Results: There was no change in peak oxygen uptake from baseline to follow-up in either group (intervention group 27.9 (±4.7) to 28.8 (±5.6) mL·kg (-1) min (−1), control group 32.0 (±6.2) to 32.8 (±5.8) mL·kg (−1) min (−1), with no between-group difference, $p = 0.22$). Quality of life and blood biomarkers remained essentially unchanged, and both self-reported and measured physical activity levels were similar between groups after 12 months.

Conclusions: A maintenance exercise program for 12 months did not improve adherence to exercise or peak oxygen uptake in CAD patients after discharge from cardiac rehabilitation compared to usual care. This suggests that infrequent supervised high intensity interval training sessions are inadequate to improve peak oxygen uptake in this patient group.

Trial Registration: ClinicalTrials.gov NCT01246570

Editor: Terence J. Quinn, University of Glasgow, United Kingdom

Funding: Authors were supported by funds from the Liaison Committee for Central Norway Regional Health Authority and the Norwegian University of Science and Technology, Funds for Medical Research at St. Olavs University Hospital, and the Norwegian Fund for Post-Graduate Training in Physiotherapy. The funders had no role in study design, data collection and analysis, decision to publish, or preparation of the manuscript.

Competing Interests: The authors have declared that no competing interests exist.

* Email: trine.moholdt@ntnu.no

Introduction

Exercise-based rehabilitation in patients with coronary artery disease (CAD) reduces mortality [1–4], and cardiorespiratory fitness is a strong, independent predictor of both cardiac- and all-cause mortality in patients with CAD [5,6]. Therefore, it is important to establish effective exercise programs that patients can adhere to in this patient group. Unfortunately, most beneficial effects from physical activity are lost quite rapidly if regular exercise is discontinued. In line with this, peak oxygen uptake (VO_{2peak}) has been found to decline at six months, and more so at 30 months, after discharge from cardiac rehabilitation in patients with CAD [7]. Thus, there is a need for studies to assess interventions that may help patients adhere to regular and effective exercise training after ending a formalized cardiac rehabilitation exercise program [8]. It is known that high intensity interval training (HIIT) is more effective than continuous training with low-to-moderate intensity with respect to increasing VO_{2peak} in patients with CAD [9], but there is a lack of knowledge regarding long-term effects of HIIT interventions.

The primary aim of this study was therefore to assess if a 12-month maintenance program following discharge from formal cardiac rehabilitation would improve adherence to physical activity and peak oxygen uptake We hypothesized that the maintenance program would lead to an attenuated decline in VO_{2peak} 12 months after ending the formal cardiac rehabilitation, compared with patients in usual care. Secondary endpoints were physical activity level, quality of life and blood markers of cardiovascular risk.

Materials and Methods

Design

The protocol for this trial and supporting CONSORT checklist are available as supporting information; see Checklist S1 and Protocol S1. This was a two-centre, open, parallel randomized controlled trial. The study was approved by the Regional Committee for Medical and Health Research Ethics in Middle-Norway (REK-Midt 2010/86), and registered at clinicaltrials.gov (NCT01246570). Patients gave their informed, written consent before entering the study, and we performed the study according to the Helsinki declaration for medical research. After acquisition of all baseline data, patients were randomized stratified by centre the same day, using a web-based randomization tool, developed and administered by Unit of Applied Clinical Research, Department of Cancer Research and Molecular Medicine, Norwegian University of Science and Technology, Trondheim. Stratified for study centre, patients were randomized either to a maintenance exercise program or to usual care for 12 months with a 1:1 allocation ratio (Figure 1).

Participants

We recruited optimal medically treated patients above 18 years of age from the cardiac rehabilitation centres at St. Olav's University Hospital in Trondheim, and Ålesund Hospital, both in central Norway. Inclusion criteria were completion of a 12-week organized in-hospital cardiac rehabilitation program, consisting of 2 exercise sessions per week, including both HIIT and moderate continuous exercise. Patients were included in the current study 1–2 weeks after ending the formal cardiac rehabilitation program. Patients were excluded if they fulfilled one or more of the following criteria; unstable angina pectoris (chest pain at light physical activity), hemodynamic significant valvular disease (valvular disease confirmed by echocardiography and dyspnoea at light physical activity), chronic obstructive pulmonary disease or chronic heart failure with symptoms at rest or in light physical activity, uncontrolled arterial hypertension (hypertension grade 2 despite medical treatment) chronic renal failure (serum creatinine>140 μmol/L), or pregnancy.

Interventions

Maintenance program group. Patients in the maintenance program group received a written exercise program with the aim of three sessions of high intensity interval training (HIIT) per week, and were invited to attend a monthly supervised exercise session at

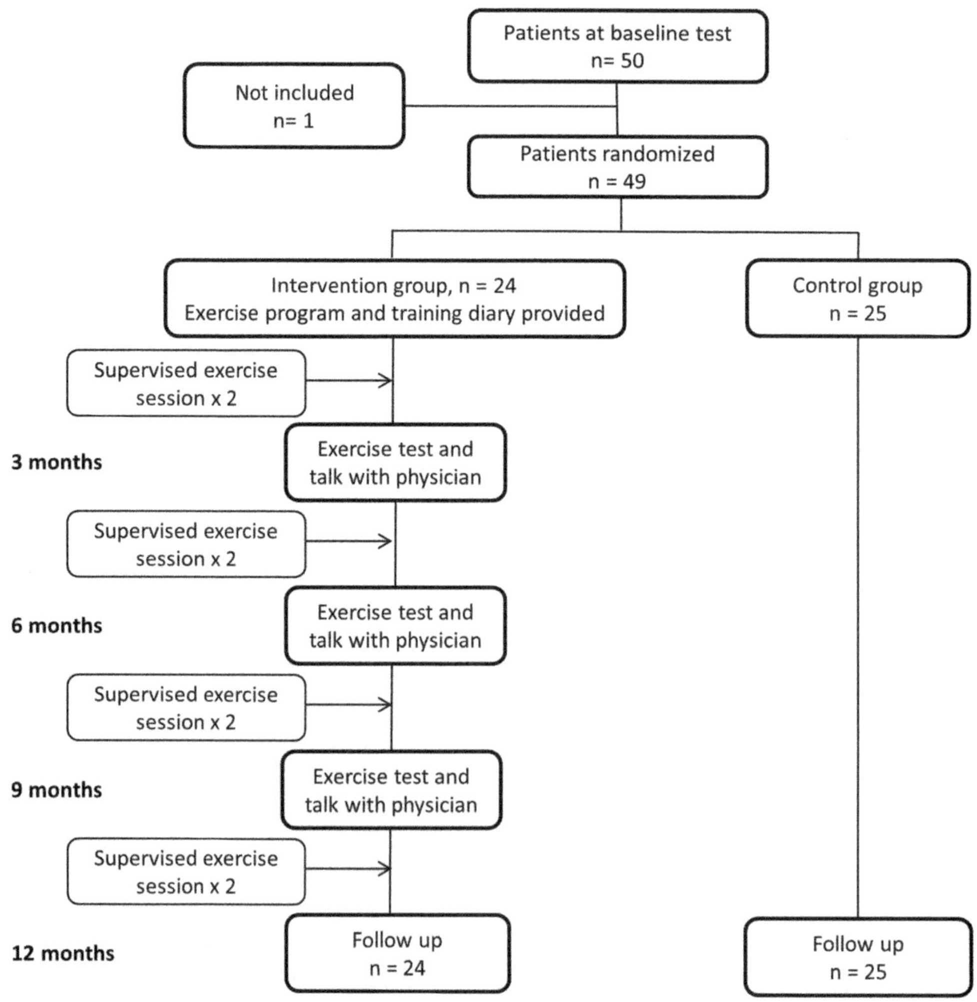

Figure 1. Flow chart of participants throughout the study.

the hospital. The HIIT program was based on protocols from previous studies [10–14], and consisted of 8–10 minutes of warm-up, followed by four times four minutes intervals, with an active pause of three minutes in-between intervals and at the end. The target heart rate was 85–95% of the maximum heart rate as measured at the initial exercise test in intervals, and 70% of maximum heart rate in the active pauses.

During the supervised exercise sessions once per month, patients walked or ran on treadmills (Woodway PPS55, Weil am Rhein, Germany), wearing heart rate monitors (Polar Electro, Kempele, Finland) to ensure that they reached target heart rate. An experienced physiotherapist and/or exercise physiologist instructed and motivated the patients on how to perform HIIT, and patients were asked about their home exercise training and encouraged to maintain a high level of activity. Such instructions have previously been found to be enough to give an acceptable adherence to exercise training during 6 months [10]. The written exercise program also explained in detail how to perform the HIIT, and patients were instructed to perform HIIT as home-based exercise training, as activities which engaged large muscle groups, i.e. walking uphill, running, cross-country skiing, or bicycling. Patients were told to either use a heart rate monitor to ensure that the intensity was adequate, or to exercise with an intensity making them breathe heavily during home exercise training. We gave no advice regarding diet or other lifestyle factors during the follow-up period.

Every third month, patients in the maintenance group did a maximum exercise test as described below. These tests were done to monitor their exercise capacity; to give patients individualized feedback on their VO_{2peak} level, and to ensure them that maximal effort was well tolerated.

Control group. Patients in the control group received no instructions in how to exercise apart from what was given by the rehabilitation staff at the hospitals as usual care. In the two participating hospitals, CAD patients are encouraged to be physically active but are not given any concise exercise prescription. The control group attended baseline and 12 months follow-up tests as described below, without any other contact with the study or hospital personnel.

Outcomes and follow-up

The primary outcome measure was change in VO_{2peak} between baseline and 12 months follow-up. Secondary outcome measures were physical activity level, resting blood pressure, health-related quality of life, cardiometabolic blood markers and anthropometric measurements. In the original study protocol, endothelial function measurements (flow mediated dilatation of the brachial artery) were described. Due to technical issues at one of the participating hospitals, endothelial function could not be included in the study. Physical activity registration was not pre-specified in the original protocol, but during the preparation phase of the study it became clear that such data would be needed and thus physical activity questionnaires and activity monitors were included into the protocol.

Peak oxygen uptake. All patients performed a treadmill cardiopulmonary maximum exercise test at baseline and at follow-up after 12 months, without discontinuation of prescribed medication. Gas exchange data was analysed (Oxycon Pro, Jaeger, Hoechberg, Germany) continuously using mixing chamber, and patients were monitored with a 12-lead electrocardiogram during maximum exercise tests. After 10 minutes of warm-up, we individually adjusted a ramp protocol, by increasing the incline and speed of the treadmill, for the test to last 8–12 minutes as recommended [15]. The test was terminated when the patients reported to be exhausted, or if clinical symptoms occurred. Peak oxygen uptake (VO_{2peak}) was calculated as the mean of the three highest VO_2 measurements during the test, each obtained over a 10-sec average. Peak heart rate was recorded at the end of the test and was not compared to age predicted values as the patients were taking betablockers. We did not use a threshold value of respiratory exchange ratio (RER) as a criterion for reaching VO_{2peak}, but average RER-values obtained during the tests are outlined in the results. Heart rate recovery was defined as the change in heart rate from the peak heart rate to the heart rate after one minute of rest standing on the treadmill.

Physical activity level. All patients reported physical activity level by questionnaires. They were asked how often they exercised ($\leq$1, 2–3, $\geq$4 sessions per week), the mean duration of each exercise session (<30, 30–45, 45–60,>60 minutes per session), and the mean intensity-level during sessions (light, medium or hard intensity). In a subgroup of patients (n = 18, 37%), everyday physical activity level was measured with an on-body activity monitoring system (Sensewear, Bodymedia Inc., Pittsburgh, PA, USA) worn for 3–7 days during the first 1–3 weeks and repeated during the last 1–3 weeks in the follow-up period. We measured the numbers of steps taken per day, and the time spent in different activity level zones defined by metabolic equivalents (METs). Sedentary time was defined as activity <3 METs, moderate physical activity was defined as activity $\geq$3 and <6 METs, and vigorous physical activity was defined as $\geq$6 METs.

Resting blood pressure and resting heart rate. Resting systolic and diastolic blood pressure was measured sitting after 10 minutes of rest with a calibrated automated blood pressure monitor (Welch Allyn, Germany). Blood pressure was automatically measured three times by the monitor, and the average value of the two last measurements was used. Resting heart rate was measured, after 10 minutes of rest in supine position, using electrocardiogram. Height was measured to the nearest centimetre and body weight was measured to the nearest 0.1 kg using a Seca 877 scale (Seca Corp, Germany). Body mass index was calculated as body weight in kilograms divided by the square of height in meter. Waist circumference was measured to the nearest half centimetre, using a measuring tape at the height of the umbilicus.

Blood markers. Venous blood samples were drawn after 12 hours of fasting, and analysed using accredited in-hospital procedures for serum glucose, total cholesterol, low-density lipoprotein cholesterol, high-density lipoprotein cholesterol, triglycerides, and high-sensitive C-reactive protein (all using standard commercial kits on a Roche Modular P, Roche, Basel, Switzerland), and glycosylated haemoglobin (Roche Cobas Integra 400).

Health related quality of life. Health related quality of life was measured by MacNew Heart Disease Health-Related Quality of Life Questionnaire [16]. This is a disease-specific questionnaire with a validated Norwegian translation [17]. The questionnaire assesses social, emotional, and physical quality of life using a 1–7 scale. Higher scores indicated better quality of life and a change of 0.5 is found to be clinically significant [16].

Sample size and statistics

A decline in VO_{2peak} of 2.0 $mL \cdot kg^{-1} \cdot min^{-1}$ (SD 4.0) could be expected after 12 months without formal rehabilitation [18]. We anticipated that the intervention program would give an increase of 2.0 $mL \cdot kg^{-1} \cdot min^{-1}$ after 12 months, giving a difference of 4.0 $mL \cdot kg^{-1} \cdot min^{-1}$ compared to usual care. This yields a standardised difference of $4/4 = 1$. With a two-tailed t-test for independent samples at a power (1-β) of 0.9 and $\alpha = 0.05$, a total of 44 subjects had to be enrolled [19]. To allow for an expected 10% drop out, we aimed at including 48 patients. The actual statistical analysis performed takes within-person correlation into account and thereby improves power.

Observed data are given as frequencies with percentages in parenthesis, or means ± standard deviation (SD). Baseline characteristics were compared using the chi square test, Mann-Whitney U-test or student t-test where appropriate. Changes from baseline to follow-up are reported with 95% confidence intervals (CI) using a univariate general linear model in the analyses. To test for differences between groups, we used a univariate general linear model analysis of covariance (ANCOVA) with Bonferroni adjustments. In the model, the change in the outcome variable (Δ-values) was the dependent variable, with group as fixed factor and baseline values of the outcome variable as covariates [20]. Between-group differences are reported with 95% CIs and p-values. Within- and between-group differences were considered significant if the 95% CI did not include zero [21]. Physical activity data are only presented as descriptive statistics. All statistical analyses were performed using SPSS (version 20.0, IBM, Chicago, IL, USA).

Results

Forty-nine patients (15 women) were recruited from January 2011 to March 2012 at St.Olav's Hospital and from November 2011 to June 2012 at Ålesund Hospital. Patient characteristics at baseline can be found in Table 1. All registered variables at baseline were comparable between groups except for age, which was lower in the control group ($p<0.05$, Table 1), and VO_{2peak}, which was higher in the control group ($p<0.01$, Table 2).

We experienced no adverse events during maximum exercise testing or training sessions. All participants completed scheduled tests, and the mean attendance at training sessions was 7.8 out of 8 sessions in the intervention group. None of the patients changed their medication use during the study period. During follow-up, two patients in each group were hospitalized. In the intervention group, one patient was diagnosed with a duodenal ulcer and atrial fibrillation, and one patient was diagnosed with chronic lymphatic leukaemia. In the control group, one patient experienced a tibia fracture and one patient underwent surgical treatment for breast carcinoma.

We found no within-group changes in VO_{2peak} from baseline to follow-up, and no between-group difference ($p = 0.22$, Table 2). In the intervention group, VO_{2peak} was at its highest at the third maximum exercise test, and declined slightly at test number four and five (Figure 2). We found no changes in resting heart rate, heart rate recovery, blood pressure, neither within- or between-groups from baseline to follow-up. Blood markers did not change during follow-up in any group (Table 2). Quality of life (social domain) was increased in the control group, but there was no between-group difference ($p = 0.39$).

Self-reported physical activity level is summarized in Table 3. In the intervention group, all patients reported some regular physical activity both at baseline and follow-up, whereas 5 patients in the control group reported no regular physical activity at follow-up. The majority of patients in both groups reported that they had been physically active 2–3 times per week, with duration of 45–60 minutes and with a medium intensity. Physical activity level was adequately monitored in 18 patients (37%). The mean number of steps taken per day was 7024 in the intervention group (10 patients), and 9338 in the control group (8 patients). The mean time spent in sedentary, moderate and vigorous activity level zones per day was 1333 minutes, 58 minutes and 3 minutes in the intervention group. The corresponding numbers in the control

Table 1. Patient characteristics and medication use at baseline.

	Intervention group (n = 24)	Control group (n = 25)
Sex, male/female	18/6	18/7
Age, years (range)	64.4 (47–78)	58.5 (42–71)*
Treatment qualifying for referral to rehabilitation		
PCI	15 (63)	15 (60)
CABG	7 (29)	7 (28)
Valve replacement	2 (8)	1 (4)
Cardiomyopathy	0 (0)	2 (8)
Co-morbidity		
Heart failure	3 (13)	4 (16)
PAD	0 (0)	1 (4)
Hypertension	11 (46)	13 (52)
Diabetes	4 (17)	3 (12)
Medication at baseline		
Aspirin	24 (100)	25 (100)
Clopidogrel	18 (75)	16 (64)
Warfarin	1 (4)	1 (4)
Betablockers	19 (79)	19 (76)
Statins	23 (96)	25 (100)
ACE/ARA	9 (38)	11 (44)

Data are given as numbers with percentages in parenthesis when not otherwise specified. PCI; percutaneous coronary intervention, CABG; coronary artery bypass grafting, PAD; peripheral artery disease, ACE; angiotensin converting enzyme inhibitors, ARA; angiotensin II receptor antagonists. * Between group difference at baseline ($p = 0.02$).

Table 2. Outcome measures at baseline and after 12 months follow-up.

	Intervention group (n = 24)			Control group (n = 25)			ANCOVA	
	Baseline	**12 months**	**Change scores (95% CI)**	**Baseline**	**12 months**	**Change scores (95% CI)**	**Between-group difference (95% CI)**	**P value**
Exercise test								
VO_{2peak}, ml·kg^{-1}·min^{-1}	27.9±4.7	28.8±5.6	0.9 (−0.6, 2.4)	32.0±6.2	32.8±5.8	0.8 (−0.5, 2.2)	0.6 (−1.5, 2.7)	0.58
VO_{2peak}, ml·min^{-1}	2405±517	2533±576	129 (−18, 275)	2535±760	2614±734	79 (−45, 203)	−0.04 (−0.2, 0.2)	0.70
RER_{peak}	1.09±0.07	1.09±0.09	0.004 (−0.03, 0.04)	1.10±0.07	1.09±0.06	−0.01 (−0.04, 0.01)	−0.01 (−0.05, 0.03)	0.71
HR_{peak}, beats	154.7±13.1	155.8±15.9	1.1 (−5.1, 7.3)	160.6±11.3	161.6±13.1	1.0 (−2.3, 4.2)	1.4 (−5.5, 8.3)	0.68
HR recovery, beats	27.7±11.2	31.2±14.6	3.5 (−1.9, 8.9)	28.9±10.0	30.1±10.2	1.2 (−2.9, 5.4)	−1.7 (−8.3, 4.9)	0.60
Resting measurements								
HR, beats/min	64.0±10.2	65.7±11.6	1.6 (−1.5, 4.8)	61.2±11.5	63.2±11.1	2.0 (−1.4, 5.4)	−0.2 (−4.8, 4.4)	0.92
Systolic BP, mmHg	132.8±14.7	133.7±16.4	0.9 (−4.4, 6.2)	131.3±14.5	134.3±14.0	3.0 (−2.3, 8.2)	1.4 (−5.9, 8.8)	0.69
Diastolic BP, mmHG	78.8±7.2	79.3±7.5	0.5 (−2.1, 3.1)	75.1±10.7	77.5±10.0	2.4 (−1.5, 6.2)	−0.08 (−4.8, 4.6)	0.97
Anthropometric measurements								
Weight, kg	86.8±15.6	89.0±16.5	2.1 (0.8, 3.5)*	79.2±17.8	79.9±17.3	0.7 (−0.8, 2.2)	−1.5 (−3.6, 0.5)	0.14
BMI, kg/m^2	28.0±3.9	28.7±4.1	0.7 (0.2, 1.1)*	25.8±3.3	26.1±3.2	0.3 (−0.2, 0.7)	−0.5 (−1.2, 0.2)	0.16
Waist, cm	101.4±12.1	103.2±11.7	1.8 (0.1, 3.5)*	92.6±9.8	93.0±9.4	0.3 (−0.8, 1.5)	−2.2 (−4.2, −0.1)‡	0.04
Quality of life								
Emotional domain	6.0±0.8	6.0±0.6	0.1 (−0.2, 0.3)	5.7±0.8	6.1±0.8	0.4 (−0.2, 0.7)	0.1 (−0.4, 0.6)	0.69
Physical domain	6.2±0.7	6.3±0.6	0.1 (−0.2, 0.4)	6.3±0.6	6.4±0.5	0.1 (−0.1, 0.3)	0.1 (−0.2, 0.5)	0.40
Social domain	6.4±0.6	6.5±0.4	0.1 (−0.1, 0.3)	6.4±0.6	6.7±0.4	0.3 (0.1, 0.5)*	0.1 (−0.1, 0.4)	0.37
Blood markers								
hsCPR, mg/L	1.09±0.9	1.07±0.6	−0.02 (−0.3, 0.3)	1.2±0.9	1.5±2.5	0.3 (−0.7, 1.3)	0.4 (−0.7, 1.4)	0.51
Cholesterol, mmol/L	4.3±1.0	4.3±0.8	−0.08 (−0.4, 0.2)	3.9±0.6	3.9±0.8	−0.02 (−0.2, 0.2)	−0.1 (−0.5, 0.3)	0.57
LDL, mmol/L	2.2±0.9	2.2±0.7	−0.03 (−0.3, 0.2)	2.0±0.5	2.0±0.6	0.01 (−0.2, 0.2)	−0.0 (−0.4, 0.2)	0.70
HDL, mmol/L	1.5±0.4	1.5±0.4	0.05 (−0.02, 0.13)	1.3±0.4	1.3±0.4	0.004 (−0.05, 0.05)	−0.04 (−0.1, 0.04)	0.34
TG, mmol/L	1.4±0.8	1.2±0.7	−0.19 (−0.4, 0.01)	1.2±0.6	1.3±1.1	0.07 (−0.3, 0.4)	0.2 (−0.2, 0.6)	0.24
Glucose, mmol/L	6.7±3.7	6.4±2.2	−0.3 (−0.6, 0.1)	6.0±1.8	6.2±2.4	0.2 (−0.2, 0.6)	0.3 (−0.4, 1.0)	0.43
HbA1c, %	6.1±1.2	6.0±1.0	−0.1 (−0.2, −0.01)*	6.1±0.7	6.2±1.4	0.1 (−0.1, 0.4)	0.2 (−0.1, 0.6)	0.21

VO_{2peak}; peak oxygen uptake, RER_{peak}; respiratory exchange ratio at peak oxygen uptake, HR_{peak}; peak heart rate, HRR, 1 min; heart rate recovery the first minute after ending an exercise test, HR; resting heart rate, SBP; systolic blood pressure, DBP; diastolic blood pressure, BMI; body mass index, hsCRP; high-sensitive C-reactive protein, LDLc; low-density lipoprotein cholesterol, HDLc; high-density lipoprotein cholesterol, TG; triglycerides, HbA1c; glycosylated haemoglobin.

* indicates within-group changes from baseline to 12 months,

‡ indicates between groups changes in mean difference.

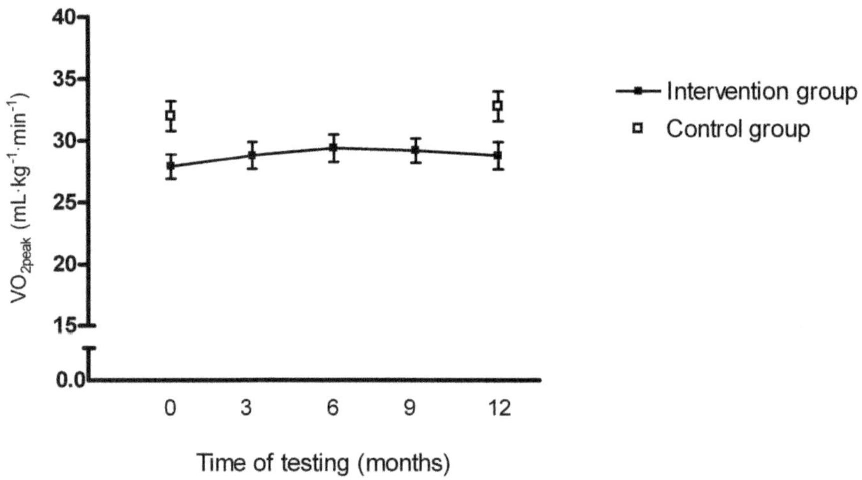

Figure 2. Peak oxygen uptake in the intervention group at baseline, after 3, 6 and 9 months, and at follow-up, and peak oxygen uptake in the control group at baseline and follow-up. The bars represent ± standard error of mean.

group were 1288 minutes, 111 minutes, and 7 minutes, respectively.

Discussion

In this randomized trial we assessed whether patients with CAD discharged from cardiac rehabilitation would benefit with respect to VO_{2peak} by attending a maintenance exercise program for 12 months compared to usual care of no formal follow-up. Our main finding was that the maintenance program did not improve VO_{2peak} compared to usual care. However, neither group deteriorated with respect to exercise capacity during follow-up. This was to us unexpected as exercise capacity has been found to decrease in CAD patients after discharge from formal rehabilitation when the patients were not aware of the last follow-up test [18].

We can only suggest some potential explanations for our findings. Participants enrolled in clinical exercise studies may be highly motivated to perform exercise, especially when they are aware of future follow-up tests. This was illustrated by Gupta et al. [22] who found an increased level of physical activity and 6-minute walking distance at 12 months after discharge from cardiac rehabilitation. Also Izawa et al. [23] demonstrated high exercise maintenance in patients with myocardial infarction 18 months

Table 3. Self-reported physical activity.

	Intervention group (n = 24)		Control group (n = 25)	
	Baseline	**Follow-up**	**Baseline**	**Follow-up**
Self-reported	**n = 19***	**n = 21***	**n = 22***	**n = 22***
Frequency				
No exercise	0 (0)	0 (0)	1 (5)	5 (23)
<1/week	1 (5)	0 (0)	0 (0)	0 (0)
1/week	0 (0)	1 (5)	0 (0)	2 (9)
2–3/week	12 (63)	16 (76)	17 (77)	14 (64)
≥4/week	6 (32)	4 (19)	4 (18)	1 (4)
Duration				
<30 min	0 (0)	1 (5)	1 (5)	0 (0)
30–45 min	6 (31.5)	6 (28.5)	2 (9)	5 (29.5)
45–60 min	10 (52.5)	8 (38)	11 (50)	5 (29.5)
>60 min	3 (16)	6 (28.5)	7 (36)	7 (41)
Intensity				
Low	1 (5)	1 (5)	1 (5)	1 (6)
Medium	16 (84)	11 (52)	13 (62)	10 (59)
High	2 (11)	9 (43)	7 (33)	6 (35)

Data are given as numbers with percentages in parenthesis.
* Valid questionnaires for 19 patients at baseline and 21 patients at follow-up in the intervention group, and 22 patients at baseline and follow-up in the control group.

after cardiac rehabilitation. Both these studies had an observational design without strategies to improve exercise adherence after ending formal rehabilitation, and with patients being aware of future follow-ups. We argue that the knowledge of future follow-up tests by cardiac rehabilitation units may act as a motivation for increased levels of physical activity. This may have also been the case in our study. In fact, the objectively measured physical activity indicated that patients in the control group spent more time in the moderate activity level zone and had a higher daily step count than the patients in the intervention group. Patients randomized to the intervention group were on average 6 years older than in the control group, possibly explaining the tendency for lower level of physical activity in the intervention group. Previous studies have found adherence to physical activity to decline with age [24,25]. However, a previous study found no significant effect of age on improvement in VO_{2peak} after HIIT in patients with CAD [26]. We therefore think that the potential effect of age was on the adherence to exercise rather than on the physiological adaptations to HIIT. Of note, all included patients had some knowledge of HIIT, as this was included in the cardiac rehabilitation program prior to study inclusion.

Several studies have demonstrated that HIIT is superior to moderate continuous exercise in improving VO_{2peak} in patients with CAD [12,27,28] without compromising safety [29]. In the current study, patients in the intervention group were invited to attend a monthly supervised HIIT session at the hospital. However, one monthly session of HIIT is obviously not enough to improve or maintain exercise capacity, and therefore patients also received a training program with the aim of three sessions of HIIT per week. A previous study [10] of home-based HIIT after coronary artery bypass grafting has shown good adherence to such exercise prescription. According to the self-reported physical activity data in the current study, however, only about one third of patients in the intervention group reported that they exercised with high-intensity 2–3 times a week. Thus, a lack of adherence to prescribed exercise at home in the maintenance group is probably the single most important explanation to the lack of VO_{2peak} improvement at 12 months.

Our study may have implications for clinical rehabilitation units. We argue that all patients with CAD enrolled in a rehabilitation program should be offered one or several follow-up sessions, and that a maximum exercise testing should preferably be a part of this follow-up. Our data implies that this type of follow-up may be sufficient to prevent deterioration with respect to VO_{2peak}. However, follow-up programs of infrequent supervised exercise sessions seemed not to be effective. It is possible that a maintenance program with more frequent supervised exercise could have resulted in improvements in VO_{2peak}. In a study of patients with congestive heart failure, Prescott et al. [30] found a small beneficial effect in patients that followed a low-cost maintenance training program with group training sessions every two weeks, indicating that supervised sessions must be more frequent than in our study to result in increased work capacity.

The complete follow-up testing of patients and the high adherence to the supervised exercise are regarded as strengths of our study. Our study is however limited by the fact that the study group consisted of relatively young patients, who probably were quite motivated to exercise without formal follow-up during 12 months. Thus, our results may not be valid for older and less motivated patients with established CAD. Also, neither investigators nor participants were blinded for the study endpoints, which could raise concerns regarding objectivity of testing. However, all patients were told to exercise to complete exhaustion at every exercise test. Further, there was no difference in peak heart rate or peak RER achieved during the baseline and the follow-up test. We also chose to inform the patients in the intervention group about their VO_{2peak} at intermediate tests as we considered it to act motivating for sustained or increase levels of exercise training.

Conclusions

A 12-month maintenance exercise program consisting of infrequent supervised HIIT sessions, a home-based HIIT program and regular exercise testing did not result in improved adherence to exercise or increased VO_{2peak} in CAD patients compared to usual care. However, both the intervention and the control group sustained their VO_{2peak} 12 months after discharge from formal cardiac rehabilitation.

Author Contributions

Conceived and designed the experiments: TM EM IA. Performed the experiments: TM EM IA LW IG. Analyzed the data: TM EM. Contributed reagents/materials/analysis tools: IG LW IA TM EM. Wrote the paper: EM TM. Collected all data at Ålesund Hospital: IG LW.

References

1. Jolliffe JA, Rees K, Taylor RS, Thompson D, Oldridge N, et al. (2001) Exercise-based rehabilitation for coronary heart disease. Cochrane Database Syst Rev: CD001800.
2. Taylor RS, Brown A, Ebrahim S, Jolliffe J, Noorani H, et al. (2004) Exercise-based rehabilitation for patients with coronary heart disease: systematic review and meta-analysis of randomized controlled trials. American Journal of Medicine 116: 682–692.
3. Clark AM, Hartling L, Vandermeer B, McAlister FA (2005) Meta-analysis: secondary prevention programs for patients with coronary artery disease. Annals of Internal Medicine 143: 659–672.
4. O'Connor GT, Buring JE, Yusuf S, Goldhaber SZ, Olmstead EM, et al. (1989) An overview of randomized trials of rehabilitation with exercise after myocardial infarction. Circulation 80: 234–244.
5. Myers J, Prakash M, Froelicher V, Do D, Partington S, et al. (2002) Exercise capacity and mortality among men referred for exercise testing. New England Journal of Medicine 346: 793–801.
6. Keteyian SJ, Brawner CA, Savage PD, Ehrman JK, Schairer J, et al. (2008) Peak aerobic capacity predicts prognosis in patients with coronary heart disease. American Heart Journal 156: 292–300.
7. Moholdt T, Aamot IL, Granoien I, Gjerde L, Myklebust G, et al. (2011) Long-term follow-up after cardiac rehabilitation: a randomized study of usual care exercise training versus aerobic interval training after myocardial infarction. International Journal of Cardiology 152: 388–390.
8. Fletcher GF (2007) Cardiac rehabilitation: Something old—something new—more to do. J Cardiopulm Rehabil Prev 27: 21–23.
9. Weston KS, Wisloff U, Coombes JS (2013) High-intensity interval training in patients with lifestyle-induced cardiometabolic disease: a systematic review and meta-analysis. Br J Sports Med. 48: 1227–1234
10. Moholdt T, Bekken Vold M, Grimsmo J, Slordahl SA, Wisloff U (2012) Home-based aerobic interval training improves peak oxygen uptake equal to residential cardiac rehabilitation: a randomized, controlled trial. PLoS One 7: e41199.
11. Moholdt T, Aamot IL, Granoien I, Gjerde L, Myklebust G, et al. (2012) Aerobic interval training increases peak oxygen uptake more than usual care exercise training in myocardial infarction patients: a randomized controlled study. Clin Rehabil 26: 33–44.
12. Rognmo O, Hetland E, Helgerud J, Hoff J, Slordahl SA (2004) High intensity aerobic interval exercise is superior to moderate intensity exercise for increasing aerobic capacity in patients with coronary artery disease. Eur J Cardiovasc Prev Rehabil 11: 216–222.

13. Wisloff U, Stoylen A, Loennechen JP, Bruvold M, Rognmo O, et al. (2007) Superior cardiovascular effect of aerobic interval training versus moderate continuous training in heart failure patients: a randomized study. Circulation 115: 3086–3094.
14. Aamot IL, Forbord SH, Gustad K, Lockra V, Stensen A, et al. (2013) Home-based versus hospital-based high-intensity interval training in cardiac rehabilitation: a randomized study. Eur J Prev Cardiol. doi: 10.1177/2047487313488299
15. Froelicher V, Myers J (2006) Exercise and the heart. 5th edn. Philadelphia: Saunders Elsevier.
16. Hofer S, Lim L, Guyatt G, Oldridge N (2004) The MacNew Heart Disease health-related quality of life instrument: a summary. Health Qual Life Outcomes 2: 3.
17. Hiller A, Helvik AS, Kaasa S, Slordahl SA (2010) Psychometric properties of the Norwegian MacNew Heart Disease health-related quality of life inventory. Eur J Cardiovasc Nurs 9: 146–152.
18. Moholdt T, Aamot IL, Granoien I, Gjerde L, Myklebust G, et al. (2011) Long-term follow-up after cardiac rehabilitation A randomized study of usual care exercise training versus aerobic interval training after myocardial infarction. Int J Cardiol 152: 388–390.
19. Machin D (1997) Sample size tables for clinical studies. 2nd edn. Oxford: Blackwell Science.
20. Vickers AJ, Altman DG (2001) Statistics notes: Analysing controlled trials with baseline and follow up measurements. BMJ 323: 1123–1124.
21. Gardner MJ, Altman DG (1986) Confidence intervals rather than P values: estimation rather than hypothesis testing. Br Med J (Clin Res Ed) 292: 746–750.
22. Gupta R, Sanderson BK, Bittner V (2007) Outcomes at one-year follow-up of women and men with coronary artery disease discharged from cardiac rehabilitation: what benefits are maintained? J Cardiopulm Rehabil Prev 27: 11–18.
23. Izawa KP, Yamada S, Oka K, Watanabe S, Omiya K, et al. (2004) Long-term exercise maintenance, physical activity, and health-related quality of life after cardiac rehabilitation. American Journal of Physical Medicine and Rehabilitation 83: 884–892.
24. Jefferis BJ, Sartini C, Lee IM, Choi M, Amuzu A, et al. (2014) Adherence to physical activity guidelines in older adults, using objectively measured physical activity in a population-based study. BMC Public Health 14: 382.
25. Lohne-Seiler H, Hansen BH, Kolle E, Anderssen SA (2014) Accelerometer-determined physical activity and self-reported health in a population of older adults (65-85 years): a cross-sectional study. BMC Public Health 14: 284.
26. Moholdt T, Madssen E, Rognmo O, Aamot IL (2013) The higher the better? Interval training intensity in coronary heart disease. J Sci Med Sport. doi: 10.1016/j.jsams.2013.07.007
27. Moholdt TT, Amundsen BH, Rustad LA, Wahba A, Lovo KT, et al. (2009) Aerobic interval training versus continuous moderate exercise after coronary artery bypass surgery: a randomized study of cardiovascular effects and quality of life. American Heart Journal 158: 1031–1037.
28. Moholdt T, Aamot IL, Granoien I, Gjerde L, Myklebust G, et al. (2012) Aerobic interval training increases peak oxygen uptake more than usual care exercise training in myocardial infarction patients: a randomized controlled study. Clinical Rehabilitation 26: 33–44.
29. Rognmo O, Moholdt T, Bakken H, Hole T, Molstad P, et al. (2012) Cardiovascular risk of high- versus moderate-intensity aerobic exercise in coronary heart disease patients. Circulation 126: 1436–1440.
30. Prescott E, Hjardem-Hansen R, Dela F, Orkild B, Teisner AS, et al. (2009) Effects of a 14-month low-cost maintenance training program in patients with chronic systolic heart failure: a randomized study. Eur J Cardiovasc Prev Rehabil 16: 430–437.

Whole Body Vibration Improves Cognition in Healthy Young Adults

G. Ruben H. Regterschot[1]*, Marieke J. G. Van Heuvelen[1], Edzard B. Zeinstra[1,3], Anselm B. M. Fuermaier[2], Lara Tucha[2], Janneke Koerts[2], Oliver Tucha[2], Eddy A. Van Der Zee[3]

1 University of Groningen, University Medical Center Groningen, Center for Human Movement Sciences, Groningen, The Netherlands, **2** Department of Clinical and Developmental Neuropsychology, University of Groningen, Groningen, The Netherlands, **3** Center of Behaviour and Neuroscience, Department of Molecular Neurobiology, University of Groningen, Groningen, The Netherlands

Abstract

This study investigated the acute effects of passive whole body vibration (WBV) on executive functions in healthy young adults. Participants (112 females, 21 males; age: 20.5±2.2 years) underwent six passive WBV sessions (frequency 30 Hz, amplitude approximately 0.5 mm) and six non-vibration control sessions of two minutes each while sitting on a chair mounted on a vibrating platform. A passive WBV session was alternated with a control session. Directly after each session, performance on the Stroop Color-Block Test (CBT), Stroop Color-Word Interference Test (CWIT), Stroop Difference Score (SDS) and Digit Span Backward task (DSBT) was measured. In half of the passive WBV and control sessions the test order was CBT-CWIT-DSBT, and DSBT-CBT-CWIT in the other half. Passive WBV improved CWIT ($p = 0.009$; effect size $r = 0.20$) and SDS ($p = 0.034$; $r = 0.16$) performance, but only when the CBT and CWIT preceded the DSBT. CBT and DSBT performance did not change. This study shows that two minutes passive WBV has positive acute effects on attention and inhibition in young adults, notwithstanding their high cognitive functioning which could have hampered improvement. This finding indicates the potential of passive WBV as a cognition-enhancing therapy worth further evaluation, especially in persons unable to perform active forms of exercise.

Editor: Reury F. P. Bacurau, University of Sao Paulo, Brazil

Funding: The authors have no support or funding to report.

Competing Interests: The authors have declared that no competing interests exist.

* E-mail: g.r.h.regterschot@umcg.nl

Introduction

There is growing evidence that physical exercise has positive effects on cognition [1]. Especially executive functions benefit from physical exercise [2]. Executive functions are a set of cognitive processes that regulate, manage and control other cognitive processes in order to achieve a goal, such as planning, working memory, mental flexibility, inhibition, attention, problem-solving and multi-tasking [3]. Executive functions are associated with the prefrontal cortex [4]. People who are not able to perform physical exercise, however, cannot fully benefit from the positive effects of physical exercise on executive functions. Therefore, whole body vibration (WBV) may be an alternative. WBV is the undergoing of mechanical vibrations produced by a vibrating platform to improve physical fitness. Often exercises are performed while standing on the vibrating platform. Besides this active form of WBV, it is also possible to undergo WBV without performing exercises. Such a passive form of WBV, referred to as passive WBV hereafter, may be a suitable physical therapy for improving executive functions in persons who are not able to perform physical exercise. However, the effects of passive WBV on executive functions have not been investigated yet. Therefore, this study investigated the acute effects of passive WBV on executive functions in healthy young adults.

It has been shown that active WBV has positive acute effects on human physiology. For example, oxygen uptake, heart rate, diastolic blood pressure and muscle activity are increased during active WBV compared to values during the performance of the same exercises without WBV [5–7]. The working mechanism behind the acute physiological effects of WBV, however, is not clear yet [6]. It is hypothesized that WBV stimulates muscle spindles, leading to a reflex response of the muscle [8]. This may enhance muscle activity, resulting in increased oxygen uptake and heart rate (both reflecting increased energy expenditure).

Besides possible excitation of muscle spindles, WBV stimulates vibration-sensitive mechanoreceptors in the skin, such as the Meissner corpuscles sensitive to 10–80 Hz vibrations and specifically to 30–40 Hz vibrations [9–11]. Afferent signals of cutaneous mechanoreceptors are transmitted to the primary somatic sensory cortex [12]. The sensory association areas have a direct and indirect connection to the prefrontal cortex [13], a region strongly involved in cognitive processing [4,14]. The indirect pathway involves the limbic system (e.g. the amygdala and the hippocampus, regions important in learning and memory), which can mediate the influence of the sensory association areas on the prefrontal cortex [13]. Furthermore, the amygdala also has projections to non-thalamic nuclei (e.g. the cholinergic nuclei of the basal forebrain) that have diffuse connections to a number of brain regions [13]. Thus, sensory stimulation may influence neurotransmission in sensory brain regions as well as the prefrontal cortex, hippocampus, amygdala and other brain regions. Therefore, a passive WBV session may have positive acute effects on cognition by sensory stimulation.

Empirical support for positive effects of WBV on cognition is provided by chronic WBV studies in animals. In these studies mice were placed in a cage connected to a vibrating platform and exposed to 10 minutes WBV (30 Hz–1.9 g) per day for five weeks. Results showed that daily exposure to WBV for five weeks significantly improved cognition (e.g. spatial memory) in young and aged mice compared to non-vibrated control mice [15,16]. Furthermore, the expression of the immediate early gene c-fos was enhanced in brain areas involved in sensorimotor and learning and memory functions (while leaving other brain regions largely unchanged) of mice exposed to WBV [17]. C-fos is up-regulated by an increase in neurotransmission and activates genes involved in the production of proteins necessary for neuronal plasticity and long-term memory [18,19]. The brain regions in which c-fos expression was enhanced are the same brain regions in which sensory stimulation is assumed to increase neurotransmission (sensory brain regions, prefrontal cortex, hippocampus). In addition, we recently demonstrated that WBV significantly increased the activity of the mouse forebrain cholinergic system (unpublished data). These findings suggest that sensory stimulation induced by WBV is an essential part of the mechanism underlying the improved cognitive performance in mice.

The neuroanatomical connections between mechanoreceptors and cognition-related brain regions (e.g. the prefrontal cortex), as well as the positive effects of WBV on cognition and neurotransmitter systems in mice, suggest that passive WBV may positively influence neurotransmission in a wide range of human brain regions. However, since the sensory brain regions have a direct and indirect connection to the prefrontal cortex, we expected that sensory stimulation by passive WBV would in particular affect executive functions. Therefore, the general aim of this study was to investigate the acute effects of passive WBV on executive functions in healthy young adults. Because sensory stimulation by passive WBV may positively influence neurotransmission in the prefrontal cortex, we hypothesized that passive WBV would improve executive functions.

Methods and Results

Ethics Statement

The Institutional Review Board (the Ethical Committee Psychology) of the Psychology Department of the University of Groningen approved the study. The study protocol conforms to the Helsinki declaration. All participants signed an informed consent before the experiment started.

2.1 Study Design

First a pilot study was performed to investigate the acute effects of passive WBV on executive functions in a small sample of young adults. An additional aim of the pilot study was to identify the optimal WBV frequency and amplitude for acute cognitive enhancement. After the pilot study, the main study was performed. The aim of the main study was to investigate the acute effects of passive WBV on executive functions in a large sample of young adults by using the optimal frequency and amplitude for acute cognitive enhancement as determined by the pilot study.

2.2 The Pilot Study

2.2.1 Participants. In the pilot study 12 healthy young adults (4 females and 8 males; age: 22.8±1.5 years; mass: 68.3±9.3 kg; height: 1.81±0.1 m; amount of exercise: 5.6±3.0 hours/week) voluntarily participated without receiving a reward for participation. The participants were students from the University of Groningen, the Netherlands. Participants did not have red-green color deficiency or any history of neurological or psychiatric disease.

2.2.2 Whole body vibration chair. A commercially available vibration device (Vibe 300 from Tonic Vibe, Nantes, France) was used in this study. A wooden plate (0.5 m×0.9 m×0.02 m) was mounted on the vibrating platform to enlarge the platform of the device (Figure 1). In order to apply passive WBV, a chair (with armrests and a seating area of soft material) was firmly mounted on the wooden plate to control activity and movement of participants (Figure 1). The vibration platform generated mainly vertical sinusoidal vibrations. According to the manufacturer, the vibration frequency could be adjusted with 1 Hz increments from 15 Hz to 60 Hz and the vertical vibration amplitude could be set at 2 mm or 4 mm. In this study accelerometers (tri-axial accelerometers, model 3093B, Dytran Instruments Inc, Chatsworth, CA, USA) were used to determine the actual frequency and amplitude of the vibration platform. With an average spectrum analysis of the acquired acceleration signal (using OR36 Signal Analyzer and NVGATE software version 7.00 from OROS SA, Grenoble, France) the actual frequency (Hz) and amplitude (mm) of the vibration platform were determined. We found that the actual frequency was equal or very similar to the frequency set on the vibration device (Table 1). However, the actual amplitude was lower than the amplitude reported by the manufacturer (Table 1).

2.2.3 Study design and procedures. Participants participated in 10 different passive WBV conditions (see Table 1 for the vibration frequency and amplitude per WBV condition) and a control condition while sitting on the WBV chair. In the control condition no vibration was applied. Three random orders of the 11 conditions were generated. By reversing these three orders three additional orders were created to counterbalance the design to avoid order effects. To obtain a total of 12 orders (one order for each participant), each of the six orders was applied twice. The 12 orders of the 11 conditions were randomly allocated to the 12 participants. Figure 2 shows an example of a condition order used in the pilot study. Each condition (passive WBV or control) lasted two minutes, immediately followed by assessment of executive functions. After the cognitive assessment participants had three minutes rest while sitting on the WBV chair (without vibration) before the next condition started.

Participants were instructed to sit in an upright position against the back of the chair throughout the whole experiment, with their arms on the armrests and their feet on the wooden plate. In addition, they were instructed to keep body movements to a minimum.

2.2.4 Measurements. In the pilot study executive functions (attention and inhibition) were assessed with the Color-Word Interference Test (CWIT) of the Stroop Color-Word Interference task [4,20]. In the CWIT a card with 20 color names (blue, red, orange, green or black printed in Dutch) was presented to the participant. Each word was printed in one of five possible colors (blue, red, orange, green or black). However, the ink color of each word was different from the color name (e.g. the word blue was printed in red). Participants were asked to name the ink color of the 20 words as fast as possible, thereby ignoring the written color name. The time (in seconds) needed to accomplish the test was measured. The participants practiced the CWIT once before the experiment started. Twelve parallel versions (one version for practice and 11 versions for assessments during the experiment) of the same CWIT (20 color names, five colors) were designed. Three random orders were generated of the 12 CWIT versions. Three additional orders were created by reversing the three random

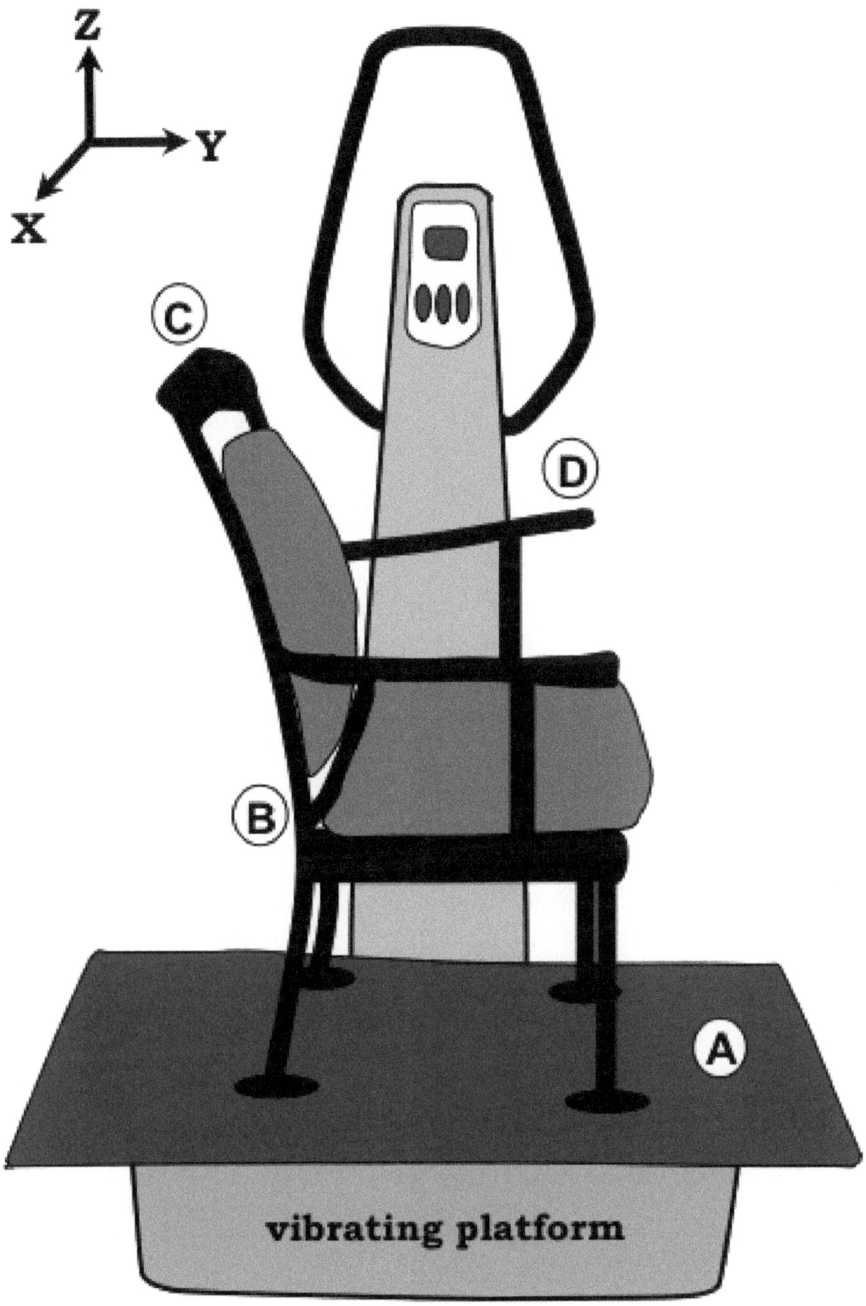

Figure 1. The WBV chair. Accelerations were measured at location A – D to determine the actual vibration frequency and amplitude (see Table 1).

orders to counterbalance the order of the 12 CWIT versions across participants. Each of the six orders was used twice to obtain a total of 12 orders. The 12 orders of the 12 CWIT versions were randomly allocated to the 12 participants.

2.2.5 Statistical analyses. CWIT (s) outcomes were not normally distributed. For that reason, Wilcoxon signed-rank tests were used to compare CWIT performance between individual WBV conditions and the control condition.

Statistical significance was set at $p<0.05$. Bonferroni's adjustment was applied to correct the statistical significance level for multiple comparisons. Moreover, effect sizes were calculated in the form of Pearson's correlation coefficient r. Effect sizes were calculated as $r=Z/\sqrt{N}$ using Wilcoxon signed-rank test statistics [21]. The N represents the total number of observations. Effect sizes were considered small when $0.10\leq r<0.30$, medium when $0.30\leq r<0.50$ and large when $r\geq 0.50$ [22]. Statistical analyses were performed with SPSS 17.0.

2.2.6 Results. WBV condition 7 (30 Hz frequency and approximately 0.5 mm amplitude, see Table 1) was the only WBV condition that significantly ($p=0.004$) improved CWIT (s) performance compared to the control condition (Table 2).

2.2.7 Conclusion. The passive WBV condition with 30 Hz frequency and approximately 0.5 mm amplitude (WBV condition 7 in Table 1) improved CWIT performance in healthy young adults. Therefore, this passive WBV condition was selected for further investigation in the main study.

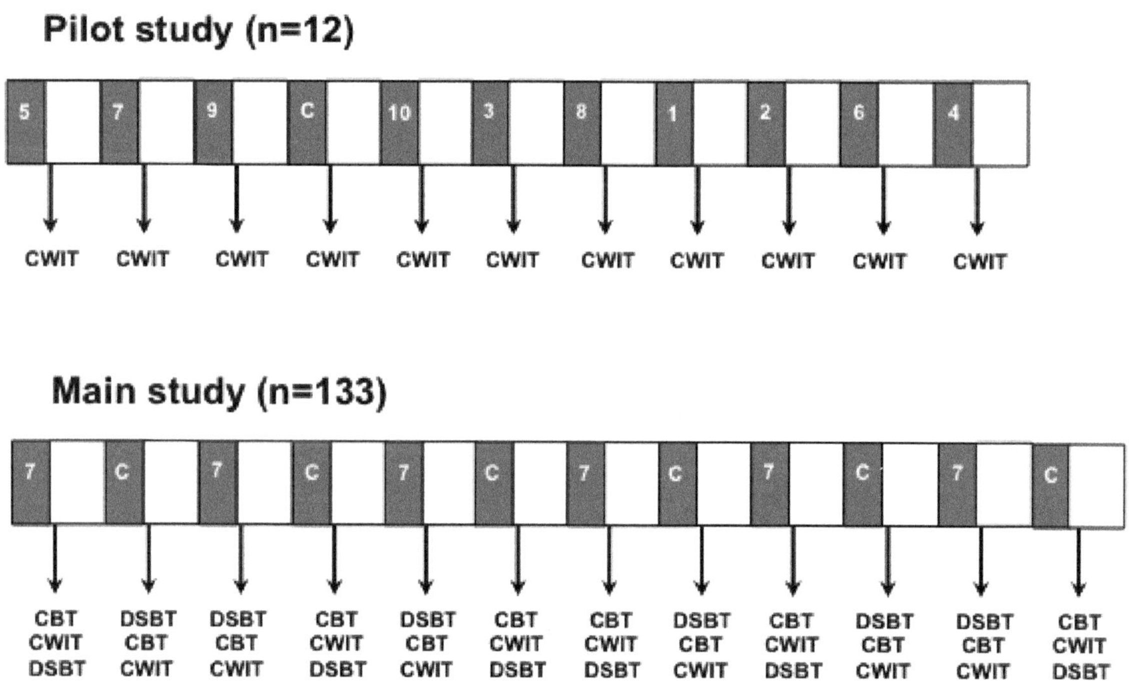

Figure 2. An example of a session order used in the pilot study and the main study. Grey blocks represent the WBV conditions (WBV conditions 1–10 in pilot study and WBV condition 7 in main study; see Table 1 for frequency and amplitude per WBV condition) or control condition (C). White blocks represent the rest periods. Executive functions were assessed immediately after each WBV and control session by using the Color-Word Interference Test (CWIT) in the pilot study, and the CWIT, Color-Block Test (CBT) and Digit Span Backward task (DSBT) in the main study.

2.3 The Main Study

2.3.1 Participants. In total, 133 healthy young adults (112 females and 21 males; age: 20.5±2.2 years; mass: 65.5±11.1 kg; height: 1.73±0.8 m; amount of exercise: 3.3±3.3 hours/week) participated. All participants were students from the University of Groningen, the Netherlands. Participation was on a voluntary basis and not paid. However, participation was rewarded towards a research requirement for undergraduate students. None of the participants reported any history of neurological or psychiatric disease and none of the participants indicated to suffer from red-green color deficiency.

2.3.2 Study design and procedures. Each participant underwent six times a passive WBV session with a frequency of 30 Hz and an amplitude of approximately 0.5 mm (WBV condition 7 in Table 1) and six times a control session while sitting on the WBV chair. The control session was without vibration. The order of the 12 sessions was counterbalanced across participants to avoid order effects. Figure 2 shows one of the two session orders used in the main study. Each session (passive WBV or control) lasted two minutes, immediately followed by assessments of executive functions and a rest period of three minutes while sitting on the WBV chair (without vibration). Following each

Table 1. The actual vibration frequency and amplitude of vertical displacement for different locations (A–D in Figure 1) and different frequency and amplitude settings on the vibration device.

WBV condition	Settings WBV device (Hz, mm)	Actual frequency and amplitude (Hz, mm)			
		Location A	*Location B*	*Location C*	*Location D*
1	20, 2	20, 0.38	20, 0.45	20, 0.38	20, 0.50
2	30, 2	30, 0.10	30, 0.19	30, 0.08	30, 0.62
3	40, 2	38, 0.16	38, 0.29	38, 0.26	38, 0.28
4	50, 2	48, 0.28	48, 0.33	48, 0.33	48, 0.33
5	60, 2	58, 0.38	58, 0.36	58, 0.45	58, 0.19
6	20, 4	20, 0.71	20, 0.72	20, 0.76	20, 0.74
7	30, 4	30, 0.44	30, 0.44	30, 0.64	30, 0.50
8	40, 4	38, 0.39	38, 0.46	38, 0.42	38, 0.47
9	50, 4	48, 0.46	48, 0.51	48, 0.53	48, 0.58
10	60, 4	58, 0.59	58, 0.60	58, 0.81	58, 0.33

The actual frequency and amplitude were calculated based upon acceleration data. Accelerations were measured without a person on the WBV chair.

Table 2. Color-Word Interference Test (CWIT) performance after the control condition and after WBV conditions 1–10 (n = 12).

Condition	CWIT (s) (mean±SD)	% change compared to control	z-value	p-value[a] (one-tailed)	Effect size (r)
Control	13.43±2.4	–	–	–	–
WBV 1	13.02±4.5	−3.1%	1.10	0.136	0.22
WBV 2	13.15±4.2	−2.1%	1.26	0.105	0.26
WBV 3	12.32±2.0	−8.3%	2.13	0.017	0.44
WBV 4	12.45±2.0	−7.3%	1.96	0.025	0.40
WBV 5	13.48±3.3	+0.3%	−0.24	0.593	−0.05
WBV 6	13.16±4.5	−2.0%	0.90	0.184	0.18
WBV 7	12.35±2.3	−8.0%	2.67	0.004*	0.54
WBV 8	12.66±2.4	−5.7%	1.96	0.025	0.40
WBV 9	12.52±2.5	−6.8%	2.04	0.021	0.41
WBV 10	12.73±2.9	−5.2%	1.65	0.050	0.33

Results of Wilcoxon signed-rank tests between WBV conditions and the control condition are also shown. [a] P-values <0.005 are significant after Bonferroni correction for multiple comparisons. *Indicates statistical significance.

rest period, participants underwent the next session (passive WBV or control).

During the whole experiment participants were sitting in an upright position against the back of the chair, with their arms positioned on the armrests and their feet on the wooden plate. Participants were asked to keep body movements to a minimum.

2.3.3 Measurements. Participants performed the Color-Block Test (CBT) and the CWIT as conditions of the Stroop Color-Word Interference task [20]. The CBT is a measure of psychomotor speed and attention. In the CBT, 20 squares printed in one of four possible colors (blue, red, yellow or green) were presented on a card. The participant's task was to name the colors of the squares as fast as possible. Time (in seconds) needed to complete the test was measured. The procedure of the CWIT was the same as in the pilot study, except that four colors (blue, red, yellow and green) were used instead of five colors. In addition, the Stroop Difference Score (SDS) was calculated as an additional measure of attention and inhibition by subtracting the time (in seconds) needed for completion of the CBT from the time (in seconds) needed for completion of the CWIT [20].

Participants also performed the Digit Span Backward task (DSBT). The DSBT is a subtest of the Wechsler Memory Scale-Revised and is a measure of executive functioning (working memory) [23]. In the DSBT a sequence of digits was read aloud to the participant with a speed of one digit per second. The task of the participant was to repeat the digits in the reversed order. Two sequences with the same number of digits were tested, one after the other. If at least one of the two sequences was recalled correctly in the reversed order, the level of difficulty was increased by adding one more digit to the length of the sequence. The first two sequences consisted of two digits. The test ended when a participant failed to recall both sequences of the same length in the reversed order. The number of correctly recalled sequences in reversed order was registered.

The participants practiced the CBT, the CWIT and the DSBT once before the start of the experiment in order to become familiar with the procedures of the tests. Immediately after each session (passive WBV or control), the CBT, the CWIT and the DSBT were performed (Figure 2). Following three passive WBV sessions and three control sessions, the CBT and the CWIT were performed before the DSBT (Figure 2). Following the other three passive WBV sessions and three control sessions, the DSBT was performed prior to the CBT and the CWIT (Figure 2). The CBT always preceded the CWIT. The order in which the Stroop tests and the DSBT were applied was counterbalanced across participants. In total 13 parallel versions (one version for practice and 12 versions for the assessments during the experiment) were designed of the CBT, the CWIT and the DSBT.

2.3.4 Statistical analyses. Two different test sequences (first the DSBT and then the two conditions of the Stroop Color-Word Interference task or vice versa) were performed three times after two different experimental sessions (passive WBV or control). Therefore, per cognitive test a mean score was calculated across the three trials for each combination of experimental session and test sequence. All outcome measures were normally distributed. Cognitive performance was compared between the passive WBV session and the control session by using dependent t-tests.

A p-value smaller than 0.05 was considered to indicate statistical significance. Pearson's correlation coefficient r was used as effect size measure and calculated as $r = \sqrt{(t^2/(t^2+df))}$ using dependent t-test statistics [21]. The effect sizes were interpreted as follows: small when $0.10 \leq r < 0.30$, medium when $0.30 \leq r < 0.50$ and large when $r \geq 0.50$ [22]. SPSS 17.0 was used to perform the statistical analyses.

2.3.5 Results. *Cognitive performance immediately after passive WBV and control session:* CBT (s) results did not reveal differences ($p = 0.16$) between the passive WBV and control session (Table 3). However, performance on the CWIT (s) and the SDS (s) improved significantly ($p = 0.009$ and $p = 0.034$ respectively) after the passive WBV session compared to the control session (Table 3). The performance on the DSBT (number of correctly recalled sequences) did not differ ($p = 0.66$) between the passive WBV and control session (Table 3).

Cognitive performance when cognitive test was preceded by another cognitive test: Performance on the CBT (s), CWIT (s) and SDS (s) did not differ ($p \geq 0.20$) between the passive WBV and control session (Table 3). Also performance on the DSBT (number of correctly recalled sequences) did not change ($p = 0.20$) by passive WBV compared to the control session (Table 3).

Discussion

The general aim of this study was to investigate the acute effects of passive WBV on executive functions in healthy young adults.

Table 3. Comparison of the performance on the Color-Block Test (CBT), Color-Word Interference Test (CWIT), Stroop Difference Score (SDS) and the Digit Span Backward task (DSBT) between the WBV and control session (n = 133).

	WBV session (mean±SD)	Control session (mean±SD)	t-value	p-value[a]	Effect size r
Performance immediately after WBV and control session					
CBT (s)	9.67±1.44	9.73±1.40	1.00	0.16	0.09
CWIT (s)	13.37±2.09	13.64±2.19	2.40	0.009*	0.20
SDS (s)	3.72±1.46	3.92±1.62	1.84	0.034*	0.16
DSBT (number)	6.24±1.92	6.29±1.76	−0.41	0.66	−0.04
Performance after another cognitive test					
CBT (s)	9.83±1.41	9.88±1.32	0.84	0.20	0.07
CWIT (s)	13.37±2.13	13.41±2.28	0.33	0.37	0.03
SDS (s)	3.54±1.44	3.53±1.58	−0.12	0.55	−0.01
DSBT (number)	6.22±1.58	6.13±1.93	0.85	0.20	0.07

[a]One-tailed p-value.
*p<0.05 indicates statistical significance.

We hypothesized that passive WBV would improve executive functions in young adults, possibly as a result of increased neurotransmission in the prefrontal cortex by sensory stimulation. Our hypothesis was based on the neuroanatomical connections between mechanoreceptors and cognition-related brain regions [12,13], and the positive effects of WBV on cognition and neurotransmitter systems in mice [15–17]. Indeed, the results of the pilot and main study showed that two minutes passive WBV with 30 Hz frequency and approximately 0.5 mm amplitude (WBV condition 7 in Table 1) improves CWIT performance in young adults, notwithstanding the already high level of cognitive functioning of the subjects. In addition, the main study demonstrated that two minutes passive WBV improved performance on the CWIT and the SDS only when the CBT and CWIT were performed immediately after passive WBV. Thus, two minutes passive WBV improved specific executive functions (attention and inhibition) measured with the CWIT and the SDS, while leaving another executive function (working memory) measured with the DSBT unchanged.

The improvement in CWIT performance by passive WBV may be explained by improved functioning of the prefrontal cortex and regions around the inferior frontal sulcus, because these brain regions are associated with CWIT performance [24]. Since afferent signals of cutaneous mechanoreceptors are transmitted to sensory brain areas [12] that are connected to prefrontal brain regions [13], passive WBV may acutely increase neurotransmission in the prefrontal cortex and in regions around the inferior frontal sulcus by sensory stimulation. Future research should investigate whether passive WBV increases neuronal activity in the mentioned brain regions, and whether sensory stimulation is indeed the mechanism underlying the positive acute effects of passive WBV on executive functions.

Only the passive WBV condition with 30 Hz frequency and approximately 0.5 mm amplitude improved executive functions (attention and inhibition). This may be explained by the specific sensitivity of Meissner corpuscles in the skin. Meissner corpuscles are especially sensitive to 30–40 Hz vibration [11]. Therefore, passive WBV with 30 Hz frequency and approximately 0.5 mm amplitude may induce a relatively strong stimulation of Meissner corpuscles in the skin, subsequently improving executive functioning. Other studies indicate that 30 Hz frequency is also optimal for stimulating oxygen uptake and muscle activity during active forms of WBV [5,6].

Evidence for a short duration of the positive acute effects of passive WBV on executive functions is provided by the main study. Passive WBV did not improve performance on the CWIT and the SDS when the CBT and the CWIT were preceded by the DSBT (the duration of the DSBT was about two minutes). Additional evidence for a short duration of the positive acute effect of passive WBV on executive functions is provided by a comparison between the results of the main study and the results of the pilot study. In the main study the CWIT showed an improvement when it was performed only after the CBT, which was approximately 10 to 25 seconds after passive WBV. In the pilot study, however, the CWIT was performed directly after passive WBV. The positive effect on the CWIT was larger in the pilot study (effect size r = 0.54 versus r = 0.20). Therefore, the results of both studies indicate that the positive acute effects of passive WBV on executive functions are of short duration and already reduced in the time interval of approximately 10 to 25 seconds after passive WBV. This may explain the absence of improvements in DSBT performance, since the duration of the DSBT was approximately two minutes. Further research should investigate the effects of passive WBV on shorter tests of verbal working memory to find out whether verbal working memory is sensitive to the effects of passive WBV.

This short duration may question the functional relevance of our findings, but it should be noted that the optimal duration of a single passive WBV session for enhancing cognitive performance is unknown. In the present study the duration of the passive WBV sessions was very short (2 minutes). A longer acute exposure to passive WBV may increase the size of the positive effects on the CWIT and the SDS as well as the duration of the positive effects on executive functions. A longer passive WBV treatment may also improve performance on the DSBT. For these reasons it is recommended that future studies investigate the acute cognitive effects of prolonged periods of passive WBV (i.e. >2 minutes). This recommendation is supported by a recent pilot study with healthy adults in which we used a duration of 4 minutes of passive WBV in a chronic treatment protocol (5 weeks, 3 days per week, n = 5). Our preliminary result revealed even stronger improvements in Stroop test performance (maximally 14% improvement) than the acute effects reported here. Moreover, the effects were still significantly present after one week without WBV treatment, illustrating the potential of passive WBV to improve cognition.

The results of this study indicate that passive WBV may be a clinically relevant therapy. We found that passive WBV enhances CWIT performance in healthy young adults with a high level of education and an age at which CWIT performance is highest across the lifespan [25]. This suggests that passive WBV may also have treatment effects in older adults and other populations with impaired attention and inhibition (such as people with attention deficit hyperactivity disorder). The forementioned pilot study on a chronic, 4 minutes passive WBV treatment in healthy adults corroborates this suggestion. Furthermore, passive WBV is easy to apply and not expensive. Therefore, passive WBV may be a relevant therapy for cognitively impaired populations unable to perform active forms of exercise, such as immobile older adults. Future studies should investigate the cognitive effects of passive WBV in older persons and clinical populations.

A limitation of this study may be the lack of an appropriate control condition. In the control sessions participants were sitting on the switched-off WBV chair, without the sound of the switched-on WBV platform. This suggests that the sound produced by the WBV platform may have contributed to the observed positive effects on cognition. However, the sound of the WBV condition that enhanced cognitive performance was very similar to the sound of other WBV conditions that did not improve cognitive performance in the pilot study. Therefore, results of the pilot study indicate that it is primarily the vibration that enhances cognitive performance and not the sound of the WBV platform. A strong point of the main study was the lack of an untreated control condition, since participants underwent passive WBV a couple of minutes before the control conditions. This is a conservative approach and strengthens the differences in cognitive performance that we found between the passive WBV and control condition. Other strong points of the main study were the use of an optimal vibration frequency and amplitude for improving executive functions based on the results of the pilot study, and the large sample size (n = 133).

In conclusion, this study demonstrated that passive WBV has positive effects on cognition in humans. Results showed that a short session of passive WBV with 30 Hz frequency and approximately 0.5 mm amplitude has a positive short-term effect on executive functions (attention and inhibition) in healthy young adults with a high level of cognitive functioning. Additional studies are in progress in young adults, (immobile) older adults and people with attention deficit hyperactivity disorder.

Acknowledgments

We thank F. Regterschot for his help with designing and constructing the WBV chair, and C. de Jong for providing the preliminary data with the chronic passive WBV protocol in healthy adults.

Author Contributions

Conceived and designed the experiments: GRHR MJGvH EBZ ABMF LT JK OT EAvdZ. Performed the experiments: GRHR EBZ ABMF LT. Analyzed the data: GRHR MJGvH EBZ ABMF LT JK OT EAvdZ. Contributed reagents/materials/analysis tools: MJGvH OT EAvdZ. Wrote the paper: GRHR MJGvH EBZ ABMF LT JK OT EAvdZ.

References

1. Kramer AF, Erickson KI, Colcombe SJ (2006) Exercise, cognition and the aging brain. J Appl Physiol 101: 1237–1242.
2. Hillman CH, Erickson KI, Kramer AF (2008) Be smart, exercise your heart: exercise effects on brain and cognition. Nat Rev Neurosci 9: 58–65.
3. Chan RC, Shum D, Toulopoulou T, Chen EY (2008) Assessment of executive functions: review of instruments and identification of critical issues. Arch Clin Neuropsychol 23: 201–216.
4. Smith EE, Jonides J (1999) Storage and executive processes in the frontal lobes. Science 283: 1657–1661.
5. Cardinale M, Lim J (2003) Electromyography activity of vastus lateralis muscle during whole-body vibrations of different frequencies. J Strength Cond Res 17: 621–624.
6. Cochrane DJ, Sartor F, Winwood K, Stannard SR, Narici MV, et al. (2008) A comparison of the physiologic effects of acute whole-body vibration exercise in young and older people. Arch Phys Med Rehabil 89: 815–821.
7. Rittweger J, Schiessl H, Felsenberg D (2001) Oxygen uptake during whole-body vibration exercise: comparison with squatting as a slow voluntary movement. Eur J Appl Physiol 86: 169–173.
8. Cardinale M, Bosco C (2003) The use of vibration as an exercise intervention. Exerc Sport Sci Rev 31: 3–7.
9. Dykes RW (1983) Parallel processing of somatosensory information: a theory. Brain Res Rev 6: 47–115.
10. Johansson RS, Vallbo AB (1983) Tactile sensory coding in the glabrous skin of the human hand. Trends Neurosci 6: 27–32.
11. Talbot WH, Darian-Smith I, Kornhuber HH, Mountcastle VB (1968) The sense of flutter-vibration: comparison of the human capacity with response patterns of mechanoreceptive afferents from the monkey hand. J Neurophysiol 31: 301–334.
12. Martin JH (2003) Neuroanatomy: text and atlas. New York: McGraw-Hill.
13. Braak H, Braak E, Yilmazer D, Bohl J (1996) Functional anatomy of human hippocampal formation and related structures. J Child Neurol 11: 265–275.
14. Kolb B, Whishaw IQ (2003) Fundamentals of human neuropsychology. New York: Worth Publishers.
15. Lahr MMH, Postema F, Venema BJ, Luiten PGM, Riedel G, et al. (2009) Whole body stimulation functions as a cognitive enhancer in young and old mice. 8th Dutch Endo-Neuro-Psycho Meeting Abstract 170.
16. Timmer M, Van der Zee EA, Riedel G (2006) Whole body vibration and behaviour: investigation of the role of various neurotransmitter systems. Federation of European Neuroscience Societies Abstract 3: 089.31.
17. Van der Zee EA, Riedel G, Rutgers EH, De Vries C, Postema F, et al. (2010) Enhanced neuronal activity in selective brain regions of mice induced by whole body stimulation. Federation of European Neuroscience Societies Abstract 5: 024.49.
18. Kang DK, Kim KO, Lee SH, Lee YS, Son H (2000) C-Fos expression by dopaminergic receptor activation in rat hippocampal neurons. Mol Cells 10: 546–551.
19. Tischmeyer W, Grimm R (1999) Activation of immediate early genes and memory formation. Cell Mol Life Sci 55: 564–574.
20. Stroop JR (1935) Studies of interference in serial verbal reactions. J Exp Psychol 18: 643–662.
21. Field A (2005) Discovering statistics using SPSS. London: Sage Publications Ltd.
22. Cohen J (1992) A power primer. Psychol Bull 112: 155–159.
23. Wechsler D (1987) Wechsler Memory Scale-Revised. New York: Psychological Corporation.
24. Zysset S, Müller K, Lohmann G, von Cramon DY (2001) Color-word matching Stroop task: separating interference and response conflict. Neuroimage 13: 29–36.
25. Uttl B, Graf P (1997) Color-Word Stroop test performance across the adult life span. J Clin Exp Neuropsychol 19: 405–420.

Single Muscle Fiber Gene Expression with Run Taper

Kevin Murach, Ulrika Raue, Brittany Wilkerson, Kiril Minchev, Bozena Jemiolo, James Bagley, Nicholas Luden, Scott Trappe*

Human Performance Laboratory, Ball State University, Muncie, Indiana, United States of America

Abstract

This study evaluated gene expression changes in gastrocnemius slow-twitch myosin heavy chain I (MHC I) and fast-twitch (MHC IIa) muscle fibers of collegiate cross-country runners (n = 6, 20±1 y, VO_{2max} = 70±1 ml•kg^{-1}•min^{-1}) during two distinct training phases. In a controlled environment, runners performed identical 8 kilometer runs (30:18±0:30 min:s, 89±1% HR_{max}) while in heavy training (~72 km/wk) and following a 3 wk taper. Training volume during the taper leading into peak competition was reduced ~50% which resulted in improved race times and greater cross-section and improved function of MHC IIa fibers. Single muscle fibers were isolated from pre and 4 hour post run biopsies in heavily trained and tapered states to examine the dynamic acute exercise response of the growth-related genes Fibroblast growth factor-inducible 14 (*FN14*), Myostatin (*MSTN*), Heat shock protein 72 (*HSP72*), Muscle ring-finger protein-1 (*MURF1*), Myogenic factor 6 (*MRF4*), and Insulin-like growth factor 1 (*IGF1*) via qPCR. *FN14* increased 4.3-fold in MHC IIa fibers with exercise in the tapered state ($P<0.05$). *MSTN* was suppressed with exercise in both fiber types and training states ($P<0.05$) while *MURF1* and *HSP72* responded to running in MHC IIa and I fibers, respectively, regardless of training state ($P<0.05$). Robust induction of *FN14* (previously shown to strongly correlate with hypertrophy) and greater overall transcriptional flexibility with exercise in the tapered state provides an initial molecular basis for fast-twitch muscle fiber performance gains previously observed after taper in competitive endurance athletes.

Editor: Stephen E. Alway, West Virginia University School of Medicine, United States of America

Funding: Funding provided by National Institutes of Health (AG 038576). The funders had no role in study design, data collection and analysis, decision to publish, or preparation of the manuscript.

Competing Interests: The authors have declared that no competing interests exist.

* Email: strappe@bsu.edu

Introduction

Athletes routinely reduce training volume prior to a major competition to help facilitate peak performance. A 3–4 week reduced training phase, known as taper, typically results in a 2–4% improvement in race performance [1–3]. In the last 30 years, taper research has identified increased power output at the whole muscle and single muscle fiber level as an important physiological basis for improved performance [1,2,4]. More specifically, tapering has been repeatedly shown to target fast-twitch muscle fibers by increasing their size [1–3] and power [1,2] with improvements in contractile performance largely accounted for by hypertrophy. However, little is known about molecular alterations that are contributing to performance gains in fast-twitch muscle fibers with tapering.

Recent methodological advances in our laboratory have established the ability to examine gene expression at the single muscle fiber level [5–7]. We sought to apply this novel approach with tapering to better understand potential molecular adaptations in fast-twitch muscle fibers. We were guided into these single muscle fiber gene studies by previous work in cross-country runners (for whom muscle biopsy samples were still available) that had an altered transcriptional response in mixed-muscle homogenate samples after identical 8 km running bouts in the heavily trained versus tapered state [2]. This alteration was intriguing since previous research has shown a blunted transcriptional response to exercise in well-conditioned skeletal muscle [6,8]. Thus, it appears that skeletal muscle of highly trained athletes may be more sensitive at the molecular level to various training phases than previously thought. Further support for conducting these single fiber gene studies was that the runners' MHC IIa fibers hypertrophied (+15%) and increased power output (+9%) with taper [2]. The combination of single muscle fiber gene measurements at strategically timed muscle biopsies after a heavily trained and tapered state 8 km run provided a unique opportunity to gauge the transcriptional flexibility of the MHC IIa fibers during these two training periods.

For the single muscle fiber gene experiments, we selected six genes that have been implicated in muscle size regulation and remodeling and included *FN14*, *MSTN*, *HSP72*, *MURF1*, *MRF4*, and *IGF1*. In developed human skeletal muscle, Fibroblast growth factor-inducible 14 (*FN14/TNFRSF12A*) was recently shown to strongly correlate with fast-twitch specific growth in response to exercise [6,9], the cytokines Myostatin (*MSTN/GDF8*) and Insulin-like growth factor 1 (*IGF1*) are components of major growth pathways [10], Myogenic factor 6 (*MRF4/MYF6*) is associated with exercise-induced remodeling [7], Muscle ring-finger protein-1 (*MURF1/TRIM63*) is a marker of ubiquitin-proteasome mediated myofibrillar breakdown [11], and Heat shock protein 72 (*HSP72/HSPA1A*) combats protein degradation [12]. We hypothesized that advantageous post exercise regulation of *HSP72*, *MURF1*, and *MRF4* previously observed in mixed-muscle with taper [2] would be more pronounced in MHC IIa fibers and that favorable *FN14*, *MSTN*, and *IGF1* expression would be targeted to the MHC IIa muscle fibers.

Materials and Methods

Subjects

Seven male runners from Taylor University's (Upland, Indiana) cross-country team volunteered to participate in a previous study [2]. Of these seven subjects, six were used for this investigation (age [y] 20±1, height [cm] 178±5, weight [kg] 66.1±5.1) (Table 1) as insufficient tissue at one time point for one subject negated molecular analysis. Details of the general study design and taper program are outlined in our previous investigation [2] and briefly profiled here (Figures 1 and 2). Subjects were competitive runners with 8 km lifetime best average performances of 26:32±0:32 (min:s). Prior to the investigation, subjects competitively participated in running for ~7 years (range: 4.5–10.0 y). Subjects were provided with written and oral information about experimental procedures and potential risks prior to providing written consent.

Ethics Statement

Support was granted by the coaching staff and all procedures were approved by the Ball State University and Taylor University Institutional Review Boards.

Experimental Design

A schematic of the study design is presented in Figure 3. Identical laboratory procedures were performed in the heavily trained (T1 and T2) and tapered (T3 and T4) conditions. Resting (heavily trained - T1, tapered - T3) and 4 h post exercise (heavily trained - T2, tapered - T4) gastrocnemius muscle biopsies were collected around an 8 km standardized indoor track run. MHC I and IIa fibers were individually isolated and pooled in order to conduct targeted fiber type specific gene expression analysis via reverse transcription quantitative real-time polymerase chain reaction (qPCR). The effect of taper was examined by conducting exercise response comparisons (T1:T2 and T3:T4) in both fiber types. Subjects were treadmill tested for aerobic capacity before and after the taper period.

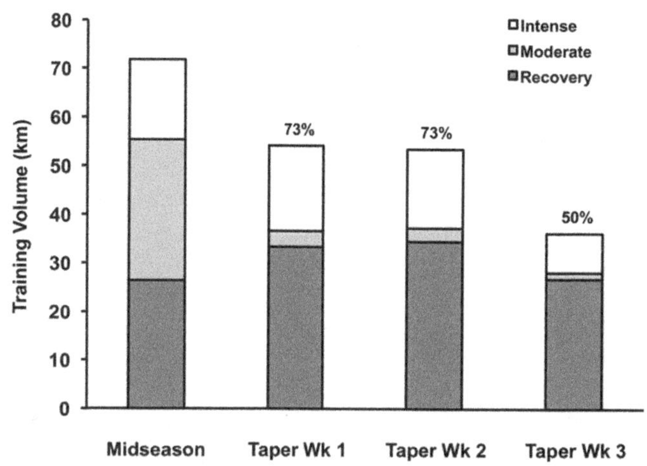

Figure 2. Summary of training volume and intensity during heavy training (11 wks) and each week of taper (3 wks), reproduced from Luden et al. [2] **with permission from the American Physiological Society.**

Training

Taylor University coaching staff prescribed the training performed throughout the 11 wk season (8 wks of midseason heavy training +3 wks of reduced-volume taper) based upon recommendations from our laboratory team. Training load was quantified using heart rate monitor data (Polar, Lake Success, NY) and self-reported running logs while mid-season training load (8 wks) was aggregated to represent one mean for heavy training. Average mid-season weekly running volume (6 d/wk) was approximately 72 km. During the 3 wk taper, weekly running volume in the moderate intensity range was progressively reduced

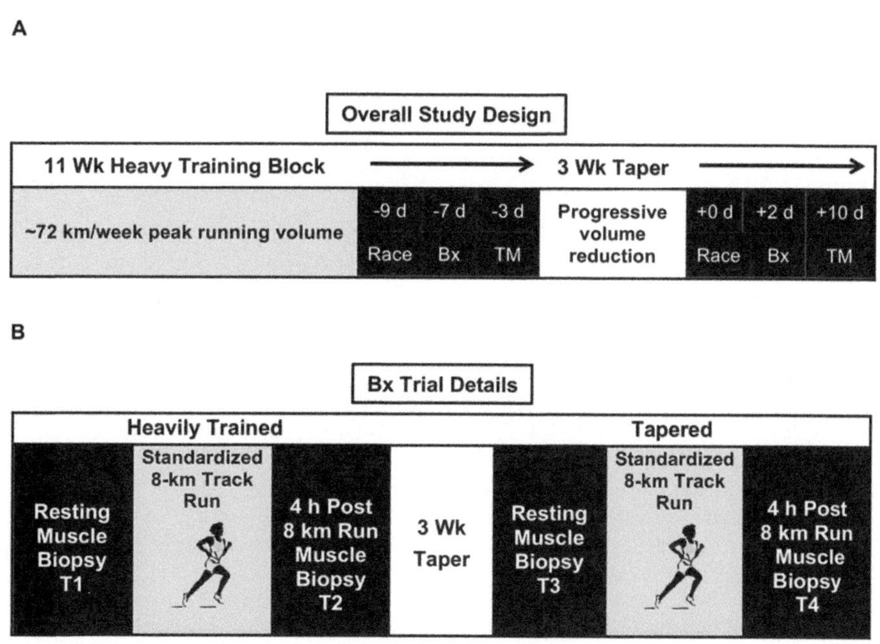

Figure 1. Overall study design (A), and Biopsy trial details (B). Bx = lateral gastrocnemius muscle biopsy, TM = Treadmill VO_{2max} testing.

Table 1. Subject characteristics and physiological data (n = 6).

	Heavily Trained	Tapered	% Δ
MHC IIa CSA (μm^2)	5812±622	6631±758	+14%
MHC IIa Power (μN•FL^{-1}•s^{-1})	58.7±6.4	63.5±7.3	+9%
VO_{2max} (ml•kg^{-1}•min^{-1})	70.0±1.1	69.1±1.1	↔
X-Country Race Performance (min:s)	27:42±0:25	27:00±0:30	−3%

Data derived from Luden et al. [2] less one subject.

to 50% of mid-season training while high intensity training volume was maintained (Figure 2).

Standardized 8 km Indoor Track Run

Subjects were instructed to run 8 km on a 200 m indoor track between 15.2 and 16.0 km/h (~45–48 s/lap) depending on talent level (30:18±0:30 min:s, 89±1% HR_{max}). This pace was chosen because it corresponded to a training velocity commonly performed by this group. Lap times were verbalized throughout the run to ensure even pacing and each lap split was recorded manually. Subjects performed identical runs in the heavily trained and tapered state and were monitored by the investigative team.

Muscle Biopsy

Four muscle biopsies (T1, T2, T3, T4) were obtained from the lateral head of the gastrocnemius. The gastrocnemius was chosen based on its documented use during running [13] and the large amount of gastrocnemius research conducted in runners over the past 40 years. Subjects reported to Taylor University having refrained from physical activity for two days (~48 h). After 30 min of supine rest, a resting muscle biopsy was obtained (T1, T3) followed by a standardized 8 km run on a 200 m indoor track. Subjects then underwent 4 h of supine rest upon which a second biopsy was obtained from the opposite leg (T2, T4). The rationale for the 4 h post exercise biopsy time point was based on previous post exercise mRNA time course investigations from our laboratory [7,14]. From each biopsy, a muscle sample weighing ~15 mg was placed in 0.5 ml of RNA*later* (Ambion, Austin, TX), stored at 4°C overnight, and subsequently stored at −20°C until fiber separation and RNA extraction.

Muscle Fiber Separation and MHC Identification

See Figure 3 for a schematic representation of the method used for fiber type-specific isolation and fiber pooling for qPCR. Individual muscle fibers were isolated in RNAlater using fine tweezers under a light microscope at room temperature as previously described [5,11,15,16]. An average of 129 fibers were isolated from each of the 24 samples (6 subjects×4 biopsies) for a total of 3,096 fibers. Approximately one quarter of each fiber was clipped and placed into 40 μl sodium dodecyl sulfate (SDS) buffer (1% SDS, 6 mg/ml ethylenediaminetetraacetic acid [EDTA], 0.06 M Tris [pH 6.8], 2 mg/ml bromophenol blue, 15% glycerol, and 5% b-mercaptoethanol) for SDS-PAGE (sodium dodecyl sulfate polyacrylamide gel electrophoresis) MHC identification as previously described by our laboratory [5,11,15,16]. The remaining fiber segment was placed into an individual well of a number-labeled 96-well plate with 75 μl RNA*later* and stored at −20°C until MHC type was confirmed and before fiber type-specific pooling. Overall MHC fiber type distribution of each subject's lateral gastrocnemius was determined using all fibers extracted from each individual.

Fiber Pooling and RNA Extraction

Following MHC isoform identification, the corresponding MHC I and IIa fiber segments were located in the 96-well plate. Muscle fibers of each type (MHC I and IIa) at each time point (T1, T2, T3, T4) were extracted from their individual wells containing RNA*later* and combined in a tube containing 500 μl TRI Reagent (Molecular Research Center, Cincinnati OH) used for RNA extraction. RNA extraction was performed according to the manufacturers protocol (MRC) and total RNA concentration (4.07±0.15 ng/μl) was determined using the Quant-iT RNA assay kit (Invitrogen, Carlsbad, CA) in conjunction with the Qubit fluorometer (Invitrogen). Forty-eight samples (24 samples×2 fiber types) were ultimately generated containing 36±6 (range 23–54) fibers, an amount sufficient to yield an RNA concentration of > 1.5 ng/μl [6,7].

Reverse Transcription and qPCR

Oligo (dT) primed first-strand cDNA was synthesized (16.5 ng of total RNA) using SuperScript II RT (Invitrogen) and quantification of mRNA levels (in duplicate) was performed in a 72-well Rotor-Gene 3000 Centrifugal Real-Time Cycler (Corbett Research, Mortlake, NSW, Australia). Ribosomal protein, large, P0 (*RPLP0*) was used as a reference gene as we have previously described [17]. All primers used in this study were mRNA-specific (on different exons and crossing over an intron) and designed for qPCR (Vector NTI Advance 9 software, Invitrogen) using SYBR Green chemistry. The primer sequences for *FN14* were: Forward -ACTTCTGCCTGGGCTGCGCT and Reverse -TCTCCTGCGGCATCGTCTCC, Genbank number: NM_016639.2. Primer sequences and characteristics for *MSTN*, *HSP72*, *MURF1*, *MRF4*, and *IGF1* as well as qPCR parameters have been reported previously from our laboratory [2,5,7,14,18]. For each qPCR run, a melting curve analysis was generated to validate the presence of only one product and a serial dilution curve (cDNA made of 500 ng total RNA from human skeletal muscle; Ambion, Austin, TX) was generated to evaluate reaction efficiencies. The amplification calculated by the Rotor-Gene software was specific and highly efficient (efficiency = 1.03±0.02; R^2 = 0.99±0.00; slope = 3.24±0.04). The gene expression response to exercise (8 km run) was examined in the heavily trained and tapered state using the $2^{-\Delta\Delta C_T}$ (fold change) quantification method [14,19,20].

Statistics

Data were checked for normality and sphericity and original or log transformed data were used for statistical analyses. Within each fiber type, the gene expression response to exercise in the heavily trained and tapered state was evaluated using a repeated measures two-way ANOVA with factors of time (T1–T4) and training state (heavily trained and tapered). Due to the minimal number of hybrids (<8%) and no IIx fibers in these highly trained runners,

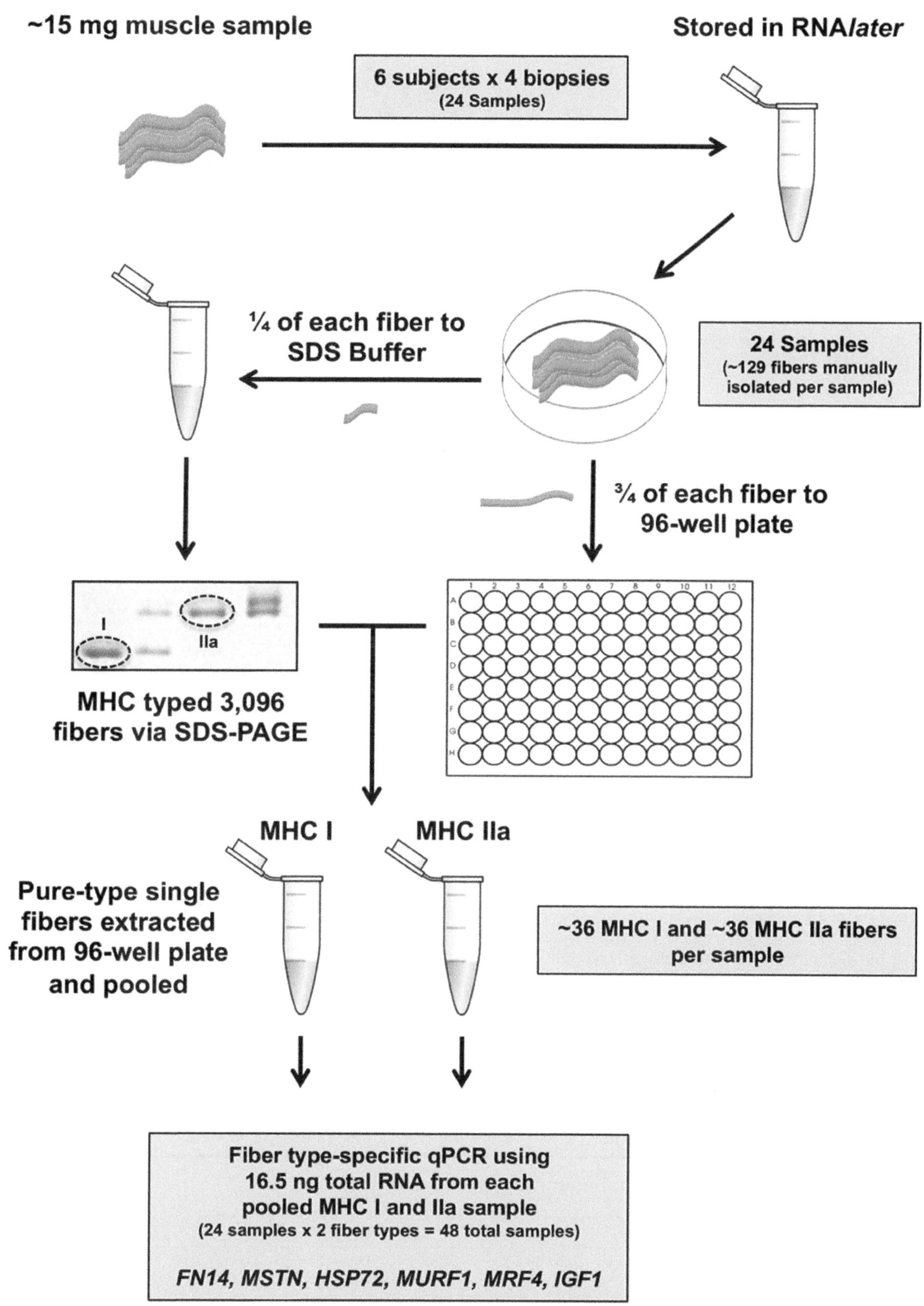

Figure 3. Schematic of method used to conduct fiber type-specific isolation of single muscle fibers for qPCR analysis.

gene expression analysis was limited to MHC I and MHC IIa fibers. All statistics were conducted in SPSS 17.0 for Windows, all data are presented as means ± SE, and significance was set at P< 0.05.

Results

Exercise-Induced (T1:T2 and T3:T4) Gene Expression in MHC IIa fibers

In the tapered state (T3:T4), *FN14* mRNA increased 4.3-fold (time and interaction effect, P<0.05, Figure 4) 4 h following the 8 km run. *MSTN* decreased 1.6-fold in the heavily trained state and 2.0-fold in the tapered state (time effect, P<0.05, Figure 5A). *MURF1* increased 2.7-fold in the heavily trained state and 4.0-fold in the tapered state (time effect, P<0.05, Figure 6). No changes were observed with exercise for *FN14* in the heavily trained state or *HSP72*, *MRF4*, or *IGF1* in the heavily trained or tapered state (Table 2).

Exercise-Induced (T1:T2 and T3:T4) Gene Expression in MHC I fibers

Exercise decreased *MSTN* 1.7-fold in the heavily trained state and 1.1-fold in the tapered state (time effect, P<0.05, Figure 5B). *HSP72* increased 1.7-fold in the heavily trained state and 2.0-fold in the tapered state (time effect, P<0.05, Figure 7). No changes occurred in *FN14*, *MURF1*, *MRF4*, or *IGF1* with exercise in the heavily trained or tapered state (Table 3).

Lateral Gastrocnemius Fiber Type

The average fiber type distribution (percentage) of the gastrocnemius in these runners was: 61.7±4.0% MHC I, 4.5±1.6% MHC I/IIa, 30.9±3.1% MHC IIa, 2.7±1.7% MHC IIa/IIx, and 0.2±0.1% MHC I/IIa/IIx. There were no MHC IIx fibers found in any subject. Fibers expressing multiple isoforms (MHC I/IIa, MHC IIa/IIx, and MHC I/IIa/IIx) comprised 7.4% of the total fiber population.

Discussion

The unique aspect of this investigation was the examination of MHC I and IIa gene responses in competitive collegiate runners after identical 8 km runs in the heavily trained versus tapered state. The 8 km running stimulus used in our study design reflects a typical weekly training run (~89% HR_{max}) these athletes performed throughout the competitive season. The post 4 h run time point coincides with anabolic and catabolic mRNA expression patterns following exercise [7,14] and captures elements of muscle remodeling. The main finding was that *FN14*, a gene strongly associated with fast-twitch hypertrophy [6,9], was robustly induced in MHC IIa fibers with exercise in the tapered state. Additionally, *MSTN* was suppressed with exercise in

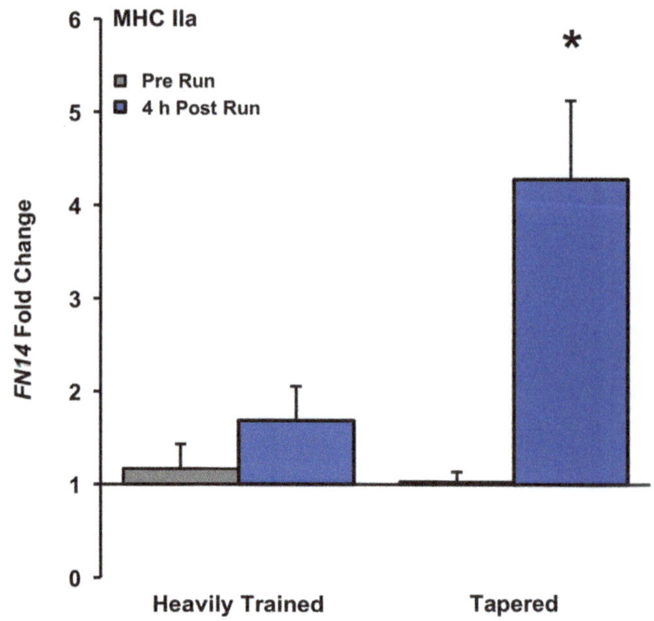

Figure 4. *FN14* gene expression response after an 8 km run in the heavily trained (T1:T2) and tapered (T3:T4) state in MHC IIa fibers, presented as fold change, *Time and interaction effect, P<0.05.

both fiber types and training states while *MURF1* and *HSP72* responded to running in MHC IIa and I fibers, respectively, regardless of training state. Contrary to the notion that exercise gene response [6,8,21,22] and adaptive potential [23] are attenuated as training status improves, these data indicate transcriptional flexibility in MHC I and IIa fibers of highly trained runners after an effective three week taper. The marked *FN14* response in MHC IIa fibers provides an initial molecular basis to support MHC IIa hypertrophy observed with taper, a stimulus that generally produces the highest calculated fast-twitch fiber growth rate in humans.

Tapered training of ≤3 weeks in aerobically fit runners [2], swimmers [1], and cyclists [3] can be calculated to confer MHC IIa growth rates of 5.0%, 8.0%, and 14.2% per week, respectively. By comparison, MHC IIa growth with progressive resistance training in young healthy individuals occurs at a maximum rate of 3.8% by 4 weeks [24] and approaches an asymptote by 12 weeks [25] as adaptation becomes more refined (see Table S1 for comprehensive review of fast-twitch growth with exercise). Despite being highly conditioned, fast-twitch muscle fibers of trained endurance athletes can rapidly change size in response to training adjustments which measurably affects whole muscle and single

Table 2. Genes not responsive to exercise in MHC IIa fibers in the heavily trained or tapered state.

	Heavily Trained		Tapered	
	T1	T2	T3	T4
HSP72	1.07±0.17	1.31±0.32	1.06±0.15	1.77±0.32
MRF4	1.03±0.12	0.84±0.09	1.15±0.28	0.9±0.11
IGF1	1.09±0.17	1.02±0.21	1.18±0.30	0.77±0.12

Presented as fold change, mean ± SE.

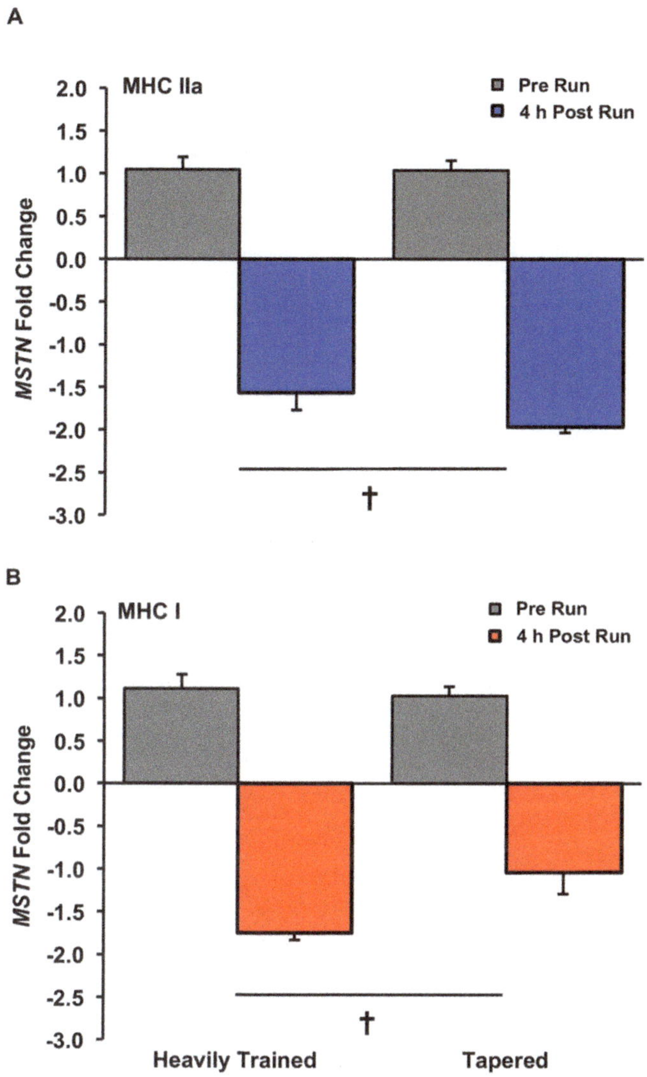

Figure 5. ***MSTN*** **gene expression response after an 8 km run in the heavily trained (T1:T2) and tapered (T3:T4) state in MHC I (A) and IIa (B) fibers, presented as fold change, Main time effect for exercise, $P<0.05$.**

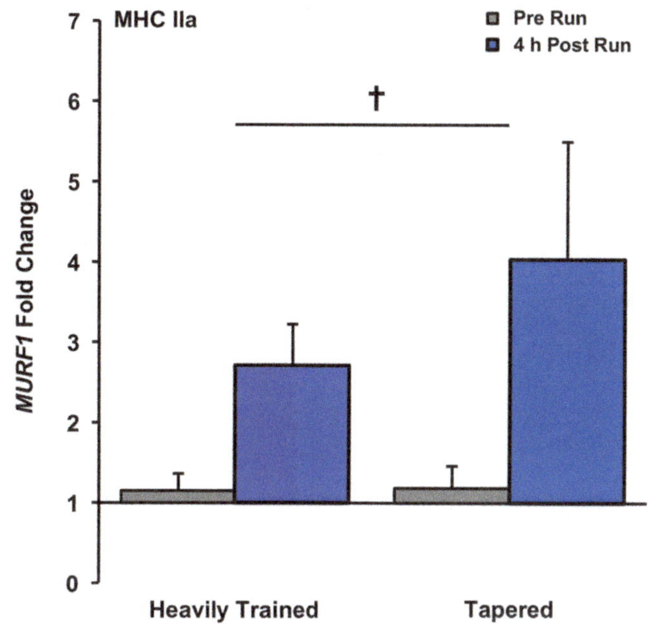

Figure 6. ***MURF1*** **gene expression response after an 8 km run in the heavily trained (T1:T2) and tapered (T3:T4) state in MHC IIa fibers, presented as fold change, Main time effect for exercise, $P<0.05$.**

fiber power [1,2,26,27]. However, the only transcript-level insight into mediators of fiber type-specific size regulation in humans has been in reference to resistance exercise. Acute resistance exercise elicits differential MHC I and IIa proteolytic mRNA responses [11] and activates a distinct MHC IIa transcriptome that precedes resistance training-induced increases in MHC IIa single fiber cross sectional area [6,9]. The current investigation reinforces the differential gene regulation concept, namely that *FN14* induction may augment the capacity of MHC IIa fibers to quickly grow and improve contractile function with taper.

The 4.3-fold *FN14* induction post run in tapered MHC IIa fibers aligns with our laboratory's recent finding that robust *FN14* expression after exercise is associated with isolated fast-twitch fiber size increases from resistance training [6,9]. A member of the TNFα superfamily, FN14 is a cell-surface receptor found on a variety of tissues including skeletal muscle [28] and appears to signal through the diverse NF-Kβ pathway [28,29]. While linked to atrophy in pathological conditions [30], FN14 also appears necessary for muscle proliferation, differentiation, and regeneration in mice and cell culture [31,32]. In this investigation, *FN14* gene induction after running in the tapered state was uniform (six of six subjects) and four responses were larger (≥4.4-fold) than the largest heavily trained response (2.8-fold). These occurrences highlight the magnitude of this fiber type-specific induction and further implicate *FN14* as an important component specific to the MHC IIa remodeling process in humans' response to exercise.

MSTN decreased post-run in both conditions and fiber types. Myostatin is a negative regulator of skeletal muscle mass that is blunted following a hypertrophic stimulus in humans [9,14,33–36]. Interestingly, Myostatin is also suppressed at the gene and protein level in humans after non-hypertrophic exercise [14,37,38]. This could signal a metabolic purpose for down-regulation [38,39] or Myostatin's supporting role in muscle remodeling and homeostasis after aerobic exercise [40]. It is worth noting, however, that the largest *MSTN* reduction observed here (2.0-fold) was in tapered MHC IIa fibers. Skeletal muscle reportedly has ~2–3 times the amount of Myostatin necessary to restrain growth [41] while animal [42–46] and human [47–49] fast-twitch muscle appears most sensitive to *MSTN* alterations. The 2.0-fold tapered state reduction in *MSTN* with running may have surpassed a physiologically significant threshold for Myostatin-mediated growth to occur and could have contributed to previously observed MHC IIa hypertrophy with taper [2].

MURF1 was responsive to run exercise in the heavily trained and tapered state in MHC IIa fibers. A marker of myofibrillar protein breakdown, *MURF1* increases after acute resistance [14,20,50] and endurance [14,51] exercise and is elevated concomitant with training-induced hypertrophy [52]. Increased *MURF1* with exercise may therefore represent a normal component of the MHC IIa remodeling process in healthy human muscle. *HSP72*, *MRF4*, and *IGF1* were not altered with exercise in MHC IIa fibers in either training state. In animals, heat shock protein is less constitutively expressed in fast-twitch than slow-twitch muscle [53–55] and is less responsive to exercise in human Type IIa fibers [56]. A lack of *HSP72* response to intense training

Table 3. Genes not responsive to exercise in MHC I fibers in the heavily trained or tapered state.

	Heavily Trained		Tapered	
	T1	T2	T3	T4
FN14	2.04±1.14	3.18±0.92	1.47±0.53	2.25±1.13
MURF1	1.12±0.19	3.94±1.88	1.17±0.29	1.04±0.27
MRF4	1.05±0.16	1.45±0.17	1.25±0.41	1.09±0.12
IGF1	1.09±0.19	1.03±0.13	1.06±0.17	0.77±0.06

Presented as fold change, mean ± SE.

and taper may therefore reflect a normal pattern of heat shock protein expression in MHC IIa fibers. *MRF4* induction after taper observed previously in mixed-muscle of these runners was relatively modest (1.4 fold) [2] and was abolished at the single fiber level in both fiber types. This discrepancy could result from a combinatorial effect of all fiber types yielding significant *MRF4* expression in mixed-muscle or the potential influence of satellite cells (express *MRF4* upon activation [57,58]). Common mRNA markers of quiescent satellite cells (*NCAM1, CD34, CDH15, CALCR*) are present in fibers mechanically dissected using the method described here [6] which suggests satellite cell presence but the extent of satellite cell adhesion has not yet been determined. IGF1 activates the Akt/mTOR pathway and is strongly implicated in exercise-induced muscle hypertrophy [10]. However, *IGF1* transcript is shown to not change appreciably in the early recovery from aerobic [18] or resistance exercise [18,59,60] which agrees with our findings.

HSP72 responded to exercise in MHC I fibers in both training states. This induction is consistent with greater HSP72 protein levels in Type I vs IIa fibers following 30 minutes of acute exercise [56]. In well-conditioned aerobic athletes, the greatest increase in

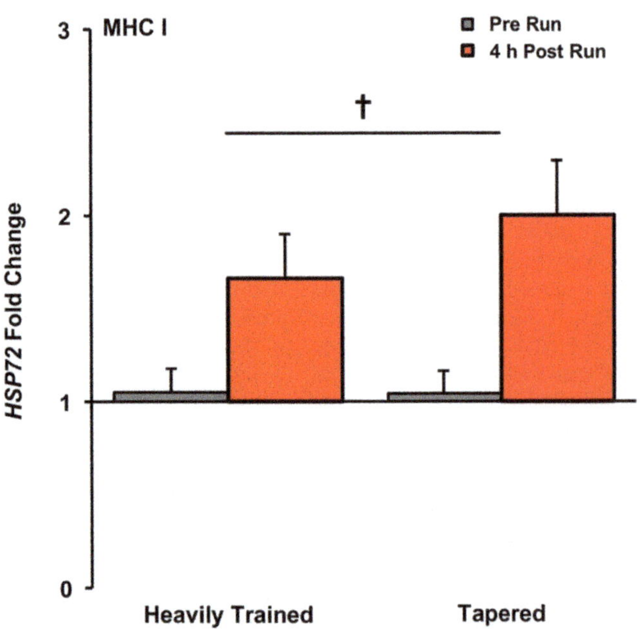

Figure 7. *HSP72* gene expression response after an 8 km run in the heavily trained (T1:T2) and tapered (T3:T4) state in MHC I fibers, presented as fold change, Main time effect for exercise, P<0.05.

basal HSP72 protein level occurs with intensified training but overall content peaks following a reduced training period [61]. While speculative, it is conceivable that improved translational efficiency in reaction to tapering along with a slightly more pronounced *HSP72* response to exercise in tapered MHC I fibers (Figure 7) of the trained runners studied here ultimately results in greater HSP72 protein levels after taper. This could be interpreted as a positive adjustment to the post run cellular environment that would aid in the localized stress tolerance of intense exercise performance [12] that coincides with peak level competition [1,2,4].

A properly conducted taper program in athletes prior to peak competition improves performance that appears to be mediated, in part, by increased power at the whole muscle and single muscle fiber level. The single muscle fiber performance gains with taper are targeted to MHC IIa fibers and are primarily driven by hypertrophy [1,2]. The current study extends these MHC IIa-specific muscle fiber adaptations with taper to the molecular level and reports a sizeable *FN14* induction in the tapered state that may have contributed to rapid fast-twitch remodeling. A potentially meaningful *MSTN* suppression with tapered state exercise may also help support a favorable fast-twitch growth environment. We speculate that intense aerobic training periods reduce MHC IIa plasticity of growth-related gene targets and that taper reverses this process. To what extent the taper-induced MHC IIa adaptations are due to super-compensation from intense training or recovery to levels prior to the heavy training phase has not been established. The current study illustrates how tapering can promote transcriptional flexibility not previously thought possible in well-conditioned muscle [6,8]. These basic alterations at the molecular level provide a framework for expanded studies (i.e. transcriptome, protein quantification, epigenetics, etc.) to further our understanding of MHC IIa plasticity with exercise training paradigms.

Supporting Information

Table S1 Summary of literature on selective fast-twitch size alterations in young healthy individuals.

Acknowledgments

We would like to thank the Taylor University cross-country team, Ted Bowers (head coach), and the coaching staff for their enthusiastic participation in this research. Thank you to Dr. David Costill for his review and comments on the manuscript. We also wish to thank Drs. Erik Hayes, Andrew Galpin, Matt Harber, and Todd Trappe for their assistance with data collection during the taper project and Dr. Holmes Finch for his invaluable insight concerning statistics.

Author Contributions

Conceived and designed the experiments: ST K. Murach NL UR. Performed the experiments: K. Murach UR BW K. Minchev BJ JB. Analyzed the data: K. Murach UR BJ ST. Contributed reagents/materials/analysis tools: ST. Wrote the paper: K. Murach ST.

References

1. Trappe S, Costill D, Thomas R (2000) Effect of swim taper on whole muscle and single muscle fiber contractile properties. Med Sci Sports Exerc 32: 48–56.
2. Luden N, Hayes E, Galpin A, Minchev K, Jemiolo B, et al. (2010) Myocellular basis for tapering in competitive distance runners. J Appl Physiol 108: 1501–1509.
3. Neary JP, Martin TP, Quinney HA (2003) Effects of taper on endurance cycling capacity and single muscle fiber properties. Med Sci Sports Exerc 35: 1875–1881.
4. Costill D, King D, Thomas R, Hagreaves M (1985) Effects of Reduced Training on Muscular Power in Swimmers. The Physician and Sports Medicine 13: 94–101.
5. Jemiolo B, Trappe S (2004) Single muscle fiber gene expression in human skeletal muscle: validation of internal control with exercise. Biochem Biophys Res Commun 320: 1043–1050.
6. Raue U, Trappe TA, Estrem ST, Qian HR, Helvering LM, et al. (2012) Transcriptome signature of resistance exercise adaptations: mixed muscle and fiber type specific profiles in young and old adults. J Appl Physiol 112: 1625–1636.
7. Yang Y, Creer A, Jemiolo B, Trappe S (2005) Time course of myogenic and metabolic gene expression in response to acute exercise in human skeletal muscle. J Appl Physiol 98: 1745–1752.
8. Schmutz S, Dapp C, Wittwer M, Vogt M, Hoppeler H, et al. (2006) Endurance training modulates the muscular transcriptome response to acute exercise. Pflugers Arch 451: 678–687.
9. Raue U, Slivka D, Minchev K, Trappe S (2009) Improvements in whole muscle and myocellular function are limited with high-intensity resistance training in octogenarian women. J Appl Physiol 106: 1611–1617.
10. Harridge SD (2007) Plasticity of human skeletal muscle: gene expression to in vivo function. Exp Physiol 92: 783–797.
11. Yang Y, Jemiolo B, Trappe S (2006) Proteolytic mRNA expression in response to acute resistance exercise in human single skeletal muscle fibers. J Appl Physiol 101: 1442–1450.
12. Yamada P, Amorim F, Moseley P, Schneider S (2008) Heat shock protein 72 response to exercise in humans. Sports Med 38: 715–733.
13. Costill DL, Sparks K, Gregor R, Turner C (1971) Muscle glycogen utilization during exhaustive running. J Appl Physiol 31: 353–356.
14. Louis E, Raue U, Yang Y, Jemiolo B, Trappe S (2007) Time course of proteolytic, cytokine, and myostatin gene expression after acute exercise in human skeletal muscle. J Appl Physiol 103: 1744–1751.
15. Dickinson JM, Lee JD, Sullivan BE, Harber MP, Trappe SW, et al. (2010) A new method to study in vivo protein synthesis in slow- and fast-twitch muscle fibers and initial measurements in humans. J Appl Physiol 108: 1410–1416.
16. Galpin AJ, Raue U, Jemiolo B, Trappe TA, Harber MP, et al. (2012) Human skeletal muscle fiber type specific protein content. Anal Biochem 425: 175–182.
17. Trappe TA, Carroll CC, Jemiolo B, Trappe SW, Dossing S, et al. (2008) Cyclooxygenase mRNA expression in human patellar tendon at rest and after exercise. Am J Physiol Regul Integr Comp Physiol 294: R192–199.
18. Coffey VG, Jemiolo B, Edge J, Garnham AP, Trappe SW, et al. (2009) Effect of consecutive repeated sprint and resistance exercise bouts on acute adaptive responses in human skeletal muscle. Am J Physiol Regul Integr Comp Physiol 297: R1441–1451.
19. Livak KJ, Schmittgen TD (2001) Analysis of relative gene expression data using real-time quantitative PCR and the 2(-Delta Delta C(T)) Method. Methods 25: 402–408.
20. Raue U, Slivka D, Jemiolo B, Hollon C, Trappe S (2007) Proteolytic gene expression differs at rest and after resistance exercise between young and old women. J Gerontol A Biol Sci Med Sci 62: 1407–1412.
21. Egan B, O'Connor PL, Zierath JR, O'Gorman DJ (2013) Time course analysis reveals gene-specific transcript and protein kinetics of adaptation to short-term aerobic exercise training in human skeletal muscle. PLoS One 8: e74098.
22. Perry CG, Lally J, Holloway GP, Heigenhauser GJ, Bonen A, et al. (2010) Repeated transient mRNA bursts precede increases in transcriptional and mitochondrial proteins during training in human skeletal muscle. J Physiol 588: 4795–4810.
23. Saltin B, Henriksson J, Nygaard E, Andersen P, Jansson E (1977) Fiber types and metabolic potentials of skeletal muscles in sedentary man and endurance runners. Ann N Y Acad Sci 301: 3–29.
24. Woolstenhulme MT, Conlee RK, Drummond MJ, Stites AW, Parcell AC (2006) Temporal response of desmin and dystrophin proteins to progressive resistance exercise in human skeletal muscle. J Appl Physiol (1985) 100: 1876–1882.
25. Hakkinen K, Alen M, Komi PV (1985) Changes in isometric force- and relaxation-time, electromyographic and muscle fibre characteristics of human skeletal muscle during strength training and detraining. Acta Physiol Scand 125: 573–585.
26. Fitts RH, Costill DL, Gardetto PR (1989) Effect of swim exercise training on human muscle fiber function. J Appl Physiol 66: 465–475.
27. Kohn TA, Essen-Gustavsson B, Myburgh KH (2011) Specific muscle adaptations in type II fibers after high-intensity interval training of well-trained runners. Scand J Med Sci Sports 21: 765–772.
28. Winkles JA (2008) The TWEAK-Fn14 cytokine-receptor axis: discovery, biology and therapeutic targeting. Nat Rev Drug Discov 7: 411–425.
29. Burkly LC, Michaelson JS, Zheng TS (2011) TWEAK/Fn14 pathway: an immunological switch for shaping tissue responses. Immunol Rev 244: 99–114.
30. Mittal A, Bhatnagar S, Kumar A, Lach-Trifilieff E, Wauters S, et al. (2010) The TWEAK-Fn14 system is a critical regulator of denervation-induced skeletal muscle atrophy in mice. J Cell Biol 188: 833–849.
31. Dogra C, Hall SL, Wedhas N, Linkhart TA, Kumar A (2007) Fibroblast growth factor inducible 14 (Fn14) is required for the expression of myogenic regulatory factors and differentiation of myoblasts into myotubes. Evidence for TWEAK-independent functions of Fn14 during myogenesis. J Biol Chem 282: 15000–15010.
32. Girgenrath M, Weng S, Kostek CA, Browning B, Wang M, et al. (2006) TWEAK, via its receptor Fn14, is a novel regulator of mesenchymal progenitor cells and skeletal muscle regeneration. EMBO J 25: 5826–5839.
33. Costa A, Dalloul H, Hegyesi H, Apor P, Csende Z, et al. (2007) Impact of repeated bouts of eccentric exercise on myogenic gene expression. Eur J Appl Physiol 101: 427–436.
34. Kim JS, Petrella JK, Cross JM, Bamman MM (2007) Load-mediated downregulation of myostatin mRNA is not sufficient to promote myofiber hypertrophy in humans: a cluster analysis. J Appl Physiol 103: 1488–1495.
35. Raue U, Slivka D, Jemiolo B, Hollon C, Trappe S (2006) Myogenic gene expression at rest and after a bout of resistance exercise in young (18–30 yr) and old (80–89 yr) women. J Appl Physiol 101: 53–59.
36. Roth SM, Martel GF, Ferrell RE, Metter EJ, Hurley BF, et al. (2003) Myostatin gene expression is reduced in humans with heavy-resistance strength training: a brief communication. Exp Biol Med (Maywood) 228: 706–709.
37. Harber MP, Crane JD, Dickinson JM, Jemiolo B, Raue U, et al. (2009) Protein synthesis and the expression of growth-related genes are altered by running in human vastus lateralis and soleus muscles. Am J Physiol Regul Integr Comp Physiol 296: R708–714.
38. Hittel DS, Axelson M, Sarna N, Shearer J, Huffman KM, et al. (2010) Myostatin decreases with aerobic exercise and associates with insulin resistance. Med Sci Sports Exerc 42: 2023–2029.
39. Chen Y, Ye J, Cao L, Zhang Y, Xia W, et al. (2010) Myostatin regulates glucose metabolism via the AMP-activated protein kinase pathway in skeletal muscle cells. Int J Biochem Cell Biol 42: 2072–2081.
40. Matsakas A, Friedel A, Hertrampf T, Diel P (2005) Short-term endurance training results in a muscle-specific decrease of myostatin mRNA content in the rat. Acta Physiol Scand 183: 299–307.
41. Welle S, Burgess K, Thornton CA, Tawil R (2009) Relation between extent of myostatin depletion and muscle growth in mature mice. Am J Physiol Endocrinol Metab 297: E935–940.
42. Arounleut P, Bialek P, Liang LF, Upadhyay S, Fulzele S, et al. (2013) A myostatin inhibitor (propeptide-Fc) increases muscle mass and muscle fiber size in aged mice but does not increase bone density or bone strength. Exp Gerontol 48: 898–904.
43. Carlson CJ, Booth FW, Gordon SE (1999) Skeletal muscle myostatin mRNA expression is fiber-type specific and increases during hindlimb unloading. Am J Physiol 277: R601–606.
44. Liu CM, Yang Z, Liu CW, Wang R, Tien P, et al. (2008) Myostatin antisense RNA-mediated muscle growth in normal and cancer cachexia mice. Gene Ther 15: 155–160.
45. Magee TR, Artaza JN, Ferrini MG, Vernet D, Zuniga FI, et al. (2006) Myostatin short interfering hairpin RNA gene transfer increases skeletal muscle mass. J Gene Med 8: 1171–1181.
46. Wehling M, Cai B, Tidball JG (2000) Modulation of myostatin expression during modified muscle use. FASEB J 14: 103–110.
47. Jespersen JG, Nedergaard A, Andersen LL, Schjerling P, Andersen JL (2011) Myostatin expression during human muscle hypertrophy and subsequent atrophy: increased myostatin with detraining. Scand J Med Sci Sports 21: 215–223.
48. Reardon KA, Davis J, Kapsa RM, Choong P, Byrne E (2001) Myostatin, insulin-like growth factor-1, and leukemia inhibitory factor mRNAs are upregulated in chronic human disuse muscle atrophy. Muscle Nerve 24: 893–899.
49. Wojcik S, Nogalska A, Engel WK, Askanas V (2008) Myostatin and its precursor protein are increased in the skeletal muscle of patients with Type-II muscle fibre atrophy. Folia Morphol (Warsz) 67: 6–12.
50. Nedergaard A, Vissing K, Overgaard K, Kjaer M, Schjerling P (2007) Expression patterns of atrogenic and ubiquitin proteasome component genes with exercise: effect of different loading patterns and repeated exercise bouts. J Appl Physiol (1985) 103: 1513–1522.

51. Harber MP, Konopka AR, Jemiolo B, Trappe SW, Trappe TA, et al. (2010) Muscle protein synthesis and gene expression during recovery from aerobic exercise in the fasted and fed states. Am J Physiol Regul Integr Comp Physiol 299: R1254–1262.
52. Leger B, Cartoni R, Praz M, Lamon S, Deriaz O, et al. (2006) Akt signalling through GSK-3beta, mTOR and Foxo1 is involved in human skeletal muscle hypertrophy and atrophy. J Physiol 576: 923–933.
53. Hernando R, Manso R (1997) Muscle fibre stress in response to exercise: synthesis, accumulation and isoform transitions of 70-kDa heat-shock proteins. Eur J Biochem 243: 460–467.
54. Larkins NT, Murphy RM, Lamb GD (2012) Absolute amounts and diffusibility of HSP72, HSP25, and alphaB-crystallin in fast- and slow-twitch skeletal muscle fibers of rat. Am J Physiol Cell Physiol 302: C228–239.
55. Locke M, Noble EG, Atkinson BG (1991) Inducible isoform of HSP70 is constitutively expressed in a muscle fiber type specific pattern. Am J Physiol 261: C774–779.
56. Tupling AR, Bombardier E, Stewart RD, Vigna C, Aqui AE (2007) Muscle fiber type-specific response of Hsp70 expression in human quadriceps following acute isometric exercise. J Appl Physiol (1985) 103: 2105–2111.
57. Cornelison DD, Wold BJ (1997) Single-cell analysis of regulatory gene expression in quiescent and activated mouse skeletal muscle satellite cells. Dev Biol 191: 270–283.
58. Yablonka-Reuveni Z, Rivera AJ (1994) Temporal expression of regulatory and structural muscle proteins during myogenesis of satellite cells on isolated adult rat fibers. Dev Biol 164: 588–603.
59. Hameed M, Orrell RW, Cobbold M, Goldspink G, Harridge SD (2003) Expression of IGF-I splice variants in young and old human skeletal muscle after high resistance exercise. J Physiol 547: 247–254.
60. Psilander N, Damsgaard R, Pilegaard H (2003) Resistance exercise alters MRF and IGF-I mRNA content in human skeletal muscle. J Appl Physiol 95: 1038–1044.
61. Liu Y, Mayr S, Opitz-Gress A, Zeller C, Lormes W, et al. (1999) Human skeletal muscle HSP70 response to training in highly trained rowers. J Appl Physiol 86: 101–104.

Resting Energy Expenditure Prediction in Recreational Athletes of 18–35 Years: Confirmation of Cunningham Equation and an Improved Weight-Based Alternative

Twan ten Haaf[1], Peter J. M. Weijs[1,2,3]*

1 Department of Nutrition & Dietetics, School of Sports and Nutrition, Amsterdam University of Applied Sciences, Amsterdam, The Netherlands, 2 Department of Nutrition & Dietetics, Internal Medicine, VU University Medical Center, Amsterdam, The Netherlands, 3 EMGO+ Institute for Health and Care Research, VU University Medical Center, Amsterdam, The Netherlands

Abstract

Introduction: Resting energy expenditure (REE) is expected to be higher in athletes because of their relatively high fat free mass (FFM). Therefore, REE predictive equation for recreational athletes may be required. The aim of this study was to validate existing REE predictive equations and to develop a new recreational athlete specific equation.

Methods: 90 (53M, 37F) adult athletes, exercising on average 9.1±5.0 hours a week and 5.0±1.8 times a week, were included. REE was measured using indirect calorimetry (Vmax Encore n29), FFM and FM were measured using air displacement plethysmography. Multiple linear regression analysis was used to develop a new FFM-based and weight-based REE predictive equation. The percentage accurate predictions (within 10% of measured REE), percentage bias, root mean square error and limits of agreement were calculated.

Results: The Cunningham equation and the new weight-based equation $REE(kJ/d) = 49.940^{*} weight(kg) + 2459.053^{*} height(m) - 34.014^{*} age(y) + 799.257^{*} sex(M=1, F=0) + 122.502$ and the new FFM-based equation $REE(kJ/d) = 95.272^{*} FFM(kg) + 2026.161$ performed equally well. De Lorenzo's equation predicted REE less accurate, but better than the other generally used REE predictive equations. Harris-Benedict, WHO, Schofield, Mifflin and Owen all showed less than 50% accuracy.

Conclusion: For a population of (Dutch) recreational athletes, the REE can accurately be predicted with the existing Cunningham equation. Since body composition measurement is not always possible, and other generally used equations fail, the new weight-based equation is advised for use in sports nutrition.

Editor: Marià Alemany, Faculty of Biology, Spain

Funding: These authors have no support or funding to report.

Competing Interests: The authors have declared that no competing interests exist.

* Email: p.j.m.weijs@hva.nl

Introduction

An optimal balance between energy intake and energy expenditure is crucial for athlete performance. Determining resting energy expenditure (REE) is essential for nutrition and exercise professionals in providing nutritional advice for athletes, since REE contributes to 60–70% of daily energy expenditure [1]. REE is the maintenance energy cost of the body in rest under steady state conditions. This is different from the minimal energy cost. Energy expenditure can for example be lower during sleep or during undernutrition [2]. REE can be measured through indirect calorimetry or estimated using REE predictive equations. The gold standard to determine the REE is measurement by indirect calorimetry. However, nutrition and exercise professionals do not usually have the necessary equipment. Moreover, indirect calorimetry [3] is expensive and requires trained personnel to guarantee the reliability. Therefore, predictive equations are most often used to estimate the REE.

In general, REE predictive equations can be considered population specific [4–8]. Because of their relatively high fat free mass (FFM), REE in athletes is underestimated by the majority of the existing equations [9]. Only a few studies have validated predictive equations in a group of athletes [10,11]. Thompson and Manore [11] concluded that the Cunningham equation was the most accurate equation, while LaForgia et al. [10] indicated the equation of De Lorenzo as the most accurate predictive equation. However, it should be noted that both studies investigated a different set of equations.

Cunninghams equation was established using 239 healthy adult subjects from the studies of Harris and Benedict [12], but they excluded 16 male subjects because they were identified as trained athletes. Moreover, the only factor included in the equation is lean body weight, but body composition measurements are not always possible in sports practice. Factors in De Lorenzo's equation are weight and height, which are better applicable in sports practice.

Moreover, the De Lorenzo equation is actually based on athletes [13]. However, the De Lorenzo equation was developed using the REE from 51 male athletes exercising at least 3 hours/day. This equation may therefore only apply to (sub) elite athletes while it may less accurately predict the REE for recreational athletes, which represent a significant part of the society. Therefore, the aim of this study was to validate existing resting energy expenditure predictive equations (Table 1) and to develop 2 new equations, specifically for recreational athletes. One equation was developed using FFM, since the body composition of (recreational) athletes differs from that of the average population. In addition, an equation was developed without FFM, since this parameter cannot always be used in sport practice. It was hypothesized that a new equation specifically developed for recreational athletes would result in better estimations of the resting energy expenditure.

Methods

103 athletes (age 18–35 y), who participated in sports for at least 3 hours a week and 2 times a week, participated in the study. Subjects were of self-reported stable weight, did not suffer from any metabolic disorders and did not take any medications affecting metabolic rate. They did not perform vigorous exercise within 12 hours before the measurement, neither did they consume food or beverages (except water) within 4 hours before the measurement. Subjects were at least 30 minutes at rest in the laboratory before the start of the measurement. 9 participants were excluded from analysis because they were in the ovulation phase of the menstrual cycle [14] and 4 were excluded because their Respiratory Exchange Ratio (RER) was below 0.7 or above 1.0 [15]. Finally, 90 athletes (Characteristics: Table 2; Sport specifications: Table 3; Age and Activity level: Figure 1) were included for validation and development of REE predictive equations. Mean (±SD) age was 23.2±4.8 year and mean REE was 7.68±1.16 MJ/day (1837±278 kcal/day). The training hours were 9.1±5.0 hours/week and the training frequency spent on sports was 5.0±1.8 times/week. Written informed consent was obtained from all subjects and the study was approved by the medical ethical committee of the VU University Medical Center (2009/302).

REE was calculated by the manufacturer's software, using oxygen consumption and carbon dioxide production measured by indirect calorimetry with a ventilated hood system (Vmax Encore n29; Viasys Healthcare, Houten, Netherlands). Calibration of the equipment with 2 different standard gases and 1 standard volume was performed on a daily basis, before starting the measurements. Additionally, an automatic recalibration of the system was done every 5 minutes. The subjects remained lying down but awake. The measurement took 30 minutes. Only steady state periods of measurement were selected according to the procedures for the ventilated hood system (<10% CV). The first 5 minutes of the measurements were discarded.

Body weight, FFM, and fat mass (FM) were determined using air displacement plethysmography (BODPOD, Life Measurement Inc, Concord, CA). Total lung volume was measured (31 were estimated) with the BODPOD system to correct total body volume. The BODPOD was calibrated on a daily basis directly before use. Height was measured by using a stadiometer (Seca 222; Seca; Hamburg; Germany).

Statistical analysis was performed using SPSS 20. Multiple linear regression analysis was used to develop 2 new REE predictive equations. Firstly, a stepwise regression approach was used with the variables FFM, FM, age, sex and a constant to verify a possible FFM-based REE equation. Weight-based equations are usually most successful when predictors of active cell mass are entered, being body weight, height, age and sex [16]. Therefore, these variables and a constant were used in a regression analysis. In both regression analyses, variables were included when the p-value for the F-test was smaller than 0.05.

The predicted REE from the 2 developed equations and from other commonly used equations (Table 4) were compared with the measured REE. Firstly, accuracy was calculated as the percentage of accurate REE predictions (within 10% of the measured REE). Secondly, the bias was calculated as the relative deviation (%) of the predicted REE from the measured REE. Thirdly, the root mean squared error (RMSE) was calculated as the expected absolute deviation (MJ/d) of the predicted REE from the measured REE. Lastly, limits of agreement were calculated as the 95% confidence interval of the bias.

Results

Using the previously described regression analyses, the following new equations were obtained (in kJ and kcal) for weight-based:

Table 1. Equations evaluated in this study.

Equation	Sample size	Remarks on population
Cunningham [17]	M=120 F=103	Healthy adults, trained athletes were excluded
De Lorenzo [13]	M=51	Athletes, exercising at least 3 hours a day
FAO [21]	N=11000	Mainly based on Schofield data, also including group mean values also
FAO (height) [21]	N=11000	Mainly based on Schofield data, also including group mean values
Harris-Benedict 1919 [21]	M=136 F=103	Mainly normal weight subject
Harris-Benedict 1984 [28]	M=168 F=169	Mainly normal weight subject
Mifflin [18]	M=251 F=247	Including obese subjects
Mifflin (FFM) [18]	M=251 F=247	Including obese subjects
Owen [19,20]	M=60 F=44	Including obese subjects
Owen (FFM) [19,20]	M=60 F=44	Including obese subjects
Schofield [29]	M=3575 F=1239	47% Italian subjects
Schofield (height) [29]	M=3575 F=1239	47% Italian subjects

Table 2. Subjects characteristics: mean ± standard deviation [range].

	Male (N = 53)		Female (N = 37)		Total (N = 90)	
Age (y)	23.1±4.7	[18–35]	23.5±5.0	[18–35]	23.2±4.8	[18–35]
Height (m)	1.82±.09	[1.63–2.05]	1.72±.05	[1.61–1.84]	1.78±.09	[1.61–2.05]
Weight (kg)	75.7±7.8	[62.1–100.3]	62.6±6.6	[52.8–78.3]	70.3±9.7	[52.8–100.3]
BMI (kg/m^2)	22.8±2.0	[18.6–27.0]	21.3±1.9	[17.9–26.7]	22.2±2.1	[17.9–27.0]
FFM (%)	88.3±4.9	[73.7–98.5]	78.4±4.7	[67.8–88.8]	84.3±6.8	[67.8–98.5]
FM (%)	11.7±4.9	[1.5–26.3]	21.6±4.7	[11.2–32.2]	15.7±6.8	[1.5–32.2]
REE (kcal/d)	2007±206	[1562–2551]	1594±162	[1111–1832]	1837±278	[1111–2551]
REE (MJ/d)	8.40±0.86	[6.53–10.67]	6.67±0.68	[4.65–7.67]	7.69±1.16	[4.65–10.67]
Activity (h/week)	10.0±5.4	[3.0–28.0]	7.9±4.0	[3.0–18.0]	9.1±5.0	[3.0–28.0]
Activity (#/week)	5.3±1.8	[2–12]	4.5±1.7	[2–9]	5.0±1.8	[2–12]

BMI: Body mass index, FFM: Fat free mass, FM: Fat mass, REE: Resting energy expenditure.

$$REE(kJ/d) = 49.940^{*} weight(kg) + 2459.053^{*} height(m) - 34.014^{*} age(y) + 799.257^{*} sex(M=1, F=0) + 122.502$$

or,

$$REE(kcal/d) = 11.936^{*} weight(kg) + 587.728^{*} height(m) - 8.129^{*} age(y) + 191.027^{*} sex(M=1, F=0) + 29.279$$

and FFM-based:

$$REE(kJ/d) = 95.272^{*} FFM(kg) + 2026.161$$

or,

$$REE(kcal/d) = 22.771^{*} FFM(kg) + 484.264$$

The weight-based equation for resting energy expenditure included body weight (kilograms), body height (meters), age (years), sex (value 1 for male, value 0 for female) and a constant. The fat free mass based equation only included fat free mass (kilograms) and a constant. The predicted REE values are plotted against measured REE values (Figure 2).

The accuracy for all equations is depicted in Figure 3B. The Cunningham equation resulted in the highest percentage accurate predicted equations (M 84.9%; F 78.4%), followed by the weight-based equation (M 83.0%; F 75.7%) and the FFM-based equation (M 83.0%; F 72.3%). The De Lorenzo equation for elite male athletes (M 77.4%; F 59.5%) had an inferior accuracy compared to the weight-based equation. All other, generally used equations showed less than 50% accuracy.

Equal to the accuracy, lowest bias was observed for Cunningham, both new equations and De Lorenzo (Figure 3A). The low bias for De Lorenzo's equation was based on opposite bias (male: negative, female: positive). Since this is not a cross-validation study, the bias for the new equations approached zero.

The FFM-based equation resulted in the lowest RMSE (M 0.62 MJ/d; F 0.57 MJ/d), and Cunningham's and the weight-based equation resulted in a comparable RMSE (Figure 3C). The RMSE for De Lorenzo was higher (M 0.74 MJ/d; F 0.77 MJ/d).

Table 3. Description of sports activity.

	Male (N = 53)	Female(N = 37)	Total (N = 90)
Athletics Long distance	5	9	14
Athletics Sprint	3	2	5
Cycling	6	4	10
Gymnastics	4	5	9
Fitness	3	5	8
Rowing/canoeing	7	5	12
Swimming	2	1	3
Team sports*	17	4	21
Remaining sports**	6	2	8

* Hockey, korfball, soccer, volleyball.
** Dancing, martial arts, skating, tennis.

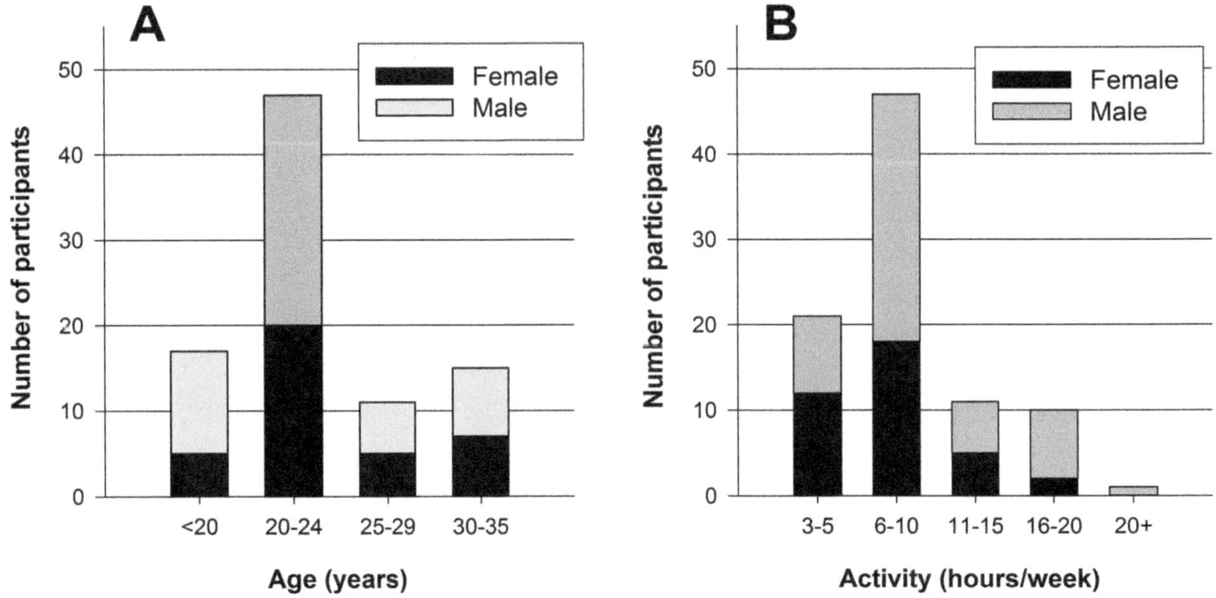

Figure 1. Description of the study participants (N = 90) for (A) age group and (B) activity level (hours per week).

The generally used equations all resulted in RMSE larger than 0.95 MJ/day.

In Figure 4 the errors are plotted against the individual measured REE for 6 equations. A negative proportional bias could be observed for all equations, meaning the equations tended to underestimate a higher REE.

Discussion

The purpose of this study was to validate existing predictive equations for REE and to develop and validate 2 new equations, specifically for recreational athletes. This study shows that the new FFM-based equation provides the best prediction of REE in recreational athletes. The weight-based equation and Cunningham's equation [17] performed equally well. De Lorenzo's equation [13] performed less, and can be improved by the new weight-based equation. The other generally used REE predictive equations have low accuracy in recreational athletes.

Although the Cunningham equation was developed in a general population, this equation performed better than the already existing equations. This suggests that FFM is an important predictor of REE for a population of recreational athletes. However, the FFM-based equations from Mifflin [18] and Owen [19,20] did perform worse than the new weight-based equation and De Lorenzo's equation [13], and not better than the other non-FFM equations. The difference of those equations with Cunningham [17] and the new FFM-based equation might be explained by the population that was used to develop the equations. Mifflin [18] and Owen [19,20] used lean and obese subjects. The mean BMI in Mifflin's study was 27.5±4.1 kg/m^2 for male and 26.2±4.9 kg/m^2 for female, with a maximum of 42 kg/m^2. In Owen's study, the BMI for male was 28.2±7.5 kg/m^2 and 27.8±8.6 kg/m^2 for female, with a maximum of 58.7 kg/m^2. Therefore, the better performance of the new FFM-based and Cunningham's equation over the weight and/or height based equations might result from the different body composition of (recreational) athletes compared with a general population.

De Lorenzo's equation [13] is the only equation which is actually based on a population of athletes. The accuracy was higher than the other generally used equations, but lower than Cunningham and the new developed equations. The participants in the study of De Lorenzo exercised at least 3 hours/day. The equation includes body weight and height and probably these factors do not predict resting energy expenditure well in recreational athletes due to a substantial different body composition. This emphasises the role of the specificity of the population. Other studies have pointed out that the accuracy of a prediction equation not only depends on activity level. For example, Henry [2] described the inaccuracy of the FAO equations [21] for many communities. The population used to develop the FAO equations consisted of a disproportional number of Italians, who seem to have a higher basal metabolic rate then people living in the tropical area, China or Australia. Another example of the specific accuracy of REE prediction equation is depicted by Weijs [5], who showed differences between US and Dutch obese adults. As a consequence of the specificity of a REE equation, a researcher always has to deal with a trade-off between internal and external validity (i.e. the more homogeneous the population, the more accurate the REE prediction but the less applicable to a heterogeneous population). Therefore, validation of the new equations in other cohorts is needed.

This study has some major limitations. Firstly, participants were instructed to not perform vigorous exercise within 12 hours before the measurement. However, Compher et al. [15] advised to perform no physical activity 14 hours prior to indirect calorimetry measurement to have energy expenditure returned to baseline levels. Physical activity will increase REE after exercise [22,23]. The time needed for REE to return to normal is called recovery time, which is dependent on the type of activity, intensity, duration and physical exercise level. In trained individuals, like in this study, recovery time is shorter than in untrained [15]. The study upon which the advice of 14 hours is based, included only 10 subjects [24]. Another small, but well designed study [25] used a 12 hour recovery time for different levels of activity, and showed no effect of physical activity on REE. Therefore, a period of 12 hours was selected for the present study.

Table 4. Resting energy expenditure prediction equations given in their original unit (kcal/day, except Schofield (MJ/day)).

Name	Equation
Cunningham	22(FFM) +500
De Lorenzo	9(wt) +1170(ht) −857
FAO	
Male (18–30 y)	15.3(wt) +679
Male (30–60 y)	11.6(wt) +879
Male (>60 y)	13.5(wt) +487
Female (18–30 y)	14.7(wt) +496
Female (30–60 y)	8.7(wt) +829
Female (>60 y)	10.5(wt) +596
FAO (height)	
Male (18–30 y)	15.4(wt) −27(ht) +717
Male (30–60 y)	11.3(wt) −16(ht) +901
Male (>60 y)	8.8(wt) + 1128(ht) −1071
Female (18–30 y)	13.3(wt) +334(ht) +35
Female (30–60 y)	8.7(wt) −25(ht) +865
Female (>60 y)	9.2(wt) + 637(ht) −302
Harris-Benedict 1919	
Male	13.75(wt) +500.33(ht) −6.76(age) +66.47
Female	9.56(wt) +184.96(ht) −4.68(age) +655.10
Harris-Benedict 1984	
Male	13.40(wt) +479.9(ht) −5.68(age) +88.36
Female	9.25(wt) +309.8(ht) −4.33(age) +477.59
Mifflin	9.99(wt) +625(ht) −4.92(age) +166(gender) −161
Mifflin (FFM)	19.7(FFM) +413
Owen	
Male	10.2(wt) +879
Female	7.18(wt) +795
Owen (FFM)	
Male	22.3(FFM) +290
Female	19.7(FFM) +334
Schofield	
Male (18–30 y)	63(wt) +2896*
Male (30–60 y)	48(wt) +3653*
Male (>60 y)	49(wt) +2459*
Female (18–30 y)	62(wt) +2036*
Female (30–60 y)	34(wt) +3538*
Female (>60 y)	38(wt) +2755*
Schofield (height)	
Male (18–30 y)	63(wt) −42(ht) +2953*
Male (30–60 y)	48(wt) −11(ht) +3670*
Male (>60 y)	49(wt) +4068(ht) −3491*
Female (18–30 y)	62(wt) +1148(ht) +411*
Female (30–60 y)	34(wt) +6(ht) +3530*
Female (>60 y)	38(wt) +1917(ht) +74*

FFM: Fat free mass (kg); wt: weight (kg); ht: height (m); age (y); gender (0: female, 1: male).
* Equation for values in MJ/day.

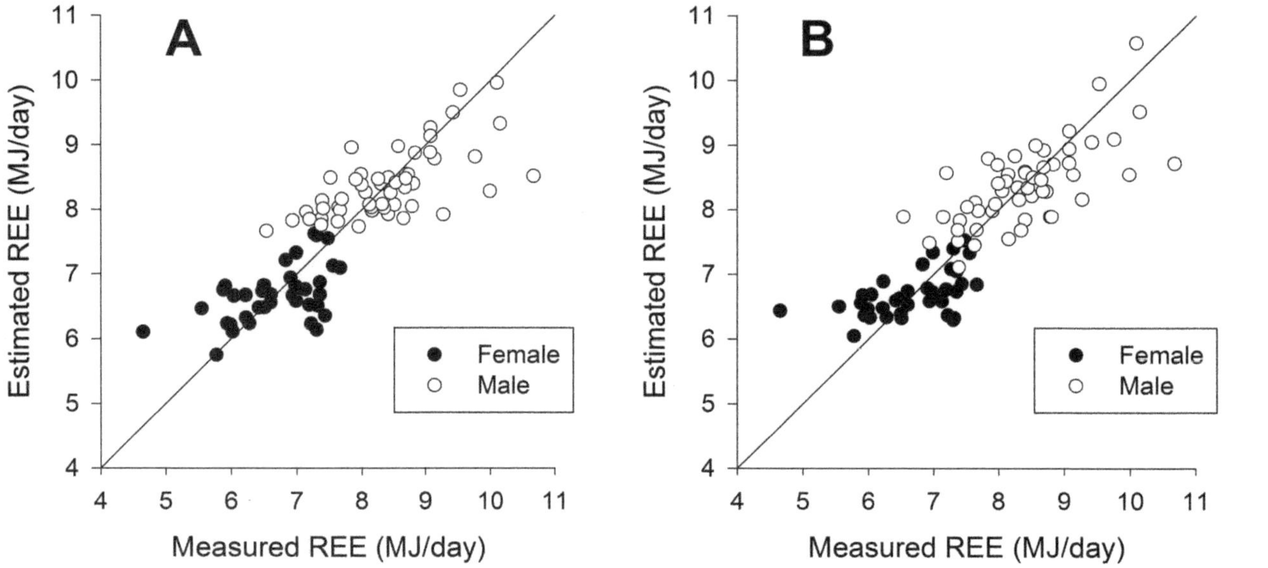

Figure 2. Predicted REE (MJ/day) plotted against REE (MJ/day) measured by indirect calorimetry for male (open dot) and female (filled dot). Graphs represent (A) the new weight-based and (B) the new FFM-based equation. The solid line is the line of identity.

Secondly, subjects were instructed to not eat within 4 hours prior to the measurement, while Compher et al. [15] recommended a minimal fast of 5 hours. However, they stated that for small meals a minimum fast of 4 hours is acceptable. Moreover, Weststrate [26,27] showed that the thermic effect of food could be nearly completed within 4 hour. The mean period of fasting by our subjects was on average 9.1±4.6 hours. Therefore, it is assumed that the thermic effect of food was negligible in this study.

Conclusions

In general, it is advised to use the REE prediction equation that is most specific for the target population. For a population of (Dutch) recreational athletes, the REE can accurately be predicted with the existing Cunningham equation. Since body composition measurement is not always possible, and other generally used equations fail, the new weight-based equation is advised for use in sports nutrition.

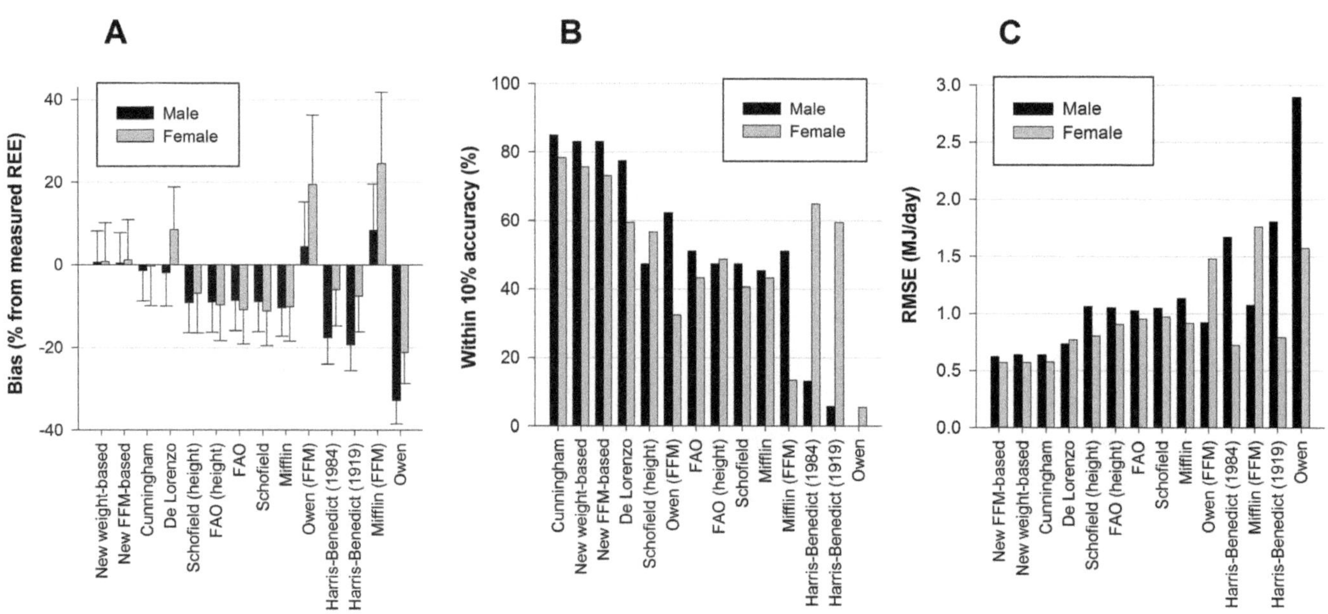

Figure 3. Outcome measures for the REE predictive equations for male (N = 53) and female (N = 37). The graphs represent (**A**) Percentage bias (±SD), (**B**) percentage accurate REE predictions and (**C**) Root mean squared error (MJ/day).

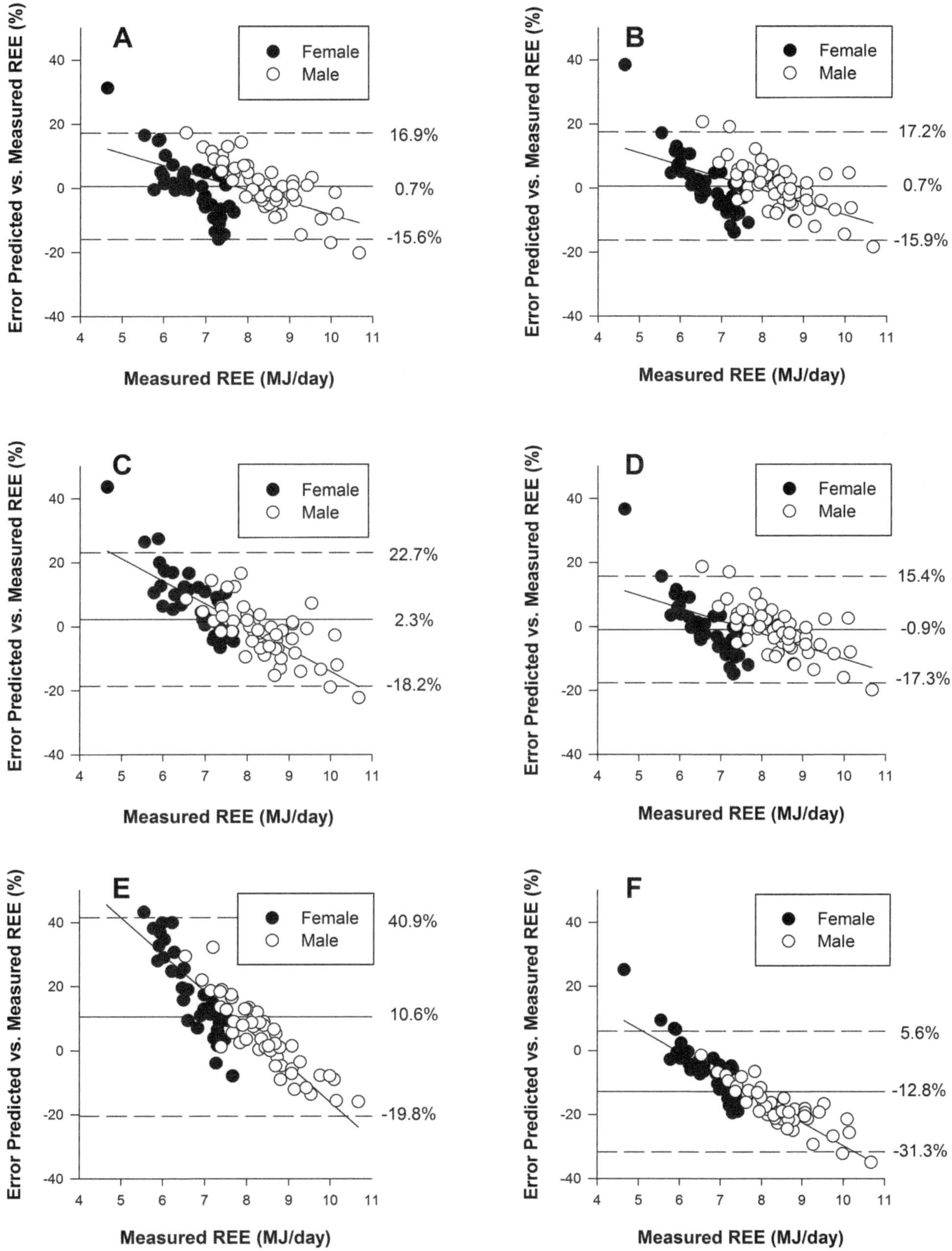

Figure 4. Limits of agreement analysis (bias: vertical solid line; 95% confidence interval: vertical dashed lines) for REE predictive equations versus measured REE (MJ/day) for male (open dot) and female (filled dot). Graphs represent equations of (**A**) new weight-based; (**B**) new FFM-based; (**C**) De Lorenzo; (**D**) Cunningham; (**E**) Owen FFM and (**F**) Harris-Benedict 1984.

Supporting Information

Dataset S1 Contains raw data used for development and testing of the prediction equations. The dataset contains information on gender; age; training volume; training frequency; weight; fat mass (%); fat mass (kg); fat free mass (kg); height; BMI; fat free mass (%) and measured REE (kJ) of the subjects.

Acknowledgments

We thank Marcel Hesseling for his help in the Nutritional Assessment Lab, all athletes for their participation, Anna Elisabeth van den Hoven, Jitske Spijker, Anne-Marijke Ambergen, Janine Reitsema, Jessica van Nieuwkerk, Maaike van Rijn, Astrid Schepers, Lisette van Wijk, Anneke Sman, Carine Bekenkamp, Antoinette Drexhage, Anousckha Severin and Martine Kampman for collecting part of the data, Amely Verreijen and Minse de Bos Kuil for their assistance.

Author Contributions

Conceived and designed the experiments: TtH PW. Analyzed the data: TtH PW. Wrote the paper: TtH PW.

References

1. Trexler ET, Smith-Ryan AE, Norton LE (2014) Metabolic adaptation to weight loss: implications for the athlete. J Int Soc Sports Nutr 11: 7–7.
2. Henry CJK (2005) Basal metabolic rate studies in humans: measurement and development of new equations. Public Health Nutr 8: 1133–1152.
3. Ferrannini E (1988) The theoretical bases of indirect calorimetry: A review. Metabolism 37: 287–301.
4. da Rocha EEM, Alves VGF, Silva MHN, Chiesa Ca, da Fonseca RBV (2005) Can measured resting energy expenditure be estimated by formulae in daily clinical nutrition practice? Curr Opin Clin Nutr Metab Care 8: 319–328.
5. Hofsteenge GH, Chinapaw MJ, Delemarre-van de Waal HA, Weijs PJ (2010) Validation of predictive equations for resting energy expenditure in obese adolescents. Am J Clin Nutr 91: 1244–1254.
6. Weijs PJM (2008) Validity of predictive equations for resting energy expenditure in US and Dutch overweight and obese class I and II adults aged 18–65 y. Am J Clin Nutr 88: 959–970.
7. Weijs PJM, Kruizenga HM, van Dijk AE, van der Meij BS, Langius JaE, et al. (2008) Validation of predictive equations for resting energy expenditure in adult outpatients and inpatients. Clin Nutr 27: 150–157.
8. Weijs PJM, Vansant GaaM (2010) Validity of predictive equations for resting energy expenditure in Belgian normal weight to morbid obese women. Clin Nutr 29: 347–351.
9. Dunford M (2006) Sports Nutrition. Chicago, USA: American Dietetic Association.
10. LaForgia J, Withers RT, Van der Ploeg GE, Gunn SM (2000) The accuracy of resting metabolic rate prediction equations in male athletes. Proc Nutr Soc Aust 24: 127–127.
11. Thompson J, Manore MM (1996) Predicted and measured resting metabolic rate of male and female endurance athletes. J Am Diet Assoc 96: 30–34.
12. Harris JA, Benedict FG (1919) A biometric study of basal metabolism in man. Washington DC: Carnegue Institution of Washington.
13. De Lorenzo A, Bertini L, Candeloro N, Piccinelli R, Innocente L, et al. (1999) A new predictive equation to calculate resting metabolic rate in athletes. J Sports Med Phys Fitness 39: 213–219.
14. Henry CJK, Lightowler HJ, Marchini J (2003) Intra-individual variation in resting metabolic rate during the menstrual cycle. Br J Nutr 89: 811–817.
15. Compher C, Frankenfield D, Keim N, Roth-Yousey L (2006) Best practice methods to apply to measurement of resting metabolic rate in adults: A systematic review. J Am Diet Assoc 106: 881–903.
16. Korth O, Bosy-Westphal A, Zschoche P, Glüer CC, Heller M, et al. (2007) Influence of methods used in body composition analysis on the prediction of resting energy expenditure. Eur J Clin Nutr 61: 582–589.
17. Cunningham JJ (1980) A reanalysis of the factors influencing basal metabolic rate in normal adults. Am J Clin Nutr 33: 2372–2374.
18. Mifflin MD, St Jeor ST, Hill LA, Scott BJ, Daugherty SA, et al. (1990) A new predictive equation for resting energy expenditure in healthy individuals. Am J Clin Nutr 51: 241–247.
19. Owen OE, Holup JL, D'Alessio Da, Craig ES, Polansky M, et al. (1987) A reappraisal of the caloric requirements of men. Am J Clin Nutr 46: 875–885.
20. Owen OE, Kavle E, Owen RS (1986) A reappraisal of caloric requirements in healthy women. Am J Clin Nutr 44: 1–19.
21. FAO/WHO/UNU (1985) Energy and protein requirements: Report of a joint FAO/WHO/UNU expert consultation. Geneva, Switzerland. pp.1–206.
22. Horton TJ, Geissler CA (1994) Effect of habitual exercise on daily energy expenditure and metabolic rate during standardized activity. Am J Clin Nutr 59: 13–19.
23. Poehlman ET, Melby CL, Badylak SF (1988) Resting metabolic rate and postprandial thermogenesis in highly trained and untrained males. Am J Clin Nutr 47: 793–798.
24. Short KR, Wiest JM, Sedlock DA (1996) The effect of upper body exercise intensity and duration on post-exercise oxygen consumption. Int J Sports Med 17: 559–563.
25. Weststrate JA, Weys P, Poortvliet E, Deurenberg P, Hautvast JG (1990) Lack of a systematic sustained effect of prolonged exercise bouts on resting metabolic rate in fasting subjects. Eur J Clin Nutr 44: 91–97.
26. Weststrate JA (1993) Original Resting metabolic a methodological Communications rate and diet-induced thermogenesis. Am J Clin Nutr 58: 592–601.
27. Weststrate JA, Weijs PJ, Poortvliet EJ, Deurenberg P, Hautvast JG (1989) Diurnal variation in postabsorptive resting metabolic rate and diet-induced thermogenesis. Am J Clin Nutr 50: 908–914.

14

Direct Proof of the *In Vivo* Pathogenic Role of the AChR Autoantibodies from Myasthenia Gravis Patients

Gregory Kordas[1], George Lagoumintzis[1], Sotirios Sideris[1], Konstantinos Poulas[1]*, Socrates J. Tzartos[1,2]*

1 Department of Pharmacy, University of Patras, Patras, Greece, 2 Department of Biochemistry, Hellenic Pasteur Institute, Athens, Greece

Abstract

Several studies have suggested that the autoantibodies (autoAbs) against muscle acetylcholine receptor (AChR) of myasthenia gravis (MG) patients are the main pathogenic factor in MG; however, this belief has not yet been confirmed with direct observations. Although animals immunized with AChR or injected with anti-AChR monoclonal Abs, or with crude human MG Ig fractions exhibit MG symptoms, the pathogenic role of isolated anti-AChR autoAbs, and, more importantly, the absence of pathogenic factor(s) in the autoAb-depleted MG sera has not yet been shown by *in vivo* studies. Using recombinant extracellular domains of the human AChR α and β subunits, we have isolated autoAbs from the sera of four MG patients. The ability of these isolated anti-subunit Abs and of the Ab-depleted sera to passively transfer experimental autoimmune MG in Lewis rats was investigated. We found that the isolated anti-subunit Abs were at least as efficient as the corresponding whole sera or whole Ig in causing experimental MG. Abs to both α- and β-subunit were pathogenic although the anti-α-subunit were much more efficient than the anti-β-subunit ones. Interestingly, the autoAb-depleted sera were free of pathogenic activity. The later suggests that the myasthenogenic potency of the studied anti-AChR MG sera is totally due to their anti-AChR autoAbs, and therefore selective elimination of the anti-AChR autoAbs from MG patients may be an efficient therapy for MG.

Editor: William Phillips, University of Sydney, Australia

Funding: This work was funded by the Muscular Dystrophy Association of USA (MDA), the Fight-MG grant of the FP7 EC program, the Association Francaise contre les Myopathies (AFM), and by the Greek national funds through the Operational Program "Education and Lifelong Learning" of the National Strategic Reference Framework (NSRF) Research Funding Program: THALES. The funders had no role in study design, data collection and analysis, decision to publish, or preparation of the manuscript.

Competing Interests: The authors have declared that no competing interests exist.

* Email: stzartos@gmail.com (ST); kpoulas@upatras.gr (KP)

Introduction

Myasthenia gravis (MG) is considered the classical organ specific, autoantibody-mediated, and T cell dependent human autoimmune disease [1–6]. MG is associated with autoantibodies (autoAbs) against the acetylcholine receptor (AChR) of the neuromuscular junction (NMJ). These autoAbs are found in approximately 85% of the patients with generalized MG (AChR-MG) [1,2], while the remaining ~15% of MG patients have autoAbs to additional NMJ proteins: MuSK (Muscle-Specific Kinase) [7–9] and LRP4 (lipoprotein receptor-related protein) [10,11] or not yet detectable autoAbs [12]. MG patients are suffering from fatigability and weakness of skeletal muscles, usually due to destruction of the AChRs in the NMJ [2–4,13].

The AChR located in the muscle endplates is a ligand-gated ion channel formed by five homologous subunits with stoichiometry $\alpha_2\beta\gamma\delta$ in the embryos and $\alpha_2\beta\varepsilon\delta$ in the adults. The subunits are arranged symmetrically around a central pore and are embedded in the postsynaptic muscle membrane, with their extracellular domains (ECDs) oriented in the synaptic space. Muscle AChRs bear one binding site per α-subunit for acetylcholine (ACh), the neurotransmitter which is responsible for the transmission of the nerve impulse to the muscle fibers [14,15].

The autoimmune nature of the MG has been proved by several observations supporting the role of anti-AChR autoAbs in the pathogenesis of MG. AChR-MG patients have serum circulating anti-AChR autoAbs, detected also at the NMJ. Moreover, patients' clinical picture improves after plasma or IgG apheresis [16,17]. Transplacental transfer of IgG (including anti-AChR autoAbs) from MG mothers to infants is thought to be responsible for the transient MG observed in the newborns [18,19]. Moreover, the disease can be reproduced in animal models (experimental autoimmune MG, EAMG) either by active immunization with AChR (whole or parts of it) [20–22], or by passive transfer of MG sera [23–25] and monoclonal Abs (mAbs) against the AChR [26,27]. However, although it is clear that animal anti-AChR autoAbs can cause EAMG, it has not yet been directly shown whether the anti-AChR Ab fraction of MG patients' sera is indeed the only or at least the main pathogenic factor in these sera.

The anti-AChR autoAbs in sera of MG patients appear heterogeneous in terms of epitope binding [28]. A large fraction of the autoAbs is directed against a specific region, located at the α-subunits called main immunogenic region (MIR) [29,30]. The MIR is believed to consist of a group of overlapping conformation-dependent epitopes around the 67–76 amino acids of the ECD of the α-subunits, but additional segments also contribute to this antigenic region [31,32]. Its antigenic structure is favored by its position near the synaptic end. In addition to the MIR region, autoAbs against the rest of the α-subunit and the other subunits have also been identified [33,34]. Moreover *E. coli*- and *P.*

pastoris-expressed ECDs of the five human AChR subunits bind anti-AChR autoAbs from various MG sera, underlying the heterogeneity and the variable antigenic specificity of these autoAbs [35].

Epitope variability may explain the lack of correlation between patients' serum autoAb titers and their clinical condition. Indeed, passive transfer experiments with MG sera have demonstrated the induction of the disease only from certain sera [36]. In addition, passive transfer of the disease with mAbs against the AChR has been observed mostly with the use of anti-MIR Abs [26]. In this paper, we isolated autoAbs from the sera of four MG patients using recombinant human α- and β-AChR ECDs. We subsequently tested the ability of the purified autoAbs as well as those of the intact and autoAb-depleted sera to induce EAMG when injected intraperitoneally (*i.p.*) to Lewis rats. Whole sera and purified AChR subunit-specific autoAbs could induce EAMG, whereas the autoAb-depleted sera could not; the latter directly shows that the myasthenic potency of AChR-MG sera is due to their anti-AChR autoAbs. In addition, we showed that the anti-α subunit autoAbs are not the only pathogenic anti-AChR autoAbs though they are much more capable in inducing MG than the anti-β ones.

Materials and Methods

Ethics Statement

Animal experiments were conducted at the Hellenic Pasteur Institute (rat injections, anesthesia and sacrificing) under a protocol approved by the Hellenic Pasteur Institute Animal Care and Use Committee. Anti-AChR auto-Abs isolation from MG sera was performed at the University of Patras. Use of human biological samples was approved by the Bioethics Committee of the Hellenic Pasteur Institute (Permit No. 1288). Written informed consent was taken from all donors participating in this study.

Animals

Lewis rats, 3–4 weeks old, were used. Animals were housed in groups of 4 animals per standard cage in a climate-controlled room on a 12:12 h light:dark cycle with water and standard rodent chow. General anesthesia during animal procedures was provided using Diethyl ether.

MG sera and evaluation of the autoAb titer

Large plasma volumes from MG patients were collected during therapeutic plasmapheresis procedure at the Department of Clinical Therapeutics, Renal Unit, Alexandra Hospital, Athens, Greece. MG serum samples used were from a large number of anti-AChR autoAb-positive sera held in our laboratory at the Hellenic Pasteur Institute for diagnostic purposes as previously described [37]. For simplicity we will use the term "serum" for both plasma and serum. All four patients whose sera were used in this study had generalized mild to moderate MG symptoms (MGFA grades II–III). Interestingly patients MG1 and MG2 (with predominantly anti-α antibodies) had not more severe symptoms than patients MG3 and MG4 (with predominantly anti-β antibodies).

The anti-AChR autoAb titers of the MG sera used in this study were determined by the anti-AChR autoAb assay kit (RSR Ltd, Cardiff, UK) according to the manufacturer's instructions with slight modifications, as previously described [38]. Briefly, the diluted sera or isolated autoAbs [supplemented with NHS (normal human serum) to total 5 μl serum] were incubated overnight at 4°C with 25 μl (about 35,000 cpm) of ^{125}I-AChR solution [^{125}I-α-Bgtx (alpha-bungarotoxin) labeled AChR], and the ^{125}I-AChR-Ab complexes were precipitated by incubation for 2 h at 4°C with 25 μl of goat anti-human IgG serum. The precipitated radioactivity was measured in a γ-counter (2470 WIZARD^2 TM). To test the cross-reactivity of the MG anti-AChR autoAbs with rat AChR, 20 μl of rat muscle extract containing 60 fmol of rat AChR was labeled with approximately 0.1 pmol of ^{125}I-α-Bgtx (~50,000 cpm). After the addition of MG sera or isolated autoAbs (supplemented with NHS to total 5 μl serum), the samples were incubated at 4°C overnight. Antibody-AChR complexes were precipitated by adding 25 μl of goat anti-human IgG serum. The pellets were washed twice with PBS, pH 7.4, 0.5% Triton X-100 and the radioactivity was counted in a γ-counter. Anti-AChR autoAb titers were expressed as nano moles of ^{125}I-α-Bgtx binding sites precipitated per liter of serum (nM).

Competition experiment of serum autoAbs and ^{125}I-α-Bgtx

Human AChR (RSR Ltd, Cardiff, UK) was added to 5 μl serum (mixture of a predetermined quantity of MG1 serum supplemented with NHS to reach the 5 μl). After incubation for 1.5 h, ^{125}I-labeled α-Bgtx (70,000 cpm) was added for 1 h at room temperature. In parallel human AChR was firstly incubated with the ^{125}I-labeled α-Bgtx for 1 h followed by the addition of the MG serum and further incubation for 1.5 h. Complexes were precipitated with goat anti-human serum and the precipitated radioactivity was measured in a γ-counter.

E. coli-expressed ECDs and construction of affinity chromatography CNBr-Sepharose beads columns

Recombinant *E. coli*-expressed human α and β ECDs (α1-210 and β1-221with N-terminal 6×His tag sequence) were produced by growing pET15b/ECD-transformed *BL21(pLysS)DE3* cells as previously described [38]. Purification was performed following the manufacturer's instructions for binding to, and elution from, Ni-NTA (Nickel- Nitrilotriacetic acid) beads (Qiagen). The purified ECDs were used for the construction of CNBr (Cyanogen bromide) -Sepharose columns, in a final concentration 1 mg ECD per mL CNBr-Sepharose according to the manufacturer (Pharmacia-Biotech) guidelines and as previously described [38].

Ig purification by saturated ammonium sulphate

A maximum of 2 ml of MG serum per animal was used for passive transfer experiments. When serum volumes greater than 2 ml had to be used, the Ig of the serum were isolated and concentrated by ammonium sulphate precipitation (40% saturation). When the needed final volume of the precipitated Ig per animal was over 2 ml, it was further concentrated by dialysis membrane covered with polyethelenglycol 40,000.

Affinity purification of the anti-ECD autoAbs

Immunoadsorption experiments were performed by incubating a certain volume of each MG serum or Ig fraction overnight at 4°C with gentle agitation with the appropriate ECD-Sepharose suspension, capable of removing all of the corresponding anti-ECD specific autoAbs (approximately 1 μg of ECD per 2.1 pmol of autoAbs). The reduction in the amount of serum autoAbs represents the fraction of autoAbs in the treated serum reactive with the ECD used. The α- or β-ECD-Sepharose beads with the bound autoAbs were washed three times with PBS and the bound autoAbs were rapidly released from the Sepharose beads by incubation for 5 to 10 seconds at room temperature with 0.2 M glycine-HCl, pH 2.8; then 1/15 volume of 1 M Tris-HCl pH 9.0 was immediately added to the isolated autoAbs to raise the pH, and the samples were extensively dialyzed against PBS, pH 7.4. Finally, the isolated autoAbs and the depleted sera or Ig fractions were tested for binding to the human and rat AChR by radioimmunoassay (RIA), using ^{125}I-α-Bgtx labeled AChR (see above).

Passive transfer of MG - Clinical assessment

Three to four weeks old Lewis rats were injected *i.p.* with MG serum or serum derivatives, as follows: groups of 3–5 animals were injected with whole serum isolated anti-subunit autoAbs (anti-α or anti-β), depleted sera (without the anti-α or anti-β autoAbs) or with NHS or PBS, as negative controls. Each animal was weighted at the beginning of the experiment and every 24 hours, unless otherwise stated. For clinical examination, rats were evaluated for myasthenic weakness and assigned clinical scores. Briefly, rats were observed on a flat platform for a total of 2 min. They were then exercised by gently dragging them suspended by the tip of the tail across a cage top grid repeatedly (20–30 times) as they attempted to grip the grid. They were then placed on a flat platform for 2 min and again observed for signs of EAMG. Clinical muscle weakness was graded as follows: grade 0, rat with normal posture, muscle strength, and mobility at baseline and after exercise; grade 1, normal at rest but with muscle weakness characteristically shown by a hunchback posture, restricted mobility, and difficulty in raising the head after exercise; grade 2, grade 1 symptoms without exercise during observation period; grade 3, dehydrated and moribund with grade 2 weakness; and grade 4, dead. The evaluator was blinded to treatment status for all clinical evaluations.

Quantification of muscle AChR content

All groups of rats injected with MG sera (MG1–MG4) and their derivatives (autoAb-depleted sera and anti-subunit isolated Abs) as well as the control groups (injected with NHS and PBS) were sacrificed 48 h post-injection. The hind limb muscles of each rat were dissected, weighed and homogenized with a commercial blender using liquid nitrogen to freeze the tissues. The homogenates were then washed twice, using two volumes per muscle net weight (ml/g) of the following buffer: 0.1 M NaCl, 0.01 M Na_2HPO_4-NaH_2PO_4, 0.01 M EDTA, 0.01 M EGTA, 0.001 M PMSF, 0.1 M iodoacetamide, 0.05% NaN_3, 5 U/ml of aprotinin and 0.5 μg/ml of pepstatin, pH 7.4. The pellet was resuspended in an equal volume of 2% Triton X-100 regarding to its weight, in the previous buffer and incubated overnight at 4°C, with gentle agitation. After centrifugation (12,000 g for 30 min) to remove insoluble material, the muscle AChR content was determined as previously described by Lindstrom *et al.*, [39]. In brief, 20 μl aliquots of each muscle extract were labelled with 0.1 pmol of ^{125}I-α-Bgtx and the complexes precipitated using an excess of a mixture of mAbs 192, 195 and 198 followed by the addition of anti-rat IgG, incubation, washing and counting the radioactivity of the pellets. The decrease in the ratio of the Δcpm of samples from autoAb treated animals *versus* Δcpm of samples from control animals was interpreted as the Ab induced AChR-loss.

Confocal microscopy

In order to examine the physical association of MG sera and their derivatives with muscle AChRs at the NMJ, we performed *in vivo* immunofluorescence studies. Twelve hours post-injection groups of rats (2 rats per group) injected with either 0.3 ml MG1 serum or its derivatives (anti-α subunit depleted serum and isolated anti-α subunit Abs), and with Ig from 15 ml of MG3 serum or its derivatives (anti-β subunit depleted serum and isolated anti-β subunit Abs) were sacrificed and the hind limb muscles were isolated from. The hind limb muscle samples were frozen in cold isopentane and stored at −80°C. Ten μm thick sections were taken, allowed to air-dry, and fixed in cold acetone for 10 min. Then the sections were washed twice for 5 min with PBS, and blocked for 25 min with PBS-BSA 3% and FBS 10% (Cappel; MP Biomedicals). After being washed with PBS, the slides were incubated with Alexa Fluor 555-α-Bgtx (1/100) (Invitrogen) for binding on AChR and therefore to identify the NMJ endplates (red) and with F(ab2) donkey anti-human IgG FITC conjugated to identify human Abs (green) for 2 h at room temperature. Then, the slides were washed three times with PBS-Tween 0.1% for 5 min and viewed under a Leica TCS SP5 confocal microscope.

Statistical analysis

AChR loss and rat weight changes were evaluated for statistical significance using a two-tailed unpaired Student's *t*-test, using the Ms Excel 7.0 program.

Results

Selection of MG sera and their Ab specificities

Induction of passive EAMG in rats with obvious clinical symptoms by human MG sera is usually not trivial and requires several injections for several days. In order to achieve MG symptoms by single injections we used young rats (3–4-weeks old), and carefully selected MG sera. In order to select potent MG sera, first we screened over 100 MG sera for binding to both rat and human AChR by RIA. We found that the MG sera showed varying degree of Ab cross-reactivity between the two AChR species (data not shown). For the selection of the most appropriate sera we also took into account their ability to bind to the α- or β-subunit ECDs in order to allow us to isolate and study the corresponding antibody fractions. We finally selected four MG patients' sera (MG1–MG4) of moderate to high titers for rat AChR, for which we had large serum volumes available (Table 1). The selected MG sera were then tested for their autoAbs subunit specificity using immunoadsorbents with α- and β-ECDs. Table 1 shows the characteristics of the four MG sera in respect of autoAb specificities to the human α- or β- AChR subunit ECDs, as well as the cross-reactivity of these MG sera and their derivatives between human and rat AChR. Table 1 shows that their differences in anti-rat AChR titer are smaller than their differences in anti-human AChR titer. Almost half (48.1%) of the MG1 autoAbs are directed against the human α-ECD and are cross-reactive with rat AChR. The remaining anti-AChR Abs (anti-α depleted sera) are not cross-reactive with rat AChR. MG2 and MG3 sera contain autoAbs that bind exclusively α- and β- ECDs, respectively. Both sera (and their isolated autoAbs) were found cross reactive with rat AChR. MG4 serum has the majority of its anti-AChR Abs against the β- ECD (71.2%), while the remaining autoAbs are mainly against the α-ECD. MG4 serum and its derivatives (anti-β Ab depleted serum and isolated anti-β Abs) were all cross-reactive with rat AChR.

Passive transfer by MG sera and their derivatives into rats

We tested the ability of the purified Abs as well as of the intact and autoAb-depleted sera in inducing EAMG when injected *i.p.* to Lewis rats in a range of volumes. Disease severity was assessed on the basis of clinical symptoms and weight change. We initially performed preliminary experiments with the 4 MG sera by which we estimated the approximate volumes of each serum likely to produce clinical symptoms (data not shown). This information was used as a starting point for the below described experiments.

Table 1. Anti-AChR autoAb specificities and autoAb titers of MG sera and their derivatives[a].

MG serum samples	MG serum samples and derivatives	Anti-human AChR Ab titer (nM)	Subunit (ECDs) specificities (% of total anti-human AChR Abs)[b]		Anti-rat AChR Ab titer (nM)
			α subunit	β subunit	
MG1	Whole serum	1150	48.1	2.4	379
	Anti-α Abs depleted serum	596	0	2.4	0
	Isolated anti-α Abs	393	100	0	235
MG2	Whole serum	262	99.8	0	279
	Anti-α Abs depleted serum	0.2	0	0	0
	Isolated anti-α Abs	170	100	0	195
MG3	Whole serum	625	0	98.2	102
	Anti-β Abs depleted serum	0	0	0	0
	Isolated anti-β Abs	455	0	100	63
MG4	Whole serum	29.3	25.3	71.2	23.2
	Anti-β Abs depleted serum	8.4	87.8	0	7.3
	Isolated anti-β Abs	13.9	0	100	12.1

[a]The four MG sera were screened for their Ab specificities for AChR subunits using immunoadsorption ECD columns and the percentages of Ab subunit specificities are shown. The titers of the depleted sera and the isolated Abs are normalized to the corresponding whole serum volumes.
[b]test sera and Ab preparations were incubated with sepharose-immobilised ECDs and the anti-AChR titers of the depleted samples were estimated by RIA with intact AChR.

EAMG by MG1 and its derivatives. MG1 serum had the highest titer for both human and rat AChR among the 4 sera tested. Figure 1A–B show the different volumes of MG1 serum and its derivatives used in the passive transfer experiments, as well as the induced clinical symptoms. A volume of 0.4 ml MG1 whole serum (0.15 nmoles anti-rat AChR Abs) was capable in inducing death to all rats 48 h post-injection. However, Fig. 1A also shows that the anti-α-subunit depleted serum, at even higher volumes (0.4–0.8 ml/animal) was totally inefficient in causing EAMG. The isolated anti-α-subunit Abs (at amounts derived from serum volumes similar with those tested in Fig. 1A) overall were at least similarly efficient with the corresponding volumes of the intact serum (Fig. 1B). Figure 2 depicts the weight change of the group of rats injected with 0.8 ml anti-α depleted MG1 serum 48 h after the injection, while all rats injected with the other MG1 serum fractions had already died. All rats of the group injected with anti-α depleted MG1 serum increased their weight similarly to the control group of rats injected with NHS.

The fact that MG1 serum could induce MG-like symptoms in such small volumes led us to investigate the possibility that the anti-α Abs of MG1 act by blocking the acetylcholine binding site. We carried out a competition experiment between anti-AChR Abs and ^{125}I-α-Bgtx for binding to the AChR. Figure 3 shows that pre-incubation of the AChR with the MG1 serum did not inhibit ^{125}I-α-Bgtx binding to the AChR, suggesting that the MG1 Abs do not interfere with ACh activity.

EAMG by MG2 and its derivatives. Rats injected with 1 and 2 ml MG2 serum or Ig from 5 ml serum did not exhibit any MG-like symptoms (data not shown). On the contrary rats injected with Ig from higher serum volumes (10 ml), equivalent to 2.79 nmoles anti-rat AChR Abs, exhibited mild to moderate EAMG symptoms (Fig. 1C). The body weight of these groups of rats increased less than that of the control groups (Fig. 2). Interestingly the rats that were given purified anti-α Abs from 10 ml serum (1.95 nmoles anti-rat AChR Abs) exhibited severe symptoms (Fig. 1D) and lost dramatically weight (Fig. 2), 48 h post injection. We also injected one rat with anti-α subunit Abs isolated from 20 ml of MG2 serum as shown in Fig. 1D. We found that this rat showed severe MG symptoms and died before the lapse of 48 hours after injection. The anti-α depleted Ab MG fraction, when injected to rats caused no EAMG symptoms.

EAMG by MG3 and its derivatives. MG3 is a high Ab titer serum (625 nM) with autoAbs targeting exclusively the β AChR subunit. The Ig fraction of 4 and 8 ml of whole MG3 serum had no effect. A group of rats were then injected with the Ig fraction of 15 ml of whole MG3 serum corresponding to 1.53 nmoles anti-rat AChR Abs. As shown in Fig. 1E, they showed ambiguous MG symptoms and 48 h after injection they had recovered. The anti-β ECD Abs of 15 ml from MG3 serum were isolated and injected into rats, with none exhibiting any MG symptoms. The isolation of the anti-AChR Abs from the sera, allows using Abs derived from very large serum volumes, which is not possible with crude Ig. We could thus clarify whether MG3 Abs can indeed induce EAMG in rat. Antibodies from 40 ml of whole serum was isolated and injected into each of 2 rats (Fig. 1F), which showed mild MG symptoms within 24 h, while 48 h after injection they fully recovered, but their weight increased less gradually than the control rats (Fig. 2). As also shown in Fig. 1E, 15 ml of anti-β-depleted MG3 serum had no obvious clinical effect when tested in rats and these rats increased their weight normally (Fig. 2).

EAMG by MG4 and its derivatives. MG4 serum had the lowest anti-rat AChR Ab titer (23.2 nM) among the four sera tested in passive transfer experiments. As shown in Fig. 1G, one group of rats was injected with Ig from 5, 10 and 15 ml serum. None exhibited any kind of MG symptoms, and their weight increased similarly with that of the control rats (Fig. 2). In addition, as shown in Fig. 1G, we injected 3 rats and 2 rats with isolated anti-β subunit Abs from 15 ml and 45 ml of MG4 serum each, respectively. No rat showed any MG symptoms.

Muscle AChR content

Using an excess of a mixture of rat AChR specific mAbs, we estimated the content of muscle AChR of each rat group treated with MG sera and derivatives as compared to the control rat group

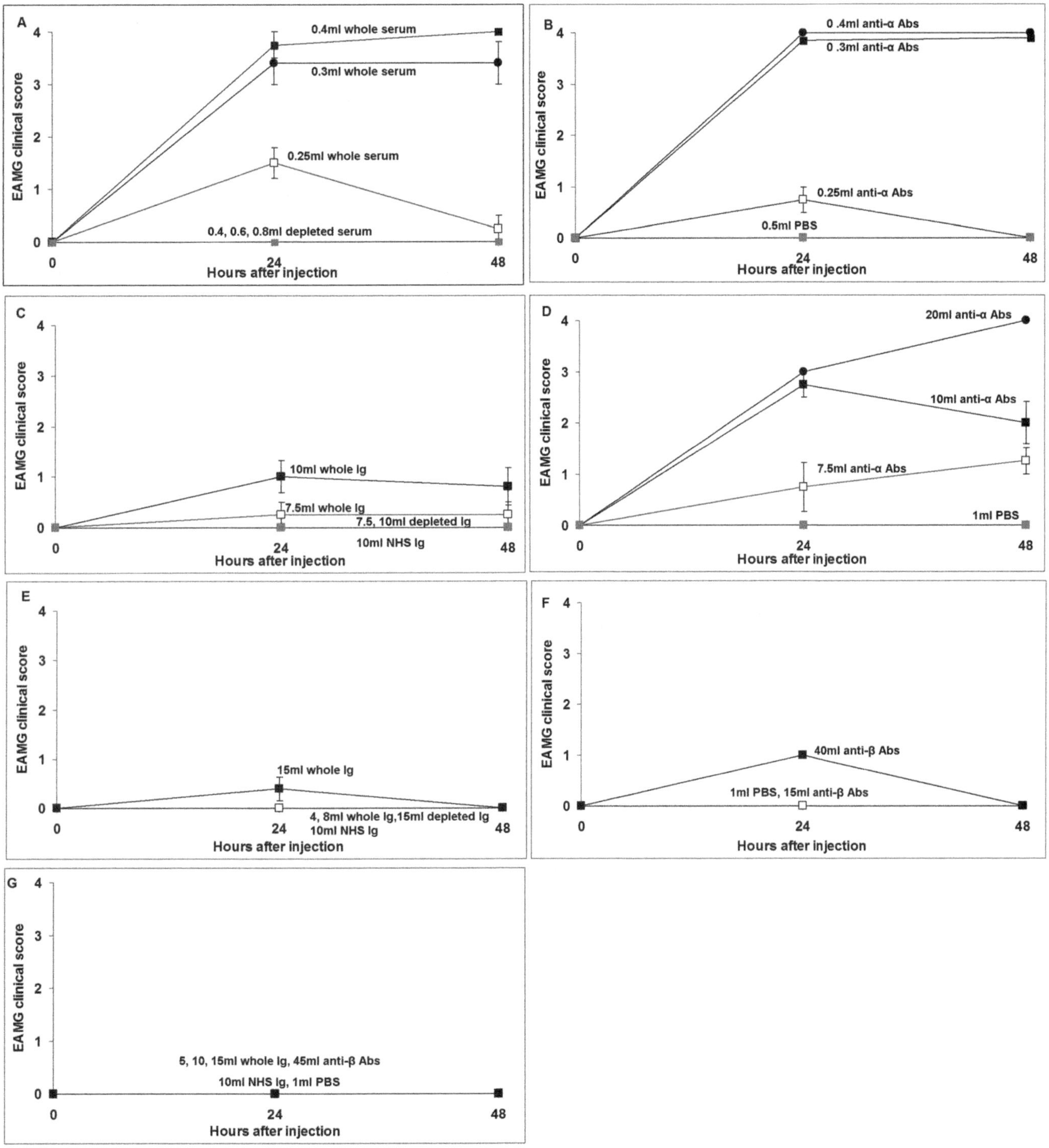

Figure 1. Clinical course of rats 24 and 48 h post-injection with MG sera and their derivatives. The figures show the clinical symptoms of groups of rats injected *i.p.* with the shown volumes of MG sera (or Ig), anti-α/β depleted sera (or Ig) and isolated autoAbs. **A–B:** EAMG-MG1; **C–D:** EAMG-MG2; **E–F:** EAMG-MG3; **G:** (EAMG-MG4). Control groups were injected with NHS and PBS. Disease severity was assessed on the basis of weakness and scored by their ability to grasp, hang and run when provoked: 0–4 (0: no clinical symptoms; 4: dead, see Methods). Points represent mean clinical scores ±SE.

(NHS or PBS) (Fig. 4). The muscle AChR content of the groups of rats injected with PBS are not represented in Fig. 4, as they had similar values to the NHS-treated rats. Administration of 0.25 ml of whole MG1 serum and anti-α subunit Abs isolated from 0.25 ml MG1, significantly reduced (~40%) the AChR molecules at the NMJ of the rats (Fig. 4a). The depleted of the anti-α AChR Abs serum and the control NHS did not cause any effect on rat AChR.

Total MG2 serum reduced the AChR content by about 40% compared to the AChR content of the controls as shown in Fig. 4b. Interestingly, the isolated anti-α Abs from 10 ml of MG2 serum reduced even more drastically the AChR content (~68%), although the actual AChR Ab amount injected to the rats was 30% lower than that of the 10 ml whole serum due to losses during Ab purification. Rats injected with anti-α depleted MG2 serum showed normal levels of AChR concentration.

Ig isolated from 15 ml whole MG3 serum and anti-β subunit Abs isolated from 40 ml MG3 serum both significantly reduced the number of AChRs compared to the anti-β MG3-depleted serum and the controls (NHS and PBS) as it is depicted in Fig. 4c. This confirms the MG symptoms, even though rather weak, induced by this anti-β-subunit serum as shown in Fig. 1E–F.

Whole MG4 serum (15 ml) and anti-β subunit isolated Abs from 45 ml MG4 serum reduced the numbers of AChR (Fig. 4d). Yet, the reduction was the lowest among the 4 MG sera (20–25%) apparently justifying the absence of symptoms in the rats (Fig. 1G).

Overall, the rats in which the antibodies induced <40% AChR loss did not exhibit significant clinical symptoms, whereas in those with >40% AChR loss, disease was observed. The rat group with the highest AChR loss (~68%) in Figure 4 (isolated Abs from MG2) suffered the most severe clinical score.

Detection of IgG deposits at the NMJ by immunofluorescence microscopy

The sections obtained from the rats injected with MG1 whole serum, pure anti-α subunit MG1 Abs, MG3 whole serum and pure anti-β subunit MG3 Abs showed considerable deposition of human IgG at the NMJs (Fig. 5, left and right upper two rows). On the contrary, the depleted MG1 and MG3 sera fractions as well as the control NHS showed little or no deposition at the neuromuscular endplates (Fig. 5, left and right bottom two rows).

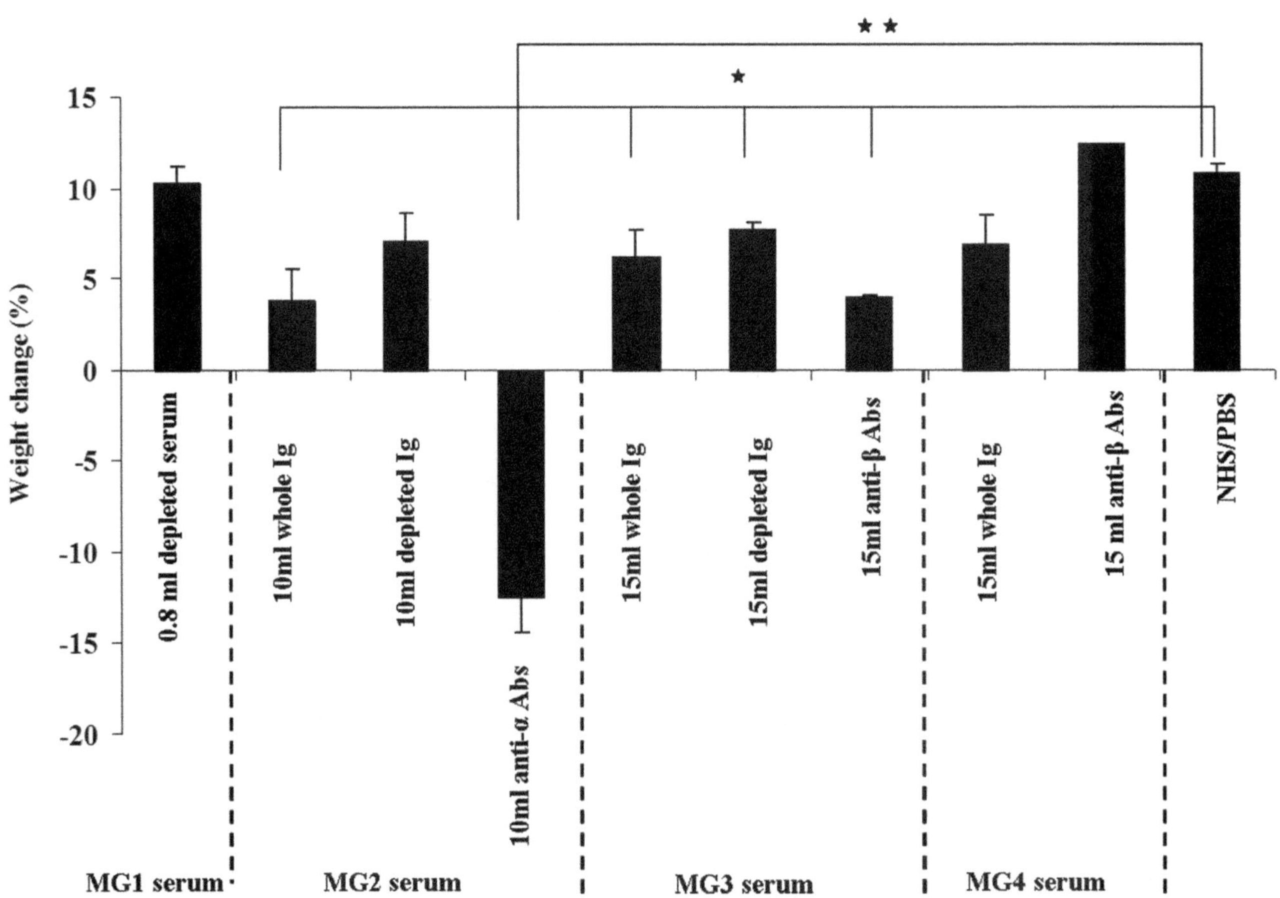

Figure 2. Weight change of rats treated with MG sera and their derivatives. The figures show the percent weight change of groups of rats injected *i.p.* with the shown volumes of MG sera, anti-α/β depleted sera and isolated autoAbs. Control groups were injected with NHS and PBS. Bars represent weight changes (% of controls) +SE, *p<0.05, **p<0.01.

Discussion

MG is an autoimmune disease usually characterized by the presence of autoAbs against the muscle AChR [2–6]. Animals' anti-AChR autoAbs have been clearly shown to cause active or passive EAMG (by immunization with AChR and injection with anti-AChR mAbs). Although MG sera and their isolated whole IgG fractions also induce MG symptoms into animal models, this does not exclude that Abs other than the anti-AChR autoAbs in these sera also contribute to the pathogenicity of the serum or even form the main pathogenic factor. Therefore, direct observation of the pathogenicity of the human MG autoAbs had yet to be achieved. Using recombinant bacterial expressed ECDs of the α and β subunits of human AChR we produced affinity chromatography columns and used them to isolate the anti-α ECD Abs from two MG sera (MG1 and MG2) and the anti-β ECD Abs from another two MG sera (MG3 and MG4). The isolated autoAbs (as well as the whole sera and the Ab-depleted sera) were tested for their ability in inducing EAMG into rats by passive transfer experiments.

Our results showed that the anti-α Abs isolated from MG1 and MG2 sera were capable of inducing severe MG symptoms and death into rats, at least as efficiently as the whole sera. Immunofluorescence studies of the rat hind limb muscles showed deposition of human IgG at muscle endplates, whereas measurements of AChR content showed that the bound anti-AChR autoAbs induced muscle AChR loss, apparently the cause of MG-like symptoms in the rats.

Here, we showed that the anti-α Abs of MG1 could induce severe MG symptoms or death, at approximately 30 times lower amount than anti-α Abs of MG2. This observation prompted us to investigate the possibility that the anti-α Abs of MG1 act by blocking the ACh binding site. We conducted a competition RIA between ^{125}I-α-Bgtx and MG serum and found that the serum autoAbs do not inhibit ^{125}I-α-Bgtx binding to the AChR. This suggests that no autoAbs of MG1 bind near or at the ACh binding site, and therefore their pathogenic effect is probably not due to inhibiting ion channel function.

The strong potency of the MG1 serum in causing EAMG was also tested in mice. Whole MG1 serum was tested in passive transfer experiments in a group of 4 Balb/c mice, 10 weeks old. The critical serum volume that caused death to mice was 0.6 ml, whereas in Lewis rats it was 0.3 ml (data not shown). Thus, although less efficient in mice than in rats (possibly because of

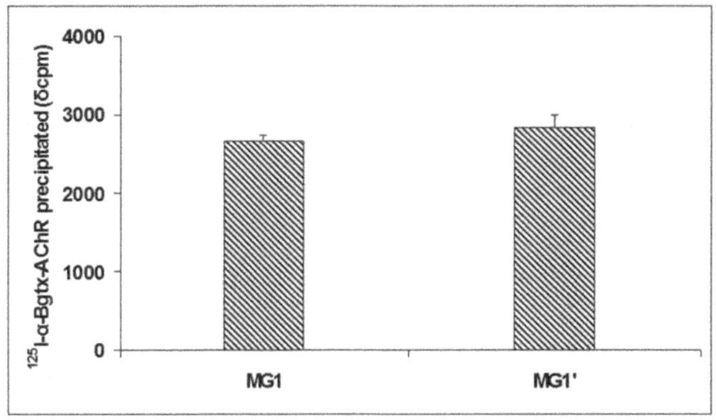

Figure 3. Competition RIA between MG1 autoAbs and ^{125}I-α-Bgtx for binding to the AChR. Anti-AChR Ab precipitation of MG1 serum by RIA and competition RIA for the detection of blocking Abs in the serum. For this, unlabeled AChR was preincubated with MG1 serum followed by the subsequent addition of ^{125}I-α-Bgtx (MG before ^{125}I-α-Bgtx); in parallel AChR was preincubated with ^{125}I-α-Bgtx followed by the subsequent addition of MG1 (MG after ^{125}I-α-Bgtx). The precipitated radioactivity, after the addition of the anti-Ab, was equal in both assays, indicating that no autoAbs of MG1 bind near or at the acetylcholine binding site.

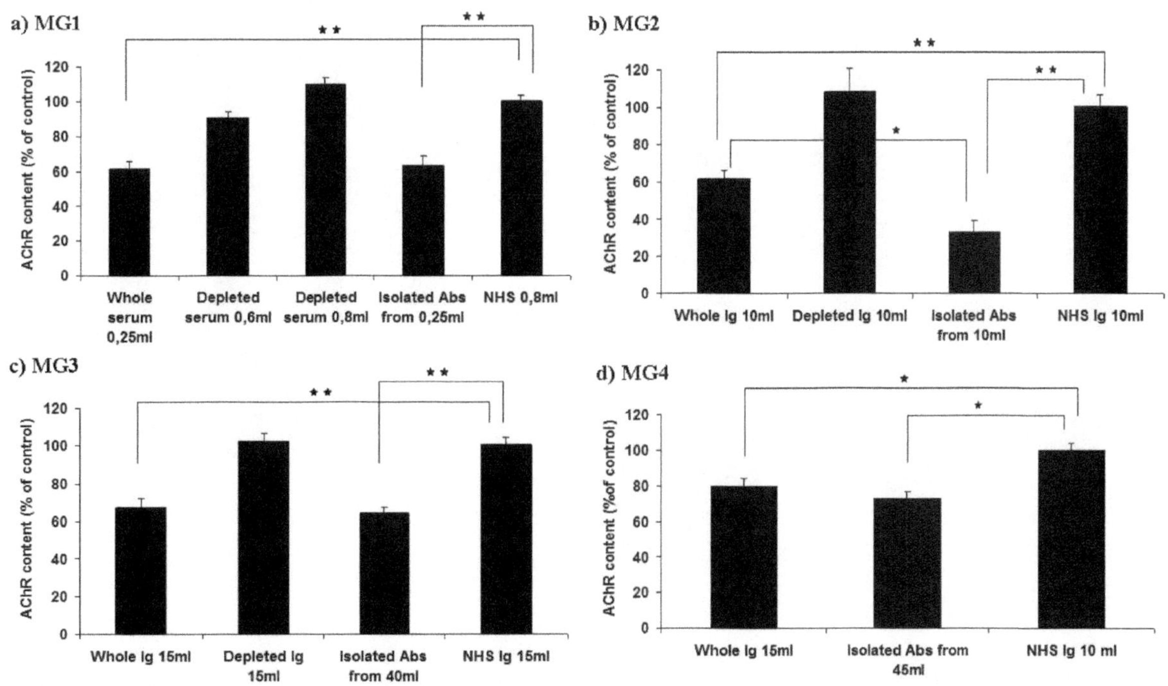

Figure 4. Muscle AChR content of treated rats. The four groups of animals injected with MG sera (MG1–MG4) and their derivatives were sacrificed 48 hours post-injection. The hind limb muscles of each rat were dissected and the extracted AChRs were estimated by RIA. Results are expressed as a percentage of the AChR of the rats receiving NHS only. Results for PBS are not shown but were very similar to the NHS. a, b, c, d: rats injected with sera and derivatives of MG1, MG2, MG3 and MG4 respectively. Bars represent mean AChR content (% of controls) +SE, *$p<0.05$, **$p<0.01$.

lower cross-reactivity) the strong potency of MG1 is not restricted to the rats.

The anti-β Abs isolated from MG3 and MG4 sera (and MG3 and MG4 total Ig) induced weak or no MG symptoms to animals, respectively. It is possible that the rat complement is not efficiently activated by the human anti-β auto-Abs (of MG3 and MG4) and that the effect on the rats injected with MG3 and MG4 and their derivatives could be mainly due to antigenic modulation of cross-linked AChR. The difference from the anti-α-subunit sera could be due to the presence of two α subunits per AChR molecule which apparently allows the anti-α antibodies to make larger AChR complexes. Since complement fixation is favored by larger antigen-antibody complexes, it would be reasonable for complement to act more strongly with the anti-α antibodies. Moreover, the α-subunits bearing the MIR region are more pathogenic than the other ones in MG patients with more than 50% of the anti-AChR autoabs are directed to the MIR [1,29]. The MIR has been shown to be located on the top of the AChR, favoring cross-linking of AChRs by the anti-MIR antibodies [31,32]. The anti-β auto-Abs in *in vitro* experiments are less capable in cross-linking the AChRs and therefore less capable in causing AChR destruction by both complement and antigenic modulation mechanisms.

This observation is in accordance with our previous studies [37], where we examined the effect of anti-α and anti-β Abs isolated from MG sera *in vitro*, in antigenic modulation experiments. Using TE671 cells we had shown that the anti-α autoAbs are about 4.3 times more effective than the anti-β Abs in internalizing membrane AChR molecules. This can explain the low potency of the anti-β subunit Abs in inducing severe symptoms into rats compared to the anti-α Abs of MG1 and MG2 sera. Nevertheless, it was shown that MG3 Abs did induce mild MG symptoms, weight and AChR loss. Finally, despite the absence of MG symptoms in rats injected with MG4 serum and its isolated anti-β Abs, the muscle AChR concentration was significantly reduced compared to the control groups. Yet, the reduction of about 20% of the total AChR molecules, as expected [40], was not sufficient to affect nerve impulse transduction. Equally important with the induction of EAMG by the isolated anti-α or anti-β Abs, was the observation that none of the depleted fractions caused any MG symptoms to the animals. MG2 and MG3 depleted sera had no anti-AChR autoAbs, as these were adsorbed by the α- and β-ECD columns, respectively. MG1 anti-α depleted serum had about 50% of the total MG1 Abs, but these Abs were not cross-reactive with rat AChR. This suggests that anti-AChR MG autoAbs not only induce EAMG but they seem to be the sole, or at least the main, pathogenic factor in anti-AChR positive MG.

Interestingly, at least in some cases, the isolated Abs seemed more potent than the whole sera. This was more apparent with MG2. The anti-α Abs from the MG2 serum induced clearly stronger clinical symptoms (Fig. 1C–D), weight loss (Fig. 2) and muscle AChR loss (Fig. 4B) than in the rats which were injected with whole MG2 serum Ig. Although this dramatic difference was observed only with MG2 serum, taking into account that the isolated Ab samples had smaller Ab titers from the whole sera or Ig (due to losses during Ab isolation) a trend for higher EAMG efficiency may be noted also for sera MG1 and MG3, overall

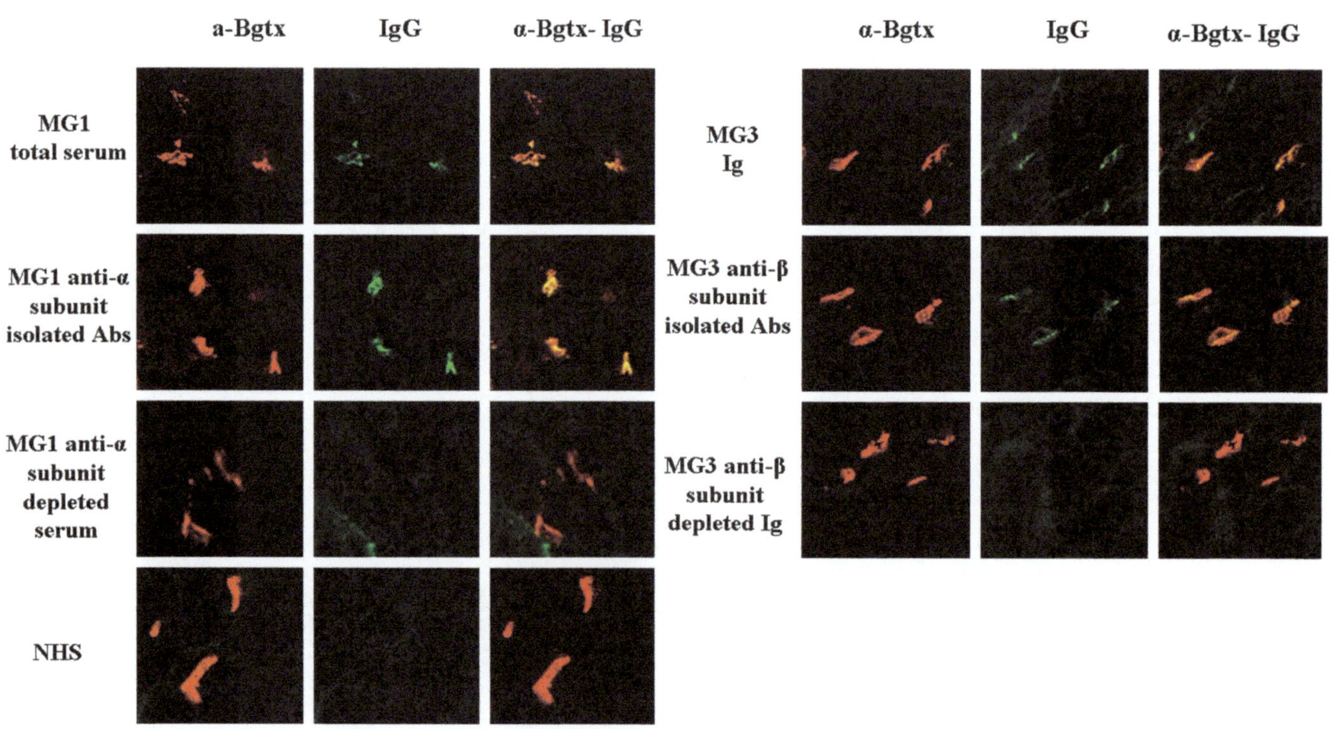

Figure 5. Deposition of IgG at the NMJ of EAMG rats detected by confocal microscopy. Hind limb muscle specimens were obtained from the rats injected with MG1 and MG3 sera and derivatives as well as from rats injected with NHS. Cryostat muscle sections were co-stained with Alexa Fluor 555-α-Bgtx to identify AChR (red) and with F(ab2) donkey anti-human IgG FITC conjugated to identify human autoAbs (green); merge on the right. The immunofluorescence data shown are representative of sections obtained from two rats of each group. Original magnification is 350×.

suggesting the possible presence of protective or suppressive factor(s) in the serum which may partially block the autoAb activity. This observation requires further study in order to identify the potential protective factors in the sera.

Elucidation of the function of anti-AChR autoAbs will help us to reveal their role in the initiation and progression of MG. Furthermore, our results also suggest that the selective removal of the anti-AChR autoAbs from the MG patients, an approach which we are pursuing with ECD-immunoadsorption columns, should be an efficient MG therapeutic approach.

Acknowledgments

The authors wish to thank Mrs. Anna Kokla for excellent technical assistance, Associate Professor Zoi Lygerou for helping with the confocal microscopy experiments, and Dr. Eirini Grapsa for MG plasmas.

Author Contributions

Conceived and designed the experiments: KP SJT. Performed the experiments: GK GL SS. Analyzed the data: GK GL SS KP SJT. Contributed to the writing of the manuscript: GK GL KP SJT.

References

1. Lindstrom JM (2000) Acetylcholine receptors and myasthenia. Muscle Nerve 23: 453–477.
2. Vincent A, Palace J, Hilton-Jones D (2001) Myasthenia gravis. Lancet 357: 2122–2128.
3. Bello-Rivero I, Cervantes M, Torres Y, Ferrero J, Rodríguez E, et al. (2004) Characterization of the immunoreactivity of anti-interferon alpha antibodies in myasthenia gravis patients. Epitope mapping. J Autoimmun 23: 63–73.
4. Infante AJ, Baillargeon J, Kraig E, Lott L, Jackson C, et al. (2003) Evidence of a diverse T cell receptor repertoire for acetylcholine receptor, the autoantigen of myasthenia gravis. J Autoimmun 21: 167–174.
5. Berrih-Aknin S, Frenkian-Cuvelier M, Eymard B (2014) Diagnostic and clinical classification of autoimmune myasthenia gravis. J Autoimmun 48–49: 143–148.
6. Berrih-Aknin S, Le Panse R (2014) Myasthenia gravis: A comprehensive review of immune dysregulation and etiological mechanisms. J Autoimmun 52: 90–100.
7. Marino M, Maiuri MT, Di Sante G, Scuderi F, La Carpia F, et al. (2014) T cell repertoire in DQ5-positive MuSK-positive myasthenia gravis patients. J Autoimmun 52: 113–121.
8. Hoch W, McConville J, Helms S, Newsom-Davis J, Melms A, et al. (2001) Autoantibodies to the receptor tyrosine kinase MuSK in patients with myasthenia gravis without acetylcholine receptor antibodies. Nat Med 7: 365–368.
9. Hoch W (2003) Molecular dissection of neuromuscular junction formation Trends Neurosci. 26: 335–337.
10. Zhang B, Tzartos JS, Belimezi M, Ragheb S, Bealmear B, et al. (2012) Autoantibodies to lipoprotein-related protein 4 in patients with double-seronegative myasthenia gravis. Arch Neurol 69: 445–451.
11. Zisimopoulou P, Evangelakou P, Tzartos J, Lazaridis K, Zouvelou V, et al. (2014) A comprehensive analysis of the epidemiology and clinical characteristics of anti-LRP4 in myasthenia gravis. J Autoimmun 52: 139–45.
12. Meriggioli MN, Sanders DB (2012) Muscle autoantibodies in myasthenia gravis: beyond diagnosis? Expert Rev Clin Immunol 8: 427–438.
13. Conti-Fine BM, Milani M, Kaminski HJ (2006) Myasthenia gravis: past, present, and future. J Clin Invest 116: 2843–2854.
14. Kalamida D, Poulas K, Avramopoulou V, Fostieri E, Lagoumintzis G, et al. (2007) Muscle and neuronal nicotinic acetylcholine receptors. Structure, function and pathogenicity. FEBS J 274: 3799–3845.
15. Albuquerque EX, Pereira EF, Alkondon M, Rogers SW (2009) Mammalian nicotinic acetylcholine receptors: from structure to function. Physiol Rev 89: 73–120.
16. Newsom-Davis J, Pinching AJ, Vincent A, Wilson SG (1978) Function of circulating antibody to acetylcholine receptor in myasthenia gravis: investigation by plasma exchange. Neurology 28: 266–272.
17. Batocchi AP, Evoli A, Di Schino C, Tonali P (2000) Therapeutic apheresis in myasthenia gravis. Ther Apher 4: 275–279.
18. Tzartos SJ, Efthimiadis A, Morel E, Eymard B, Bach JF (1990) Neonatal myasthenia gravis: antigenic specificities of antibodies in sera from mothers and their infants. Clin Exp Immunol 80: 376–380.
19. Vernet-der Garabedian B, Eymard B, Bach JF, Morel E (1989) Alpha-bungarotoxin blocking antibodies in neonatal myasthenia gravis: frequency and selectivity. J Neuroimmunol 21: 41–47.
20. Patrick J, Lindstrom J (1973) Autoimmune response to acetylcholine receptor. Science 180: 871–872.
21. Christadoss P, Poussin M, Deng C (2000) Animal models of myasthenia gravis. Clin Immunol 94: 75–87.
22. De Baets M, Stassen MH (2002) The role of antibodies in myasthenia gravis. J Neurol Sci 202: 5–11.
23. Toyka KV, Brachman DB, Pestronk A, Kao I (1975) Myasthenia gravis: passive transfer from man to mouse. Science 190: 397–399.
24. Toyka KV, Drachman DB, Griffin DE, Pestronk A, Winkelstein JA, et al. (1977) Myasthenia gravis. Study of humoral immune mechanisms by passive transfer to mice. N Engl J Med 296: 125–131.
25. Buschman E, van Oers N, Katz M, Murgita RA (1987) Experimental myasthenia gravis induced in mice by passive transfer of human myasthenic immunoglobulin. Evidence for an ameliorating effect by alpha-fetoprotein. J Neuroimmunol 13: 315–330.
26. Tzartos S, Hochschwender S, Vasquez P, Lindstrom J (1987) Passive transfer of experimental autoimmune myasthenia gravis by monoclonal antibodies to the main immunogenic region of the acetylcholine receptor. J Neuroimmunol 15: 185–194.
27. Tzartos SJ (1988) Myasthenia gravis studied by monoclonal antibodies to the acetylcholine receptor. In Vivo 2: 105–110.
28. Berrih-Aknin S (1995) Myasthenia gravis, a model of organ-specific autoimmune disease. J Autoimmun 8: 139–143.
29. Tzartos SJ, Barkas T, Cung MT, Mamalaki A, Marraud M, et al. (1998) Anatomy of the antigenic structure of a large membrane autoantigen, the muscle-type nicotinic acetylcholine receptor. Immunol Rev 163: 89–120.
30. Lindstrom J, Luo J, Kuryatov A (2008) Myasthenia gravis and the tops and bottoms of AChRs: antigenic structure of the MIR and specific immunosuppression of EAMG using AChR cytoplasmic domains. Ann N Y Acad Sci 1132: 29–41.
31. Lindstrom J, Luo J (2012) Myasthenogenicity of the main immunogenic region. Ann N Y Acad Sci 1274: 9–13.
32. Beroukhim R, Unwin N (1995) Three-dimensional location of the main immunogenic region of the acetylcholine receptor. Neuron 15(2): 323–331.
33. Tzartos SJ, Seybold ME, Lindstrom JM (1982) Specificities of antibodies to acetylcholine receptors in sera from myasthenia gravis patients measured by monoclonal antibodies. Proc Natl Acad Sci U S A 79: 188–192.
34. Ragheb S, Mohamed M, Lisak RP (2005) Myasthenia gravis patients, but not healthy subjects, recognize epitopes that are unique to the epsilon-subunit of the acetylcholine receptor. J Neuroimmunol 159: 137–145.
35. Kostelidou K, Trakas N, Tzartos SJ (2007) Extracellular domains of the beta, gamma and epsilon subunits of the human acetylcholine receptor as immunoadsorbents for myasthenic autoantibodies: a combination of immunoadsorbents results in increased efficiency. J Neuroimmunol 190: 44–52.
36. Mossman S, Vincent A, Newsom-Davis J (1988) Passive transfer of myasthenia gravis by immunoglobulins: lack of correlation between AChR with antibody bound, acetylcholine receptor loss and transmission defect. J Neurol Sci 84: 15–28.
37. Sideris S, Lagoumintzis G, Kordas G, Kostelidou K, Sotiriadis A, et al. (2007) Isolation and functional characterization of anti-acetylcholine receptor subunit-specific autoantibodies from myasthenic patients: receptor loss in cell culture. J Neuroimmunol 189: 111–117.
38. Zisimopoulou P, Lagoumintzis G, Poulas K, Tzartos SJ (2008) Antigen-specific apheresis of human anti-acetylcholine receptor autoantibodies from myasthenia gravis patients' sera using Escherichia coli-expressed receptor domains. J Neuroimmunol 200: 133–141.
39. Lindstrom JM, Einarson BL, Lennon VA, Seybold ME (1976) Pathological mechanisms in experimental autoimmune myasthenia gravis. Immunogenicity of syngeneic muscle acetylcholine receptor and quantitative extraction of receptor and antibody-receptor complexes from muscles of rats with experimental automimmune myasthenia gravis. J Exp Med 144: 726–738.
40. Christadoss P, Lindstrom J, Munro S, Talal N (1985) Muscle acetylcholine receptor loss in murine experimental autoimmune myasthenia gravis: correlated with cellular, humoral and clinical responses. J Neuroimmunol 8: 29–41.

Long-Term Aerobic Exercise Protects against Cisplatin-Induced Nephrotoxicity by Modulating the Expression of IL-6 and HO-1

Mariana Yasue Saito Miyagi[1], Marilia Seelaender[2], Angela Castoldi[1], Danilo Candido de Almeida[1], Aline Villa Nova Bacurau[3], Vinicius Andrade-Oliveira[1], Lucas Maceratesi Enjiu[2], Marcus Pisciottano[2], Caroline Yuri Hayashida[1], Meire Ioshie Hiyane[1], Patricia Chakur Brum[3], Niels Olsen Saraiva Camara[1], Mariane Tami Amano[1]*

1 Laboratory of Immunobiology of Transplants, Department of Immunology, Institute of Biomedical Sciences, University of Sao Paulo, Sao Paulo, SP, Brazil, **2** Cancer Metabolism Research Group, Department of Cell Biology, Institute of Biomedical Sciences, University of Sao Paulo, Sao Paulo, SP, Brazil, **3** Laboratory of Molecular and Cellular Exercise Physiology, School of Physical Education and Sport, University of Sao Paulo, Sao Paulo, SP, Brazil

Abstract

Nephrotoxicity is substantial side effect for 30% of patients undergoing cancer therapy with cisplatin and may force them to change or even abandon the treatment. Studies regarding aerobic exercise have shown its efficacy for the treatment of many types of diseases and its capacity to reduce tumors. However, little is known about the impact of physical exercise on cisplatin-induced acute kidney injury (AKI). In the present study, our aim was to investigate the role of physical exercise in AKI induced by cisplatin. We submitted C57Bl6 male mice to seven weeks of chronic exercise on a training treadmill and treated them with single i.p. injection of cisplatin (20 mg/kg) in the last week. Exercise efficacy was confirmed by an increased capillary-to-fiber ratio in the gastrocnemius muscle of exercised groups (EX and CIS-EX). The group submitted to exercise before cisplatin administration (CIS-EX) exhibited less weight loss and decreased serum urea levels compared to the cisplatin group (CIS). Exercise also showed a protective role against cisplatin-induced cell death in the kidney. The CIS-EX group showed a lower inflammatory response, with less TNF and IL-10 expression in the kidney and serum. In the same group, we observed an increase of IL-6 and HO-1 expression in the kidney. Taken together, our results indicate that chronic aerobic exercise is able to attenuate AKI by inducing IL-6 and HO-1 production, which results in lower inflammatory and apoptotic profiles in the kidney.

Editor: Ivan C. Moura, Institut national de la santé et de la recherche médicale (INSERM), France

Funding: This work was supported by Fundação de Amparo à Pesquisa do Estado de São Paulo (FAPESP: 11/10349-5, 12/02270-2, 12/10435-1, 12/50079-0) and Conselho Nacional de Desenvolvimento Científico e Tecnológico (CNPq, INCT Complex Fluids and Renal Immunopathology Laboratory INSERM/CNPq). The funders had no role in study design, data collection and analysis, decision to publish, or preparation of the manuscript.

Competing Interests: The authors have declared that no competing interests exist.

* Email: marianeamano.usp@gmail.com

Introduction

Cisplatin is a potent chemotherapy drug widely used for the treatment of many types of cancers, including ovarian, head and neck cancers, and is especially effective for testicular cancer, with a cure rate greater than 90% [1,2]. It is believed that cisplatin crosses through the plasma membrane, mostly through passive diffusion, and that once the chlorine atoms are hydrolyzed, the molecule becomes very reactive and binds to the DNA, blocking the replication of cancer cells and leading to cell death [1]. Nevertheless, cisplatin use is limited by cisplatin-acquired resistance and side effects such as acute kidney injury (AKI) [1,3] and cachexia [4]. The latter is a catabolic syndrome that results in the involuntary weight loss involving the loss of muscle mass and of adipose tissue [5].

Unbound cisplatin molecules are filtered and actively transported, primarily by proximal tubular epithelial cells [6]. The mechanisms of its nephrotoxic remain unclear, but it is known that it involves reactive oxygen species (ROS)-mediated oxidative stress, extrinsic and intrinsic apoptosis pathways, inflammation and fibrogenesis. These factors lead to tubular damage, sodium and potassium dysfunction, and magnesium wasting [6,7]. The inflammation process is orchestrated by tumor necrosis factor alpha (TNF), which binds to the TNFR1 and TNFR2 receptors and leads to the recruitment of two complexes. Complex 1 activates the transcription of nuclear factor–kB (NF-kB) and several inflammation and survival-related genes, while complex 2 promotes the activation of caspase-8 and -10, resulting in the induction of apoptosis [6]. TNF, normally undetectable in healthy kidneys, is produced by most renal cells in response to stimuli such as cisplatin [8,9]. To restrain TNF damage, regulatory molecules are also produced under stress conditions. IL-10 has been described as an anti-inflammatory cytokine and plays an important role in AKI protection [10,11]. Cisplatin treatment induces IL-10 and IL-10 receptor expression, and this endogenous production is essential for preventing damage to the renal tissue [10].

In response to endurance exercise, skeletal muscle releases cytokines such as IL-6, that promote the release of other anti-inflammatory cytokines such as IL-10 and IL-1 receptor antagonist (IL-1ra) and inhibit IL-1b and TNF production [12]. IL-6 has also been shown to protect against cisplatin-induced AKI [13–15].

The enzyme heme oxygenase (HO)-1 is a known regulator of the inflammatory response. It catalyzes heme degradation, thus releasing biliverdin, iron and carbon monoxide. HO-1 is associated with cytoprotection in several kidney diseases, including AKI induced by drugs [16]. Skeletal muscle cells are able to express HO-1 [17] and endurance training induces HO-1 expression in multiple immune cells [18]. Although physical exercise is able to induce HO-1, thus far, the correlation between exercise and the prevention of kidney diseases has not been established.

Physical exercise has been always recognized for its health benefits. Only in recent decades has a better understanding developed of the health benefits of physical exercise regarding the immune system and the alleviation of disability from various diseases, including obesity, diabetes mellitus, cardiovascular disease and cancer [19,20]. Recently, the favorable effects of exercise on the efficacy of oncologic therapies and the role of exercise in the palliative care of patients with cancer have been investigated most intensively [19].

Because physical exercise contributes to a decreased inflammatory response and improves cachexia symptoms, we intended to verify whether physical exercise in mice could diminish cisplatin-induced AKI. This study could suggest new approaches for patients under cisplatin treatment.

Objectives

Our aim was to investigate whether physical exercise was able to diminish cisplatin-induced AKI and to elucidate the possible mechanisms involved in this protection.

Methods

Aerobic exercise and cisplatin administration

C57Bl6 male mice, provided by UNIFESP-CEDEME, between 6 and 8 weeks of age were kept in individual cages in a vivarium with a light/dark cycle of 12/12 hours at 25±2°C, with food and water *ad libitum*. The experimental procedures were carried out according to the ethical principles for animal experimentation adopted by the Guide for the Care and Use of Laboratory Animals of the National Institutes of Health. Protocols were approved by The Ethics Committee of The Institute of Biomedical Sciences of the University of Sao Paulo – "Comissão de Ética no Uso de Animais" (CEUA) (number 046 over sheet 102 of the book 02, on April 20th, 2011). All efforts were made to minimize suffering. The aerobic exercise was performed on a training treadmill adapted for mice at the Laboratory of Cancer Metabolism, at the Institute of Biomedical Sciences of the University of Sao Paulo. All animals participated in exercise training for one week and were divided into four groups. Animals with best performances during the first week were selected to exercised groups. Cisplatin groups were picked randomly. These groups were: a sedentary control group (CT, $n = 9$), an exercised group (EX, $n = 10$), a cisplatin sedentary group (CIS, $n = 8$) and a cisplatin exercised group (CIS-EX, $n = 11$) according to their training. To evaluate the effects of chronic exercise, we adapted the protocol from Bacurau *et al.* [21], as shown in Table 1.

Cisplatin treatment

Acute kidney injury and cachexia are known side effects of cisplatin treatment. To analyze the effects of chronic exercise in this model, a single intraperitoneal (i.p.) dose of cisplatin (20 mg/kg – "Citoplax" Bergamo©) was administered. Mice were weighed and sacrificed 96 hours after drug administration by i.p. anesthesia of ketamine-xylazine and cervical dislocation. Immediately after sacrifice, blood, muscle and kidney were collected, frozen in liquid nitrogen, and stored at −80°C until subsequent measurements. Urea levels in the blood were verified using colorimetric assay (Labtest, Brazil) read with a Synegy microplate reader (BioTek, USA).

Muscle capillarity

After deparaffinization, slides of gastrocnemius muscle were washed in water for 10 min and then oxidized with 0.5% periodic acid for 10 min. They were washed second time, treated with the Schiff reagent and incubated for 15 min. A third wash was performed, and the sections then were stained with hematoxylin. Briefly, capillary-to-fiber ratio was quantified by a 10×10 grid optically superimposed on each of 5 nonoverlapping fields at x400 magnification, distributed in a random manner using a computer-assisted morphometric system (Quantimet 500; Leica, Cambridge, UK). For calculating capillary-to-fiber ratio, the total number of capillaries was divided by the total number of fibers counted in the same field. Only vessels with a diameter <10 μm were counted, which would largely comprise capillaries but might also include terminal arterioles or venules. All analyses were conducted by a single observer blinded to mouse identity.

RNA extraction and quantitative PCR (qPCR)

The gene expressions of Bcl2, Bax, TNF, IL-6, IL-10 and HO-1 were analyzed by qPCR. RNA was isolated with TRIzol Reagent (LifeTechnologies, USA) according to the manufacturer's protocol, and RNA concentrations were determined by NanoDrop (Thermo Scientific, USA). cDNA synthesis was performed using a SuperScript III RT (Life Technologies). qPCR was performed in triplicate on each sample, using a TaqMan PCR assay (Life-Technologies), with a ABI Prism 7300 sequence detection system (Life Technologies). Gene expression of each molecule was normalized to HPRT.

Cytometric Bead Array – CBA

CBA was performed with Mouse, Th1/Th2/Th17 BD Biosciences CBA Kit, following the manufacturer's instructions. We used a BD FACSCanto II flow-cytometer (BD Biosciences, USA) for cell acquisition, and FCAP array software was utilized for the data analysis.

Western Blot

Kidney cells were lysed in RIPA buffer, quantified, run on a 10% SDS-polyacrylamide electrophoresis gel and transferred onto a nitrocellulose membrane, which was incubated with primary rabbit anti–mouse Nrf2 (Santa Cruz Biotechnology, USA), HO-1 (Abcam, USA) or β-actin (Sigma-Aldrich, USA) antibodies overnight, followed by a secondary goat anti-rabbit antibody. For each molecule, the membrane was stripped and probed with the aforementioned antibodies. The bands were analyzed with the software GeneSnap (Syngene, USA) and Gene Tools (Syngene, USA).

Table 1. Chronic training.

	Monday	Tuesday	Wednesday	Thursday	Friday
Speed	**10 m/min**	**10 m/min**	**15 m/min**	**15 m/min**	**20 m/min**
Adaptation week	-	-	30 min	35 min	30 min
1st week	30 min	45 min	50 min	55 min	60 min
2nd week	60 min	60 min	60 min	60 min	60 min
3rd week	50 min	55 min	60 min	60 min	60 min
4th week	60 min	60 min	60 min	60 min	60 min
5th week	50 min	55 min	60 min	60 min	60 min
6th week	60 min*	60 min	-	-	**harvest**

*Cisplatin administration.

TUNEL assay

After deparaffinization and rehydration, kidney sections were incubated with 20 µg/mL proteinase K (Life Technologies), and washed in PBS. They were incubated with labeling solution for 1 h at 37°C. After washing, the sections were covered with 2 drops of slow fade. Image capture was performed with a Nikon ECLIPSE Ti microscope, and the analysis was performed with NS-Elements AR software.

Immunohistochemistry

Tissue section slides were deparaffinized and were incubated in a 95°C water bath for 30 min in a 0.01 M citrate solution. After drying, we added H_2O_2 for 15 min and the slides were washed twice with Tris Buffered Saline with Tween 20 (TBS-T). After blocking with non-fat dry milk 5% for 30 min, anti-HO-1 (Abcam) 1:1200 was added, and they were incubated overnight at 4°C. We washed the slides and then incubated them with secondary antibody conjugated with peroxidase (Evision-DAKO) for 30 min. They were then treated with 3-3′ diaminobenzidine tetrahydrochloride (DAB) 1:100 (DAKO) for 40 s. Image capture was performed with a Nikon ECLIPSE Ti microscope, and the analysis was performed with NS-Elements AR software.

Statistical analysis

One-way analysis of variance (ANOVA) with the Bonferroni post-test was used to analyze the statistical significance of the results with GraphPad Prism 5 software.

Results

Chronic exercise protected against renal dysfunction and cachexia

Because chronic exercise training causes physiological and metabolic stress, it is a strong proangiogenic stimulus in skeletal muscle [22]. We therefore evaluated the exercise efficiency by muscle capillary growth in gastrocnemius muscle (Figure 1A and B), and we observed an increase of capillary-muscle fiber ratio in animals submitted to exercise (EX and CIS-EX, $n = 10$ and 11, respectively). We then analyzed the influence of exercise training against the side effects of cisplatin, such as cachexia and nephrotoxicity. As depicted in Figure 1C, we observed that aerobic exercise could attenuate cisplatin-induced body weight loss, the most prominent symptom of cachexia. CIS-EX showed a lower percentage of weight loss compared to CIS ($n = 8$). After 96 h of cisplatin injection, blood was collected to evaluate renal function by determining the serum urea levels. As shown in Figure 1C, the serum urea levels increased approximately seven-fold in cisplatin-treated animals (CIS), while exercise attenuated renal dysfunction, decreasing urea levels 1.6-fold compared to CIS group. Groups not treated with cisplatin (CT and EX, $n = 9$ and 10, respectively) did not show cachexia-related weight loss or nephrotoxicity under both the sedentary and exercised conditions (Figure 1C and D).

Exercise reduced cell death in the kidney

To determine if aerobic exercise also had an impact on cisplatin-induced cell death, we analyzed apoptosis in the kidney. As shown in Figure 2 (A and B), cisplatin induced kidney cells apoptosis in the sedentary CIS group, while exercised mice (CIS-EX) were protected from this cell death in the kidney, as no difference was observed when compared to control groups (CT or EX). In the attempt to better understand the mechanism of this protection, we analyzed gene expression of the anti-apoptotic molecule Bcl2 and of the pro-apoptotic molecule Bax. But we found no difference among the groups (Figure 2C) by evaluating the ratios of these molecules.

Exercise attenuated inflammation by down-modulation of TNF

To determine that exercise was able to modulate inflammation, we analyzed the gene expression of TNF (Figure 3A) and IL-10 (Figure 3B) in the kidney as well as the levels of these two cytokines in serum (Figures 3C and D). Cisplatin increased the levels of both cytokines in the kidney and in the serum. Moreover, animals previously exposed to exercise showed decreased levels of these cytokines, indicating lower level of inflammation (Figure 3A and C). Also, a reduced need to control inflammation was observed, represented by the low levels of IL-10 (Figure 3B and D), a known regulatory cytokine.

Exercise increased IL-6 gene expression after cisplatin administration

IL-6 is usually associated with inflammatory response and promotes inflammation. In acute kidney injury induced by cisplatin, this cytokine seems to reduce inflammation. It was demonstrated that IL-6 plays a protective role in this model [13–15]. We investigated whether IL-6 plays a role in exercise-induced protection. We observed that IL-6 was expressed to a greater extent in muscle cells in the presence of cisplatin (Figure 4A), although no difference was observed between the CIS to CIS-EX groups. When we analyzed the expression of this cytokine in the

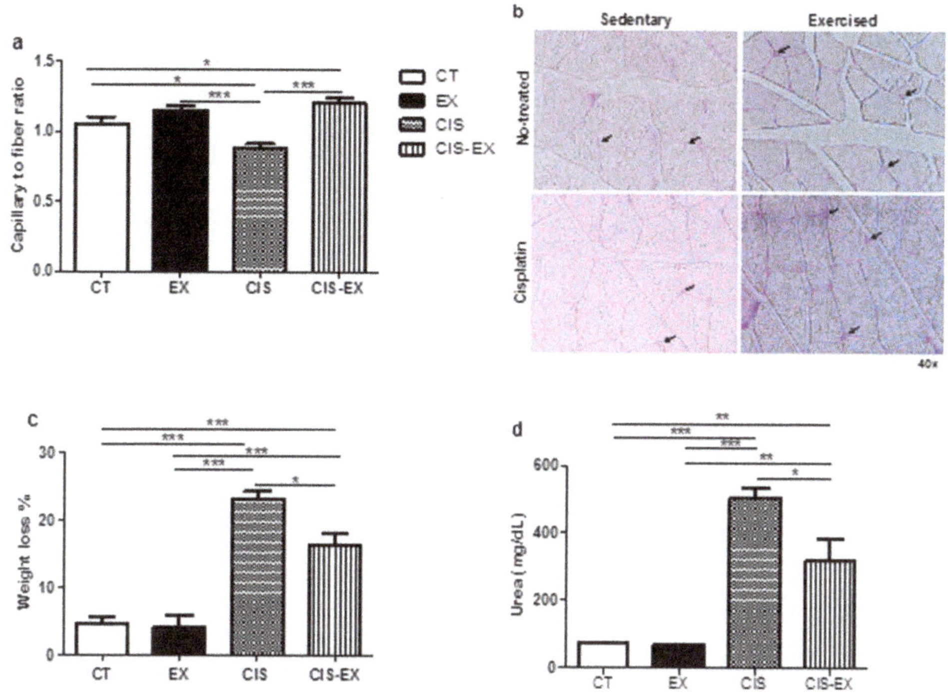

Figure 1. Aerobic exercise minimizes cisplatin-induced cachexia and renal damage. Exercise efficacy was confirmed by an increase in muscle angiogenesis in the exercised (EX) and exercised with cisplatin injection (CIS-EX) groups (**A** and **B**). Decreased weight loss (**C**) and lower levels of serum urea (**D**) in the CIS-EX group compared to the sedentary goup injected with cisplatin (CIS) indicate the protective effect of exercise. The sedentary group without cisplatin injection was used as the control (CT). *P<0.05; **P<0.01; ***P<0.001.

kidney, we noticed that IL-6 was expressed to a greater extent in the CIS groups compared to the sedentary groups (CT and EX). However, the CIS-EX group showed even higher expression of IL-6 compared to sedentary groups (Figure 4B). This result suggests

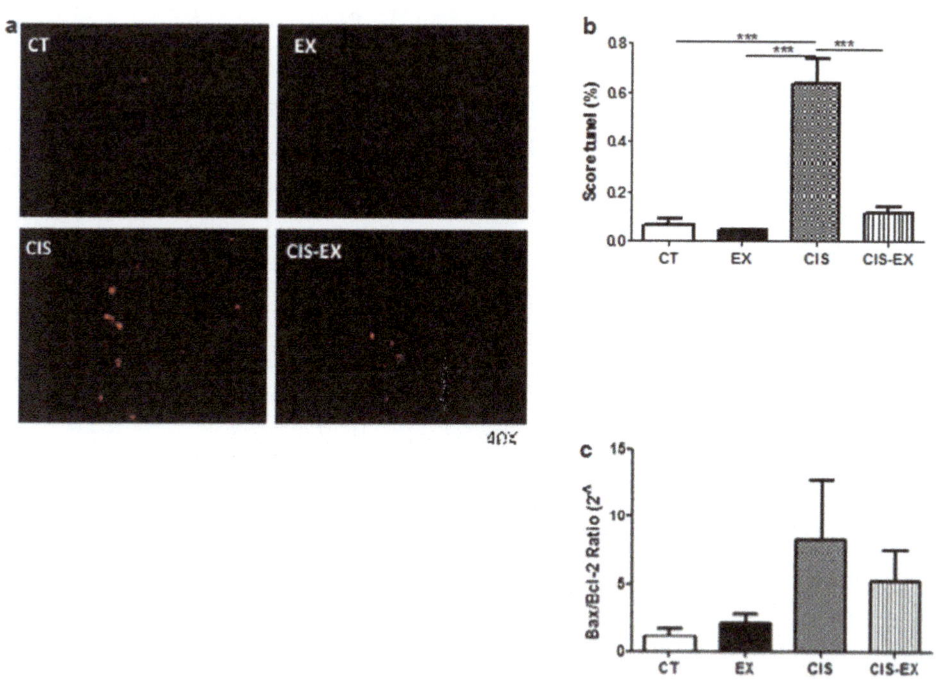

Figure 2. Aerobic exercise reduces cell death in the kidney. Representative TUNEL staining (**A**) and quantification (**B**) showed a significantly reduced percentage of TUNEL-positive cells (dead cells) in the CIS-EX group. The expression of Bcl2 and Bax genes was evaluated by qPCR and is represented by the ratio of the pro- to the anti-apoptotic molecule (Bax/Bcl2) (**C**) the CIS group was more likely to exhibit a pro-apoptotic profile, confirming the protective role of exercise. ***P<0.001.

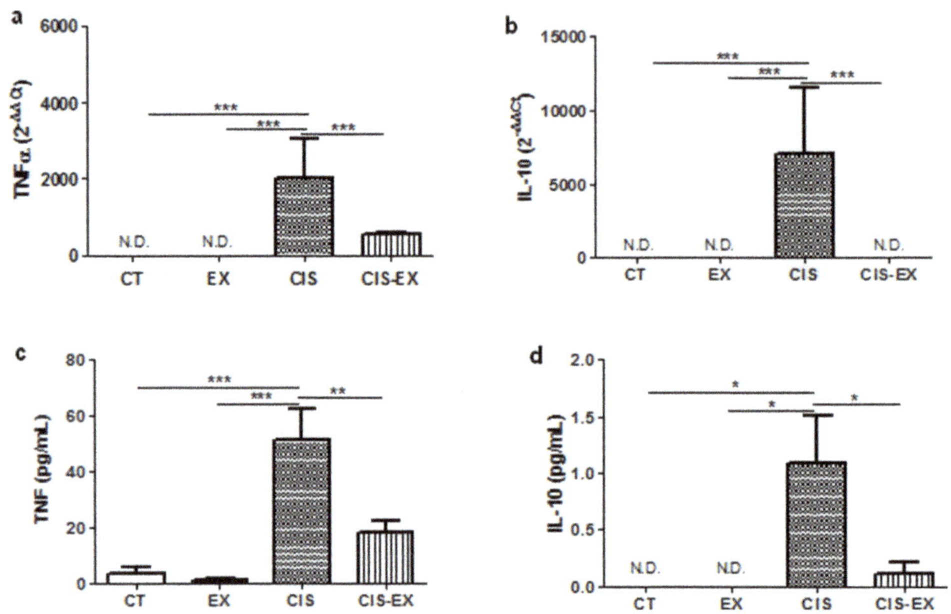

Figure 3. Exercise attenuates inflammation. qPCR analysis revealed that the CIS group showed higher expressions of TNF (**A**) and IL-10 (**B**) in the kidney, while CIS-EX did not exhibit significant differences compared to CT. The serum concentrations of TNF (**C**) and IL-10 (**D**), determined by CBA, appeared to decrease in the CIS-EX group. *P<0.05; **P<0.01; ***P<0.001; N.D. - non detected cytokine.

that exercised animals could result in higher levels of IL-6 in the kidney under stress conditions, promoting protection of the organ.

Exercise increases HO-1 mRNA and protein expression in the kidney

Because we observed less apoptosis and inflammation in the kidney of exercised animals, we questioned whether the enzyme HO-1 could be involved in the reported protective effect of chronic exercise. We first analyzed the nuclear factor erythroid-2-like 2 (Nrf2), which is a transcription factor that regulates the antioxidant response elements genes and shows effects in several inflammatory models. Nrf2 is known to induce both IL-6 [23] and HO-1 [24]. We analyzed Nrf2 production in kidney of exercised groups (Figure 5A), but no statistical significance was observed. We expected to find an increase of HO-1 in the CIS group because this enzyme is expressed during oxidative stress responses [25]. We observed increased gene expression and protein levels of HO-1 in the CIS group (Figure 5B and C). However, the exercised group (CIS-EX) showed even higher levels of HO-1 in the kidney (Figure 5A–C). Thus, we may suggest that HO-1 plays an important role in the protection induced by aerobic exercise training, by diminishing cell death and the inflammatory response in the kidney.

Discussion

Nephrotoxicity is the primary toxic side effect of cisplatin administration, and approximately 20–30% of patients develop renal dysfunction following a single dose of cisplatin, necessitating a reduction in the dose or the treatment to be abandoned [26]. Herein, we showed that exercise in mice resulted in less chemotherapy-induced cachexia (comprising weight loss and local and systemic inflammation), a frequent consequence of cisplatin treatment, and protected the kidneys from AKI (Figure 1). These results suggest that long-term aerobic exercise might be a good

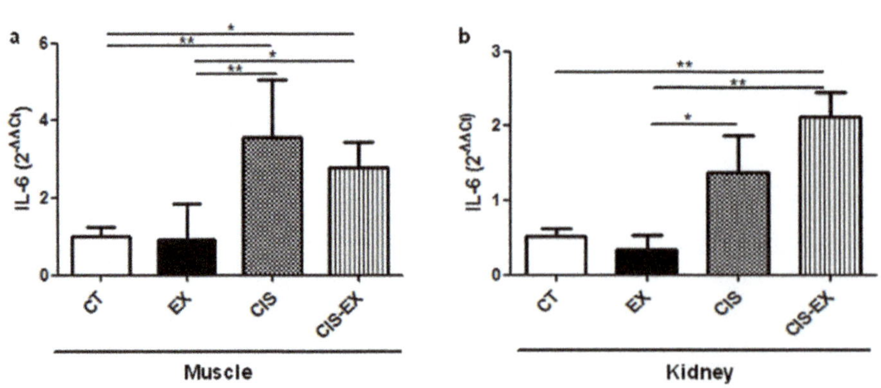

Figure 4. IL-6 contributes to kidney protection induced by exercise. The expression of the cytokine IL-6 was determined by qPCR in the muscle (**A**) and the kidney (**B**). The CIS group showed increased levels of IL-6 in both tissues compared to sedentary groups (CT and EX). However, CIS-EX showed increased IL-6 expression in the kidney, which indicates the protective role of IL-6 in this model. *P<0.05; **P<0.01.

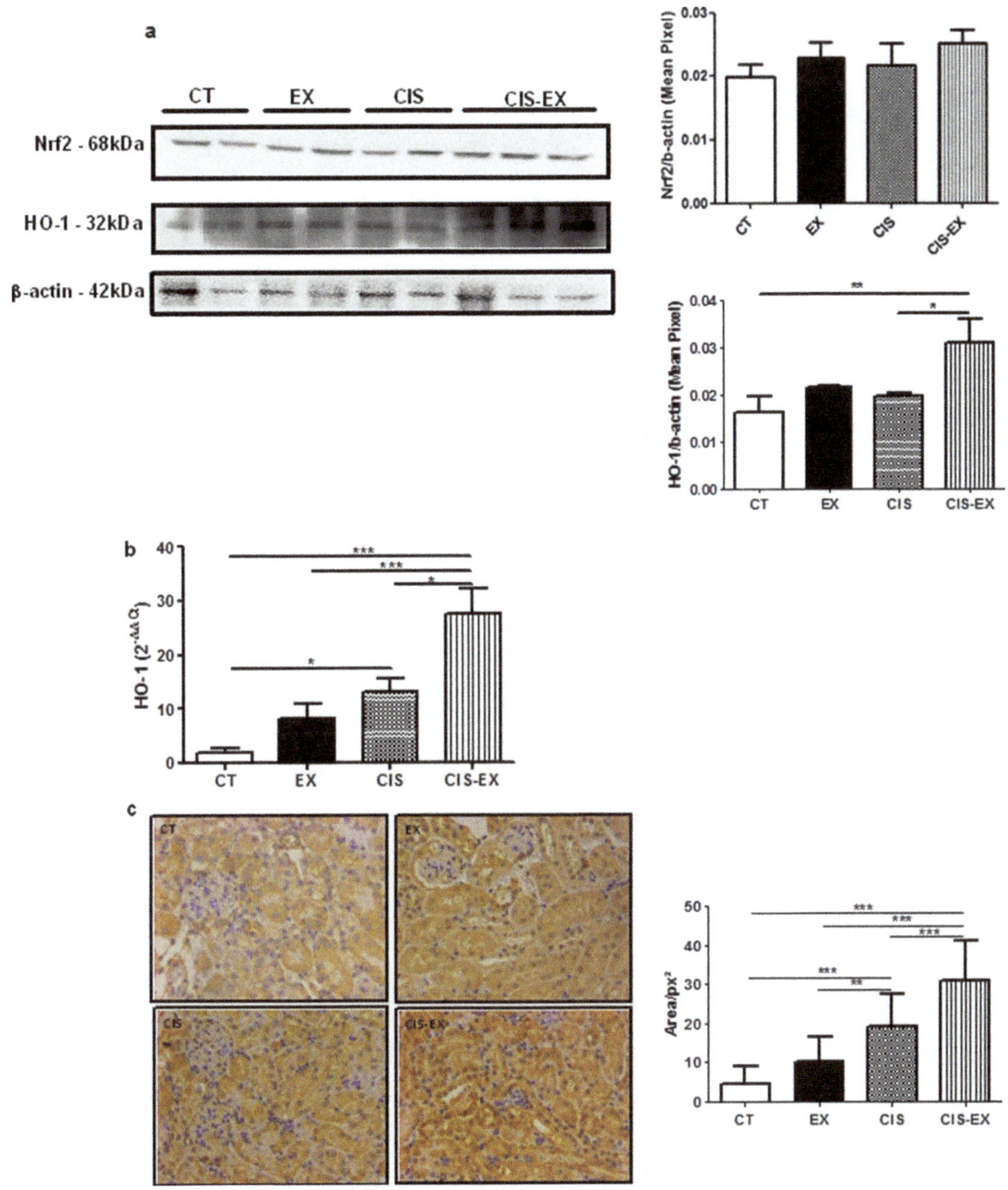

Figure 5. Exercise promotes increased HO-1 expression. Nrf2 and HO-1 expression in the kidney were evaluated by Western Blot (**left** – representative image and **right** – quantification). Exercise induced HO-1 gene expression, as confirmed by qPCR (**B**), and the levels of HO-1 in the renal tissue were analyzed by immunohistochemistry (**C, left** – representative image and **right** – quantification). *$P<0.05$; **$P<0.01$; ***$P<0.001$.

strategy to improve the quality of life for chemotherapy-treated patients. Other groups have demonstrated that moderate-intensity regular exercise can efficiently attenuate fatigue in women receiving chemotherapy [17] and that resistance and aerobic exercise in patients with gastrointestinal cancer undergoing chemotherapy resulted in low scores for pain and fatigue [18]. Although studies have shown the beneficial influence of physical exercise in several diseases, the mechanisms involved are not clear, which shows the need for further study in this field.

To clarify how exercise could be contributing to kidney protection, we analyzed cell death in the renal tissue of exercised mice given cisplatin. Apoptosis in cisplatin-induced AKI occurs mainly in tubular cells as a result of ERK-dependent signalization [20]. The intrinsic pathway of apoptosis activation involves molecules such as Bax and Bad, whereas Bcl2 is an anti-apoptotic component [27]. Analyzing TUNEL staining (Figure 2A and B), we observed that CIS-EX exhibited a dramatically decreased percentage of apoptotic cells in the kidney, which contributes to decreased compromising of renal function following cisplatin treatment. The diminished cell death could be due to an increased expression of anti-apoptotic Bcl2 compared with the pro-apoptotic Bax, but in this case we found no difference on the expression of these molecules (Figure 2C), suggesting another mechanism involved.

One key protein associated with cisplatin-induced AKI is TNF, which induces apoptosis and is also a well-known pro-inflammatory cytokine [28]. TNF is produced in the kidney by many types of cells, including parenchymal cells [8], or by infiltrating cells such as T lymphocytes [29]. TNF can also be produced in response to various stimuli and binds to TNFR1 and TNFR2, thus promoting the expression of a variety of chemokines and cytokines [6]. In the present study, we observed that exercise significantly reduced TNF levels locally in the kidney as well as systemically, as observed in the serum (Figures 3A and C). We believe that this contributes to a reduction in apoptosis and a decreased inflammatory response, which also correlates with decreased weight loss due to cachexia.

IL-10 is an anti-inflammatory cytokine that shows increased levels after cisplatin injection and controls AKI progression [10,11]. Although IL-10 is produced by adipocytes under treadmill training conditions [30] and the increased IL-10/TNF ratio indicates attenuated inflammation in cancer associated cachexia [31], no difference in IL-10 serum levels between the sedentary and exercised groups was observed. Kidneys from exercised mice did not show increased IL-10 expression (Figures 3B and D), whereas cisplatin did induce IL-10 expression in the sedentary group. Therefore, the control mechanism involved in exercised-induced protection in AKI is not associated with the IL-10 levels. We believe that the control of AKI in exercised animals occurs before the classical inflammatory response in this model, which explains the lower levels of TNF and, consequently, the decreased need for controlling the inflammation characterized by IL-10 production. These results inspired us to look for other possible mechanisms involved in this protection.

Primarily known as a pro-inflammatory cytokine, IL-6 is involved in several inflammatory disorders [32]. In acquired immunity, it plays a major role in Th17 polarization, which contributes to autoimmune diseases [33]. Although unexpected, Mitazaki *et al.* have demonstrated that IL-6 is essential for the control of cisplatin-induced injury [13–15]. In one study, they showed that IL-6 levels were increased in proximal tubular cells after cisplatin treatment and that IL-6 knockout (IL-6$^{-/-}$) mice presented more severe AKI with Bax followed by an increase in Bcl-2 and Bcl-xL [15]. This same group demonstrated that IL-6$^{-/-}$ mice showed more oxidative stress with increased cox-2 expression and ERK phosphorylation, while superoxide dismutase activity was decreased [14]. More recently, the use of dimethylthiourea (DMTU), a hydroxyl radical scavenger, was shown to protect mice from cisplatin-induced AKI by increasing IL-6, Bcl-xL and Nrf2 [13]. Thus, these data indicate that IL-6 is involved in AKI protection by controlling cell death and through upregulation of anti-oxidative stress factors. Our results support this mechanism, as elevated IL-6 expression is observed in the kidneys of the exercised group (CIS-EX), as shown in Figure 4B. Cisplatin seems to induce IL-6 on its own, which may be acting as negative feedback for the inflammatory response, and exercised mice express even greater levels of IL-6 (Figure 4B), as if they were more prone to produce this cytokine. In the liver, IL-6 is responsible for liver regeneration, hepatoprotection, antiapoptosis and anti-necrosis via STAT3 [34]. This cytokine is also produced by skeletal muscle fibers in response to physical exercise and associated with the anti-inflammatory response [35]. It has been reported that an increase in IL-6 levels depends on the intensity and duration of exercise [36] and is more pronounced in animals exposed to an overtraining protocol than to a moderate training protocol. Here, we did not notice any difference in IL-6 expression in muscle cells (Figure 4A) from exercised animals. This could be explained by the fact that samples were harvested three days after the cessation of training. According to Gholamnezhad *et al.*, a slight decrease in IL-6 is observed even 24 hours after exercise [37]. Therefore, it is very likely that local IL-6 production is responsible for the AKI protection.

We then decided to investigate Nrf2, the most potent inducer of antioxidant responsive element (ARE). This transcription factor is also able to induce IL-6 via ARE within its promoter [23]. In this study, we noticed no difference of Nrf2 level in the kidneys from exercised mice (Figure 5A). Nevertheless, another antioxidant enzyme that also contains ARE in its promoter, HO-1, was shown to be overexpressed in the kidneys of exercised mice compared to sedentary groups (Figures 5B, C and D). Several studies have demonstrated the importance of HO-1 in kidney protection. HO-1-deficient mice were shown to be more susceptible to renal injury caused by cisplatin [38], while metalloporphyrins and other inducers of HO-1 induced an anti-apoptotic response, protecting kidneys from cisplatin-induced injury [39–42]. Accordingly, our data suggest that exercise increases HO-1 expression in the kidney, possibly contributing to the protective phenotype.

Conclusions

In summary, we showed that aerobic exercise was able to diminish cisplatin-induced AKI by promoting IL-6 and HO-1 expression in the kidney, which decreases inflammation and cell death in that organ. This study suggests that the introduction of physical exercise before and during chemotherapy could attenuate the side effects caused by the drug and improve quality of life for patients.

Author Contributions

Conceived and designed the experiments: MTA NOSC MS. Performed the experiments: MYSM AC DCA AVNB VAO LME MP CYH MIH PCB MTA. Analyzed the data: MYSM AC DCA AVNB PCB MS NOSC MTA. Contributed reagents/materials/analysis tools: MS PCB NOSC MTA. Contributed to the writing of the manuscript: MYSM MS AVNB NOSC MTA.

References

1. Pabla N, Dong Z (2008) Cisplatin nephrotoxicity: mechanisms and renoprotective strategies. Kidney Int 73: 994–1007.
2. Verstappen CC, Heimans JJ, Hoekman K, Postma TJ (2003) Neurotoxic complications of chemotherapy in patients with cancer: clinical signs and optimal management. Drugs 63: 1549–1563.
3. Wensing KU, Ciarimboli G (2013) Saving ears and kidneys from cisplatin. Anticancer Res 33: 4183–4188.
4. Garcia JM, Scherer T, Chen JA, Guillory B, Nassif A, et al. (2013) Inhibition of cisplatin-induced lipid catabolism and weight loss by ghrelin in male mice. Endocrinology 154: 3118–3129.
5. Arruda AP, Milanski M, Romanatto T, Solon C, Coope A, et al. (2010) Hypothalamic actions of tumor necrosis factor alpha provide the thermogenic core for the wastage syndrome in cachexia. Endocrinology 151: 683–694.
6. Benedetti G, Fredriksson L, Herpers B, Meerman J, van de Water B, et al. (2013) TNF-alpha-mediated NF-kappaB survival signaling impairment by cisplatin enhances JNK activation allowing synergistic apoptosis of renal proximal tubular cells. Biochem Pharmacol 85: 274–286.
7. Yao X, Panichpisal K, Kurtzman N, Nugent K (2007) Cisplatin nephrotoxicity: a review. Am J Med Sci 334: 115–124.
8. Zhang B, Ramesh G, Norbury CC, Reeves WB (2007) Cisplatin-induced nephrotoxicity is mediated by tumor necrosis factor-alpha produced by renal parenchymal cells. Kidney Int 72: 37–44.
9. Ramesh G, Brian Reeves W (2006) Cisplatin increases TNF-alpha mRNA stability in kidney proximal tubule cells. Ren Fail 28: 583–592.
10. Tadagavadi RK, Reeves WB (2010) Endogenous IL-10 attenuates cisplatin nephrotoxicity: role of dendritic cells. J Immunol 185: 4904–4911.
11. Deng J, Kohda Y, Chiao H, Wang Y, Hu X, et al. (2001) Interleukin-10 inhibits ischemic and cisplatin-induced acute renal injury. Kidney Int 60: 2118–2128.
12. Hopps E, Canino B, Caimi G (2011) Effects of exercise on inflammation markers in type 2 diabetic subjects. Acta Diabetol 48: 183–189.

13. Mitazaki S, Hashimoto M, Matsuhashi Y, Honma S, Suto M, et al. (2013) Interleukin-6 modulates oxidative stress produced during the development of cisplatin nephrotoxicity. Life Sci 92: 694–700.
14. Mitazaki S, Honma S, Suto M, Kato N, Hiraiwa K, et al. (2011) Interleukin-6 plays a protective role in development of cisplatin-induced acute renal failure through upregulation of anti-oxidative stress factors. Life Sci 88: 1142–1148.
15. Mitazaki S, Kato N, Suto M, Hiraiwa K, Abe S (2009) Interleukin-6 deficiency accelerates cisplatin-induced acute renal failure but not systemic injury. Toxicology 265: 115–121.
16. Correa-Costa M, Amano MT, Camara NO (2012) Cytoprotection behind heme oxygenase-1 in renal diseases. World J Nephrol 1: 4–11.
17. Schwartz AL, Mori M, Gao R, Nail LM, King ME (2001) Exercise reduces daily fatigue in women with breast cancer receiving chemotherapy. Med Sci Sports Exerc 33: 718–723.
18. Jensen W, Baumann FT, Stein A, Bloch W, Bokemeyer C, et al. (2014) Exercise training in patients with advanced gastrointestinal cancer undergoing palliative chemotherapy: a pilot study. Support Care Cancer.
19. Eickmeyer SM, Gamble GL, Shahpar S, Do KD (2012) The role and efficacy of exercise in persons with cancer. PM R 4: 874–881.
20. Wang S, Wei Q, Dong G, Dong Z (2013) ERK-mediated suppression of cilia in cisplatin-induced tubular cell apoptosis and acute kidney injury. Biochim Biophys Acta 1832: 1582–1590.
21. Bacurau RF, Belmonte MA, Seelaender MC, Costa Rosa LF (2000) Effect of a moderate intensity exercise training protocol on the metabolism of macrophages and lymphocytes of tumour-bearing rats. Cell Biochem Funct 18: 249–258.
22. Roudier E, Forn P, Perry ME, Birot O (2012) Murine double minute-2 expression is required for capillary maintenance and exercise-induced angiogenesis in skeletal muscle. FASEB J 26: 4530–4539.
23. Wruck CJ, Streetz K, Pavic G, Gotz ME, Tohidnezhad M, et al. (2011) Nrf2 induces interleukin-6 (IL-6) expression via an antioxidant response element within the IL-6 promoter. J Biol Chem 286: 4493–4499.
24. Li N, Alam J, Venkatesan MI, Eiguren-Fernandez A, Schmitz D, et al. (2004) Nrf2 is a key transcription factor that regulates antioxidant defense in macrophages and epithelial cells: protecting against the proinflammatory and oxidizing effects of diesel exhaust chemicals. J Immunol 173: 3467–3481.
25. Choi AM, Alam J (1996) Heme oxygenase-1: function, regulation, and implication of a novel stress-inducible protein in oxidant-induced lung injury. Am J Respir Cell Mol Biol 15: 9–19.
26. Miller RP, Tadagavadi RK, Ramesh G, Reeves WB (2010) Mechanisms of Cisplatin nephrotoxicity. Toxins (Basel) 2: 2490–2518.
27. Pereira WO, Amarante-Mendes GP (2011) Apoptosis: a programme of cell death or cell disposal? Scand J Immunol 73: 401–407.
28. Ramesh G, Reeves WB (2002) TNF-alpha mediates chemokine and cytokine expression and renal injury in cisplatin nephrotoxicity. J Clin Invest 110: 835–842.
29. Liu M, Chien CC, Burne-Taney M, Molls RR, Racusen LC, et al. (2006) A pathophysiologic role for T lymphocytes in murine acute cisplatin nephrotoxicity. J Am Soc Nephrol 17: 765–774.
30. Jenkins NT, Padilla J, Arce-Esquivel AA, Bayless DS, Martin JS, et al. (2012) Effects of endurance exercise training, metformin, and their combination on adipose tissue leptin and IL-10 secretion in OLETF rats. J Appl Physiol (1985) 113: 1873–1883.
31. Lira FS, Rosa JC, Zanchi NE, Yamashita AS, Lopes RD, et al. (2009) Regulation of inflammation in the adipose tissue in cancer cachexia: effect of exercise. Cell Biochem Funct 27: 71–75.
32. Kishimoto T (2010) IL-6: from its discovery to clinical applications. Int Immunol 22: 347–352.
33. Bettelli E, Carrier Y, Gao W, Korn T, Strom TB, et al. (2006) Reciprocal developmental pathways for the generation of pathogenic effector TH17 and regulatory T cells. Nature 441: 235–238.
34. Taub R (2003) Hepatoprotection via the IL-6/Stat3 pathway. J Clin Invest 112: 978–980.
35. Pedersen BK, Steensberg A, Schjerling P (2001) Muscle-derived interleukin-6: possible biological effects. J Physiol 536: 329–337.
36. Petersen AM, Pedersen BK (2006) The role of IL-6 in mediating the anti-inflammatory effects of exercise. J Physiol Pharmacol 57 Suppl 10: 43–51.
37. Gholamnezhad Z, Boskabady MH, Hosseini M, Sankian M, Khajavi Rad A (2014) Evaluation of immune response after moderate and overtraining exercise in wistar rat. Iran J Basic Med Sci 17: 1–8.
38. Shiraishi F, Curtis LM, Truong L, Poss K, Visner GA, et al. (2000) Heme oxygenase-1 gene ablation or expression modulates cisplatin-induced renal tubular apoptosis. Am J Physiol Renal Physiol 278: F726–736.
39. Pan H, Shen K, Wang X, Meng H, Wang C, et al. (2014) Protective effect of metalloporphyrins against cisplatin-induced kidney injury in mice. PLoS One 9: e86057.
40. Tayem Y, Green CJ, Motterlini R, Foresti R (2014) Isothiocyanate-cysteine conjugates protect renal tissue against cisplatin-induced apoptosis via induction of heme oxygenase-1. Pharmacol Res 81C: 1–9.
41. Sahin K, Orhan C, Tuzcu M, Muqbil I, Sahin N, et al. (2014) Comparative in vivo evaluations of curcumin and its analog difluorinated curcumin against Cisplatin-induced nephrotoxicity. Biol Trace Elem Res 157: 156–163.
42. Sahin K, Tuzcu M, Sahin N, Ali S, Kucuk O (2010) Nrf2/HO-1 signaling pathway may be the prime target for chemoprevention of cisplatin-induced nephrotoxicity by lycopene. Food Chem Toxicol 48: 2670–2674.

16

Can Exercise Capacity Assessed by the 6 Minute Walk Test Predict the Development of Major Adverse Cardiac Events in Patients with STEMI after Fibrinolysis?

Ayman K. M. Hassan*, Salwa R. Dimitry, George W. Agban

Department of Cardiovascular Medicine, Faculty of Medicine, Assiut University, Assiut, Egypt

Abstract

Background: To assess the added value of the 6 minute walk test distance (6MWTD) in the risk-stratification methods for patients with ST -segment elevation myocardial infarction (STEMI) treated with fibrinolysis.

Methodology/Principal Findings: This is a prospective cohort study of one hundred consecutive patients with STEMI, who had received fibrinolysis, at Assuit University Hospital. All patients underwent 6MWT pre- discharge and were followed up for 3 months to monitor the incidence of major adverse cardiac events (MACE). Patients were divided into 3 groups according to the level of 6MWTD (level I>450 m, level II = 300–450 m and level III<300 m). Among the study population, the median 6MWT distance was 370 meters (interquartile range 162–462). The mean age was 60.9±10.7 years, 71.9% of them were males, 2/3 had anterior MI. only 10.5% had successful thrombolysis. Compared to patients in level I (>450 m), patients in level III (<300 m) were more likely to have clinical risk factors as hypertension, diabetes and impaired renal function. The patient's mean TIMI score was 3.4±2.2, the mean GRACE score was 150.5±27.7. There was a significant negative correlation between the 6 MWTD and GRACE risk score ($r = -0.80$, $p<0.001$). At 3 months of follow-up, 51% had MACE including 16% were dead. Multivariate logistic regression analysis identified that the GRACE risk score and 6MWT distance levels were the best predictors of the MACE at 3 month of follow up. The incidence of MACE was 4 times higher in patients with high GRACE risk score who couldn't walk more than 300 meters (OR = 4.66, 95% CI = 1.1–14.5, $p = 0.006$).

Conclusions/Significance: In patients with STEMI treated with fibrinolysis, the addition of 6MWTD assessment pre-discharge to the traditional GRACE risk score improved the risk prediction of cardiovascular events at 3 month follow up.

Editor: John Calvert, Emory University, United States of America

Funding: These authors have no support or funding to report.

Competing Interests: The authors have declared that no competing interests exist.

* E-mail: aymankhairy11@gmail.com

Introduction

The six-minute walk test (6MWT) is a simple, easy-to-perform, low tech, safe and well established self-paced assessment tool to quantify functional exercise capacity in different patients categories [1]. The 6MWT is performed by instructing the participant to march as fast as possible (without running) on a horizontal surface in 6 minutes, the distance walked (6MWD) is recorded [1].

The 6MWD is a good predictor for morbidity and mortality in patients with heart failure [1–6], pulmonary hypertension [7], and pulmonary disease [8]. Normal values available for the 6MWD are based on different adult cohorts [9,10]. However, there is no evidence regarding the ability of the 6MWT to predict outcomes in patients with ST-elevation myocardial infarction (STEMI).

Despite the improvement of different therapeutic modalities for patients with STEMI, major adverse cardiac events (MACE) are still 8.7% [11]. The prognostic models based on traditional cardiovascular disease risk factors do not fully explain the risk of future cardiovascular events in these patients. This clarifies why various risk scores have been introduced for STEMI patients with time. In the era of fibrinolysis, several different clinical scores have been used, including the GRACE [12], PAMI [13] and TIMI-STEMI [14] scores. For the current era where primary percutanious coronary intervention (PPCI) is the gold standard, new risk scores have been introduced including Zwolle score (Zs) [15], CADILLAC score[16], EuroSCORE and SYNTAX scores [17]. However, not all patients had the facility to do PPCI. So for those undergoing fibrinolysis and cannot proceed for PPCI due to financial restraints, we still need to risk stratify these patients pre-discharge. In Upper Egypt, we need to provide our patients with the best available and affordable treatment modality.

Exercise treadmill testing although provides information regarding prognosis in STEMI patients, but it is woefully underutilized [18]. This can be explained partly by patients overly cautious or reluctant to participate in exercise after STEMI, and also testing is expensive, not widely available, and time consuming.

In the present study, we evaluated the ability of the 6MWT to predict MACE in patients with STEMI treated with fibrinolysis.

Methods

Ethics Statement

The study protocol was approved by the ethical committee of Assuit faculty of medicine. A written informed consent was obtained from all participants. The consent form was designed with an explanation on the purpose and conduction of this research project. This form was to be explained to each participant; then a written consent was given. Participation was only proceeded after written consent of the participant. The full text of the form was approved by the Ethical Review Committee of Assuit faculty of medicine.

Patient's selection

Patients were included if they met the following criteria: (i) they presented typical anginal pain lasting for >30 min; (ii) there was ST-segment elevation of at least 1 mm in at least two contiguous electrocardiography (ECG) leads or new onset of complete left bundle-branch block; and (iii) they had Fibrinolysis. Exclusion criteria were absolute contraindication for fibrinolysis, primary PCI, morbid obesity or handicapped patients who cannot walk, chronic obstructive pulmonary disease, patients with clinical hemodynamic or electrical instability.

Study design

This is a prospective cohort study. Between September 2011 and March 2012, 369 patients were enrolled in the coronary care unit of Assuit university hospital (AUH). We were not able to offer the 6MWT to all patients for logistical reasons (e.g., not enough time prepare the protocol, busy nurses, obstruction of the 6MWT corridor, study staff unavailable). Of the 115 patients who were offered the 6MWT, 4 were unable to complete the 6MWT (recently experiencing unusual chest pain, or did not think they were able to walk for 6 minutes due to shortness of breath or musculoskeletal barrier), 10 refused, and 1 had incomplete data. These 15 were excluded from this analysis because they did not complete the 6MWT, leaving 100 participants for this analysis.

Study population

We enrolled 100 consecutive patients, who fulfilled the inclusion and exclusion criteria for this study. Demographic characteristics, medical history, and smoking status were assessed. We measured weight, resting blood pressure and heart rate. The mean time in minutes from symptoms onset (the maximum intensity of the pain felt by the patients) to the start of fibrinolysis in CCU (symptoms – to-needle time) was documented. Before taking the fibrinolysis, we calculated the TIMI risk score [14,19] which include (age (years), weight (kg), DM, HTN, UA, heart rate (bpm), systolic BP (mmHg), ST elevation, LBBB, Killip class and time to treatment) and the GRACE risk score which include (age (years), heart rate (bpm), systolic BP (mmHg), creatinine (mg/dL), Killip class, cardiac arrest at admission, elevated cardiac markers and ST segment deviation) [12,20,21]. After initial event, all patients received asprin (150 mg/day) indefinitely, clopidogrel (75 mg/day) for one year, other medications including beta blocker, angiotensin converting enzyme inhibitors, nitrates and statins, were prescribed according to STEMI standard guidelines [22].

Six-Minute Walk Test (6MWT)

The 6MWT was administered according to standard guidelines just before the discharge of the patients from CCU [1]. A single walk test without practice was administered. Participants were instructed to walk continuously on a CCU corridor 40 m. in length, covering as much ground as they could during six minutes. The test was performed under the control of a physician who encouraged the patients using phrases like 'You are doing well' or 'You are doing a good job'. At the end of the 6-min, the physician measured the total distance walked by the patient. On the basis of the distance walked, performance was grouped into three different levels (level I>450 m, level II = 300–450 m and level III<300 m) [1,23].

Laboratory data

Creatine kinase (CK) activity (Dimension Xpand Plus, Siemens Diagnostics; upper limit of normal (ULN) = 308 U/L). The cumulative release of CK in the first 48 hours was calculated as a measure of infarct size in each patient by an investigator blinded to the assigned treatment [24]. Serum creatinine level (Dimension Xpand Plus, Siemens Diagnostics; upper limit of normal (ULN) = 115 μmol/L).

Electrocardiographic data analysis

ST segment elevation was measured manually 20 ms after the end of the QRS complex (the J point) using a hand-held caliper. The sum of ST-segment elevation in leads V1 to V6, I, and aVL was added to the sum of ST-segment depression in leads II, III, and aVF for anterior MI. For inferior MI, the sum of ST-segment elevation in leads II, III, and aVF (and I, aVL, V5, and V6; if present) were added to the sum of ST-segment depression in leads V1 to V4. All ECGs were collected and analyzed by an investigator blinded to the assigned treatment. Total ST-segment deviation at inclusion was compared to that taken within 90 minutes after PPCI. ST-segment resolution ≥50% of the initial ST-segment deviation was calculated [25,26].

Outcome Ascertainment

All patients were followed up for 3 months. Clinical outcome was evaluated through the monitoring of major adverse cardiac events (MACE) occurring at any time during the follow up. Death was defined as "all-cause" death at follow-up. Myocardial re-infarction was defined using standard diagnostic criteria [27]. Heart failure was defined as hospitalization or emergency department visit for signs and symptoms of heart failure. The primary outcome was incidence of MACE during follow up. Secondary outcomes were the individual components of heart failure, myocardial infarction, and death from any cause.

Statistical analysis

Patients were divided into 3 groups according to level of 6MWT distance. Baseline patient's characteristics were compared using analysis of variance (ANOVA) for continuous variables, a chi-squer (X^2) test for dichotomous variables, and fisher exact test for dichotomous variables with fewer than 5 patients in a category. Correlation between different variables was evaluated using Pearson correlation coefficient analysis. Univariate analysis was performed using X^2test with Yates' correction when necessary. Multivariate logistic and linear regression analyses were performed using all potentially relevant variables to identify baseline independent predictors of MACE. All p-values are two-tailed, and statistical significance was defined if $p<0.05$. All analyses were performed with SPSS version 16.0 statistical software (SPSS Inc., Chicago, IL, USA).

Results

Patient characteristics

The study population consists of 100 patients with STEMI received fibrinolysis. Patients were divided into 3 groups according to level of 6MWT distance. Baseline characteristics of our study population are summarized in table 1. The 3 groups were comparable, with no significant differences in baseline characteristics. In our study the patient's mean age was 60.9±10.7 years (ranging from 25–83 years) and the patient's mean weight was 73.7±9.7 (ranging from 49–100 kg).

Among the study population, the median 6MWT distance was 370 meters (interquartile range 162–462). Compared to patients in level I (>450 m), patients in level III (<300 m) were more likely to have clinical risk factors of hypertension, diabetes and impaired renal function test (Table 1). Electrocardiographic and infarct size results are summarized in TABLE 2, 60% of our study population had failure of thrombolytic therapy with ST segment resolution < 50% at 90 min post fibrinolysis. The baseline levels of CK were similar in all groups. The infarct size assessed by the cumulative 48-h CK release was not statistically different across groups. Patients in level III had more failure of thrombolytic therapy by ECG analysis and higher risk grade in GRACE score (Table 2).

Six-minute walk test was compared with GRACE risk score. There was a significant negative correlation between 6 MWT distance and GRACE risk score ($r = -0.80$, $p<0.001$) (Figure 1).

All patients were followed up for 90 days. Cumulative MACE occurred in 51 patients. 12 patients had heart failure hospitalization, 10 patients had re-infarction, 13 patients had post MI angina and 16 patients died (table 3). Incidence of MACE was higher in

Table 1. Baseline characteristics of the study population by levels of sex-minute walk test distance.

		6MWT levels (m)			
	All group	**Level I (>450 m)**	**Level II (300–450 m)**	**Level III (<300 m)**	**P**
Number of pt.	*10 pt*	**40 pt**	**32 pt**	**28 pt**	
Demographics					
Age (years)	60.9±10.7	58.5±11	62.5±10	62.3±8	NS*
Gender (Males)	72 (72%)	26	28	18	NS†
Smoking	47 (47%)	18	17	12	NS†
Medical history					
Hypertension	46(46%)	16	10	20	0.08†
Diabetes mellitus	35 (35%)	5	11	19	0.01†
Known to be Ischemic	33 (33%)	9	12	12	NS†
previous PCI	4 (4%)	0	2	2	NS†
previous CABG	7 (7%)	2	2	3	NS†
Dyslipidemia	25 (25%)	7	10	8	NS†
Previous admission to CCU	25 (25%)	9	7	9	NS†
Family history	16 (16%)	4	5	7	NS†
Clinical measurements					
Weight (kg)	73.7±9.7	73.5±8	72.4±9	75.2±12	NS*
Systolic BP (mmHg)	134±30	131±19	122±62	126±41	NS*
Diastolic BP (mmHg)	77±25	80±14	74±33	77±26	NS*
Pulse (bpm)	88±24	89±18	81±31	91±23	NS*
Symptoms -to-Needle Time (min)	276±37	169±35	318±75	332±85	NS*
Arrest on admission	3 (3%)	0	1	2	NS†
Infarction location					NS†
Anterior MI	67 (67%)	15	24	26	
Inferior MI	14 (14%)	5	2	7	
Infro-posterior MI	16 (16%)	7	5	4	
Lateral MI	3 (3%)	2	1	0	
KILLIP SCORE					NS†
SCORE 1	77 (77%)	33	25	19	
SCORE 2	18 (18%)	7	4	7	
SCORE≥3	5(5%)	0	2	3	
Duration till doing 6MWT (Days)	3.5±2	3.2±1	3.5±1	4.2±2	NS*
6MWT by meters	329±153	466±25	352±40	106±53	<001*

Data are presented as mean ± standard deviation, number (%) of patients.
*Compared using ANOVA test.
†Compared using Chi-square or Fisher exact test. BP= blood pressure; MI= myocardial infarction; TIMI= Thrombolysis In Myocardial Infarction; CK= creatine kinase; 6MWT= sex-minute walk test; PCI= percutaneous coronary intervention; CABG=coronary artery bypass graft; NS=not significant.

Table 2. Laboratory, electrocardiographic and risk scoring results of the study population by levels of sex-minute walk test distance.

		6MWT levels (m)			
	All group	**Level I (>450 m)**	**Level II (300–450 m)**	**Level III (<300 m)**	**P**
Number of pt.	*100 pt*	**40 pt**	**32 pt**	**28 pt**	
Basal CK (U/L)	*1616±195*	*1454±262*	*1211±270*	*2160±437*	*NS**
Cumulative 48-h CK release (U/L)	*9085 (5976–14593)*	*8174 (4135–13482)*	*8465 (4558–14466)*	*9296 (6013–15012)*	*NS**
Serum creatinine levels (μmol/L)					***0.002****
0.4–0.79	*21(21%)*	*14*	*4*	*3*	
0.8–1.1	*46(46%)*	*22*	*15*	*9*	
1.2–1.59	*19(19%)*	*3*	*7*	*9*	
1.6–1.99	*7(7%)*	*0*	*3*	*4*	
2–3.99	*7(7%)*	*0*	*3*	*4*	
Success of fibrinolysis using ECG ST resolution					***0.04†***
<50%	*60 (60%)*	*12*	*22*	*26*	
50–75%	*30 (30%)*	*14*	*14*	*2*	
>75%	*10 (10%)*	*6*	*3*	*1*	
TIMI risk score	*3.4±2*	*2.9±2*	*3.6±2*	*3.6±2*	*NS**
GRACE risk score	*147±29*	*123±17*	*161±27*	*166±21*	***<0.001****
Low risk (49–125)	*25 (25%)*	*25*	*0*	*0*	
Intermediate risk (126–154)	*33 (33%)*	*15*	*14*	*4*	
High risk (155–319)	*42 (42%)*	*0*	*17*	*25*	

Data are presented as mean ± standard deviation, number (%) of patients.
*Compared using ANOVA test.
†Compared using Chi-square or Fisher exact test. TIMI = Thrombolysis In Myocardial Infarction; CK = creatine kinase; 6MWT = sex-minute walk test; *GRACE* = Global Registry of Acute Coronary Events; NS = not significant.

patients with level III compared to other levels of 6MWT distance (Figure 2).

Prediction of MACE after STEMI using logistic regression analysis

Success of fibrinolysis, Anterior MI, Infarction size using 48 h CK and TIMI risk score were positively related to incidence of MACE (Table 4). Symptom to Needle time was not significantly related to MACE.

GRACE risk score and 6MWT distance levels were the strongest univariable predictors and the only significant predictors in multivariable logistic regression analysis for the incidence of MACE (Table 4). The incidence of MACE were 2 times higher in patients with a level III 6MWTand GRACE risk scores (OR = 2.66, 95% CI = 1.15–4.9 & OR = 2.46, 95% CI = 1.15–5.9). According to temporal sequence of events, GRACE risk score can be assessed early just after STEMI diagnosis, but 6MWT score

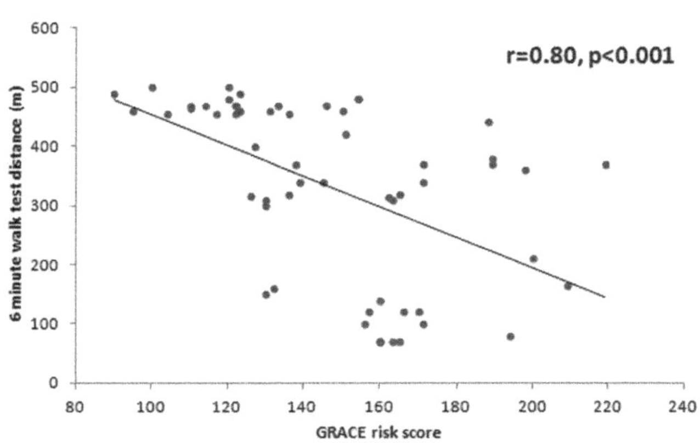

Figure 1. Six-minute walk test distance by GRACE risk score.

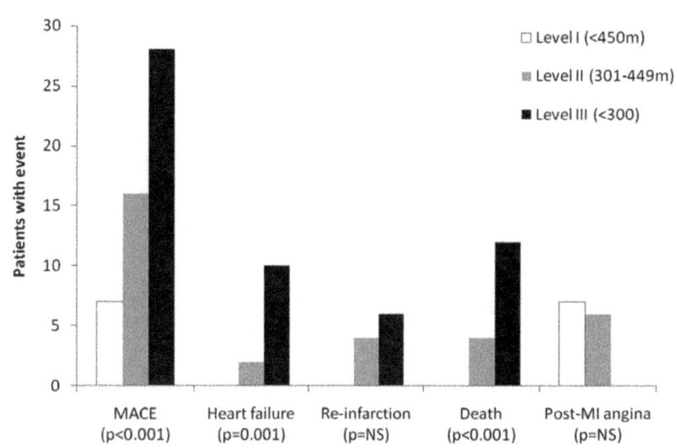

Figure 2. Cardiovascular events by levels of six-minute walk test distance.

Table 3. Clinical outcomes and complications at 90 days follow-up in the study population by levels of sex-minute walk test distance.

		6MWT levels (m)			
	All group	Level I (>450 m)	Level II (300–450 m)	Level III (<300 m)	P
Number of pt.	*100 pt*	40 pt	32 pt	28 pt	
MACE	51 (51%)	7	16	28	<0.001†
Heart failure	12 (12%)	0	2	10	0.001†
Re-infarction	10 (10%)	0	4	6	0.09†
Post-MI angina	13 (13%)	7	6	0	NS†
Death	16 (16%)	0	4	12	<0.001†

Data are presented as number (%) of patients.
†Compared using Chi-square or Fisher exact test. MACE = major adverse cardiac events; MI = myocardial infarction.

is only done pre-discharge. So after combining both scores in the multivariable analysis model, we identified only combination of 2 scores as an independent predictor of MACE (OR = 4.66, 95% CI = 1.1–14.5, p = 0.006). So it is reasonable to assume that adding 6MWT score to GRACE risk score will support the prediction of MACE in patients with STEMI treated with fibrinolysis.

Discussion

In a cohort of patients with STEMI treated with fibrinolysis, we found that shorter distance walked on 6MWT was associated with higher rates of heart failure, myocardial re-infarction, and death, independent of traditional cardiovascular disease risk factors and scoring systems. The 6MWT provided additional predictive information beyond traditional risk factors and scores. The ability of the 6MWT to predict cardiovascular events was similar to traditional GRACE risk score. These findings suggest that a simple 6MWT is a useful prognostic marker for identifying STEMI patients treated with fibrinolysis at low risk who may not need further interventions.

There has been limited evidence regarding the prognostic ability of 6MWT in patients with STEMI treated with fibrinolysis. One study evaluated patients with chronic stable coronary heart disease and found 6MWT to be predictor of cardiovascular events [28]. Another study evaluated patients with recent coronary artery bypass surgery undergoing cardiac rehabilitation and found 6MWT to be a predictor of mortality [29]. Our findings extend the evidence that the 6MWT predicts cardiovascular events to patients with STEMI treated with fibrinolysis. The results of our

Table 4. Logistic regression analysis for prediction of MACE.

	Univariable analysis			Multivariable analysis		
	OR	95%CI	P	OR	95%CI	P
Age	**1.03**	**0.98–1.09**	**0.26**	-	-	-
Male gender	**0.52**	**0.16–1.61**	**0.27**	-	-	-
Smoking	**0.65**	**0.22–1.91**	**0.44**	-	-	-
Hypertension	**0.99**	**0.33–2.88**	**0.98**	-	-	-
Diabetes	**0.79**	**0.25–2.44**	**0.68**	-	-	-
Previous MI	**0.54**	**0.05–3.58**	**0.44**	-	-	-
Dyslipidemia	**1.16**	**0.53–2.50**	**0.70**	-	-	-
Positive family history	**0.95**	**0.44–2.07**	**0.91**	-	-	-
Killip class ≥2	**2.21**	**0.19–25.14**	**0.91**	-	-	-
Symptom to Needle time	**1.00**	**0.99–7.74**	**0.88**	-	-	-
Anterior MI	**2.04**	**0.9–4.5**	**0.07**	-	-	-
Infarction size using CK	**0.93**	**0.88–0.99**	**0.07**	-	-	-
Success of fibrinolysis using ECG	**0.94**	**0.88–0.99**	**0.04**	**0.96**	**0.86–1.01**	**0.11**
GRACE risk score	**7.23**	**3.4–15.1**	**0.004**	**2.46**	**1.15–5.90**	**0.07**
TIMI score	**3.08**	**1.1–8.1**	**0.07**	**1.33**	**0.86–3.90**	**0.12**
6MWT risk score	**7.14**	**3.3–17.1**	**0.005**	**2.66**	**1.15–4.90**	**0.07**
Combination of GRACE+6MWT	**8.14**	**3.3–19.1**	**<0.001**	**4.66**	**1.15–14.90**	**0.006**

MI: myocardial infarction, PPCI: primary percutanious coronary intervention, TIMI = Thrombolysis In Myocardial Infarction; CK = creatine kinase; 6MWT = sex-minute walk test; *GRACE* = Global Registry of Acute Coronary Events.

study also expand beyond previous studies that have investigated 6MWT in patients with heart failure [1–6]. Although 6MWT distance did not reliably correlate with cardiopulmonary exercise testing measures in previous studies [30,31], most studies found that 6MWT still predicted heart failure hospitalizations and death in patients with systolic heart failure [2,5,6].

In addition, Beatty et.al. [28] revealed that the 6MWTD can predicts MACE in a broader population of patients with stable CHD, independent of traditional risk factors and markers of cardiac disease severity. More over they suggest that 6MWT is a potential alternative to treadmill exercise testing for assessment of prognosis in those patients.

Treadmill exercise testing will remain the preferred modality for evaluating patients with suspected ischemia. However, for STEMI patients undergoing risk stratification for further intervention, the 6MWT offers potential advantages. The 6MWT can be conducted with little equipment other than a hallway marked for distance and a stopwatch. Due to the self-paced nature of the test, side effects of chest pain, dyspnea, or musculoskeletal pain are usually mild; serious adverse events have not been described [1]. Further, the 6MWT is less expensive than treadmill exercise testing. The ability of the 6MWT, a simple office-based test of functional exercise capacity, to predict outcomes in patients with stable CHD is especially relevant because the 6MWT addresses physical activity, a modifiable risk factor for secondary prevention of CHD [28]. While we have demonstrated in the present work that the 6MWTD can predict cardiovascular events in STEMI patients, however, its use for improving prognosis merits further study.

Study Limitations

Our study is a single center prospective study, the level of 6MWTD was predetermined based on heart failure protocols, this consensus was taken mainly to allow comparison with other studies. The use of Treadmill exercise stress test as a control group was not valid in this study however, we recommend adding it in future studies. We cannot exclude the possibility of selection bias in the main cohort of participants, since many CCU admitted patients were not enrolled in the study for logistical reasons (eg. study staff unavailable, not enough time to prepare the protocol, busy nurses). Patients were excluded from the study if they were unable to walk. Thus, the results may not extend to patients with significant angina or other limitations in walking.

Conclusions

In patients with STEMI treated with fibrinolysis, the addition of the distance walked on 6MWT pre-discharge to traditional GRACE risk score improved risk prediction of cardiovascular events at 3 month follow up.

Author Contributions

Conceived and designed the experiments: AKMH GWA SRD. Performed the experiments: GWA. Analyzed the data: AKMH. Contributed reagents/materials/analysis tools: AKMH SRD. Wrote the paper: AKMH. Revision of the manuscript: AKMH SRD.

References

1. ATS statement: guidelines for the six-minute walk test (2002) Am J Respir Crit Care Med 166: 111–117.
2. Bittner V, Weiner DH, Yusuf S, Rogers WJ, McIntyre KM, et al. (1993) Prediction of mortality and morbidity with a 6-minute walk test in patients with left ventricular dysfunction. SOLVD Investigators. JAMA 270: 1702–1707.
3. Cahalin LP, Mathier MA, Semigran MJ, Dec GW, DiSalvo TG (1996) The six-minute walk test predicts peak oxygen uptake and survival in patients with advanced heart failure. Chest 110: 325–332.
4. Ingle L, Shelton RJ, Rigby AS, Nabb S, Clark AL, et al. (2005) The reproducibility and sensitivity of the 6-min walk test in elderly patients with chronic heart failure. Eur Heart J 26: 1742–1751.
5. Rostagno C, Olivo G, Comeglio M, Boddi V, Banchelli M, et al. (2003) Prognostic value of 6-minute walk corridor test in patients with mild to moderate heart failure: comparison with other methods of functional evaluation. Eur J Heart Fail 5: 247–252.
6. Shah MR, Hasselblad V, Gheorghiade M, Adams KF, Swedberg K, et al. (2001) Prognostic usefulness of the six-minute walk in patients with advanced congestive heart failure secondary to ischemic or nonischemic cardiomyopathy. Am J Cardiol 88: 987–993.
7. Swiston JR, Johnson SR, Granton JT (2010) Factors that prognosticate mortality in idiopathic pulmonary arterial hypertension: a systematic review of the literature. Respir Med 104: 1588–1607.
8. Rasekaba T, Lee AL, Naughton MT, Williams TJ, Holland AE (2009) The six-minute walk test: a useful metric for the cardiopulmonary patient. Intern Med J 39: 495–501.
9. Casanova C, Celli BR, Barria P, Casas A, Cote C, et al. (2011) The 6-min walk distance in healthy subjects: reference standards from seven countries. Eur Respir J 37: 150–156.
10. Chetta A, Zanini A, Pisi G, Aiello M, Tzani P, et al. (2006) Reference values for the 6-min walk test in healthy subjects 20–50 years old. Respir Med 100: 1573–1578.
11. Raber L, Kelbaek H, Ostojic M, Baumbach A, Heg D, et al. (2012) Effect of biolimus-eluting stents with biodegradable polymer vs bare-metal stents on cardiovascular events among patients with acute myocardial infarction: the COMFORTABLE AMI randomized trial. JAMA 308: 777–787.
12. Granger CBM, Goldberg RJP, Dabbous OMM, Pierper KSM, Eagle KAM, et al. (2003) Predictors of Hospital Mortality in the Global Registry of Acute Coronary Events for the Global Registry of Acute Coronary Events for the Global Registry of Acute Coronary Events Investigations. Archives of Internal Medicine 163: 2345–2353.
13. Addala S, Grines CL, Dixon SR, Stone GW, Boura JA, et al. (2004) Predicting mortality in patients with ST-elevation myocardial infarction treated with primary percutaneous coronary intervention (PAMI risk score). Am J Cardiol 93: 629–632.
14. Morrow DA, Antman EM, Charlesworth A, Cairns R, Murphy SA, et al. (2000) TIMI risk score for ST-elevation myocardial infarction: A convenient, bedside, clinical score for risk assessment at presentation: An intravenous nPA for treatment of infarcting myocardium early II trial substudy. Circulation 102: 2031–2037.
15. De Luca G, Suryapranata H, van 't Hof AW, de Boer MJ, Hoorntje JC, et al. (2004) Prognostic assessment of patients with acute myocardial infarction treated with primary angioplasty: implications for early discharge. Circulation 109: 2737–2743.
16. Halkin A, Singh M, Nikolsky E, Grines CL, Tcheng JE, et al. (2005) Prediction of mortality after primary percutaneous coronary intervention for acute myocardial infarction: the CADILLAC risk score. J Am Coll Cardiol 45: 1397–1405.
17. Capodanno D, Miano M, Cincotta G, Caggegi A, Ruperto C, et al. (2010) EuroSCORE refines the predictive ability of SYNTAX score in patients undergoing left main percutaneous coronary intervention. Am Heart J 159: 103–109.
18. Boden WE, Franklin BA, Wenger NK (2013) Physical activity and structured exercise for patients with stable ischemic heart disease. JAMA 309: 143–144.
19. Selvarajah S, Fong AY, Selvaraj G, Haniff J, Uiterwaal CS, et al. (2012) An Asian Validation of the TIMI Risk Score for ST-Segment Elevation Myocardial Infarction. PLoS One 7: e40249.
20. Bonnefoy E, Kirkorian G (2011) Mortality of myocardial infarction. Ann Cardiol Angeiol (Paris) 60: 311–316.
21. bu-Assi E, Garcia-Acuna JM, Pena-Gil C, Gonzalez-Juanatey JR (2010) Validation of the GRACE risk score for predicting death within 6 months of follow-up in a contemporary cohort of patients with acute coronary syndrome. Rev Esp Cardiol 63: 640–648.
22. Steg PG, James SK, Atar D, Badano LP, Blomstrom-Lundqvist C, et al. (2012) ESC Guidelines for the management of acute myocardial infarction in patients presenting with ST-segment elevation. Eur Heart J 33: 2569–2619.
23. Stevens D, Elpern E, Sharma K, Szidon P, Ankin M, et al. (1999) Comparison of hallway and treadmill six-minute walk tests. Am J Respir Crit Care Med 160: 1540–1543.
24. Bruschke AV, van der Laarse A, van der Wall EE (1990) Assessment of the size of acute myocardial infarction. I: Biochemical methods. Cleve Clin J Med 57: 547–550.
25. Taher T, Fu Y, Wagner GS, Goodman SG, Fresco C, et al. (2004) Aborted myocardial infarction in patients with ST-segment elevation: insights from the Assessment of the Safety and Efficacy of a New Thrombolytic Regimen-3 Trial Electrocardiographic Substudy. J Am Coll Cardiol 44: 38–43.
26. Hassan AKM, Liem SS, van der Kley F, Bergheanu SC, Wolterbeek R, et al. (2009) In-ambulance abciximab administration in STEMI patients prior to primary PCI is associated with smaller infarct size, improved LV function and

lower incidence of heart failure: Results from the Leiden MISSION! acute myocardial infarction treatment optimization program. Cathet Cardiovasc Intervent 74: 335–343.
27. Luepker RV, Apple FS, Christenson RH, Crow RS, Fortmann SP, et al. (2003) Case definitions for acute coronary heart disease in epidemiology and clinical research studies: a statement from the AHA Council on Epidemiology and Prevention; AHA Statistics Committee; World Heart Federation Council on Epidemiology and Prevention; the European Society of Cardiology Working Group on Epidemiology and Prevention; Centers for Disease Control and Prevention; and the National Heart, Lung, and Blood Institute. Circulation 108: 2543–2549.
28. Beatty AL, Schiller NB, Whooley MA (2012) Six-minute walk test as a prognostic tool in stable coronary heart disease: data from the heart and soul study. Arch Intern Med 172: 1096–1102.
29. Cacciatore F, Abete P, Mazzella F, Furgi G, Nicolino A, et al. (2012) Six-minute walking test but not ejection fraction predicts mortality in elderly patients undergoing cardiac rehabilitation following coronary artery bypass grafting. Eur J Prev Cardiol 19: 1401–1409.
30. Guazzi M, Dickstein K, Vicenzi M, Arena R (2009) Six-minute walk test and cardiopulmonary exercise testing in patients with chronic heart failure: a comparative analysis on clinical and prognostic insights. Circ Heart Fail 2: 549–555.
31. Pollentier B, Irons SL, Benedetto CM, Dibenedetto AM, Loton D, et al. (2010) Examination of the six minute walk test to determine functional capacity in people with chronic heart failure: a systematic review. Cardiopulm Phys Ther J 21: 13–21.

Efficacy of High Intensity Exercise on Disease Activity and Cardiovascular Risk in Active Axial Spondyloarthritis: A Randomized Controlled Pilot Study

Silje Halvorsen Sveaas[1,2*¶], Inger Jorid Berg[3¶], Sella Aarrestad Provan[3], Anne Grete Semb[3], Kåre Birger Hagen[1,2], Nina Vøllestad[2], Camilla Fongen[1], Inge C. Olsen[3], Annika Michelsen[4], Thor Ueland[4,6], Pål Aukrust[4,5,6,7], Tore K. Kvien[3], Hanne Dagfinrud[1,2]

1 National Advisory Unit on Rehabilitation in Rheumatology, Department of Rheumatology, Diakonhjemmet Hospital, Oslo, Norway, **2** Department of Health Sciences, University of Oslo, Oslo, Norway, **3** Department of Rheumatology, Diakonhjemmet Hospital, Oslo, Norway, **4** Research Institute of Internal Medicine, Oslo University Hospital, Rikshospitalet, Oslo, Norway, **5** Section of Clinical Immunology and Infectious Diseases, Oslo University Hospital, Rikshospitalet, Oslo, Norway, **6** Institute of Clinical Medicine, University of Oslo, Oslo, Norway, **7** K.G. Jebsen Inflammatory Research Center, University of Oslo, Oslo, Norway

Abstract

Background: Physical therapy is recommended for the management of axial spondyloarthritis (axSpA) and flexibility exercises have traditionally been the main focus. Cardiovascular (CV) diseases are considered as a major health concern in axSpA and there is strong evidence that endurance and strength exercise protects against CV diseases. Therefore, the aim of this study was to investigate the efficacy of high intensity endurance and strength exercise on disease activity and CV health in patients with active axSpA.

Methods: In a single blinded randomized controlled pilot study the exercise group (EG) performed 12 weeks of endurance and strength exercise while the control group (CG) received treatment as usual. The primary outcome was the Ankylosing Spondylitis (AS) Disease Activity Score (ASDAS). Secondary outcomes included patient reported disease activity (Bath AS Disease Activity Index [BASDAI]), physical function (Bath AS Functional Index [BASFI]), and CV risk factors measured by arterial stiffness (Augmentation Index [AIx]) and Pulse Wave Velocity [PWV]), cardiorespiratory fitness (VO_2 peak) and body composition. ANCOVA on the post intervention values with baseline values as covariates was used to assess group differences, and Mann Whitney U-test was used for outcomes with skewed residuals.

Results: Twenty-eight patients were included and 24 (EG, n = 10, CG, n = 14) completed the study. A mean treatment effect of −0.7 (95%CI: −1.4, 0.1) was seen in ASDAS score. Treatment effects were also observed in secondary outcomes (mean group difference [95%CI]): BASDAI: −2.0 (−3.6, −0.4), BASFI: −1.4 (−2.6, −0.3), arterial stiffness (estimated median group differences [95% CI]): AIx (%): −5.3 (−11.0, −0.5), and for PVW (m/s): −0.3 (−0.7, 0.0), VO_2 peak (ml/kg/min) (mean group difference [95%CI]: 3.7 (2.1, 5.2) and trunk fat (%): −1.8 (−3.0, −0.6). No adverse events occurred.

Conclusion: High intensity exercise improved disease activity and reduced CV risk factors in patients with active axSpA. These effects will be further explored in a larger trial.

Trial Registration: ClinicalTrials.gov NCT01436942

Editor: Shervin Assassi, University of Texas Health Science Center at Houston, United States of America

Funding: The present study was supported by grants from the Norwegian Foundation for Postgraduate Physiotherapist. The funders had no role in study design, data collection and analysis, decision to publish, or preparation of the manuscript.

Competing Interests: The authors have declared that no competing interests exist.

* Email: silje.halvorsen@medisin.uio.no

¶ These authors are shared first authors on this work.

Introduction

Axial spondyloarthritis (axSpA) including ankylosing spondylitis (AS) is characterized by inflammatory back pain and reduced spinal mobility [1]. Over the past decades, the management of many rheumatic diseases has been revolutionized by improvements in diagnostic techniques and medication leading to a more active treatment approach for patients with axSpA [2]. Physical therapy with supervised exercise is a cornerstone in the treatment of axSpA together with anti-inflammatory medications such as non-steroidal anti-inflammatory drugs (NSAIDs) and tumor necrosis factor (TNF)-inhibitors [2]. There are no definite recommendations on type of exercise and intensity, and traditionally flexibility exercises at a low intensity level have been recommended [3].

A Cochrane review concluded that physical therapy interventions, mainly consisting of flexibility exercises, have beneficial effects on pain, spinal mobility, physical function and patient global assessment in AS patients, but the effect sizes are small [4]. Additional support for exercise as a part of the treatment repertoire in axSpA is the evidence of increased risk of cardiovascular diseases (CVD) in these patients [5–7]. For healthy adults, cardiorespiratory exercise is recommended in guidelines for CVD prevention [8], and high intensity endurance exercise has been shown to be more effective than low intensity endurance exercise [9]. In addition, the health benefits of strength exercise in CVD prevention are well established [10]. However, the evidence for effects of high intensity endurance and strength exercise on disease activity and cardiovascular (CV) -risk is limited in patients with axSpA.

Therefore, the aim of this study was to investigate the efficacy of high intensive endurance and strength exercise on disease activity and CV-risk in patients with active axSpA.

Methods

The protocol for this trial and supporting CONSORT checklist are available as supporting information; se Checklist S1 and Protocol S1.

Design

This study was a single blinded randomized controlled pilot study comparing an exercise group (EG) with a treatment as usual control group (CG). The intervention lasted for 12 weeks, and participants were examined at baseline and post intervention. All the participants provided written informed consent to participate, and all procedures followed the Helsinki declaration. The study was approved by the Regional Committee for medical and health research Ethics of South East Norway (reference: 2011/1468) and is listed in ClinicalTrials.gov (NCT01436942).

Participants

Patients fulfilling the following criteria were considered eligible: axSpA according to the Assessment of SpA International Society (ASAS) classification criteria [11], age 18–70 years, no change in TNF-inhibitor use during the last 3 months, moderate to high disease activity (Bath AS Disease Activity Index [BASDAI] $\geq$3.5) and not performed regular endurance or strength exercise during the last year (>1 hour per week). Exclusion criteria were established CVD, other co-morbidity involving reduced exercise capacity, inability to participate in weekly exercise sessions in Oslo and pregnancy. The study was carried out at Diakonhjemmet Hospital in Oslo between October 2011 and June 2012, with recruitment of patients during the first six months. No formal sample size consideration was performed for this intervention due to the exploratory design of the study.

Intervention

The exercise program followed the American college of sports medicine (ACSM) recommendations for maintenance and improvement of cardiorespiratory- and muscular fitness [10]. Patients in the EG were encouraged to exercise 40–60 minutes three times a week for twelve weeks. Twice a week the exercise sessions were carried out at a fitness center with individual supervision from a physical therapist (SHS). These sessions consisted of both endurance and strength training. The endurance training was high intensity interval training on a treadmill for 40 minutes (four minutes walking/running at 90–95% of maximal heart rate [HR] followed by three minutes of active resting at 70% of maximal HR repeated four times) [12]. The strength training was 20 minutes with external load for major muscle groups (individually adapted, six exercises, eight to ten repetitions maximum, two to three sets). The strength program consisted of the following exercises: bench press with weight manuals or seated in a chest press machine, squat with weight or leg press machine, rowing exercise with weight manuals, exercises for triceps and biceps in a fitness machine and an abdominal stabilization exercise (abdominal bridge).

Once a week the participants exercised individually minimum 40 minutes of endurance training, either an additional session with interval training or a session with long-distance training (above 70% of maximal HR). The exercise program was individually adapted to the participant's fitness level and a physical therapist (SHS) was responsible for an adequate progression of the intensity level during the exercise period.

The maximal HR of each participant was determined during the baseline test and the HR was controlled with a HR monitor to individually tailor the intensity. Attendance at the supervised exercise sessions was recorded by the physical therapist (SHS). The weekly self-imposed exercise session was first recorded in the pulse watch and thereafter weekly reported to the physical therapist. To fulfill the exercise protocol the participants had to attend at least 80% of the planned exercise sessions.

Participants in the CG were asked to not start exercising during the intervention period. The CG was introduced to the exercise program post-intervention to reduce drop out.

Procedures of assessments

Assessments for efficacy and safety were performed at baseline and after 12 weeks (end of study) and included questionnaires, clinical examinations and laboratory measurements.

Personal characteristics, comorbidities and medication were self-reported in a questionnaire. All physical (spinal mobility, body weight/height, waist circumference and body composition) and performance (VO_2 peak) based measures were recorded by an experienced physical therapist (CF). The assessments of blood pressure (BP), HR and arterial stiffness were performed by an experienced rheumatologist (IJB).

Primary outcome measure

The primary outcome was disease activity assessed by the AS Disease Activity Score (ASDAS) [13]. ASDAS is reported to be a valid measure of disease activity as it has shown acceptable concurrent validity with both patients and physicians global assessments. ASDAS is a composite continuous score consisting of three patient reported items in addition to C-reactive protein (CRP).

Secondary outcomes measures

Disease specific measures. Disease activity was also measured by the patient reported index BASDAI [14]. The BASDAI consists of six items related to major symptoms in AS (fatigue, spinal pain, joint pain, tenderness and degree and length of morning stiffness). BASDAI is reported to be valid as it reflects the entire spectrum of the disease and is sensitive to changes over time [14]. Physical function was measured with Bath AS Functional Index (BASFI) which is a disease specific index that consists of eight questions regarding physical functioning and two questions reflecting the patient's ability to cope with everyday life [15]. For both BASDAI and BASFI each question was answered on a 10 point numeric rating scale, and a sum score was calculated (0–10, 10 = worst). Spinal mobility was measured by Bath AS Metrology Index (BASMI) [16]. BASMI includes five objective measurements of spinal mobility, and the score is 0–10 for each component, and the mean of the five scores produced a BASMI score from 0–10 (10 = worst).

Cardiorespiratory fitness. Cardiorespiratory fitness was assessed with a maximal walking treadmill test for estimation of peak oxygen uptake (VO_2 peak) as previously described [17]. Resting HR was measured after at least five minutes rest in a supine position and several recordings were made until two measurements differed by ≤5 heart beats, and the mean was then calculated.

Arterial stiffness. We measured arterial stiffness after at least five minutes of rest in a supine position, using the Sphygmocor apparatus (AtCor, Sidney, Australia). Several recordings were made from each patient and only those of high quality, according to standardized criteria [18], were chosen for further analyses. Augmentation Index (AIx) was estimated through pulse wave recordings at the radial artery. The pulse waves of the central arteries were derived by applying a validated transfer factor [19]. For measurements of Pulse Wave Velocity (PWV), we recorded the pulse at the carotid artery and the femoral artery. The distance between these points was measured (subtracting the distance between carotid artery and sternal notch from distance between femoral artery and sternal notch). The time of wave travel was simultaneously recorded with electrocardiogram. PWV was calculated by dividing the distance with the time, expressed in m/s.

Body composition. Body weight and body height were measured with calculation of body mass index (BMI) (kg/m^2). Waist circumference was measured with a measuring tape at the height of umbilicus with the patient lying in supine position. Dual-energy X-ray absorptiometry (DXA) was used to assess body composition (body fat) and DXA is reconized as a validated reference method for assessing body composition [20].

Blood pressure. Brachial BP was measured in a supine position after at least five minutes rest using Omron M7 (Kyoto, Japan). Several measurements were performed until two differed by ≤5 mmHg in both systolic and diastolic BP and the average of these two measurements were calculated.

Inflammatory markers, cytokines and lipids. Blood samples were drawn after at least four hours fasting, and at least 48 hours after the last exercise session, and then analyzed for CRP, total cholesterol (TC) and high density lipoprotein cholesterol (HDL-c) by COBAS 6000 (Roche Diagnostics, Basel, Switzerland). Low density lipoprotein cholesterol (LDL-c) was calculated from Freidewalds formula [21]. Erythrocyte sedimentation rate (ESR) was measured using the Westergren method. In addition, blood samples were collected in EDTA containing vacutainer tubes, plasma were isolated and frozen at −80°Celsius and batch analyzed by enzyme immunoassays (EIAs). The following were analyzed: interleukin (IL)-6, IL-23 (Abcam, Cambridge, UK), IL-17a (Peprotec, Rocky Hill, NJ, USA), IL-18 and soluble TNF receptor 1 (sTNF-R1) and 2 (sTNF-R2) (RnDsystems, Stillwater, MN) at the end of the study. The inter- and intra-assay coefficients of variation were less than 10% for all EIAs.

Safety. Safety was considered as absence of a flare up in disease activity and was defined in terms of stable or decreased self-reported disease activity (ASDAS and BASDAI) and acute phase reactants (CRP and ESR). Further, we included the report of any adverse events in the definition of safety.

Randomization and blinding

Allocation to EG or CG followed a computer-generated randomization list prepared by a study-independent statistician. Block-randomization with a block-size of four was used. The group assignment was concealed in envelopes and revealed consecutively after baseline testing. The recruiting investigator was unaware of the next participant's allocation. The assessors were blinded for group assignment and participants were instructed not to reveal any information regarding their group attachment or treatment program to the assessors.

Statistical analyses

Statistical analyses were performed using SPSS version 21. The main statistical analyses were performed on the per-protocol population since this was an explanatory study [22]. The per-protocol population consisted of all randomized patients following the exercise protocol (at least 80% exercise attendance in EG and no exercise in CG). We used analysis of covariance (ANCOVA) on the post-intervention values to assess the group differences with p-values, mean difference and 95% CI. Baseline values were included as covariates. We assessed the normality assumptions of the ANCOVA models by pp-plots of the residuals. The residuals for ESR, CRP, IL-6, AIx and PWV were not normally distributed, and group differences in change from baseline were analyzed using the Mann-Whitney U-test with median and corresponding 95% confidence limits by the Hodges-Lehman estimator. P-values < 0.05 were considered to be statistically significant. We considered all analyses to be exploratory, and did not adjust for multiple testing.

Results

Participant flow

Thirty-four patients were assessed for eligibility (Figure 1). Six patients were excluded or withdrawn before randomization. Twenty-eight patients were randomized, 13 in EG, 15 in CG. One patient in the EG withdrew immediately after randomization due to hospitalization. Three patients dropped out during the intervention period (EG = 2, CG = 1). In the EG, one patient dropped out because of a streptococcal infection in the throat and one patient dropped out because the intervention was physically challenging and time consuming. In the CG, one patient did not perform testing after 12 weeks.

All the completing participants in the EG followed ≥80% of the exercise protocol, and reached their targeted HR during the endurance exercise sessions. In the CG, none of the completing participants reported that they had exercised during the intervention period, but one patient in the CG started with TNF-inhibitor four weeks after the baseline assessment. Following this, the per-protocol population consisted of 24 patients, 10 in the EG and 14 in the CG.

Characteristics

There were significantly more males in the CG compared to the EG ($p = 0.01$), and the groups differed in weight ($p = 0.01$) and height ($p = 0.01$), presumable due to the gender difference (Table 1). Baseline characteristics were similar across the groups for other variables (Table 1).

Efficacy on disease activity

Although not statistically significant, there was an improvement in the primary outcome ASDAS score in the EG compared to the CG (adjusted mean between group difference −0.66, 95%CI [−1.37, 0.05], $p = 0.07$) (Table 2), whereas patient reported

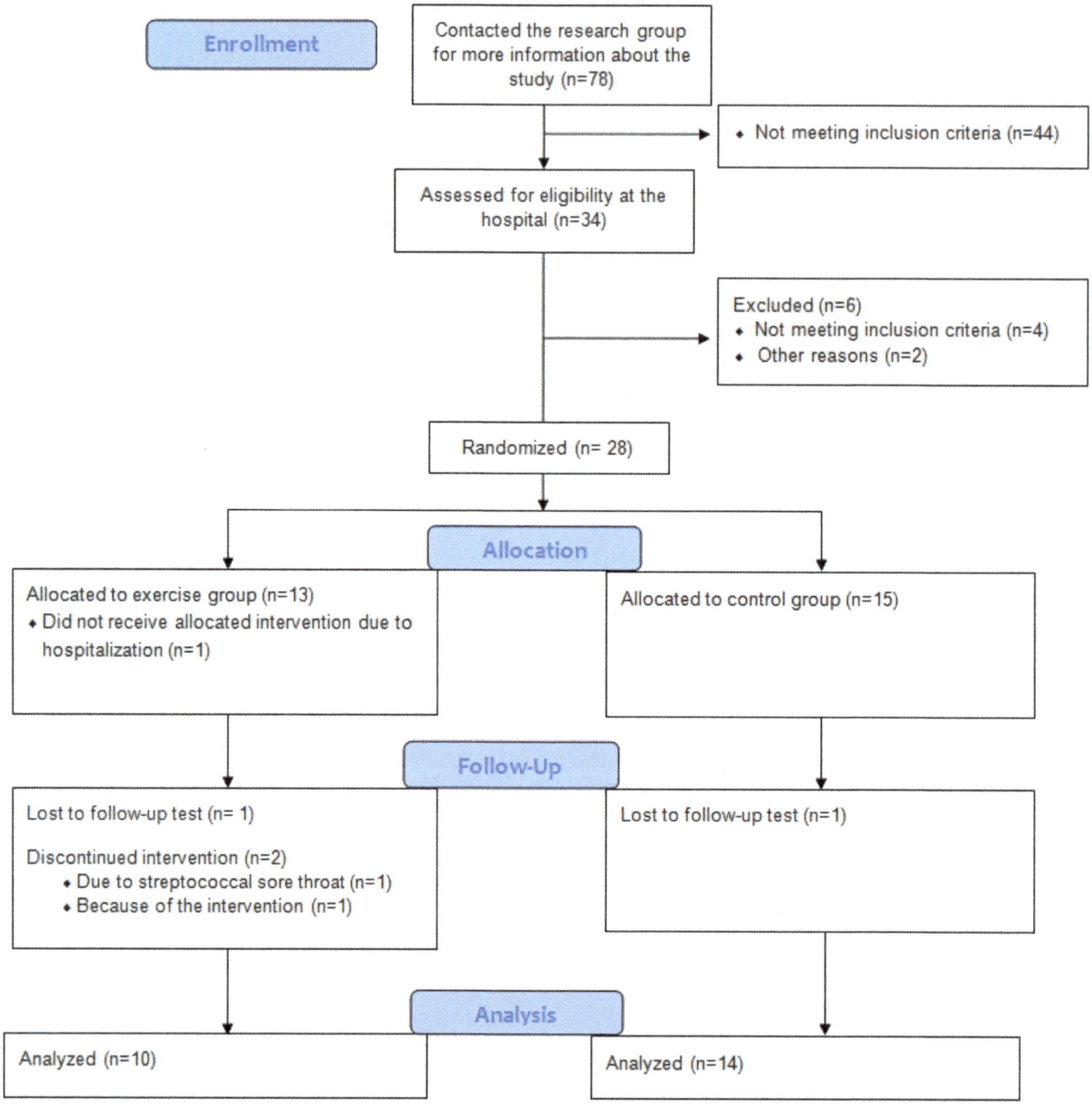

Figure 1. Flow of participants through the randomized controlled pilot study. EG: exercise group. CG: control group.

disease activity, BASDAI, improved significantly (adjusted mean between group difference −2.0, 95%CI [−3.6, −0.4], p = 0.02).

Efficacy on cardiovascular risk factors

Arterial stiffness was significantly reduced in the EG compared to CG. The median changes in AIx and PWV for the EG and CG are presented in Figure 2. All changes were in favor of the EG. Further, significant treatment effects were seen for VO_2 peak, resting HR, total body fat and abdominal fat (Table 3). A significant reduction in waist circumference was observed for subjects who had an increased waist circumference at baseline (males ≥94 cm and females ≥80 cm, analyzed: EG n = 6 and CG n = 12) in the EG compared to CG.

Efficacy on other secondary outcome measures

Significant treatment effects were seen for patient reported physical function, BASFI, but not for spinal mobility (BASMI) (Table 2). In general, there were no differences between the groups in change in inflammatory markers, although there was a trend towards a reduction in IL-17a and IL-23 in the EG compared to the CG (Table 2).

Safety

Seven of 10 subjects in the EG had decreased disease activity, one had a stable disease activity and two increased their disease activity (+0.2 and +0.5 in ASDAS) from baseline to post intervention. There were no differences in change in inflammatory markers (CRP and ERS) between the groups. Furthermore, no

Table 1. Baseline descriptive of all patients, exercise group and control group.

	All patients, n = 24	Exercise group, n = 10	Control group, n = 14
Age, years, mean (SD)	48.5 (12.0)	46.6 (13.6)	49.9 (11.1)
Gender, male, n (%)	12 (50)	2 (20)[a]	10 (71)[a]
Current smoking, n (%)	3 (13)	1 (10)	2 (14)
Height, m, mean (SD)	1.75 (0.07)	1.71 (0.06)[a]	1.78 (0.07)[a]
Weight, kg, mean (SD)	79.5 (15.7)	70.0 (12.3)[a]	86.3 (14.6)[a]
Disease duration, years, mean (SD)	24.9 (15.8)	19.2 (19.8)	28.6 (11.9)
ASDAS, mean (SD)	2.6 (0.6)	2.3 (0.6)	2.7 (0.8)
BASDAI, mean (SD)	5.3 (1.4)	5.3 (1.4)	5.3 (1.4)
CRP, median (range)	2 (1, 23)	1 (1, 9)	2 (1, 23)
ERS, median (range)	7(1, 41)	10 (2, 41)	6 (1, 24)
Diabetes, n (%)	1 (4)	1 (10)	0 (0)
Hypertension, n (%)	4 (17)	1 (10)	3 (21)
NSAIDs, n (%)	18 (75)	8 (80)	10 (71)
TNF-inhibitor, n (%)	7 (29)	1 (10)	6 (43)
Anti-hypertensives, n (%)	4 (17)	0 (0)	4 (29)
Statins, n (%)	5 (21)	2 (20)	3 (21)

ASDAS, Ankylosing Spondylitis Disease Activity Score; BASDAI, Bath Ankylosing Spondylitis Disease Activity Index (0–10, 10= worst); CRP, C-reactiv protein; ESR, erythrocyte sedimentation rate NSAIDs, non-steroidal anti-inflammatory drugs; TNF, tumor necrosis factor, SD; standard deviation.
[a]Statistically significant differences between groups. Analysed with bivariate test as appropriate.

Table 2. Effects of high intensity exercise on disease activity, inflammatory markers and cytokines.

	Exercise group, n = 10		Control group, n = 14		Estimated mean group difference (95% CI)[a]	p-value
	Baseline	3 months	Baseline	3 months		
Disease activity						
ASDAS, mean (SD)	2.3 (0.6)	1.8 (0.9)	2.7 (0.8)	2.6 (0.8)	−0.7 (−1.4, 0.1)[a]	0.07
BASDAI, mean (SD)	5.3 (1.4)	3.3 (2.0)	5.3 (1.3)	5.2 (2.0)	−2.0 (−3.6, −0.4)[a]	0.02
BASFI, mean (SD)	2.6 (2.2)	1.5 (1.5)	3.1 (1.6)	3.1 (1.4)	−1.4 (−2.6, −0.3)[a]	0.02
BASMI, mean (SD)	2.3 (1.5)	2.0 (1.6)	3.0 (1.8)	2.9 (1.8)	−0.3 (−0.9, 0.3)[a]	0.32
Inflammatory markers						
ESR (mm/h), median (range)	10 (2, 41)	9 (5, 26)	6 (1, 24)	7 (1, 46)	−1 (−6, 2)[b]	0.40[c]
CRP (mg/L), median (range)	1 (1,9)	1 (1,12)	2 (1, 23)	3 (1, 13)	0 (−1, 2)[b]	0.89[c]
Cytokines						
IL-6 (pg/mL), median (range)	0.3 (0.2, 5.0)	0.3 (0.2, 16.2)	0.4 (0.2, 2.8)	0.3 (0.2, 2.4)	0.0 (−0.3, 0.5)[b]	0.95[c]
IL-17a (pg/mL), mean (SD)	82 (53)	72 (27)	103 (90)	105 (80)	−16 (−34, 2)[a]	0.08
IL-18 (pg/mL), mean (SD)	95 (20)	86 (15)	97 (37)	101 (43)	−13 (−30, 4)[a]	0.12
IL-23 (pg/ml), mean (SD)	123 (39)	103 (25)	95 (47)	113 (39)	−24 (−49, 1)[a]	0.06
sTNFr1 (ng/mL), mean (SD)	0.87 (0.23)	0.87 (0.16)	0.98 (0.20)	1.03 (0.31)	−0.05 (−0.18, 0.09)[a]	0.46
sTNFr2 (ng/mL), mean (SD)	3.0 (2.5)	3.0 (2.5)	3.9 (3.3)	4.0 (3.3)	−0.1 (−0.3, 0.2)[a]	0.64

Differences between the groups in post intervention (3 months) values, analyzed with ANCOVA with baseline values as covariates.
All BAS-instruments 0–10, 10= worst.
ASDAS, Ankylosing Spondylitis Disease Activity Score; BASDAI, Bath Ankylosing Spondylitis Disease Activity Index; BASFI, Bath Ankylosing Spondylitis Functional Index; BASMI, Bath Ankylosing Spondylitis Metrology Index; CRP, C-reactive protein; ESR, erythrocyte sedimentation rate; IL, interleukin; sTNFR, soluble tumor necrosis factor receptor.
[a]Estimated regression coefficients,
[b]Hodges-Lehman median estimator,
[c]Mann-Whitney U-test.

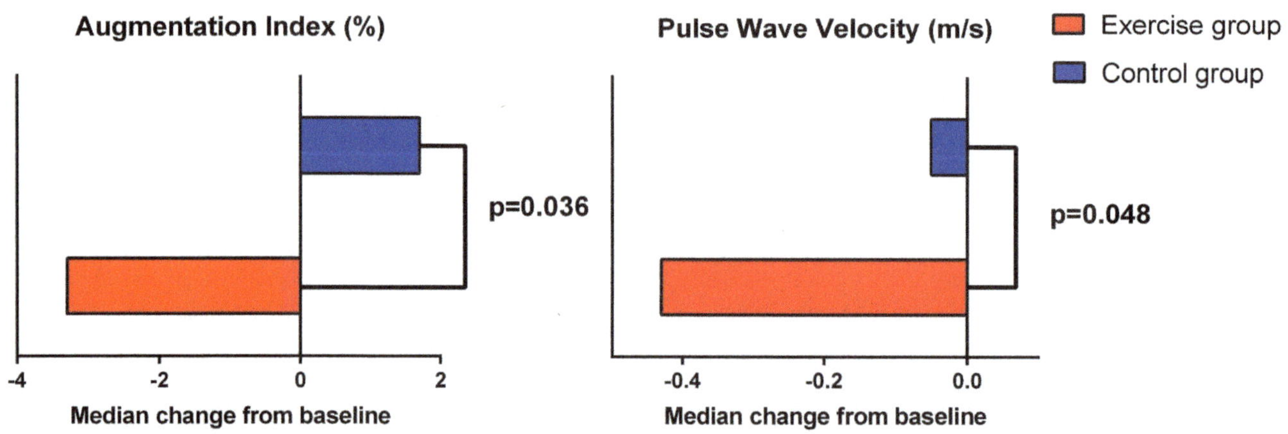

Figure 2. Median change in arterial stiffness after 3 months intervention of high intensity exercise, compairsons between control group and exercise group using Mann-Whitney U-test.

Table 3. Effects of high intensity exercise on cardiovascular risk.

	Exercise group, n = 10		Control group, n = 14		Estimated mean group difference (95% CI)[a]	p-value
	baseline	3 month	baseline	3 month		
Cardiorespiratory fitness						
VO_2 peak (ml/kg/min) mean (SD)	36.0 (5.1)	39.4 (4.5)	36.8 (4.9)	36.3 (3.8)	3.7 (2.1, 5.2)[a]	<0.001
Resting HR, mean (SD)	64 (7)	59 (6)	59 (8)	62 (9)	−6 (−11, −1)[a]	0.02
Body composition						
Body weight total (kg), mean (SD)	70.0 (12.3)	70.6 (12.5)	86.3 (14.6)	86.8 (15.3)	0.5 (−1.1, 2.1)[a]	0.49
BMI (kg/m^2), mean (SD)	24.0 (3.8)	24.2 (3.8)	27.1 (3.9)	27.2 (4.0)	0.0 (−0.6, 0.6)[a]	0.89
Waist circumference (cm)^2, mean (SD)	94.7 (7.9)[b]	91.2 (6.8)[b]	101.3 (9.8)[b]	101.3 (10.1)[b]	−3.8 (−6.9, −0.8)[a,b]	0.02[b]
Fat, total (%), mean (SD)	32.2 (7.4)	30.8 (7.2)	29.9 (6.2)	29.8 (6.2)	−1.4 (−2.1, −0.6)[a]	<0.001
Fat, abdominal (%), mean (SD)	29.8 (8.3)	27.5 (8.2)	29.6 (7.2)	29.2 (7.1)	−1.8 (−3.0, −0.6)[a]	<0.001
Lipids						
TC (mmol/L), mean (SD)	5.7 (1.2)	5.4 (1.2)	5.7 (1.0)	5.6 (0.7)	−0.2 (−0.8, 0.4)[a]	0.60
LDL-c, (mmol/L), mean (SD)	3.1 (1.3)	2.8 (0.9)	3.6 (0.9)	3.6 (0.9)	−0.5 (−1.1, 0.1)[a]	0.10
HDL-c, (mmol/L), mean (SD)	2.1 (0.3)	2.0 (0.5)	1.3 (0.4)	1.3 (0.5)	−0.3 (−0.7, 0.1)[a]	0.11
TC/HDL-c, (mmol/L), mean (SD)	2.8 (0.9)	2.9 (1.1)	4.9 (1.7)	4.6 (1.5)	−0.1 (−0.8, 0.7)[a]	0.88
Blood pressure						
Brachial SBP (mmHg), mean (SD)	126 (17)	126 (24)	130 (13)	124 (9)	7 (−3, 16)[a]	0.15
Brachial DBP (mmHg), mean (SD)	80 (8)	77 (11)	81 (7)	79 (8)	−1 (−8, 6)[a]	0.68
Arterial stiffness					**Estimated median group difference (95%CI)[c]**	
AIx (%), median (range)	21.5 (−8.7, 34.5)	18.5 (−17, 34.5)	16.4 (−5.0, 29,5)	15.5 (5, 30)	−5.3 (−11.0, −0.5)[c]	0.04[d]
PWV (m/s), median (range)	7.2 (5.8, 11.0)	6.2 (4.4, 10.4)	7.4 (5.3, 8.8)	6.6 (5.1, 8.1)	−0.3 (−0.7, 0.0)[c]	0.048[d]

Differences between the groups in post intervention (3 months) values, analyzed with ANCOVA with baseline values as covariates.
AIx, Augmentation Index; BMI, body mass index; DBP, diastolic blood pressure; HR, heart rate; HDL-c, high density lipoprotein cholesterol; LDL-c, low density lipoprotein cholesterol; PWV, Pulse Wave Velocity; SBP, systolic blood pressure; TC, total cholesterol; VO_2 peak, peak oxygen uptake.
[a]Estimated regression coefficients;
[b]analyzing only subjects with an increased waist circumference at baseline (males ≥94 cm and females ≥80 cm, EG n = 6, CG n = 12),
[c]Hodges-Lehman median estimator,
[d]Mann-Whitney U-test.

adverse events were reported during the intervention, indicating that high intensity exercise was safe and well tolerated in patients with active axSpA.

Discussion

This pilot study showed that high intensity endurance and strength exercise improved disease activity and reduced CV-risk factors in axSpA patients with active disease.

To our knowledge this is the first study aiming to examine whether patients with active axSpA could participate in a high intensity exercise program without a flare up in disease activity. Given the treatment effect of improved patient reported disease activity and stable inflammatory markers, the concept of high intensity exercise for axSpA-patients with active disease seems to be applicable. Our results are in accordance with a recently published case matched study by Stavropoulos-Kalinoglou et al. reporting that high intensity exercise significantly improved disease activity in patient with rheumatoid arthritis (RA) [23].

BASDAI has commonly been used as disease activity outcome measure in studies of effects of medication or exercise in patients with AS. Systematic reviews have reported treatment effects of TNF-inhibitors with effect size (ES) between 0.3 and 1.5 [24], and ES of exercise therapy (mainly flexibility exercises) to be between 0 and 0.8 in BASDAI [25]. In comparison, we found an ES of 1.4, suggesting that the intervention may have beneficial effects on patient reported disease symptoms. Thus, the improvement in BASDAI in our study supports that high intensity exercise may serve as an effective supplement to a pharmacological intervention.

Increased CV risk is an important factor for increased morbidity and mortality in patients with rheumatic diseases including those with axSpA. In the present study we found improvements in several CV risk factors. Central arterial stiffness measured as PWV is a validated marker of CV risk and has been used as a surrogate endpoint of CVD [26]. AIx is an estimation of central arterial pressure and has also been shown to predict CV mortality [27]. This is the first study to demonstrate improvements of arterial stiffness after exercise intervention in patients with axSpA, and in rheumatic diseases in general. However, improvement in arterial stiffness after an exercise intervention has been reported in young and middle aged healthy men [28,29], and a cross-sectional study on RA patients reported that a higher level of self-reported physical activity was associated with lower arterial stiffness [30]. The magnitude of the reduction in arterial stiffness in the exercise group was AIx 3% and PWV 0.4 m/s, which is comparable to the reduction reported in studies on other populations [28,29,31]. A population study has shown that in young men, 10 years of vascular aging corresponds to an increase in PWV of 0.48 m/s and AIx of 9%, and in elderly men an increase in PWV of 1.36 m/s and AIx 1% [32]. Thus, the improvement in arterial stiffness in our study seems to be clinically meaningful in reducing CV risk. Arterial stiffness is determined by elastic properties of the artery wall (composition of elastin and collagen) and vasoconstrictor tone exerted by the smooth muscle cells [33]. The structural composition of elastin and collagen is believed to develop over years, and thus it seems unlikely that this would change after a short term intervention. Exercise can however alter arterial stiffness over a short period by modulation of the sympathetic-adrenergic tone either directly or through nitric oxide [29,33,34]. In addition, arterial stiffness can be affected by alterations of CV risk factors such as lipids, inflammation and especially BP [26]. In the present study these parameters showed no significant treatment effects. Our findings are supported by a study on healthy men, demonstrating favorable effects of exercise on arterial stiffness without changes in traditional CV risk factors, thus indicating a direct effect of exercise on the arterial stiffness [29].

In addition to arterial stiffness, the EG group improved VO_2 peak and reduced resting HR, and hereby confirm that the exercise intervention was effective in improving cardiorespiratory fitness. In the exercise study by Stavropoulos-Kalinoglou et al., the RA patients showed similar improvements in VO_2 peak [35]. Physical fitness is inversely related to CV risk in the general population [36]. Even small improvements in cardiorespiratory fitness are recognized as significant in reducing CV morbidity and mortality [37], and a prospective study reported that an increase in VO_2 peak of 3.5 ml/kg/min corresponded to a substantial decrease in cardiac events in a broad heterogeneous cohort of middle-aged men [38]. We found a mean 3.7 ml/kg/min difference in change in VO_2 peak in favor of the EG, thus indicating that the improvement in cardiorespiratory fitness seen in this study is of clinically importance in preventing CVD.

In addition, this study demonstrated significant treatment effects on total body fat and abdominal fat, although there were no differences in change in total body weight between the groups. Abdominal fat is associated with CV risk [39], and adipose tissue is described as an endocrine organ secreting inflammatory mediators like adipokines which play relevant roles in the pathophysiology of both CVD and inflammatory diseases [40]. Thus, the significant treatment effect on abdominal fat underline the potential of intensive exercise as a disease modifying treatment modality in patients with axSpA.

In contrast to these effects, and as mentioned above, we found no differences between the groups in change the plasma lipids and brachial BP. Two different meta-analyses concluded that exercise interventions have beneficial effects on BP, HDL-c and to some extend TC in the general population [41,42]. Furthermore, Stavropoulos-Kalinoglou et al. found significant reductions in BP and improvement of lipid profile after three months and six months of exercise in RA patients [35]. In contrast and in line with our results, a recent RCT on a 12 week moderate intensity exercise intervention in AS did not show any significant reductions in TC [43]. The lack of effect on lipids and brachial BP in our study might be due to a small sample size, a short intervention period and that most patients were within the normal range of BP and lipids at baseline.

Enhanced inflammation is an important pathogenic mediator in various rheumatic disorders including axSpA. For healthy adults, an anti-inflammatory effect of exercise is reported [44], but to our knowledge, this has not been investigated in patients with axSpA. We found no significant effects of high intensity endurance and strengths exercise on plasma levels of a wide range of cytokines or cytokine modulators. However, the EG showed a trend towards a decrease in IL-17a and IL-23 as compared with the CG, and notably both these cytokines have recently been suggested to be major players in the pathogenesis of axSpA [45]. Interestingly, treatment with inhibitors of IL-17 [46] and IL-23/IL-12 [47] has recently shown promising results in reducing disease activity in patients with active AS. In order to obtain more insight in the effects of exercise on the inflammatory process in axSpA patients, exercise-response of relevant inflammatory markers should be further explored.

Our findings support a favourable effect of exercise on CV risk in an axSpA population. Whether these results may be extrapolated to other inflammatory diseases with increased CV risk, e.g. suchs as HIV infections [48], should be investigated.

A strength of the present study was the randomized controlled design. Further, the intervention was in accordance with the ASCMs exercise recommendations, was individualized and the patients were supervised in order to obtain the optimal dose of exercise as prescribed in the protocol. The intervention was individually adapted and the intensity was controlled, ensuring that the intended physiological goals were met. Thus, the results of this study may be considered as measures of efficacy, and the adherence to the program was confirmed by the physiological response in terms of increased cardiorespiratory fitness. The main limitation is that this was a small explanatory study carried out under close to optimal conditions. Further, the participants and the therapist were not blinded to treatment allocation, and lack of blinding is likely to exaggerate treatment effects on subjective outcomes [49]. The sample size is small, and negative results may not be true negative due to the insufficient power to show significant differences. Moreover, based on its explorative nature, a large number of parameters were compared in a relative small study population without correcting for multiple comparisons further underscoring that secondary outcomes should be interpreted with some caution.

Conclusions

The results of the present study showed that high intensity cardiorespiratory and strength exercises improved disease activity and reduced CV risk factors in patients with active axSpA. The promising results of this pilot study will be further explored in a larger randomized controlled trial.

Author Contributions

Conceived and designed the experiments: SHS IJB KB NV AGS SAP HD CF. Performed the experiments: SHS IJB CF. Analyzed the data: SHS IJB SAP AGS ICO TU PA AM TKK HD KB. Contributed reagents/materials/analysis tools: SHS IJB SAP AGS AM TU PA TKK HD. Wrote the paper: SHS IJB SAP AGS KBH NV CF ICO AM TU PA TKK HD. Final approval of the manuscript to be published: SHS IJB SAP AGS KBH NV CF ICO AM TU PA TKK HD.

References

1. Dougados M, Baeten D (2011) Spondyloarthritis. Lancet 377: 2127–2137.
2. Braun J, van den Berg, Baraliakos X, Boehm H, Burgos-Vargas R, et al. (2011) 2010 update of the ASAS/EULAR recommendations for the management of ankylosing spondylitis. Ann Rheum Dis 70: 896–904.
3. Corrigan B, Kannangra S (1978) Rheumatic disease: exercise or immobilization? Aust Fam Physician 7: 1007–1014.
4. Dagfinrud H, Kvien TK, Hagen KB (2008) Physiotherapy interventions for ankylosing spondylitis. Cochrane Database Syst Rev CD002822.
5. Szabo SM, Levy AR, Rao SR, Kirbach SE, Lacaille D, et al. (2011) Increased risk of cardiovascular and cerebrovascular disease in individuals with ankylosing spondylitis: A population-based study. Arthritis Rheum 63: 3294–304.
6. Bremander A, Petersson IF, Bergman S, Englund M (2011) Population-based estimates of common comorbidities and cardiovascular disease in ankylosing spondylitis. Arthritis Care Res (Hoboken) 63: 550–556.
7. Mathieu S, Gossec L, Dougados M, Soubrier M (2011) Cardiovascular profile in ankylosing spondylitis: A systematic review and meta-analysis. Arthritis Care Res (Hoboken) 63: 557–563.
8. Perk J, De BG, Gohlke H, Graham I, Reiner Z, et al. (2012) European Guidelines on cardiovascular disease prevention in clinical practice (version 2012): The Fifth Joint Task Force of the European Society of Cardiology and Other Societies on Cardiovascular Disease Prevention in Clinical Practice (constituted by representatives of nine societies and by invited experts). Atherosclerosis 223: 1–68.
9. Rehn TA, Winett RA, Wisloff U, Rognmo O (2013) Increasing physical activity of high intensity to reduce the prevalence of chronic diseases and improve public health. Open Cardiovasc Med J 7: 1–8.
10. Garber CE, Blissmer B, Deschenes MR, Franklin BA, LaMonte MJ, et al. (2011) American College of Sports Medicine position stand. Quantity and quality of exercise for developing and maintaining cardiorespiratory, musculoskeletal, and neuromotor fitness in apparently healthy adults: guidance for prescribing exercise. Med Sci Sports Exerc 43: 1334–1359.
11. Rudwaleit M, van der Heijde D, Landewe R, Listing J, Akkoc N, et al. (2009) The development of Assessment of SpondyloArthritis international Society classification criteria for axial spondyloarthritis (part II): validation and final selection. Ann Rheum Dis 68: 777–783.
12. Helgerud J, Høydal K, Wang E, Karlsen T, Berg P, et al. (2007) Aerobic high-intensity intervals improve VO2max more than moderate training. Med Sci Sports Exerc 39: 665–671.
13. van der Heijde D, Lie E, Kvien TK, Sieper J, Van den Bosch F, et al. (2009) ASDAS, a highly discriminatory ASAS-endorsed disease activity score in patients with ankylosing spondylitis. Ann Rheum Dis 68: 1811–1818.
14. Garrett S, Jenkinson T, Kennedy LG, Whitelock H, Gaisford P, et al. (1994) A new approach to defining disease status in ankylosing spondylitis: the Bath Ankylosing Spondylitis Disease Activity Index. J Rheumatol 21: 2286–2291.
15. Calin A, Garrett S, Whitelock H, Kennedy LG, O'Hea J, et al. (1994) A new approach to defining functional ability in ankylosing spondylitis: the development of the Bath Ankylosing Spondylitis Functional Index. J Rheumatol 21: 2281–2285.
16. van der Heijde D, Landewe R, Feldtkeller E (2008) Proposal of a linear definition of the Bath Ankylosing Spondylitis Metrology Index (BASMI) and comparison with the 2-step and 10-step definitions. Ann Rheum Dis 67: 489–493.
17. Halvorsen S, Vøllestad NK, Fongen C, Provan SA, Semb AG, et al. (2012) Physical fitness in patients with ankylosing spondylitis: comparison with population controls. Phys Ther 92: 298–309.
18. AtCor Medical (2013) Available: http://atcormedical.com/technical_notes.html. Accessed December.
19. Pauca AL, O'Rourke MF, Kon ND (2001) Prospective evaluation of a method for estimating ascending aortic pressure from the radial artery pressure waveform. Hypertension 38: 932–937.
20. Andreoli A, Scalzo G, Masala S, Tarantino U, Guglielmi G (2009) Body composition assessment by dual-energy X-ray absorptiometry (DXA). Radiol Med 114: 286–300.
21. Friedewald WT, Levy RI, Fredrickson DS (1972) Estimation of the concentration of low-density lipoprotein cholesterol in plasma, without use of the preparative ultracentrifuge. Clin Chem 18: 499–502.
22. Armijo-Olivo S WS, Magee D (2009) Intention to treat analysis, compliance, drop-outs an how to deal with missing data in clinical research: a review. Physical Therapy Reviews 14: 36–49.
23. Stavropoulos-Kalinoglou A, Metsios GS, Veldhuijzen van Zanten JJ, Nightingale P, Kitas GD, et al. (2012) Individualised aerobic and resistance exercise training improves cardiorespiratory fitness and reduces cardiovascular risk in patients with rheumatoid arthritis. Ann Rheum Dis 72: 1819–25.
24. Baraliakos X, van den Berg R, Braun J, van der Heijde D (2012) Update of the literature review on treatment with biologics as a basis for the first update of the ASAS/EULAR management recommendations of ankylosing spondylitis. Rheumatology (Oxford) 51: 1378–1387.
25. van den Berg R, Baraliakos X, Braun J, van der Heijde D (2012) First update of the current evidence for the management of ankylosing spondylitis with non-pharmacological treatment and non-biologic drugs: a systematic literature review for the ASAS/EULAR management recommendations in ankylosing spondylitis. Rheumatology (Oxford) 51: 1388–1396.
26. Laurent S, Cockcroft J, Van BL, Boutouyrie P, Giannattasio C, et al. (2006) Expert consensus document on arterial stiffness: methodological issues and clinical applications. Eur Heart J 27: 2588–2605.
27. Vlachopoulos C, Aznaouridis K, O'Rourke MF, Safar ME, Baou K, et al. (2010) Prediction of cardiovascular events and all-cause mortality with central haemodynamics: a systematic review and meta-analysis. Eur Heart J 31: 1865–1871.
28. Heydari M, Boutcher YN, Boutcher SH (2013) High-intensity intermittent exercise and cardiovascular and autonomic function. Clin Auton Res 23: 57–65.
29. Tanaka H, Dinenno FA, Monahan KD, Clevenger CM, DeSouza CA, et al. (2000) Aging, habitual exercise, and dynamic arterial compliance. Circulation 102: 1270–1275.
30. Crilly MA, Wallace A (2013) Physical inactivity and arterial dysfunction in patients with rheumatoid arthritis. Scand J Rheumatol 42: 27–33.
31. Edwards DG, Schofield RS, Magyari PM, Nichols WW, Braith RW (2004) Effect of exercise training on central aortic pressure wave reflection in coronary artery disease. Am J Hypertens 17: 540–543.
32. McEniery CM, Yasmin, Hall IR, Qasem A, Wilkinson IB, et al. (2005) Normal vascular aging: differential effects on wave reflection and aortic pulse wave

velocity: the Anglo-Cardiff Collaborative Trial (ACCT). J Am Coll Cardiol 46: 1753–1760.
33. Zieman SJ, Melenovsky V, Kass DA (2005) Mechanisms, pathophysiology, and therapy of arterial stiffness. Arterioscler Thromb Vasc Biol 25: 932–943.
34. Schuler G, Adams V, Goto Y (2013) Role of exercise in the prevention of cardiovascular disease: results, mechanisms, and new perspectives. Eur Heart J 34: 1790–1799.
35. Stavropoulos-Kalinoglou A, Metsios GS, Veldhuijzen van Zanten JJ, Nightingale P, Kitas GD, et al. (2012) Individualised aerobic and resistance exercise training improves cardiorespiratory fitness and reduces cardiovascular risk in patients with rheumatoid arthritis. Ann Rheum Dis.
36. Kodama S, Saito K, Tanaka S, Maki M, Yachi Y, et al. (2009) Cardiorespiratory fitness as a quantitative predictor of all-cause mortality and cardiovascular events in healthy men and women: a meta-analysis. JAMA 301: 2024–2035.
37. Aspenes ST, Nilsen TI, Skaug EA, Bertheussen GF, Ellingsen O, et al. (2011) Peak oxygen uptake and cardiovascular risk factors in 4631 healthy women and men. Med Sci Sports Exerc 43: 1465–1473.
38. Laukkanen JA, Kurl S, Salonen R, Rauramaa R, Salonen JT (2004) The predictive value of cardiorespiratory fitness for cardiovascular events in men with various risk profiles: a prospective population-based cohort study. Eur Heart J 25: 1428–1437.
39. Pischon T, Boeing H, Hoffmann K, Bergmann M, Schulze MB, et al. (2008) General and abdominal adiposity and risk of death in Europe. N Engl J Med 359: 2105–2120.
40. Scotece M, Conde J, Gomez R, Lopez V, Pino J, et al. (2012) Role of adipokines in atherosclerosis: interferences with cardiovascular complications in rheumatic diseases. Mediators Inflamm 2012: 125458.
41. Cornelissen VA, Fagard RH (2005) Effects of endurance training on blood pressure, blood pressure-regulating mechanisms, and cardiovascular risk factors. Hypertension 46: 667–675.
42. Leon AS, Sanchez OA (2001) Response of blood lipids to exercise training alone or combined with dietary intervention. Med Sci Sports Exerc 33: S502–S515.
43. Niedermann K, Sidelnikov E, Muggli C, Dagfinrud H, Hermann M, et al. (2013) Cardiovascular training improves fitness in patients with ankylosing spondylitis. Arthritis Care Res (Hoboken).
44. Walsh NP, Gleeson M, Shephard RJ, Gleeson M, Woods JA, et al. (2011) Position statement. Part one: Immune function and exercise. Exerc Immunol Rev 17: 6–63.
45. Sherlock JP, Joyce-Shaikh B, Turner SP, Chao CC, Sathe M, et al. (2012) IL-23 induces spondyloarthropathy by acting on ROR-gammat+ CD3+CD4-CD8- entheseal resident T cells. Nat Med 18: 1069–1076.
46. Baeten D, Baraliakos X, Braun J, Sieper J, Emery P, et al. (2013) Anti-interleukin-17A monoclonal antibody secukinumab in treatment of ankylosing spondylitis: a randomised, double-blind, placebo-controlled trial. Lancet 382: 1705–1713.
47. Poddubnyy D, Hermann KG, Callhoff J, Listing J, Sieper J (2014) Ustekinumab for the treatment of patients with active ankylosing spondylitis: results of a 28-week, prospective, open-label, proof-of-concept study (TOPAS). Ann Rheum Dis 73: 817–823.
48. D'Ascenzo F, Cerrato E, Biondi-Zoccai G, Moretti C, Omede P, et al. (2012) Acute coronary syndromes in human immunodeficiency virus patients: a meta-analysis investigating adverse event rates and the role of antiretroviral therapy. Eur Heart J 33: 875–880.
49. Wood L, Egger M, Gluud LL, Schulz KF, Juni P, et al. (2008) Empirical evidence of bias in treatment effect estimates in controlled trials with different interventions and outcomes: meta-epidemiological study. BMJ 336: 601–605.

18

Suprathreshold Heat Pain Response Predicts Activity-Related Pain, but Not Rest-Related Pain, in an Exercise-Induced Injury Model

Rogelio A. Coronado[1]*, Corey B. Simon[1], Carolina Valencia[2], Jeffrey J. Parr[3], Paul A. Borsa[4], Steven Z. George[1,5]*

1 Department of Physical Therapy, University of Florida, Gainesville, Florida, United States of America, **2** Department of Applied Medicine and Rehabilitation, Indiana State University, Terra Haute, Indiana, Unites States of America, **3** Department of Sports Medicine and Nutrition, University of Pittsburgh, Pittsburgh, Pennsylvania, United States of America, **4** Department of Applied Physiology and Kinesiology, University of Florida, Gainesville, Florida, United States of America, **5** Center for Pain Research and Behavioral Health, University of Florida, Gainesville, Florida, United States of America

Abstract

Exercise-induced injury models are advantageous for studying pain since the onset of pain is controlled and both pre-injury and post-injury factors can be utilized as explanatory variables or predictors. In these studies, rest-related pain is often considered the primary dependent variable or outcome, as opposed to a measure of activity-related pain. Additionally, few studies include pain sensitivity measures as predictors. In this study, we examined the influence of pre-injury and post-injury factors, including pain sensitivity, for induced rest and activity-related pain following exercise induced muscle injury. The overall goal of this investigation was to determine if there were convergent or divergent predictors of rest and activity-related pain. One hundred forty-three participants provided demographic, psychological, and pain sensitivity information and underwent a standard fatigue trial of resistance exercise to induce injury of the dominant shoulder. Pain at rest and during active and resisted shoulder motion were measured at 48- and 96-hours post-injury. Separate hierarchical models were generated for assessing the influence of pre-injury and post-injury factors on 48- and 96-hour rest-related and activity-related pain. Overall, we did not find a universal predictor of pain across all models. However, pre-injury and post-injury suprathreshold heat pain response (SHPR), a pain sensitivity measure, was a consistent predictor of activity-related pain, even after controlling for known psychological factors. These results suggest there is differential prediction of pain. A measure of pain sensitivity such as SHPR appears more influential for activity-related pain, but not rest-related pain, and may reflect different underlying processes involved during pain appraisal.

Editor: Ruth Landau, University of Washington, United States of America

Funding: Funding for this study was received by a NIAMS/NIH grant AR055899. RAC was supported by NIH T32 Interdisciplinary Training in Rehabilitation and Neuromuscular Plasticity grant (5T32HDO43730). CBS was supported in part by the NIH/NCATS Clinical and Translational Science Awards to the University of Florida (TL1 TR000066 and UL1 TR000064). The funders had no role in study design, data collection and analysis, decision to publish, or preparation of the manuscript.

Competing Interests: The authors have declared that no competing interests exist.

* Email: rogelio.coronado@vanderbilt.edu (RAC); szgeorge@phhp.ufl.edu (SZG)

Introduction

Pain ratings are commonly queried during the assessment of individuals with musculoskeletal pain. In clinical studies, current or rest-related pain intensity is most often assessed [1], while pain ratings with specific activity (e.g., activity-related pain) are less frequently reported. A recent systematic review of post-surgical trials by Srikandarajah and Gilron [2] found that only 39% (281/726) of published trials included a measurement of activity-related pain as a clinical outcome. Failure to include a measure of activity-related pain is noteworthy as activity-related pain may have a stronger association with functional limitations, or greater sensitivity in assessing therapeutic response, than measures of rest-related pain [3,4].

Differentiating rest and activity-related pain can be difficult in clinical studies. Exercise-induced injury models may better control comparisons of rest and activity-related pain. In a study by Dannecker and Sluka [5], the authors showed that following eccentric exercise for the elbow flexors, higher pain ratings occurred with elbow extension than at rest. This study is relevant as it suggests exercise-induced injury models can induce higher levels of pain dependent on activity, and may be appropriate models for studying the prediction of rest and activity-related pain.

Predictive models have been generated to determine which factors influence pain outcomes following exercise-induced injury [6–9]. Similar to clinical studies, most exercise-induced injury studies focus on predicting rest-related pain rather than activity-related pain. Factors shown to be predictive of rest-related pain are predominantly psychological in nature, such as pain catastrophizing [9,10]. However, current limitations in the prediction of pain following exercise-induced injury are twofold. First, it is unclear whether psychological factors are predictors of activity-related pain. Second, measures of pain sensitivity have not been widely considered within predictive models for pain following exercise-induced injury [6,7]. Pain sensitivity measures are thought to reflect pain processing within the nervous system and are receiving attention as potential prognostic variables [11,12]. Pain sensitivity can potentially improve prediction models that already include psychological factors and, therefore, may allow better evaluation of different processes relevant to the perception of rest or activity-related pain. Furthermore, pain sensitivity, if found to be an important predictor, could be considered a relevant factor to include in clinical assessment, especially as it is not commonly assessed in a clinical context [13].

Thus, further investigation is needed to ascertain the influence pain sensitivity has on an individual's pain perception at rest or during activity. Specifically, we sought primarily to assess the predictive ability of 1) baseline, pre-injury pain sensitivity on post-injury rest and activity-related pain at 48 and 96-hours and 2) 48-hours post-injury pain sensitivity on post-injury rest and activity-related pain at 96-hours. We used an exercise-induced injury model in a group of healthy volunteers, as these models are standardized induced-pain methods to study the development and progression of chronic pain. In these models, the overall pain experience is shorter in duration, yet generates similar pain and impairment characteristics observed in clinical pain conditions [14–16]. Moreover, the influence of both pre-injury (e.g., pre-clinical) and post-injury (e.g., clinical) factors on the painful episode can be examined as the onset of injury is controlled within the model. We hypothesized that pain sensitivity factors would be predictive of rest and activity-related pain, even after controlling for psychological factors. We did not have a specific hypothesis on a differential influence of pain sensitivity on pain outcome.

Materials and Methods

Ethics Statement

This study was approved by the University of Florida Institutional Review Board. Prior to enrollment, all participants provided written informed consent.

Participants

Participants were recruited from the campus of the University of Florida and the surrounding community. All participants were between the ages of 18 and 85 years old and not performing strength training exercises for the upper extremity either currently or during the previous 6 weeks. Participants were not included if they 1) were currently experiencing neck or shoulder pain, 2) had neurological impairments of the upper extremity, such as loss of sensation, muscle weakness, or reflex changes, 3) were currently taking pain medication, or 4) had previous shoulder surgery.

Procedure

After providing written informed consent at the initial assessment session, all participants completed standardized questionnaires and underwent pain sensitivity testing. Testing was conducted in the same private laboratory environment controlled for room temperature and humidity, and where distractions were minimized. Next, participants performed an eccentric exercise protocol on their dominant shoulder to induce pain [8] using a Kin-Com isokinetic dynamometer (Chattanooga Group, Chattanooga, TN). Participants were seated according to manufacturer's recommendations and straps were affixed across the torso to minimize trunk motion. The dominant shoulder was placed in a standardized position within the scapular plane. After determining maximum voluntary isometric contraction (MVIC) for each individual, participants completed repetitions of isokinetic concentric/eccentric external rotation actions to induce shoulder pain. Specifically, participants performed a standard bout of 3 sets of 10 repetitions at 60°/sec with a goal of fatiguing participants so they generated 50% or less of their initial MVIC. If necessary, additional repetitions (e.g., 1 set of 8 repetitions) were performed until the standard fatigue level was reached. After completing the initial session which lasted approximately one hour, participants were then scheduled for 2 follow-up sessions. Follow-up sessions occurred at 48- and 96-hours after the initial session, where repeat measurements of psychological variables, pain sensitivity, and outcome occurred at 48-hours and outcome alone at 96-hours.

Measures

Demographics. Demographic information included age, sex, height, weight, and dominant arm. Height and weight information were used to compute body mass index (BMI) as a covariate for exercise-induced injury.

Shoulder Pain Intensity. Using a 101-point numeric pain rating scale (0 = "no pain," 100 = "worst pain imaginable"), participants verbally indicated their intensity of shoulder pain [17]. Shoulder pain intensity was asked during three states: 1) at rest (e.g., upper extremity held at side); 2) during active motion (e.g., shoulder abduction); 3) during isometric activation (e.g., resisted external rotation).

Pain Catastrophizing. Pain catastrophizing was assessed using the Pain Catastrophizing Scale (PCS) as this variable has been shown to influence pain-related outcomes [9,18,19]. The PCS is a 13-item questionnaire (score ranges from 0 to 52) that measures thoughts on various pain experiences where higher scores reflect higher levels of pain catastrophizing [20].

Fear of Movement. Fear of movement was assessed using the shortened version of the Tampa Scale of Kinesiophobia (TSK-11) and has shown to be associated with shoulder injury outcome [21,22]. The TSK-11 is a 17-item questionnaire (score ranges from 11 to 44) that measures fear of movement where higher scores reflect higher levels of fear of movement [23].

Pressure Pain Threshold. Pressure pain threshold (PPT) was measured at the tip of the acromion of the dominant shoulder using a hand-held algometer (Pain Diagnostics & Treatment, Great Neck, NY) with a 1 cm^2 diameter probe. PPT is a single stimulus threshold measure of static pain sensitivity, and is commonly used in laboratory and clinical research trials [24]. Our assessment of PPT for the shoulder undergoing exercise-induced injury is a marker of local pain sensitivity. [25,26] A trained examiner applied a standard pressure force with a target rate of approximately 1 kg/sec until the pressure sensation was first reported by the participant to be painful [25–28]. Lower PPT values were indicative of higher pain sensitivity. A total of 3 trials were obtained with rest in between each testing trial. The average of the 3 trials was used for analyses.

Suprathreshold Heat Pain Response. Suprathreshold heat pain response (SHPR) was measured at the thenar aspect of both hands using a contact thermode with 2.5 cm^2 surface area connected to a computer-controlled PATHWAY Model Contact Heat Evoked Potential Stimulator (CHEPS) (Medoc Advanced Medical Systems). SHPR is a dynamic measure of pain sensitivity and thought to be predominantly mediated by C-fiber activity [24,29]. A series of 5 consecutive heat pulses at a rate of 30°C/sec with interstimulus interval of 2.5 seconds was delivered with a peak temperature of 48°C. We used 48°C as this temperature elicits a moderate level of pain (e.g., pain ratings near 50/100 on pain rating scale) for a majority of participants [30]. Each heat pulse was rated by the participant using the same 101-point numeric pain rating scale. SHPR was identified as the pain intensity rating of the fifth heat pulse in a train of 5 heat pulses and has been used as a clinically meaningful dynamic measure of pain sensitivity [30,31]. Higher pain ratings on SHPR indicate higher pain sensitivity. The average SHPR rating of both hands was used for analyses.

Conditioned Pain Modulation. Conditioned pain modulation (CPM) was measured using the same CHEPS setup as SHPR. The CPM protocol included a measured response of a test stimulus before and after application of a conditioning stimulus [32]. The test stimulus was delivered to the thenar aspect of the non-dominant hand and involved a sequence of 5 heat pulses at a temperature that induced a moderate level of pain intensity (e.g., 50/100 on pain scale) with the same parameters as SHPR. Participants rated each heat pulse with the same 101-point numeric pain rating scale used in the SHPR protocol. The pain rating of the fifth heat pulse was used as the test stimulus response. For the conditioning stimulus, participants immersed their dominant hand into a cold water bath for up to 60 seconds. The water temperature was maintained at a constant temperature of 8°C using a refrigeration unit (NESLAB RTE 7 Digital One, Thermo Scientific Co., Massachusetts, USA) which circulated water to prevent warming. Participants were instructed to keep their hand in the cold water bath for a minimum of 30 seconds, at which time they could remove their hand, if needed. After the 60 second cold water time period, a second bout of the same test stimulus was conducted. CPM was computed as the absolute difference in SHPR before and after the conditioning stimulus [32]. Like SHPR, CPM is a dynamic measure of pain sensitivity and indicative of central sensitivity. Moreover, CPM is a behavioral correlate of endogenous pain inhibition [33]. Larger differences (e.g., larger reductions in SHPR) were indicative of greater degrees of pain modulation.

Data Analysis

We used IBM SPSS Statistics for Windows (version 21.0, SPSS, Inc., Chicago, IL) for all data analyses. Alpha was set a priori at the 0.05 level for statistical significance.

Descriptive statistics were computed for all pertinent baseline and follow-up measures. To assess whether the exercise-induced injury model induced changes in relevant factors, baseline and 48-hour psychological variables (PCS, TSK-11) and pain sensitivity (PPT, SHPR, CPM) comparisons were made using a paired samples t-test.

The primary dependent variables (e.g., outcomes) for all analyses were the exercise-induced 1) rest-related shoulder pain (pain intensity with shoulder at rest); 2) shoulder pain with motion (pain intensity during active shoulder abduction); and 3) isometric shoulder pain (pain during isometric resisted external rotation of the shoulder). The latter two dependent variables were considered measures of activity-related pain. These variables were measured at 48- and 96-hours after exercise-induced shoulder pain.

Zero-order correlation coefficients were computed for independent variables (e.g., predictors) measured at baseline (pre-injury: age, sex, BMI, PCS, TSK-11, PPT, SHPR, CPM) with dependent variables at 48- and 96-hours, and independent variables measured at 48-hours (post-injury: PCS, TSK-11, PPT, SHPR, CPM) with dependent variables at 96-hours. All variables were analyzed as continuous variables, except for sex which was a dichotomous variable (0 for female, 1 for male). These correlations coefficients express the simple relationship between each independent and dependent variable.

Subsequently, we examined the unique relationship between independent and dependent variables after controlling for other variables, using hierarchical linear regression. Hierarchical linear regression modeling allows us to account for other factors in an a-priori, theoretical fashion. Separate hierarchical linear regression models were created using 1) baseline, pre-injury independent variables for each of the three dependent variables at 48- and 96-hours and 2) baseline demographic (age, sex, BMI) and 48-hour, post-injury independent variables (PCS, TSK-11, PPT, SHPR, CPM) for each of the three dependent variables at 96-hours.

In each of the hierarchical linear regression models, demographic variables of age, sex, and BMI were entered into the first block, psychological variables of PCS and TSK-11 were entered into the second block, and pain sensitivity variables of PPT, SHPR, and CPM were entered into the third and final block. In the 96-hour prediction model, each respective independent variable outcome measured at 48-hours was entered in the first block. We built these models in this fashion to assess the unique contribution of pain sensitivity factors after accounting for relevant demographic and psychological variables.

Correlation values between independent variables were examined prior to entering into regression models in order to prevent significant inter-correlation (i.e., multicollinearity). An a-priori correlation of 0.7 or greater was used to reflect potential multicollinearity [34]. Additional multicollinearity tests were tolerance and variance inflation, which should be greater than.2 and less than 10, respectively [35]. All tests indicated a lack of multicollinearity, and therefore, confirmed the stability of our models. Overall model statistics were examined along with changes in r-squared and p-value for each model step. Relative individual predictor strength was assessed with β estimates.

Sample Size Determination

To determine the minimum acceptable sample size needed for these analyses, we used estimation criteria from Green [36], as well as the general rule of thumb of 10–15 cases per predictor, as guidelines [35,37]. Since we were interested in assessing both the overall fit of our regression modeling and testing individual predictors ($n = 8$) we used the larger of the two sample sizes needed from Green's criteria. In this case, the minimum total sample size needed was 114 participants and was approximate to the more stringent rule of thumb criteria of 120 participants (e.g., 15 cases per predictor with 8 predictors).

Results

Sample Characteristics

Descriptive data from 143 individuals who participated in this study are presented in Table 1. All enrolled participants, except for one (illness), completed study. Participants ranged in age from 18 to 58 years (mean age = 23.7 years, SD = 6.7 years) and the 59% were female (85 female, 58 male). Comparison of baseline and 48-hour values for psychological variables and pain sensitivity showed that exercise-induced shoulder pain resulted in significantly lower PPT (higher local pain sensitivity) and PCS (lower pain catastrophizing) values and higher TSK-11 values (higher fear of movement) ($p<0.05$).

Association between Predictor and Outcome Variables

Table 2 lists correlation coefficients for each pre-injury and post-injury variable and 48- and 96-hour pain outcome. For pain sensitivity predictors, pre-injury SHPR was positively associated with both measures of activity-related pain at 48- and 96-hours ($p<0.05$), but not rest-related pain at these time points ($p>0.05$). Furthermore, post-injury SHPR, along with post-injury PPT, was associated with 96-hour activity-related pain ($p<0.05$). The

Table 1. Baseline, 48-hour, and 96-hour Descriptive Data (N = 143).

	Pre-injury	Post-injury	
Variable	**Baseline**	**48-hour**	**96-hour**
Demographic			
Age (years)	23.7 (6.7)	-	-
Sex (N of females)	85	-	-
Dominant arm (N of right)	126	-	-
BMI	23.5 (4.0)		
Psychological			
PCS	9.9 (7.9)	8.0 (8.0)	-
TSK-11	18.0 (4.4)	18.8 (5.0)	-
Pain Sensitivity			
PPT (kg)	5.5 (2.0)	4.8 (1.8)	-
SHPR (x/100)	23.2 (24.4)	20.9 (22.7)	-
CPM (x/100)	−8.6 (12.8)	−7.8 (13.6)	-
Shoulder Pain Intensity (x/100)			
At Rest	-	22.2 (20.5)	7.5 (10.1)
With Active Motion	-	15.5 (16.4)	4.2 (7.4)
With Isometric Contraction	-	20.6 (18.8)	10.5 (16.3)

Values are expressed as mean (SD) unless otherwise indicated.
Abbreviations: BMI = body mass index, CPM = conditioned pain modulation, N = number, PCS = Pain Catastrophizing Scale, PPT = pressure pain threshold, SHPR = suprathreshold heat pain response, TSK-11 = Tampa Scale of Kinesiophobia.

relationship of SHPR and PPT with pain outcome was such that the more pain sensitive an individual was (e.g., higher SHPR or lower PPT), the higher the report of shoulder pain.

Prediction of Rest- and Activity-Related Pain at 48 Hours

Table 3 includes results from the hierarchical regression models predicting 48-hour rest-related shoulder pain and shoulder pain with activity using pre-injury predictors. The final regression model for 48-hour rest-related shoulder pain indicated that none of the covariate variables were predictive of outcome ($F_{8,133} = 1.145$, $p = 0.338$, $r^2 = 0.064$). In contrast, the final regression models for shoulder pain with motion ($F_{8,132} = 2.360$, $p < 0.05$) and isometric shoulder pain ($F_{8,130} = 5.159$, $p < 0.001$) demonstrated predictive ability explaining 12.5% and 24.1% of the variance in pain outcome, respectively. In these models, pre-injury SHPR ($\beta = 0.285$, $p < 0.05$) was the strongest predictor of 48-hour shoulder pain with motion, even after accounting for psychology (PCS: $\beta = 0.209$, $p < 0.05$). In addition, pre-injury SHPR ($\beta = 0.472$, $P < 0.05$) was the sole predictor of 48-hour isometric shoulder pain.

Prediction of Rest- and Activity-Related Pain at 96 Hours

Table 4 includes results from the hierarchical regression models predicting 96-hour resting shoulder pain and shoulder pain with activity using pre-injury predictors. The final regression model predicting 96-hour rest-related shoulder pain was not statistically significant, and therefore, was not predictive of outcome ($F_{8,131} = 0.683$, $p = 0.706$, $r^2 = 0.040$). The final regression models for shoulder pain with motion ($F_{8,130} = 2.259$, $p = 0.027$) and isometric shoulder pain ($F_{8,128} = 3.102$, $p = 0.003$) demonstrated predictive ability, explaining 12.2% and 16.2% of the variance in pain outcome, respectively. Despite lack of significance, pre-injury SHPR ($\beta = 0.172$, $p = 0.067$) was the strongest predictor of 96-hour shoulder pain with motion. Moreover, pre-injury SHPR was a unique predictor ($\beta = 0.387$, $p < 0.001$) of 96-hour isometric shoulder pain.

Table 5 includes results from the hierarchical regression models predicting 96-hour rest and activity-related pain using 48-hour post-injury predictors. The final regression model for 96-hour rest-related shoulder pain was predictive of outcome ($F_{9,129} = 4.700$, $p < 0.001$), explaining 24.7% of the variance. The final regression models for shoulder pain with motion ($F_{9,128} = 9.338$, $p < 0.001$) and isometric shoulder pain ($F_{9,126} = 13.266$, $p < 0.001$) were also predictive, explaining 39.6% and 48.7% of the variance in pain outcome, respectively. Pain outcome measured at 48-hours was the strongest predictor across all models (i.e., rest pain at 48-hours for rest pain at 96-hours, etc.), however, post-injury PPT ($\beta = -0.164$, $p < 0.05$) and post-injury SHPR ($\beta = 0.154$, $p < 0.05$) also predicted 96-hour shoulder pain with motion. Furthermore, post-injury SHPR ($\beta = 0.164$, $p < 0.05$) was a predictor of 96-hour isometric shoulder pain.

Discussion

We induced shoulder pain using an eccentric exercise protocol and evaluated the influence of pre-injury and post-injury factors, namely pain sensitivity, on rest and activity-related shoulder pain measured at 48- and 96-hours. We did not observe consistent predictors across both rest and activity-related pain. However, SHPR, a pain sensitivity measure, was a consistent and oft-times the sole predictor of activity-related pain. These findings suggest that rest and activity-related pain may be modulated by different underlying processes and mechanisms [10]. Specifically, the results of our study indicate that activity-related pain is more likely to be modulated by factors related to pain sensitivity. The relevance of these findings for pain research and clinical practice is further considered in subsequent sections.

Table 2. Correlation of Pre-Injury and Post-Injury Predictors with Shoulder Pain Outcome at 48 and 96-Hours.

	48-Hours			96-Hours		
		Activity-Related Pain			Activity-Related Pain	
Variable	**Rest-Related Pain**	**Motion Pain**	**Isometric Pain**	**Rest-Related Pain**	**Motion Pain**	**Isometric Pain**
Pre-injury						
Age	−0.014	0.011	−0.053	−0.123	−0.084	−0.096
Sex	−0.171*	0.066	−0.039	−0.066	0.050	0.040
BMI	−0.051	0.033	−0.062	−0.020	0.042	0.005
PCS	0.096	0.125	0.128	0.175*	0.179*	0.145
TSK-11	−0.015	−0.044	−0.003	0.073	0.073	0.091
PPT	−0.131	−0.076	−0.162*	−0.048	−0.051	−0.079
SHPR	0.045	0.251*	0.437*	0.073	0.222*	0.320*
CPM	0.091	−0.051	−0.118	−0.056	−0.197*	−0.039
Post-Injury						
48 Pain	-	-	-	0.423*	0.568*	0.670*
PCS	-	-	-	0.253*	0.176*	0.095
TSK-11	-	-	-	0.139	0.201*	0.050
PPT	-	-	-	−0.129	−0.233*	−0.203*
SHPR	-	-	-	0.162*	0.286*	0.418*
CPM	-	-	-	−0.023	−0.087	0.017

*p-value<0.05.
Values are correlation coefficients.
Abbreviations: BMI = body mass index, CPM = conditioned pain modulation, PCS = Pain Catastrophizing Scale, PPT = pressure pain threshold, SHPR = suprathreshold heat pain response, TSK = Tampa Scale of Kinesiophobia.

Relevance to Pain Research

Exercise-induced injury paradigms like the one in our study have been used to model the pain experience [5–9,11,15,16,18,19,38–42]. In general, pre-injury psychological factors have been shown to be predictive of post-injury resting pain reports [7–9,18,19]. Pain sensitivity, however, predicted activity-related pain, even after controlling for selected psychological factors. These findings are consistent with results reported by Rakel et al. [10] that examined pre-operative psychological and pain sensitivity predictors of rest and activity-related pain following total knee replacement. These authors found pre-operative pain sensitivity measures (e.g., cutaneous mechanical and thermal threshold) to be predictive of activity-related movement pain, but not rest-related pain. Additionally, PPT had limited predictive ability on either rest or activity-related pain [10], which is concordant with our PPT findings.

Our study advances current evidence by including both static (PPT) and dynamic (SHPR, CPM) pain sensitivity measures in predicting pain. In doing so, we show that a dynamic measure of pain sensitivity, SHPR, is an important predictor of clinical pain outcome in a novel pain model (e.g., exercise-induced shoulder injury model) and corroborates a previously published trial of exercise-induced pain [6,7]. Bishop et al [6] examined the influence of static and dynamic thermal pain sensitivity on exercise-induced low back pain and reported a significant association between dynamic thermal pain sensitivity (e.g., temporal summation of pain) and daily muscle pain intensity. While the authors did not specifically examine activity-related pain, measures of daily muscle pain intensity may include appraisals of activity-related pain within their metric, especially if activity-related pain coincides with moments of worst pain during the day. This may explain why we found no association between pain sensitivity and resting pain intensity, because resting pain only assesses current pain when no movement is occurring at the shoulder.

The lack of consistent predictors across rest and activity-related pain aligns with current models on the pain experience or pain perception [43,44]. Pain sensation appraisal is context-dependent and involves influence from cognitive, sensory and affective components, and is likely processed in serial, parallel, and cyclical fashion. Conceptually, individuals may appraise pain differently when at rest and during activity [45,46], and possible explanations include the following mechanisms. First, rating pain during a controlled activity (i.e., lifting arm in controlled fashion like in our study), may not be as threatening as pain during either unpredictable or uncontrollable moments (e.g., daily events or at rest when not anticipating pain). Second, evoked pain may be seen as a challenge to the sensory system and result in activity-dependent responses. Thus, pain sensitivity may be suited to reflect these underlying activity-dependent states more so than during basal states such as rest.

Relevance to Clinical Practice

While our findings are consistent with findings across pre-clinical (i.e., healthy participant) and postoperative studies [6,7,10,47–49], we used an exercise-induced injury model which is advantageous for the assessment of pre-injury influence. We are unaware of studies that assessed the association between pain sensitivity and the transition of pre-injury to post-injury states and this was one of our primary aims [47,48]. Measuring pre-injury states is difficult to conduct in clinical studies where the future development of pain is uncertain. While our findings are

Table 3. Hierarchical Regression Models Predicting 48-hour Shoulder Pain at Rest, with Motion, and with Isometric Action Using Baseline, Pre-injury Predictors.

					Activity-Related Pain							
	Rest-Related Pain				Motion Pain				Isometric Pain			
	Beta	P	Δ R^2	P	Beta	P	Δ R^2	P	Beta	P	Δ R^2	P
1			0.027	0.281			0.006	0.850			0.005	0.889
Age	0.025	0.785			<0.001	0.996			−0.027	0.771		
Sex	−0.163	0.065			0.071	0.423			−0.011	0.902		
BMI	−0.016	0.867			0.013	0.890			−0.049	0.605		
2			0.020	0.249			0.043	0.232			0.029	0.461
Age	0.061	0.512			0.054	0.564			0.013	0.893		
Sex	−0.157	0.076			0.079	0.367			−0.005	0.955		
BMI	−0.021	0.819			0.004	0.968			−0.053	0.577		
PCS	0.170	0.095			**0.247**	**0.015**			**0.202**	**0.048**		
TSK-11	−0.099	0.323			−0.149	0.135			−0.088	0.382		
3			0.017	0.338			0.076	0.021			0.207	<0.001
Age	0.071	0.449			0.054	0.552			0.011	0.899		
Sex	−0.137	0.140			0.107	0.232			0.040	0.632		
BMI	0.017	0.855			0.051	0.579			0.023	0.789		
PCS	0.170	0.100			**0.209**	**0.036**			0.133	0.149		
TSK-11	−0.074	0.466			−0.144	0.142			−0.080	0.378		
PPT	−0.057	0.533			−0.061	0.494			−0.084	0.311		
SHPR	0.083	0.384			**0.285**	**0.002**			**0.472**	**<0.001**		
CPM	0.128	0.186			0.041	0.665			0.056	0.527		

All predictor variables measured at baseline (pre-injury).
Abbreviations: BMI = body mass index, CPM = conditioned pain modulation, PCS = Pain Catastrophizing Scale, P = p-value, PPT = pressure pain threshold, SHPR = suprathreshold heat pain response, TSK = Tampa Scale of Kinesiophobia.

Table 4. Hierarchical Regression Models Predicting 96-hour Shoulder Pain at Rest, with Motion, and with Isometric Action Using Baseline, Pre-Injury Predictors.

					Activity-Related Pain							
	Rest-Related Pain				**Motion Pain**				**Isometric Pain**			
	Beta	**P**	**Δ R^2**	**P**	**Beta**	**P**	**Δ R^2**	**P**	**Beta**	**P**	**Δ R^2**	**P**
1			0.022	0.379			0.016	0.541			0.014	0.607
Age	−0.138	0.134			−0.119	0.201			−0.116	0.215		
Sex	−0.068	0.446			0.060	0.506			0.061	0.501		
BMI	0.050	0.592			0.070	0.463			0.031	0.746		
2			0.016	0.379			0.036	0.205			0.025	0.393
Age	−0.111	0.240			−0.071	0.455			−0.084	0.382		
Sex	−0.058	0.512			0.070	0.430			0.068	0.452		
BMI	0.052	0.580			0.072	0.445			0.037	0.699		
PCS	0.139	0.179			**0.204**	**0.048**			0.139	0.179		
TSK-11	−0.018	0.859			−0.012	0.900			0.038	0.702		
3			0.002	0.706			0.070	0.027			0.124	0.003
Age	−0.111	0.249			−0.087	0.348			−0.092	0.312		
Sex	−0.049	0.601			0.094	0.303			0.102	0.257		
BMI	0.059	0.541			0.121	0.193			0.088	0.340		
PCS	0.134	0.203			0.166	0.100			0.100	0.311		
TSK-11	−0.016	0.876			−0.039	0.694			0.054	0.573		
PPT	−0.024	0.794			−0.046	0.604			−0.040	0.652		
SHPR	0.033	0.736			0.172	0.067			**0.387**	**<0.001**		
CPM	0.005	0.960			−0.145	0.123			0.127	0.172		

All predictor variables measured at baseline (pre-injury).
Abbreviations: BMI = body mass index, CPM = conditioned pain modulation, PCS = Pain Catastrophizing Scale, P = p-value, PPT = pressure pain threshold, SHPR = suprathreshold heat pain response, TSK = Tampa Scale of Kinesiophobia.

Table 5. Hierarchical Regression Models Predicting 96-hour Shoulder Pain at Rest, with Motion, and with Isometric Action using 48-Hour, Post-Injury Predictors.

					Activity-Related Pain							
	Rest-Related Pain				Motion Pain				Isometric Pain			
	Beta	P	ΔR^2	P	Beta	P	ΔR^2	P	Beta	P	ΔR^2	P
1			0.216	<0.001			0.334	<0.001			0.458	<0.001
Age	−0.149	0.074			−0.111	0.150			−0.075	0.284		
Sex	0.001	0.986			0.040	0.596			0.071	0.295		
BMI	0.055	0.520			0.067	0.395			0.063	0.379		
48 Pain	**0.445**	**<0.001**			**0.563**	**<0.001**			**0.669**	**<0.001**		
2			0.018	<0.001			0.011	<0.001			0.001	<0.001
Age	−0.129	0.123			−0.103	0.190			−0.074	0.300		
Sex	0.009	0.913			0.036	0.629			0.073	0.287		
BMI	0.043	0.614			0.075	0.341			0.059	0.412		
48 Pain	**0.410**	**<0.001**			**0.566**	**<0.001**			**0.667**	**<0.001**		
PCS	0.148	0.122			−0.062	0.482			0.032	0.684		
TSK-11	−0.016	0.866			0.125	0.148			−0.034	0.665		
3			0.013	<0.001			0.052	<0.001			0.027	<0.001
Age	−0.129	0.130			−0.106	0.172			−0.086	0.232		
Sex	0.022	0.791			0.100	0.188			0.084	0.234		
BMI	0.051	0.553			0.113	0.150			0.060	0.404		
48 Pain	**0.398**	**<0.001**			**0.497**	**<0.001**			**0.594**	**<0.001**		
PCS	0.146	0.130			−0.070	0.421			0.037	0.638		
TSK-11	−0.010	0.913			0.135	0.110			−0.031	0.689		
PPT	−0.039	0.642			**−0.164**	**0.032**			−0.011	0.874		
SHPR	0.101	0.213			**0.154**	**0.041**			**0.164**	**0.035**		
CPM	0.054	0.499			<0.001	0.996			0.114	0.087		

All predictor variables except age, sex, and BMI measured at 48 hours (post-injury).
Abbreviations: 48 Pain = Pain report of each respective outcome variable at 48 hours, BMI = body mass index, CPM = conditioned pain modulation, PCS = Pain Catastrophizing Scale, P = p-value, PPT = pressure pain threshold, SHPR = suprathreshold heat pain response, TSK = Tampa Scale of Kinesiophobia.

preliminary, our results suggest that early indication of individuals at risk for persistent activity-related pain may be identified by pre-injury pain sensitivity. This has potential implications for clinical management or screening as pain sensitivity assessment may be an additional tool to predict individuals at risk for chronic pain [47]. Recommendations such as these have been made in populations including postoperative pain [50,51] and there are ongoing efforts for the identification of pain sensitivity profiles or phenotypes for improved pain management [52]. If our findings are replicated in patients with musculoskeletal pain, then current recommendations may be extended to suggest phenotypes of pain-free individuals at risk of activity-evoked pain after musculoskeletal injury.

In a well-conducted meta-analysis, Hubscher et al [53] reported a weak association between pain sensitivity responses and clinical pain intensity. Rather than reflect poor clinical validity of pain sensitivity, the apparent weak association with pain sensitivity and clinical pain potentially may suggest a more complex relationship between measures of pain sensitivity and clinical outcome. Pain sensitivity, in general, may in fact be weakly associated to resting pain ratings, but may show stronger associations when evoked pain (as occurs during movement) is considered the clinical outcome of interest. Not apparent in the review by Hubscher et al [53] is whether a distinction between rest and activity-related pain was made when assessing outcome. But, perhaps in future clinical studies the utility of pain sensitivity will not be in predicting rest-related pain, but in activity-related pain.

Furthermore, select pain sensitivity responses may yield better association or prediction than others. Hubscher et al [53] reported relatively stronger correlations between clinical pain intensity and dynamic pain sensitivity (e.g., temporal summation), as compared to static pain sensitivity. This is consistent with our current findings where SHPR showed stronger relative prediction than PPT. Interestingly, we did not find CPM to be predictive of activity-related pain and that may be because our exercise-induced injury model is a model of acute pain. Evidence suggests that a lack of inhibitory mechanisms, as inferred through CPM, is more often shown in chronic pain syndromes [54,55], so these results may be expected and future studies in clinical populations should continue to use CPM until this issue is explored further.

Study Limitations

This study has several limitations. First, we standardized the initial bout of exercise for injury induction, but allowed continued exercise performance if our fatigue criterion was not met. Thus, we did not include the dosage of exercise to induce injury into our models for those individuals requiring a larger volume to induce the same injury criterion. Second, our study results can only be generalized to a population of younger, healthy individuals with induced shoulder pain following eccentric exercise. Although similar results have been observed in experimental and clinical trials [6,7,10], further validation of these findings to older and clinical populations is warranted. Third, our results are limited to those predictive factors included in our models. Other known predictors of resting pain such as depression were not included in these analyses. Furthermore, we did not include interaction terms within our model as we did not have specific hypotheses for interactions. Our models assessed only the main effects from each of the included predictors.

Additionally, we included only select measures of pressure and heat pain sensitivity and no other modalities. Currently, there is no consensus for pain sensitivity assessment, however multiple modality testing is encouraged and we included both static and dynamic pain sensitivity [13]. We did not include assessments of pain beyond 96-hours post-injury, but it is common for resolution of pain to occur for most individuals within this timeframe. Our pain outcome assessment was limited to pain intensity as compared to unpleasantness or other pain dimension measures. We did find some discrepancy in pain outcome between our study and the study by Dannecker and Sluka [5] where our activity-related pain measures did not elicit higher pain ratings than pain at rest. This may be due to the lack of specificity in our activity. In other words, we did not selectively stress the musculoskeletal tissue that was fatigued as was done by Dannecker and Sluka [5]. Further studies should assess whether induced shoulder pain can elicit higher pain ratings with selective movements as opposed to a general active or resisted motion.

Conclusion

Our prediction models within an exercise-induced injury paradigm allowed us to assess whether pain sensitivity was related to pain outcome as a risk (pre-injury) factor or prognostic (post-injury) factor. Based on our findings, pain sensitivity and SHPR specifically is associated with activity-related pain, however further investigations are needed to validate these findings and their potential translation into clinical practice.

Acknowledgments

We wish to acknowledge Dr. Kelly Larkin Kaiser for assisting with data collection.

Author Contributions

Conceived and designed the experiments: PAB SZG. Performed the experiments: RAC CBS CV JJP SZG. Analyzed the data: RAC SZG. Wrote the paper: RAC CBS CV JJP PAB SZG.

References

1. Litcher-Kelly L, Martino SA, Broderick JE, Stone AA (2007) A systematic review of measures used to assess chronic musculoskeletal pain in clinical and randomized controlled clinical trials. J Pain 8: 906–913.
2. Srikandarajah S, Gilron I (2011) Systematic review of movement-evoked pain versus pain at rest in postsurgical clinical trials and meta-analyses: a fundamental distinction requiring standardized measurement. Pain 152: 1734–1739.
3. Kehlet H, Dahl JB (2011) Assessment of postoperative pain–need for action! Pain 152: 1699–1700.
4. Wu CL, Rowlingson AJ, Partin AW, Kalish MA, Courpas GE, et al. (2005) Correlation of postoperative pain to quality of recovery in the immediate postoperative period. Reg Anesth Pain Med 30: 516–522.
5. Dannecker EA, Sluka KA (2011) Pressure and activity-related allodynia in delayed-onset muscle pain. Clin J Pain 27: 42–47.
6. Bishop MD, George SZ, Robinson ME (2012) Dynamic, but not static, pain sensitivity predicts exercise-induced muscle pain: covariation of temporal sensory summation and pain intensity. Neurosci Lett 526: 1–4.
7. Bishop MD, Horn ME, George SZ (2011) Exercise-induced pain intensity predicted by pre-exercise fear of pain and pain sensitivity. Clin J Pain 27: 398–404.
8. George SZ, Dover GC, Fillingim RB (2007) Fear of pain influences outcomes after exercise-induced delayed onset muscle soreness at the shoulder. Clin J Pain 23: 76–84.
9. George SZ, Dover GC, Wallace MR, Sack BK, Herbstman DM, et al. (2008) Biopsychosocial influence on exercise-induced delayed onset muscle soreness at the shoulder: pain catastrophizing and catechol-o-methyltransferase (COMT) diplotype predict pain ratings. Clin J Pain 24: 793–801.

10. Rakel BA, Blodgett NP, Bridget Zimmerman M, Logsden-Sackett N, Clark C, et al. (2012) Predictors of postoperative movement and resting pain following total knee replacement. Pain 153: 2192–2203.
11. Ayles S, Graven-Nielsen T, Gibson W (2011) Vibration-induced afferent activity augments delayed onset muscle allodynia. J Pain 12: 884–891.
12. Cruz-Almeida Y, Fillingim RB (2014) Can quantitative sensory testing move us closer to mechanism-based pain management? Pain Med 15: 61–72.
13. Backonja MM, Attal N, Baron R, Bouhassira D, Drangholt M, et al. (2013) Value of quantitative sensory testing in neurological and pain disorders: NeuPSIG consensus. Pain 154: 1807–1819.
14. Henriksen M, Alkjaer T, Lund H, Simonsen EB, Graven-Nielsen T, et al. (2007) Experimental quadriceps muscle pain impairs knee joint control during walking. J Appl Physiol (1985) 103: 132–139.
15. Bishop MD, Horn ME, George SZ, Robinson ME (2011) Self-reported pain and disability outcomes from an endogenous model of muscular back pain. BMC Musculoskelet Disord 12: 35.
16. Slater H, Arendt-Nielsen L, Wright A, Graven-Nielsen T (2003) Experimental deep tissue pain in wrist extensors–a model of lateral epicondylalgia. Eur J Pain 7: 277–288.
17. Price DD, McGrath PA, Rafii A, Buckingham B (1983) The validation of visual analogue scales as ratio scale measures for chronic and experimental pain. Pain 17: 45–56.
18. Parr J, Borsa P, Fillingim R, Kaiser K, Tillman MD, et al. (2014) Psychological influences predict recovery following exercise induced shoulder pain. Int J Sports Med 35: 232–237.
19. Parr JJ, Borsa PA, Fillingim RB, Tillman MD, Manini TM, et al. (2012) Pain-related fear and catastrophizing predict pain intensity and disability independently using an induced muscle injury model. J Pain 13: 370–378.
20. Sullivan MJL, Bishop SR, Pivik J (1995) The Pain Catastrophizing Scale: Development and validation. Psychological Assessment 7: 524–532.
21. Mintken PE, Cleland JA, Whitman JM, George SZ (2010) Psychometric properties of the Fear-Avoidance Beliefs Questionnaire and Tampa Scale of Kinesiophobia in patients with shoulder pain. Arch Phys Med Rehabil 91: 1128–1136.
22. Lentz TA, Barabas JA, Day T, Bishop MD, George SZ (2009) The relationship of pain intensity, physical impairment, and pain-related fear to function in patients with shoulder pathology. J Orthop Sports Phys Ther 39: 270–277.
23. Woby SR, Roach NK, Urmston M, Watson PJ (2005) Psychometric properties of the TSK-11: a shortened version of the Tampa Scale for Kinesiophobia. Pain 117: 137–144.
24. Arendt-Nielsen L, Yarnitsky D (2009) Experimental and clinical applications of quantitative sensory testing applied to skin, muscles and viscera. J Pain 10: 556–572.
25. Coronado RA, Kindler LL, Valencia C, George SZ (2011) Thermal and pressure pain sensitivity in patients with unilateral shoulder pain: comparison of involved and uninvolved sides. J Orthop Sports Phys Ther 41: 165–173.
26. Coronado RA, Simon CB, Valencia C, George SZ (2014) Experimental pain responses support peripheral and central sensitization in patients with unilateral shoulder pain. Clin J Pain 30: 143–151.
27. Chesterton LS, Sim J, Wright CC, Foster NE (2007) Interrater reliability of algometry in measuring pressure pain thresholds in healthy humans, using multiple raters. Clin J Pain 23: 760–766.
28. Persson AL, Brogardh C, Sjolund BH (2004) Tender or not tender: test-retest repeatability of pressure pain thresholds in the trapezius and deltoid muscles of healthy women. J Rehabil Med 36: 17–27.
29. Price DD, Mao J, Frenk H, Mayer DJ (1994) The N-methyl-D-aspartate receptor antagonist dextromethorphan selectively reduces temporal summation of second pain in man. Pain 59: 165–174.
30. Valencia C, Fillingim RB, George SZ (2011) Suprathreshold heat pain response is associated with clinical pain intensity for patients with shoulder pain. J Pain 12: 133–140.
31. Valencia C, Kindler LL, Fillingim RB, George SZ (2012) Investigation of central pain processing in shoulder pain: converging results from 2 musculoskeletal pain models. J Pain 13: 81–89.
32. Valencia C, Kindler LL, Fillingim RB, George SZ (2013) Stability of conditioned pain modulation in two musculoskeletal pain models: investigating the influence of shoulder pain intensity and gender. BMC Musculoskelet Disord 14: 182.
33. Kong JT, Schnyer RN, Johnson KA, Mackey S (2013) Understanding central mechanisms of acupuncture analgesia using dynamic quantitative sensory testing: a review. Evid Based Complement Alternat Med 2013: 187182.
34. Dormann CF, Elith J, Bacher S, Buchmann C, Carl G, et al. (2013) Collinearity: a review of methods to deal with it and a simulation study evaluating their performance. Ecography 36: 27–46.
35. Field AP (2009) Discovering statistics using SPSS. Los Angeles: SAGE Publications. xxxii, 821 p. p.
36. Green SB (1991) How Many Subjects Does It Take to Do a Regression-Analysis. Multivariate Behavioral Research 26: 499–510.
37. Babyak MA (2004) What you see may not be what you get: a brief, nontechnical introduction to overfitting in regression-type models. Psychosom Med 66: 411–421.
38. Dannecker EA, Hausenblas HA, Kaminski TW, Robinson ME (2005) Sex differences in delayed onset muscle pain. Clin J Pain 21: 120–126.
39. Dannecker EA, Koltyn KF, Riley JL 3rd, Robinson ME (2003) Sex differences in delayed onset muscle soreness. J Sports Med Phys Fitness 43: 78–84.
40. Frey Law LA, Evans S, Knudtson J, Nus S, Scholl K, et al. (2008) Massage reduces pain perception and hyperalgesia in experimental muscle pain: a randomized, controlled trial. J Pain 9: 714–721.
41. Slater H, Arendt-Nielsen L, Wright A, Graven-Nielsen T (2005) Sensory and motor effects of experimental muscle pain in patients with lateral epicondylalgia and controls with delayed onset muscle soreness. Pain 114: 118–130.
42. Torisu T, Wang K, Svensson P, De Laat A, Tanaka M, et al. (2010) Effects of eccentric jaw exercise on temporal summation in jaw-closing muscles of healthy subjects. Eur J Pain 14: 719–724.
43. Price DD (2002) Central neural mechanisms that interrelate sensory and affective dimensions of pain. Mol Interv 2: 392–403, 339.
44. Melzack R, Katz J (2013) Pain. Wiley Interdisciplinary Reviews-Cognitive Science 4: 1–15.
45. Parks EL, Geha PY, Baliki MN, Katz J, Schnitzer TJ, et al. (2011) Brain activity for chronic knee osteoarthritis: dissociating evoked pain from spontaneous pain. Eur J Pain 15: 843 e841–814.
46. Trost Z (2012) All pain is not created equal: differentiating between pain during movement versus pain at rest following total knee arthroplasty. Pain 153: 2161–2162.
47. Yarnitsky D, Crispel Y, Eisenberg E, Granovsky Y, Ben-Nun A, et al. (2008) Prediction of chronic post-operative pain: pre-operative DNIC testing identifies patients at risk. Pain 138: 22–28.
48. Valencia C, Fillingim RB, Bishop M, Wu SS, Wright TW, et al. (2013) Investigation of Central Pain Processing in Post-Operative Shoulder Pain and Disability. Clin J Pain.
49. Granot M, Weissman-Fogel I (2012) The effect of post-surgical neuroplasticity on the stability of systemic pain perception: a psychophysical study. Eur J Pain 16: 247–255.
50. Landau R, Kraft JC, Flint LY, Carvalho B, Richebe P, et al. (2010) An experimental paradigm for the prediction of Post-Operative Pain (PPOP). J Vis Exp.
51. Granot M (2009) Can we predict persistent postoperative pain by testing preoperative experimental pain? Curr Opin Anaesthesiol 22: 425–430.
52. Yarnitsky D, Granot M, Granovsky Y (2014) Pain modulation profile and pain therapy: between pro- and antinociception. Pain 155: 663–665.
53. Hubscher M, Moloney N, Leaver A, Rebbeck T, McAuley JH, et al. (2013) Relationship between quantitative sensory testing and pain or disability in people with spinal pain-a systematic review and meta-analysis. Pain 154: 1497–1504.
54. Lautenbacher S, Rollman GB (1997) Possible deficiencies of pain modulation in fibromyalgia. Clin J Pain 13: 189–196.
55. Pielsticker A, Haag G, Zaudig M, Lautenbacher S (2005) Impairment of pain inhibition in chronic tension-type headache. Pain 118: 215–223.

19

Sprint Interval and Sprint Continuous Training Increases Circulating CD34$^+$ Cells and Cardio-Respiratory Fitness in Young Healthy Women

Emma Harris[1], **Mark Rakobowchuk**[2], **Karen M. Birch**[1]*

1 Multidisciplinary Cardiovascular Research Centre, University of Leeds, Leeds, United Kingdom, **2** School of Sport and Education, Brunel University, Middlesex, United Kingdom

Abstract

Introduction: The improvement of vascular health in the exercising limb can be attained by sprint interval training (SIT). However, the effects on systemic vascular function and on circulating angiogenic cells (CACs) which may contribute to endothelial repair have not been investigated. Additionally, a comparison between SIT and sprint continuous training (SCT) which is less time committing has not been made.

Methods: 12 women (22±2 yrs) completed 12 sessions of either SIT (n = 6) or work-matched SCT (n = 6) on 3 days/week. Pre and post-training assessments included brachial artery endothelial function and peripheral blood analysis for CAC number (CD34$^+$/CD34$^+$CD45^{dim}). CAC function was measured by migration and adhesion assays. Cardio-respiratory fitness, carotid arterial stiffness and carotid-radial and brachial-foot pulse wave velocity (PWV) were also evaluated.

Results: CD34$^+$ CACs increased following training in both groups but CD34$^+$CD45^{dim} did not (Pre CD34$^+$: 40±21/10^5 leukocytes, Post CD34$^+$: 56±24/10^5 leukocytes, main time effect $p<0.05$). Brachial artery flow-mediated dilation (FMD) increased following SIT but SCT had no effect (Pre SIT: 5.0±3.4%, Post SIT: 5.9±3.0%, Pre SCT: 7.2±2.7%, Post SCT: 6.5±2.9%; group x time interaction $p = 0.08$). $\dot{V}O_{2max}$ increased in both training groups (Pre: 34.6±4.6 ml•kg•ml^{-1}, Post: 36.9±5.4 ml•kg•ml^{-1}, main time effect $p<0.05$). CAC function, carotid arterial stiffness and PWV did not change after training ($p>0.05$).

Discussion: SCT involving little time commitment is comparable to SIT in increasing CD34$^+$ cell number and $\dot{V}O_{2max}$. An increased mobilisation of CD34$^+$ CACs suggests that sprint training may be an effective method to enhance vascular repair.

Editor: Tim Lahm, Indiana University, United States of America

Funding: The work was supported by the University of Leeds. The funders had no role in study design, data collection and analysis, decision to publish, or preparation of the manuscript.

Competing Interests: The authors have declared that no competing interests exist.

* Email: k.m.birch@leeds.ac.uk

Introduction

Cardiovascular disease (CVD) is the main cause of mortality in the UK, responsible for one third of all deaths [1]. The pathogenesis of atherosclerosis, a key component in the development of CVD, is initiated by endothelial dysfunction [2]. This dysfunction is thought to indicate reduced nitric oxide bioavailability, a factor present in atherosclerotic vessels before vascular structural changes occur [3]. Endothelial dysfunction determined via an impaired brachial artery flow-mediated dilation (FMD) reflects nitric oxide bioavailability [4] and is both indicative of coronary artery endothelial dysfunction [5,6] and predictive of CVD [7]. Thus, improved endothelial function offers a target for CVD preventative strategies.

A potential method to sustain healthy endothelial function involves the mobilisation of circulating angiogenic cells (CACs). CACs represent a heterogeneous population of haematopoietic stem cells that aid in vascular repair, either through the secretion of angiogenic growth factors [8] or directly by maturation into endothelial cells and incorporation into the endothelium [9]. The mobilisation and function of CACs are impaired in patients with CVD [10] with low numbers of CD34$^+$ CAC associated with an increased CVD risk [11]. Improved CAC mobilisation and function [12–14] and enhanced endothelial function in central and peripheral arteries can be achieved through exercise [15,16] thus, exercise training offers a method for endothelial repair and CVD risk reduction.

However, only 6% of men and 4% of women in England meet the recommended guidelines for exercise participation when assessed using accelerometers, with the main barrier to exercise cited as a lack of time [17]. This has led to an increasing number of studies focusing on the benefits of high-intensity training interventions with reduced weekly time commitment. One type of high-intensity exercise emerging within the literature is sprint interval training (SIT), consisting of multiple bursts of maximal exertion separated by rest periods. Few studies have assessed the effects of SIT upon the cardiovascular system, although Rakobowchuk *et al.*, (2008) reported an increased endothelial function and distensibility of the popliteal artery in healthy individuals after only 6 weeks of SIT. A possible mechanism for this improvement is an increased expression of endothelial nitric oxide synthase (eNOS) as observed in rodents following SIT [16]. Additionally, 6 weeks of SIT in sedentary males increased eNOS content in the muscle microvasculature in the exercising limb [18]. However, the effects on systemic endothelial function such as the brachial artery and on CAC number and function have not been investigated following SIT. Additionally, due to the recovery periods involved in SIT sessions, total session duration is not much shorter than the recommended government guidelines of 30 min of moderate-intensity continuous exercise. A less time committing approach would be the performance of a single continuous sprint which would serve to shorten the total training session duration.

Sprint continuous training (SCT) sessions involve one sustained maximal effort sprint without rest periods. This type of training may be more appealing for training purposes than SIT as the time commitment is less. An acute bout of SCT has beneficial effects on metabolic health in overweight/obese men, with immediate increases in insulin sensitivity and reductions in insulin resistance evident [19]. However, the chronic effects of SCT on systemic endothelial function and repair are unknown and have not been compared with SIT. Therefore, the aims of the present study were to determine and compare the effects of work-matched SIT with a less time committing SCT protocol on brachial artery endothelial function, arterial stiffness, cardio-respiratory fitness and CAC number and function. In this first investigation comparing the effects of SIT and SCT on parameters of vascular health, pre-menopausal women will be studied, to determine whether exercise of a high-intensity might alter the vascular phenotype in a young healthy group, likely to undergo vascular changes with ageing.

Methods

Ethics statement

Informed written consent and a physical activity readiness questionnaire were completed prior to participation by all participants. The study was approved by the University Of Leeds Faculty Of Biological Sciences Ethics Committee, which conformed to the Declaration of Helsinki.

Participants

Twelve healthy eumenorrheic females (age: 22±2 yrs; BMI: 23.6±1.8 kg·m^{-2}) who were low-moderately active defined as attending between 0–2 structured exercise sessions per week, volunteered for the study. Exclusion criteria included any known cardiovascular, pulmonary or metabolic disease, use of hormonal contraceptives in the last 6 months, pregnancy, smoking, and medication and vitamin use.

Experimental protocol

Pre-training measurements were undertaken prior to the completion of a 4-week sprint training programme. The exercise training programme duration was chosen to ensure participants were assessed in the same phase of their individual menstrual cycle, and to determine if changes in vascular health can occur as quickly as those reported in skeletal muscle oxidative capacity [20]. For both pre and post-testing assessments, participants attended the laboratory on two separate days. On the first visit the vascular measures were undertaken prior to a fasted venous blood sample collection. Blood was collected in EDTA tubes and separated into two samples for CAC enumeration (1 ml) and functional assessments (30 ml). Participants were instructed not to exercise or consume alcohol in the previous 24 hrs and to refrain from consuming food or caffeine in the 8 to 12 hrs prior to testing. A cardio-respiratory exercise test was completed on the second visit which participants attended in a non-fasted state. Participants were matched for relative maximal oxygen uptake ($\dot{V}O_{2max}$) and assigned to either a SIT (n = 6) or SCT (n = 6) training group. Post-testing measures were acquired 4 weeks later between 48 and 72 hrs after the last training session.

Assessment of brachial artery endothelial function

Assessment of endothelial function was completed in a temperature controlled laboratory (20–24°C) after 20 min of supine rest. An electrocardiograph (ECG) was fitted via a three-lead setup for heart rate (HR) acquisition. Resting HR was calculated as an average over a 5 min period using LabChart software (Labchart 7.0, ADInstruments Pty Ltd, Australia). Brachial artery endothelial-dependent vasodilation was assessed according to established guidelines [21,22]. A 7 MHz linear array ultrasound probe (Aspen, Acuson; Siemens Medical, Camberley, UK) was used to obtain 20 consecutive ECG gated (end-diastolic) longitudinal images of the brachial artery in the right arm. A 5 min period of forearm ischemia was created by cuff inflation (>50 mmHg above systolic blood pressure; SBP) distal to the ultrasound probe to occlude arterial flow, and 180 end-diastolic images and blood velocity were recorded consecutively from 30 s before cuff release onwards (~2 min). Images were recorded using vascular imaging software (Vascular Imager, Medical Imaging Applications, Coralville, Iowa, USA) and analysed using semi-automated edge-detection software (Brachial Tools v.5, Medical Imaging Applications) to determine brachial artery diameters. Resting arterial diameter was calculated from an average of 20 consecutive images recorded prior to cuff inflation and peak diameter calculated as the highest value post cuff release from a 3 consecutive cardiac cycle rolling average. Relative FMD was calculated as follows:

$$\text{FMD}\ (\%) = \frac{\text{Peak diameter} - \text{Resting diameter}}{\text{Resting diameter}} \times 100$$

The area under the shear rate curve from cuff release to peak dilation (AUC_{peak}) and to 60 s post (AUC_{60}) were calculated from $(8 \times \text{VTI}) \div \text{resting diameter}$, where VTI is the velocity time integral for each period. Peak reactive hyperaemia and shear rate was determined from the highest velocity in the first 10 s post cuff release. FMD was not normalised to shear rate/AUC as not all the assumptions for the use of ratios were met [22].

Carotid arterial stiffness and structure

Brachial artery blood pressure was measured 3 times (at 5 min intervals) using an automated oscillometric device (Omron M5-I, Omron Healthcare, Europe B.V., The Netherlands) and an average was calculated to determine SBP, diastolic blood pressure (DBP), mean arterial pressure (MAP) and pulse pressure (PP). Carotid arterial stiffness measures were obtained using a combination of ultrasound imaging to determine vessel diameters, and applanation tonometry to estimate carotid artery SBP, as previously described [23]. The ultrasound probe was placed on the right common carotid artery in the longitudinal direction and two video clips were captured for a duration of 20 s at a rate of 15 frames per second (Vascular Imager, Medical Imaging Applications). Immediately post recordings a tonometer (model SPT-301B, Millar Instruments Inc., Texas, USA) was held against the left common carotid artery to capture 20 carotid artery pulse pressure waveforms. These signals were acquired and analysed using a data acquisition system (Powerlab model ML845, ADInstruments) and software (Labchart 7.0, ADInstruments). Video clips were analysed using semi-automated edge-detection software (Carotid Tools Analysis; Medical Imaging Applications) to determine average carotid artery minimum and maximum diameters and end-diastole far-wall intima-media thickness (IMT) from 20 cardiac cycles. End-diastole was identified as the point at which the carotid artery diameter was at a minimum.

As differences in DBP and MAP in different conduit arteries are negligible when in a supine position [24], carotid artery SBP was estimated from an average of 20 carotid artery pulse pressure waveforms (recorded using the tonometer) using linear extrapolation. This equates minimum and mean carotid artery waveform blood pressure values to brachial artery DBP and MAP respectively, and uses maximum carotid artery waveform values as an extrapolation point to estimate carotid artery SBP. Carotid artery PP, cross-sectional compliance (CSC), distensibility and β-stiffness index (SI) were calculated from the following equations [25]:

$$\text{PP (mmHg)} = \text{carotid SBP} - \text{brachial DBP}$$

$$\text{CSC } (\text{mm}^2/\text{mmHg}) = \frac{\pi(d_{max}/2)^2 - \pi(d_{min}/2)^2}{\text{PP}}$$

$$\text{Distensibility (mm/mmHg)} = \frac{\text{CSC}}{\pi(d_{min}/2)^2}$$

$$\text{SI (a.u.)} = \ln\frac{(\text{carotid SBP/brachial DBP})}{(d_{max} - d_{min})/d_{min}}$$

Where d_{max} and d_{min} are the average carotid artery maximum and minimum diameters, respectively.

Assessment of pulse wave velocity (PWV)

Carotid-radial (PWV_{cr}) and brachial-foot pulse wave velocities (PWV_{bf}) were measured to assess the effects of SIT and SCT on both peripheral and central arterial stiffness. Given that a strong positive correlation ($r = 0.87$) exists between PWV_{bf} and aortic PWV [26], PWV_{bf} was used as an estimate of central PWV. Additionally, brachial arterial stiffness is reflected by PWV_{cr} as a measure of peripheral artery stiffness [27,28], and was therefore used as a measure of upper limb PWV. Pulse pressure waveforms were recorded for 20 s at the carotid, radial, brachial and dorsal pedis arteries using the tonometer described above which was connected to a SphygmoCor PWV system (SCOR-Vx, AtCor Medical Pty Ltd) that enabled simultaneous ECG and pulse pressure waveform recordings. The distance between the sternal notch to these arterial sites were measured in the supine position using a standard tape measure at pre-testing. The distance between the sternal notch and the brachial and radial arteries were measured with the left arm held at a 90° angle to the body. PWV was calculated automatically by the SphygmoCor PWV system by inputting the arterial distances and selecting the intersecting tangents method for determining the pulse transit times (PTT) [29]. The PTT were calculated as the time difference between the peak of the R-wave on the ECG and the foot of the pulse pressure waveforms.

Enumeration of CACs

CACs were enumerated using a modified ISHAGE (International Society of Hematotherapy and Graft Engineering) protocol [30]. Briefly, 1 ml of peripheral blood was collected in EDTA tubes and mixed with 1 ml Phosphate buffered saline (PBS). The sample was incubated with 20 μl of Fc-receptor blocker (Miltenyi Biotec, Bergisch Gladbach, Germany) for 10 min, before incubation with fluorochrome-conjugated antibodies, CD34-PE (10 μl) and CD45-FITC (10 μl; Miltenyi Biotec, Bergisch Gladbach, Germany). The sample was lysed, centrifuged at 300 g for 10 min and the pellet resuspended in 1 ml of fluorescence activated cell sorting (FACS) buffer (PBS with 0.5% bovine serum albumin and 0.4% EDTA) before final centrifugation at 300 g for 10 min. The remaining pellet was resuspended in 500 μl of FACS buffer and immediately enumerated by flow cytometry using a FACSCalibur cytometer and CellQuest software (Becton Dickinson, Oxford, UK). Samples were analysed within 2 hrs of blood collection and at least 100,000 events recorded in gate R1 (Figure 1). Cells were enumerated using commercially available analysis software (FlowJo7 6.4). Two subsets of CACs were enumerated as previously described [30]. Cells that were positive for both CD45 and CD34 were termed $CD34^+$ cells and measured from gate R5 (Figure 1). CD34+ cells that expressed CD45 at a low intensity (R3, Figure 1), and were found in the lymphocyte region (for exclusion of mature circulating endothelial cells; R4, Figure 1), were termed $CD34^+/CD45^{dim}$ cells (R5, Figure 1). Isotype controls were not required as other cells and debris (i.e. red blood cells and platelets) that may bind to CD34 antibodies are excluded in R1 [30]. Due to flow cytometer failure, one result at post-testing was not reliable and was excluded from analysis. Cells were expressed as an absolute number per 100,000 leukocytes.

Functional assessment of CACs

Mononuclear cells were separated from a 30 ml blood sample by ficoll density-gradient centrifugation according to the manufacturer's instructions, (Ficoll Paque PLUS, GE Healthcare) and suspended in endothelial basal medium (EBM) supplemented with 20% fetal calf serum, growth factors and antibiotics (EBM-2, Bullet kit; Lonza, Inc). Cells were plated on 6-well fibronectin coated plates (5×10^6 per well) and cultured for 7 days at 37°C in 5% CO_2. On days 2, 4 and 6, non-adherent cells were removed by washing with PBS and fresh medium was added. After 7 days of culture, adherent CACs were detached using trypsin and their adhesive and migratory ability were assessed. At post-testing 1 participant from the SCT group was excluded from the adhesion and migration assays, and 1 participant from the SIT group excluded from the migration assay due to low cell number at harvest.

The ability of CACs to adhere to fibronectin can be used to assess the adhesive ability of CACs *in vitro* [31,32]. CACs were plated in 24-well fibronectin coated plates (5×10^4 per well) in 1 ml of supplemented EBM. After incubation for 24 hrs, non-adherent cells were removed by gently washing with PBS and 10 random microscopic images (×200 magnification) were collected for quantification of adherent cells. Assays were performed in triplicate and an average calculated, however in 3 participants at pre-training and 1 participant at post-testing; assays were performed in duplicate due to insufficient cell numbers.

The migratory ability of CACs towards vascular endothelial growth factor (VEGF) can be measured *in vitro* using a Boyden chamber assay [10]. The 8 μm pore Boyden chambers were placed into wells of a 24-well plate containing either 750 μl unsupplemented EBM only (negative control) or combined with VEGF (50 ng/ml). CACs at a density of 4×10^4 per 500 μl were

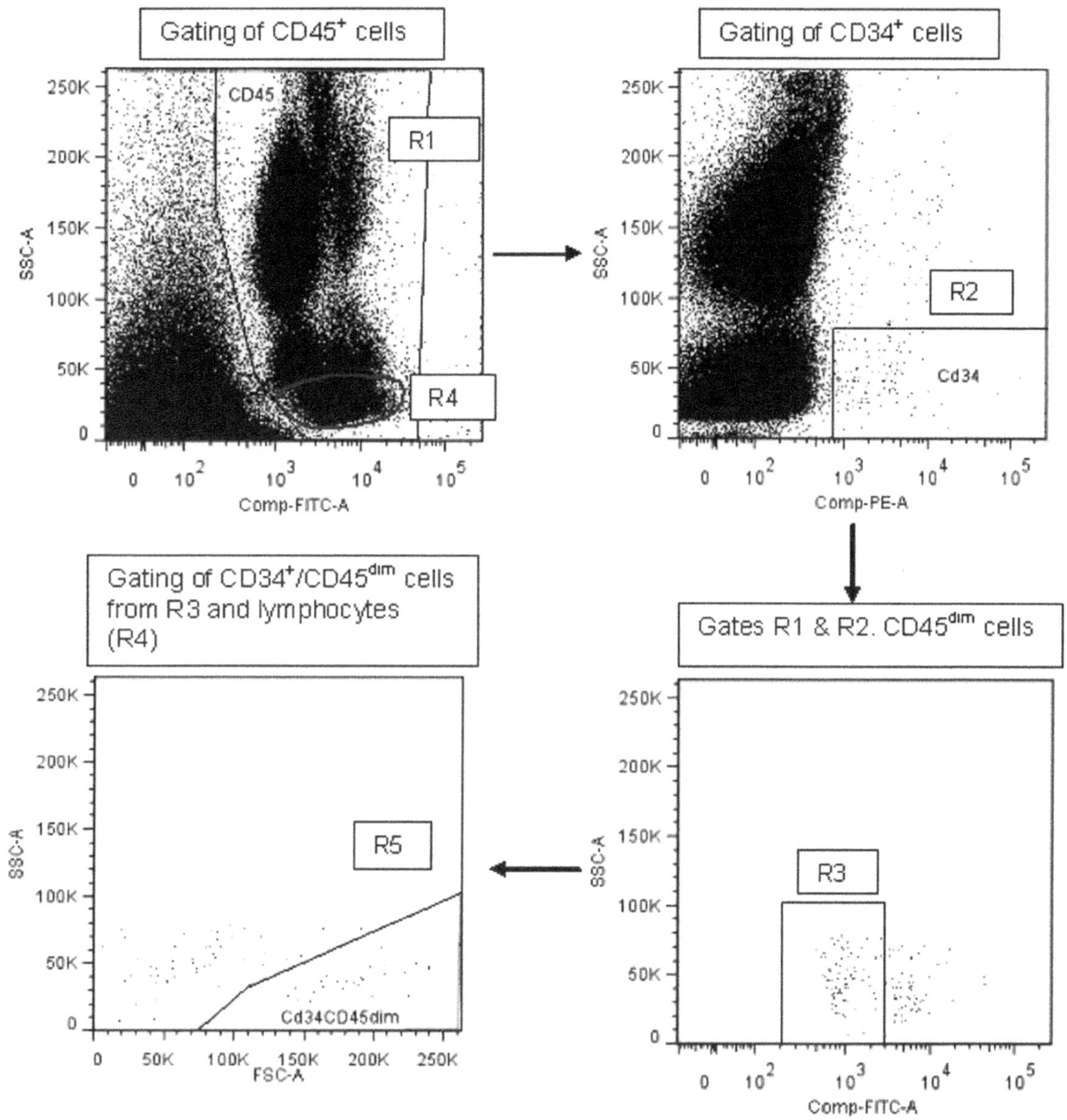

Figure 1. Enumeration of CACs. ISHAGE gating strategy for CAC enumeration. Cells positive for CD45 and therefore leukocytes were gated in R1. Cells in R1 that were positive for CD34 and had low side scatter characteristics were plotted in R2 and defined as $CD34^+$ cells. Cells from R2 were gated on a further plot to determine the $CD45^{dim}$ population. Subsequently cells from R3 were back-gated from R4 and gated on a further plot (R5) to define $CD34^+CD45^{dim}$ cells that are located within the lymphocyte population.

placed into the Boyden chambers and incubated for 24 hours. Cells were fixed with ethanol and non-migrated cells were removed from the upper surface of the Boyden chamber with a cotton swab. Migrated cells on the lower surface of the chamber were stained with haematoxylin and eosin and 10 random microscopic images (×200 magnification) were collected for quantification of migrated cells. The ability of cells to migrate to a chemoattractant was calculated as the difference between the number of migrated cells to VEGF and the number of migrated cells to unsupplemented EBM. The assay was performed in triplicate in each condition if sufficient cell numbers were available.

Assessment of cardio-respiratory fitness

Participants performed a seated ramp incremental step exercise test (RISE-105) on an electronically braked cycle ergometer (Excalibur Sport V2.0; Lode BV, Groningen, The Netherlands) for the assessment of $\dot{V}O_{2max}$ and the lactate threshold (LT). A mouthpiece and nose clip was fitted for breath by breath analyses of pulmonary gas exchange and ventilatory variables (Breeze suite v. 5.0, Medgraphics D-series; Medgraphics, Medical Graphics Corporation, St Paul, MN, USA). Briefly, a 2 min rest period was followed by 2 min of seated cycling at 20 W before initiation of the ramp incremental (RI) test (1 W/4s). The exercise was ended when the participant could no longer maintain a cycling cadence of 50 rpm despite verbal encouragement. The cessation of the RI exercise was followed by a 5 min period of cycling at 20 W before initiation of the step exercise (SE) test at 105% of the work-rate attained at the end of the RI test. The RISE-105 test is an established protocol to confirm that $\dot{V}O_{2max}$ has been achieved rather than $\dot{V}O_{2peak}$ [33]. As previously described, breath-by-breath data were exported and edited in data analysis software (OriginPro 8, OriginLab, Northampton, MA). Breaths were eliminated if $\dot{V}O_2$ values fell outside four standard deviations around the local mean. A 12-breath rolling average of $\dot{V}O_2$ was calculated for both the RI and SE phases of the test, to determine the $\dot{V}O_{2peak}$ of each phase. A paired t-test determined that the RI and SE $\dot{V}O_{2peak}$ values were not significantly different. Therefore, $\dot{V}O_{2max}$ was reported as the average of the $\dot{V}O_{2peak}$ values. The estimated LT was determined using the V-slope method which uses the inflection point of the $\dot{V}O_2$ against $\dot{V}CO_2$ curve as an estimation of LT [34]. This point was further confirmed by a rise in end tidal O_2 and a plateau in end-tidal CO_2 [35].

Exercise training protocol

Participants completed 3 supervised sprint training sessions per week in the laboratory for a 4 week period. All sprints were performed on a cycler ergometer (Ergomedic 874E Peak bike, Monark Exercise AB, Sweden) connected to software (Monark anaerobic test software, Monark Exercise AB HUR OY, Karleby, Finland) for the calculation of average power. In each training session participants in the SIT group completed four 30 s maximal effort sprints (Wingate test) at a resistance equivalent to 7.5% of body weight. The resistance was applied when the participant reached a cadence of 140–150 rpm and each Wingate test was separated by 4.5 min of unloaded pedalling. SIT sessions were based on a previous study [36] whereby vascular function was seen to improve with SIT training.

Participants in the SCT group completed a full SIT session as their first training session for the purpose of calculating the total work achieved from the four 30 s sprints. Total work was calculated in kJ as the sum of the work in each of the 4 Wingate tests from the recording of average power. The total number of revolutions performed on the cycle ergometer to achieve this total work was also recorded. For the remaining training sessions the SCT group completed a single continuous maximal effort sprint. To enable a sustained sprint, the cycle ergometer resistance was reduced by a third of the SIT session resistance to 5% of body mass. Each SCT session was stopped once the participant had completed the equivalent total number of revolutions attained in the 4 Wingate tests in their first SIT session. In this way the SCT and SIT sessions were work-matched. As the resistance was reduced by one third, the total number of revolutions was increased by one third. Thus, both training groups were matched for work relative to their own fitness level. In both groups' sessions, strong verbal motivation was provided to encourage participants to maintain a fast cadence throughout the sprints. All sessions were followed by a short cool-down that was similar between the groups. Thus, the training groups by design both involved maximal exertion sprints, were matched for relative work but differed in regards to session duration and the interval vs. continuous nature of the exercise. Participants in the SCT group completed an extra 30 s Wingate test at the end of training to assess changes in peak power from pre to post-training.

Statistical analysis

Statistical analysis was performed using statistical software (SPSS version 19.0; IBM Corporation, Somers, NY, USA). Data were assessed for normal distribution using the Kolmogorov-Smirnov test. Pre-testing data were evaluated for training group differences via a Student's independent t-test. The effect of the training interventions was analysed using a mixed model repeated measures ANOVA with time (pre vs. post-training) and training group (SIT vs. SCT) factors. Pearson correlations were performed to establish relationships between variables. Significance was accepted as $p<0.05$ and values were presented as mean ± standard deviation. The between-day reproducibility of relative FMD was calculated from a separate group of 8 young healthy moderately active participants. The participants attended the laboratory on two separate days under the same testing conditions as the trained participants (i.e. fasted, no exercise in the previous 24 hrs). The coefficient of variation was 12.4% and the absolute difference in relative FMD was 0.18%. Given the lack of knowledge on CACs and exercise training in a healthy population, CAC number was selected as the primary outcome. Using the previously reported increase of 8.7 $CD34^+$ cells/µl with a standard deviation of 3.0, following a supramaximal bout of exercise in a healthy population [37], a minimum of 8 participants in total were required to obtain 80% power ($\alpha = 0.05$), in a two-treatment parallel-design study.

Results

Participants and training effect

Participant characteristics are displayed in Table 1. There were no pre-training differences present between the training groups in any variable ($p>0.05$). BMI, resting HR and brachial artery BP did not change following training ($p>0.05$). By design both the training groups' session duration (SIT: 20 min, SCT: 3.5±0.2 min) and resistance applied to the cycle ergometer (SIT: 5.1±0.6 kg, SCT: 3.4±0.4 kg) were greater in the SIT group. Work completed per session did not significantly differ between the groups (SIT: 45.9±6.3 kJ vs. SCT: 47.6±6.2 kJ). Peak and average power calculated for a single 30 s Wingate test did not increase from session 1 to post-training ($p>0.05$). Both absolute ($p = 0.048$) and relative $\dot{V}O_{2max}$ ($p = 0.046$) increased with training with no interaction between group x time ($p>0.05$, Table 1, Figure 2a). The estimated LT also increased with training in both groups (Figure 2b); although significance was not reached ($p = 0.08$) the 95% confidence interval (CI) for pre to post-training difference ranged from −11 to 164 ml/min. The RI test duration and work-rate achieved at the end of the RI stage (WRpeak) significantly increased following training in both groups ($p<0.001$) with a greater increase following SIT (group x time interaction for both $p = 0.05$; Table 1, Figure 2c).

Brachial artery endothelial function

Resting brachial artery diameter and time from cuff release to peak dilation were unchanged following training in both groups ($p>0.05$, Table 1). However, absolute and relative FMD showed a trend for an increase (FMD_{rel} by ~19%, FMD_{abs} by ~23%) following SIT but no change following SCT (Table 1, Figure 3). Although the main time effect was not significant ($p = 0.81$), the group x time interaction showed a trend ($p = 0.08$), with 67% of participants in the SIT increasing FMD (FMD_{rel}: 95% CI for pre to post-training difference: −0.59 to 2.43%) and 67% of SCT participants exhibiting reduced FMD (FMD_{rel}: 95% CI for pre to post-training difference: −2.29 to 0.86%). Larger increases in absolute FMD occurred in participants with lower pre-training levels of absolute FMD ($r = -0.57$, $p = 0.06$). Peak reactive hyperaemia, peak shear rate, AUC_{peak} and AUC_{60} did not change in either training groups ($p>0.05$, Table 1).

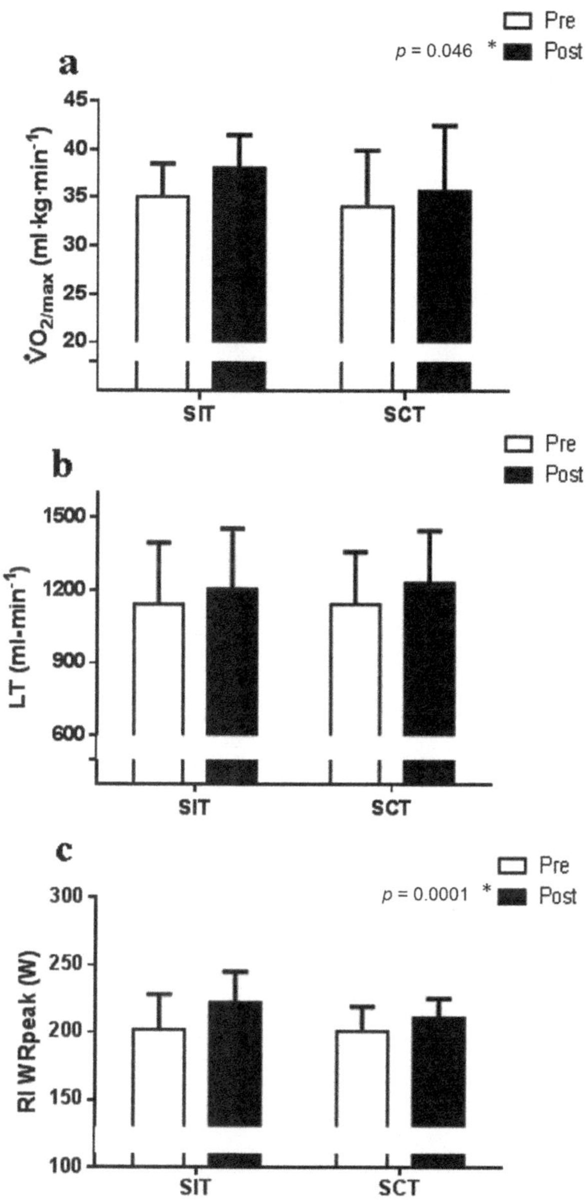

Figure 2. Cardio-respiratory fitness. * indicates a significant pre to post-training difference in both groups (time effect $p<0.05$). a) Relative maximal oxygen uptake ($\dot{V}O_{2max}$) increased following both SIT (n = 6) and SCT (n = 6; main time effect $p = 0.046$) with no group x time interaction ($p = 0.49$). b) The estimated lactate threshold (LT) followed a trend to increase in both training groups (main time effect $p = 0.08$) with no group x time interaction ($p = 0.30$). c) The ramp incremental (RI) test work-rate peak (WRpeak) significantly increased in both groups (main time effect $p = 0.0001$) with a greater increase following SIT (group x time interaction $p = 0.05$).

Arterial stiffness

Carotid to radial and brachial to foot PWV did not alter following training in either group ($p>0.05$) indicating that sprint training did not affect upper limb or central PWV (Table 2). Carotid artery IMT, distensibility, cross-sectional compliance and stiffness index were also unaltered following both types of training ($p>0.05$; Table 2).

Training effect on CAC number

Circulating $CD34^+$ cells increased following both SIT (by ~44%; n = 6) and SCT (by ~28%; n = 5; main time effect $p = 0.02$) with no group x time interaction ($p = 0.83$; Figure 4a). However, $CD34^+/CD45^{dim}$ did not change following either type of training (main time effect $p = 0.21$, group x time interaction $p = 0.67$; Figure 4b). Changes in $CD34^+$ cells with training did not correlate with pre-training or changes in FMD (Pre FMD r = 0.14, pre to post-training delta FMD r = 0.34, $p>0.05$).

CAC function

The function of CACs did not significantly improve with either type of training (main time effect, adhesion $p = 0.47$, migration $p = 0.63$; group x time interaction $p>0.05$; Table 1). However, whilst training induced changes in CAC adhesion were not related to pre-training levels ($p>0.05$), changes in CAC migration were greater in participants with lower pre-training levels of CAC migration (r = −0.67, $p = 0.03$).

Discussion

The present study to our knowledge is the first to examine the effects of sprint training on brachial artery function as an indicator of systemic vascular function, and the mobilisation and function of circulating cells that may contribute to endothelial repair. Furthermore, novel comparisons were made between SIT and SCT to explore whether sprint training involving a continuous work-rate stimulus has differential effects on the vasculature than work-matched sprinting of an interval nature. The main findings were that despite the lower training time commitment, SCT improved cardio-respiratory fitness to a similar extent as SIT. Furthermore, increased mobilisation of circulating $CD34^+$ cells was observed following both types of training, but arterial stiffness, $CD34^+/CD45^{dim}$ mobilisation and CAC function remained unchanged. Additionally, there was a trend in brachial artery FMD to increase following SIT but no change following SCT.

Improvements in exercise tolerance

Recently, a "lack of time" has been highlighted as the general publics' main barrier to exercise thus, several studies have focused on how supramaximal but less time committing exercise can be equally as beneficial to health and fitness as longer methods of exercise training. Improvements in $\dot{V}O_{2max}$ by ~10% have been observed following as little as 6 weeks of Wingate test based SIT [38], and the current study has observed similar changes. Additionally, following both training types, there was a near significant improvement in the LT and a significant increase in the RI test duration and WR_{peak}, with greater improvements following SIT. Since $\dot{V}O_{2max}$ is a strong predictor of future cardiac events [39], and the LT and WR_{peak} are markers of exercise tolerance that are associated with poorer cardiac outcomes [40], this type of training may be favourable to those who wish to rapidly increase their cardio-respiratory fitness and/or cardiovascular health. However, given that our results are in a population of young healthy females, further studies are required to investigate whether these findings can be translated to populations that have poor cardiovascular health.

Differential effects of SIT and SCT on brachial artery endothelial function

Our results indicated a close to significant trend for an increase in brachial artery FMD following SIT but no change after SCT, without any changes in peak reactive hyperaemia, peak shear rate,

Table 1. Participant characteristics at pre and post 4 weeks of either sprint interval (SIT) or sprint continuous training (SCT).

	SIT (n = 6)		SCT (n = 6)	
	PRE	POST	PRE	POST
Body mass index (kg·m^{-2})	23.6±1.8	23.8±1.6	23.1±2.3	22.9±2.6
Resting heart rate (bpm)	55±10	56±6	62±8	64±12
Brachial artery SBP	115±7	117±11	112±12	111±11
Brachial artery DBP	73±5	72±11	76±9	72±7
Brachial artery MAP	87±5	87±10	88±10	85±8
Absolute $\dot{V}O_{2max}$ (L·min^{-1})*	2.34±0.37	2.55±0.31	2.24±0.22	2.30±0.21
RI test duration (min)*	12.14±1.74	13.44±1.55	12.06±1.18	12.73±0.9
Lactate threshold (%)	48.4±7.4	46.4±5.4	49.0±6.4	51.9±8.1
Peak reactive hyperaemia (cm·s^{-1})	98.8±23.6	97.3±19.4	82.0±14.7	90.1±8.7
Peak shear rate (s^{-1})	2629±1064	2564±803	2126±449	2395±301
AUC_{peak} (a.u.)	31325±11174	30406±13875	27646±6595	31396±6366
AUC_{60} (a.u.)	39815±14654	39648±16146	39596±5261	43901±6012
Insonation angle (°)	69±1	68±2	68±2	68±1
Brachial artery baseline diameter (mm)	3.2±0.8	3.2±0.8	3.1±0.5	3.1±0.5
Absolute FMD (mm)	0.15±0.09	0.18±0.07	0.22±0.08	0.20±0.08
Time from cuff release to peak diameter (s)	38±8	35±4	34±9	34±6
CAC adhesion per microscopic image (SIT: n = 6; SCT: n = 5)	11±8	8±6	13±8	11±12
CAC migration per 10 microscopic images (SIT: n = 5; SCT: n = 5)	2±3	4±7	1±4	2±2

* indicates a significant main time effect ($p<0.05$).
No group differences at baseline or group x time interactions were observed ($p>0.05$). Absolute FMD group x time interaction was close to significant ($p = 0.08$). RI test duration group x time interaction was close to significant ($p = 0.05$). Bpm = beats per minute, SBP = systolic blood pressure, DBP = diastolic blood pressure, MAP = mean arterial pressure, $\dot{V}O_{2max}$ = maximal oxygen uptake, RI = ramp incremental, AUC = area under the shear rate curve, FMD = flow-mediated dilation and CAC = circulating angiogenic cell.

AUC_{60} or AUC_{peak}. Given that brachial artery FMD is largely nitric oxide dependent [4], this result suggests that SIT provides a greater stimulus for increased nitric oxide bioavailability than SCT. Improvements in brachial artery endothelial function following lower limb exercise training in healthy populations have occurred as early as 2 weeks and begun to return to baseline at 4 weeks due to arterial remodelling [41]. This may explain why other studies assessing upper limb endothelial function in healthy young participants following longer training protocols have not observed a change [42]. Therefore, it is plausible that if brachial artery endothelial function in the present study had been assessed after 2 weeks, a larger magnitude of change may have been present.

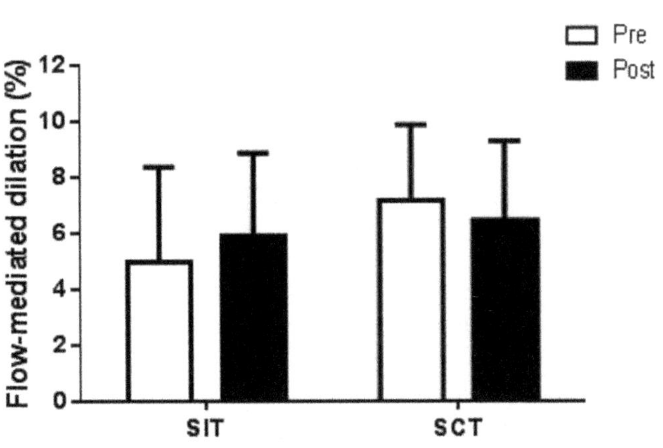

Figure 3. Brachial artery endothelial function. Brachial artery FMD displayed a trend for an increase following SIT (n = 6) but no change following SCT (n = 6; main time effect $p = 0.81$; group x time interaction $p = 0.08$).

Increases in brachial artery FMD following exercise training are believed to be caused by increases in brachial artery blood flow antegrade shear stress during exercise sessions [43], which induce nitric oxide release through activation of eNOS [15,44]. However, in the initial 5 min following lower limb cycling onset, mean brachial artery blood flow decreases due to an increase in retrograde flow caused by forearm resistance vessel vasoconstriction [45,46]. As opposed to antegrade shear stress, retrograde shear stress is pro-atherogenic as it increases reactive oxygen species and the expression of adhesion molecules which reduce nitric oxide bioavailability [47]. Additionally, greater oscillatory and retrograde shear rate in the brachial artery, activates the endothelium and induces damage, evidenced by significantly higher levels of circulating endothelial microparticles during and acutely after a period of induced disturbed flow [48]. Furthermore, retrograde shear stress reduces brachial artery FMD in a dose-dependent manner [49]. Since SCT duration was less than 5 min in our study, it is possible that the brachial artery endothelium experienced elevated retrograde shear stress unopposed by increases in antegrade shear stress, which may have negated improvements in endothelial function by reducing nitric oxide bioavailability. In contrast, SIT duration was 20 min which allowed sufficient time for antegrade shear stress to increase and for retrograde shear stress to return to baseline due to reductions in downstream peripheral resistance caused by thermoregulatory

Table 2. Arterial stiffness pre and post either sprint interval (SIT) or sprint continuous training (SCT).

	SIT (n = 6)		SCT (n = 6)	
	PRE	POST	PRE	POST
PWV_{cr} (m·s^{-1})	6.0±0.8	6.2±0.5	6.6±0.8	7.4±0.7
PWV_{bf} (m·s^{-1})	7.4±0.9	7.8±1.4	8.2±1.6	7.4±1.1
Carotid artery IMT (mm)	0.31±0.10	0.36±0.07	0.33±0.09	0.35±0.06
Carotid artery PP (mmHg)	29±4	31±5	25±3	27±5
Carotid ΔCSA within heart cycle (mm^2)	6.2±1.3	6.0±0.7	6.2±1.5	6.2±1.5
Carotid artery CSC (mm^2/mmHg)	0.22±0.05	0.19±0.03	0.25±0.06	0.24±0.08
Carotid artery DD (mm/mmHg)	0.01±0.002	0.01±0.002	0.01±0.002	0.01±0.002
Carotid artery SI (a.u.)	3.3±0.8	3.6±0.8	3.0±0.6	3.4±1.2

No group differences at pre-training, training effects or group x time interactions were found ($p>0.05$). PWV_{cr} = carotid-radial pulse wave velocity, PWV_{bf} = brachial-foot pulse wave velocity, IMT = intima-media thickness, PP = pulse pressure, CSA = cross-sectional area, CSC = cross-sectional compliance, DD = distensibilty, SI = β-stiffness index.

cutaneous vasodilation [46]. Thus, SIT may be more beneficial for brachial artery adaptations due to increases in antegrade shear stress that augment nitric oxide production, whereas SCT duration may be too short to induce the increases in antegrade shear stress required for improvements in FMD. However, further studies investigating blood flow responses to SIT and SCT are required to validate this suggestion.

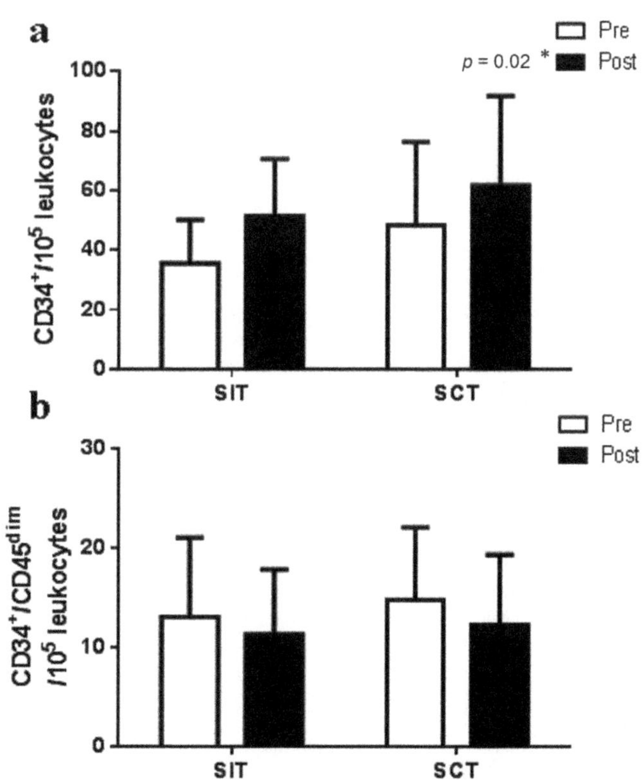

Figure 4. Circulating angiogenic cells. * indicates a significant pre to post-training difference in both groups (time effect $p<0.05$). a) CD34$^+$ cells increased following both SIT (n = 6) and SCT (n = 5; main time effect $p = 0.02$) with no group x time interaction ($p = 0.83$). However, b) CD34$^+$/CD45^{dim} cells did not change following either type of training (main time effect $p = 0.21$; group x time interaction $p = 0.67$).

Superior health benefits have been reported following interval exercise training compared to continuous exercise training, which have often been related to a higher exercise intensity, shear stress and work done experienced during interval exercise [50]. In the present study, SCT and SIT were both of a high intensity and matched for work. Therefore, it may be that the profile of the repeated increments and decrements in work-rate provided a greater stimulus for vascular adaptations than a continuous work-rate. Evidence from *in vitro* studies on endothelial cells suggests that the temporal gradients in shear stress are more important than the magnitude of the shear for eNOS activation and nitric oxide production. A rapid increase in shear stress from a pre-existing level creates a burst in nitric oxide production [51]. Subsequently, exposure to a sustained magnitude of this shear stress reduced the rate of nitric oxide production. Additionally, repeated impulses in shear stress have been seen to produce a large increase in nitric oxide production, whereas a slow ramp increase in flow to the equivalent magnitude had no effect [52]. This was thought to be due to the activation of eNOS by platelet endothelial cell activation molecule-1 (PECAM-1) which may only sense shear stress when rapid changes occur due to its sheltered position at cell-cell junctions [52]. Therefore, given that our SIT sessions involved 4 periods of rapid increases in shear stress compared to a single increase in the SCT, it seems reasonable to suggest that SIT provided a greater stimulus for nitric oxide synthesis. Furthermore, it is likely that the elevation in shear stress would have occurred for longer during SIT due to a longer session duration. The measurement of shear stress during SIT and SCT and further *in vitro* studies examining endothelial cell responses to continuous and periodic fluctuations in shear stress are required to validate these suggestions.

Unaltered arterial stiffness following sprint training

PWV, a measure of arterial stiffness associated with increased CVD risk [24], did not change with training both centrally and in the upper limb, indicating an unaltered arterial stiffness. Conversely, a previous study has observed an increased popliteal arterial distensibility following 6 weeks of SIT [36]. This suggests that sprint training can reduce arterial stiffness in the exercising limbs but not centrally or in the untrained upper limbs in a healthy population.

Carotid arterial distensibility and IMT are linked to CVD progression [53]. In the present study, carotid arterial stiffness and

IMT did not change following SIT or SCT, in agreement with a previous study following SIT in healthy individuals [36]. Healthy pre-training vasculature may explain the lack of a training effect, as carotid distensibility and IMT are similar to previously reported values in a healthy population [36,54].

Training effect on CAC mobilisation and function

The present study is the first to evaluate the effects of sprint training on CAC mobilisation and function and demonstrated an increase in circulating $CD34^+$ cells following SIT and SCT but no change in its subpopulation $CD34^+/CD45^{dim}$, suggesting that a different subpopulation of $CD34^+$ cells were mobilised. The enhanced $CD34^+$ cells did not correlate with FMD at pre-training or training induced changes in FMD, indicating that these cells may not have been directly involved in the increase in brachial artery endothelial function. It is possible that the elevated numbers of $CD34^+$ cells were recruited to other parts of the body such as the arteries supplying blood to the exercising muscles. Furthermore, cultured CACs adhesive and migratory ability did not alter following both training programmes. Conversely, increases in CAC function following exercise training have been documented in populations with or at risk of CVD [12,13,55]. However, healthy individuals do not exhibit impaired CAC function [10], which likely explains why an increase in CAC function was not observed in the present study. Furthermore, increases in CAC migratory ability occurred in those with lower pre-training levels in the present study, supporting the suggestion that exercise training increases CAC function, only when an impairment in CAC function is present at pre-training.

$CD34^+$ haematopoietic cells have been reported to migrate towards arterial injury [32], adhere to implanted grafts [56] and restore circulation to the ischemic limb of mice [57], providing evidence for their role in endothelial repair and angiogenesis. The present study is the first to show elevated numbers of CACs following exercise training in a healthy population and suggests an increased reparative potential if required. In contrast, no change in CACs was observed following 8 weeks of continuous endurance training in healthy older men [58] and in our lab following 6 weeks of moderate intensity interval training in healthy young adults [42]. Although in the latter study, some participants exhibited a sustained mobilisation of CACs following heavy intensity interval training, which may have been a result of the higher exercise intensity. This evidence combined with the sustained mobilisation of CACs following both SIT and SCT in the present study, suggests that the high intensity nature and not the duration or the interval vs. continuous nature of the exercise, was the main contributor to increased CACs. This supports the theory that a greater metabolic stress during exercise leads to a sustained upregulation of CACs in healthy individuals, as both training programmes in the present study involved maximal exertion sprints that have been shown to achieve $\dot{V}O_{2max}$ (unpublished data from our laboratory). With increases in exercise intensity, greater levels of oxidative stress are produced [59], which activates the endothelium, leading to secretion of vascular endothelial growth factor and stromal cell-derived factor-1 alpha from endothelial cells that aid in the mobilisation and homing of CACs [60]. Conversely, acute bouts of moderate intensity exercise below the LT in healthy individuals have been shown to elevate CACs [14,61] via a nitric oxide mediated pathway, with levels returning to baseline after 24 hrs. Taken together, these data suggest that for chronic increases in CACs following exercise training in healthy individuals, a higher level of oxidative and metabolic stress is required during exercise sessions.

Study limitations

Comparisons between studies examining exercise induced CAC mobilisation are difficult due to the different antigens used to define cells and the various methods and gating strategies used for cell enumeration. This may explain why previous studies have shown no change in CAC number following exercise training in healthy individuals, whereas the present study reported an elevation. We chose to examine $CD34^+$ cells since out of all its subpopulations, $CD34^+$ cells were the best predictor of CVD [11]. We observed no alteration in CAC function following training, however, the paracrine function of these cells was not assessed. Addition of this measurement may have given insight into the impact the increase in $CD34^+$ cells had on the vasculature.

The population studied were young, healthy and free from cardiovascular disease. Therefore, further studies are required to adapt this type of training to make it appropriate for individuals with or at risk of CVD. Additionally, sprint training requires motivation and specialised equipment that is not accessible to the public. Thus, future work should focus on how this type of training can be made applicable for the general public. A recent study has started progress by adapting SIT for patients with coronary artery disease, and found increases in brachial artery FMD [62]. Training sessions were 2/week for 12 weeks and involved cycling at 90% of maximal HR for 60 s with a 60 s recovery period, repeated 10 times. However, other measures of vascular health such as arterial stiffness and CAC number and function following this type of training in CVD at risk populations have not been studied. Finally, the duration of the training programme was relatively short (4 weeks); therefore, it is unknown whether greater increases in the parameters measured may occur with further training.

Conclusions

Sprint continuous training elicits similar increases in cardiorespiratory fitness and stem cell mobilisation as work-matched sprint interval training in a young healthy population, even though on average SCT session duration was only 3.5 min. However, brachial artery endothelial-dependent FMD may benefit more so following SIT due to the type or profile of shear stress experienced during the exercise. Increases in these variables in CVD populations may be of great benefit as these individuals exhibit impaired vascular function. Therefore, future studies are warranted to adapt this type of training and determine whether those with or at risk of CVD can gain the same benefits as a healthy population.

Author Contributions

Conceived and designed the experiments: EH MR KB. Performed the experiments: EH MR. Analyzed the data: EH. Wrote the paper: EH MR KB.

References

1. British Heart Foundation Coronary heart disease statistics (2010) London: British Heart Foundation Health Promotion Research Group.
2. Ross R (1999) Atherosclerosis — An Inflammatory Disease. New England Journal of Medicine 340: 115–126.
3. Naseem KM (2005) The role of nitric oxide in cardiovascular diseases. Molecular Aspects of Medicine 26: 33–65.

4. Doshi SN, Naka KK, Payne N, Jones CJ, Ashton M, et al. (2001) Flow-mediated dilatation following wrist and upper arm occlusion in humans: the contribution of nitric oxide. Clin Sci 101: 629–635.
5. Takase B, Uehata A, Akima T, Nagai T, Nishioka T, et al. (1998) Endothelium-dependent flow-mediated vasodilation in coronary and brachial arteries in suspected coronary artery disease. The American Journal of Cardiology 82: 1535–1539.
6. Neunteufl T, Katzenschlager R, Hassan A, Klaar U, Schwarzacher S, et al. (1997) Systemic endothelial dysfunction is related to the extent and severity of coronary artery disease. Atherosclerosis 129: 111–118.
7. Green DJ, Jones H, Thijssen D, Cable NT, Atkinson G (2011) Flow-Mediated Dilation and Cardiovascular Event Prediction. Hypertension 57: 363–369.
8. Rehman J, Li J, Orschell CM, March KL (2003) Peripheral Blood "Endothelial Progenitor Cells" Are Derived From Monocyte/Macrophages and Secrete Angiogenic Growth Factors. Circulation 107: 1164–1169.
9. Crosby JR, Kaminski WE, Schatteman G, Martin PJ, Raines EW, et al. (2000) Endothelial Cells of Hematopoietic Origin Make a Significant Contribution to Adult Blood Vessel Formation. Circulation Research 87: 728–730.
10. Vasa M, Fichtlscherer S, Aicher A, Adler K, Urbich C, et al. (2001) Number and Migratory Activity of Circulating Endothelial Progenitor Cells Inversely Correlate With Risk Factors for Coronary Artery Disease. Circ Res 89: e1–7.
11. Fadini GP, de Kreutzenberg SV, Coracina A, Baesso I, Agostini C, et al. (2006) Circulating CD34+ cells, metabolic syndrome, and cardiovascular risk. European Heart Journal 27: 2247–2255.
12. Sandri M, Adams V, Gielen S, Linke A, Lenk K, et al. (2005) Effects of Exercise and Ischemia on Mobilization and Functional Activation of Blood-Derived Progenitor Cells in Patients With Ischemic Syndromes. Circulation 111: 3391–3399.
13. Steiner S, Niessner A, Ziegler S, Richter B, Seidinger D, et al. (2005) Endurance training increases the number of endothelial progenitor cells in patients with cardiovascular risk and coronary artery disease. Atherosclerosis 181: 305–310.
14. Cubbon RM, Murgatroyd SR, Ferguson C, Bowen TS, Rakobowchuk M, et al. (2010) Human Exercise-Induced Circulating Progenitor Cell Mobilization Is Nitric Oxide-Dependent and Is Blunted in South Asian Men. Arterioscler Thromb Vasc Biol 30: 878–884.
15. Hambrecht R, Adams V, Erbs S, Linke A, Krankel N, et al. (2003) Regular Physical Activity Improves Endothelial Function in Patients With Coronary Artery Disease by Increasing Phosphorylation of Endothelial Nitric Oxide Synthase. Circulation 107: 3152–3158.
16. Laughlin MH, Woodman CR, Schrage WG, Gute D, Price EM (2004) Interval sprint training enhances endothelial function and eNOS content in some arteries that perfuse white gastrocnemius muscle. Journal of Applied Physiology 96: 233–244.
17. British Heart Foundation Physical Activity Statistics (2012) London: British Heart Foundation Health Promotion Research Group.
18. Cocks M, Shaw CS, Shepherd SO, Fisher JP, Ranasinghe AM, et al. (2013) Sprint interval and endurance training are equally effective in increasing muscle microvascular density and eNOS content in sedentary males. The Journal of Physiology 591: 641–656.
19. Whyte LJ, Ferguson C, Wilson J, Scott RA, Gill JMR (2013) Effects of single bout of very high-intensity exercise on metabolic health biomarkers in overweight/obese sedentary men. Metabolism-Clinical and Experimental 62: 212–219.
20. Gibala MJ, Little JP, van Essen M, Wilkin GP, Burgomaster KA, et al. (2006) Short-term sprint interval versus traditional endurance training: similar initial adaptations in human skeletal muscle and exercise performance. The Journal of Physiology 575: 901–911.
21. Corretti MC, Anderson TJ, Benjamin EJ, Celermajer D, Charbonneau F, et al. (2002) Guidelines for the ultrasound assessment of endothelial-dependent flow-mediated vasodilation of the brachial artery: a report of the International Brachial Artery Reactivity Task Force. J Am Coll Cardiol 39: 257–265.
22. Thijssen DHJ, Black MA, Pyke KE, Padilla J, Atkinson G, et al. (2011) Assessment of flow-mediated dilation in humans: a methodological and physiological guideline. American Journal of Physiology - Heart and Circulatory Physiology 300: H2–H12.
23. Rakobowchuk M, Harris E, Taylor A, Cubbon R, Birch K (2012) Moderate and heavy metabolic stress interval training improve arterial stiffness and heart rate dynamics in humans. European Journal of Applied Physiology: 1–11.
24. Nichols WW, O'Rourke MF (2005) McDonald's Blood Flow in Arteries: Theoretical, Experimental and Clinical Principles. London: Oxford University Press.
25. O'Rourke MF, Pauca A, Jiang XJ (2001) Pulse wave analysis. British Journal of Clinical Pharmacology 51: 507–522.
26. Yamashina A, Tomiyama H, Takeda K, Tsuda H, Arai T, et al. (2002) Validity, Reproducibility, and Clinical Significance of Noninvasive Brachial-Ankle Pulse Wave Velocity Measurement. Hypertension Research 25: 359–364.
27. McEleavy OD, McCallum RW, Petrie JR, Small M, Connell JMC, et al. (2004) Higher carotid-radial pulse wave velocity in healthy offspring of patients with Type 2 diabetes. Diabetic Medicine 21: 262–266.
28. Mitchell GF, Hwang S-J, Vasan RS, Larson MG, Pencina MJ, et al. (2010) Arterial Stiffness and Cardiovascular Events. Circulation 121: 505–511.
29. Chiu YC, Arand PW, Shroff SG, Feldman T, Carroll JD (1991) Determination of pulse wave velocities with computerized algorithms. American Heart Journal 121: 1460–1470.
30. Schmidt-Lucke C, Fichtlscherer S, Aicher A, Tschöpe C, Schultheiss H-P, et al. (2010) Quantification of Circulating Endothelial Progenitor Cells Using the Modified ISHAGE Protocol. PLoS ONE 5: e13790.
31. George J, Herz I, Goldstein E, Abashidze S, Deutch V, et al. (2003) Number and Adhesive Properties of Circulating Endothelial Progenitor Cells in Patients With In-Stent Restenosis. Arteriosclerosis, Thrombosis, and Vascular Biology 23: e57–e60.
32. Walter DH, Rittig K, Bahlmann FH, Kirchmair R, Silver M, et al. (2002) Statin Therapy Accelerates Reendothelialization: A Novel Effect Involving Mobilization and Incorporation of Bone Marrow-Derived Endothelial Progenitor Cells. Circulation 105: 3017–3024.
33. Rossiter HB, Kowalchuk JM, Whipp BJ (2006) A test to establish maximum O2 uptake despite no plateau in the O2 uptake response to ramp incremental exercise. Journal of Applied Physiology 100: 764–770.
34. Beaver WL, Wasserman K, Whipp BJ (1986) A new method for detecting anaerobic threshold by gas exchange. Journal of Applied Physiology 60: 2020–2027.
35. Whipp BJ, Ward SA, Wasserman K (1986) Respiratory markers of the anaerobic threshold. Adv Cardiol 35: 47–64.
36. Rakobowchuk M, Tanguay S, Burgomaster KA, Howarth KR, Gibala MJ, et al. (2008) Sprint interval and traditional endurance training induce similar improvements in peripheral arterial stiffness and flow-mediated dilation in healthy humans. Am J Physiol Regul Integr Comp Physiol 295: R236–242.
37. Morici G, Zangla D, Santoro A, Pelosi E, Petrucci E, et al. (2005) Supramaximal exercise mobilizes hematopoietic progenitors and reticulocytes in athletes. American Journal of Physiology - Regulatory, Integrative and Comparative Physiology 289: R1496–R1503.
38. Burgomaster KA, Howarth KR, Phillips SM, Rakobowchuk M, MacDonald MJ, et al. (2008) Similar metabolic adaptations during exercise after low volume sprint interval and traditional endurance training in humans. The Journal of Physiology 586: 151–160.
39. Laukkanen JA, Kurl S, Salonen R, Rauramaa R, Salonen JT (2004) The predictive value of cardiorespiratory fitness for cardiovascular events in men with various risk profiles: a prospective population-based cohort study. European Heart Journal 25: 1428–1437.
40. Myers J, Gullestad L, Vagelos R, Do D, Bellin D, et al. (1998) Clinical, Hemodynamic, and Cardiopulmonary Exercise Test Determinants of Survival in Patients Referred for Evaluation of Heart Failure. Annals of Internal Medicine 129: 286–293.
41. Birk GK, Dawson EA, Atkinson C, Haynes A, Cable NT, et al. (2012) Brachial artery adaptation to lower limb exercise training: Role of shear stress. J Appl Physiol 8: 8.
42. Rakobowchuk M, Harris E, Taylor A, Baliga V, Cubbon RM, et al. (2012) Heavy and moderate interval exercise training alters low-flow-mediated constriction but does not increase circulating progenitor cells in healthy humans. Experimental Physiology 97: 375–385.
43. Tinken TM, Thijssen DHJ, Hopkins N, Dawson EA, Cable NT, et al. (2010) Shear Stress Mediates Endothelial Adaptations to Exercise Training in Humans. Hypertension 55: 312–318.
44. Boo YC, Sorescu G, Boyd N, Shiojima I, Walsh K, et al. (2002) Shear Stress Stimulates Phosphorylation of Endothelial Nitric-oxide Synthase at Ser1179 by Akt-independent Mechanisms. Journal of Biological Chemistry 277: 3388–3396.
45. Green DJ, Bilsborough W, Naylor LH, Reed C, Wright J, et al. (2005) Comparison of forearm blood flow responses to incremental handgrip and cycle ergometer exercise: relative contribution of nitric oxide. The Journal of Physiology 562: 617–628.
46. Simmons GH, Padilla J, Young CN, Wong BJ, Lang JA, et al. (2011) Increased brachial artery retrograde shear rate at exercise onset is abolished during prolonged cycling: role of thermoregulatory vasodilation. Journal of Applied Physiology 110: 389–397.
47. Laughlin MH, Newcomer SC, Bender SB (2008) Importance of hemodynamic forces as signals for exercise-induced changes in endothelial cell phenotype. Journal of Applied Physiology 104: 588–600.
48. Jenkins NT, Padilla J, Boyle LJ, Credeur DP, Laughlin MH, et al. (2013) Disturbed Blood Flow Acutely Induces Activation and Apoptosis of the Human Vascular Endothelium. Hypertension 61: 615–621.
49. Thijssen DHJ, Dawson EA, Tinken TM, Cable NT, Green DJ (2009) Retrograde Flow and Shear Rate Acutely Impair Endothelial Function in Humans. Hypertension 53: 986–992.
50. Wisloff U, Stoylen A, Loennechen JP, Bruvold M, Rognmo O, et al. (2007) Superior Cardiovascular Effect of Aerobic Interval Training Versus Moderate Continuous Training in Heart Failure Patients: A Randomized Study. Circulation 115: 3086–3094.
51. Kuchan MJ, Frangos JA (1994) Role of calcium and calmodulin in flow-induced nitric oxide production in endothelial cells. American Journal of Physiology - Cell Physiology 266: C628–C636.
52. Dusserre N, L'Heureux N, Bell KS, Stevens HY, Yeh J, et al. (2004) PECAM-1 interacts with nitric oxide synthase in human endothelial cells: implication for flow-induced nitric oxide synthase activation. Arteriosclerosis, Thrombosis & Vascular Biology 24: 1796–1802.
53. Simons PCG, Algra A, Bots ML, Grobbee DE, van der Graaf Y, et al. (1999) Common Carotid Intima-Media Thickness and Arterial Stiffness. Circulation 100: 951–957.

54. Tanaka H, Seals DR, Monahan KD, Clevenger CM, DeSouza CA, et al. (2002) Regular aerobic exercise and the age-related increase in carotid artery intima-media thickness in healthy men. Journal of Applied Physiology 92: 1458–1464.
55. Sarto P, Balducci E, Balconi G, Fiordaliso F, Merlo L, et al. (2007) Effects of Exercise Training on Endothelial Progenitor Cells in Patients With Chronic Heart Failure. Journal of cardiac failure 13: 701–708.
56. Shi Q, Rafii S, Wu MH-D, Wijelath ES, Yu C, et al. (1998) Evidence for Circulating Bone Marrow-Derived Endothelial Cells. Blood 92: 362–367.
57. Hur J, Yoon C-H, Kim H-S, Choi J-H, Kang H-J, et al. (2004) Characterization of Two Types of Endothelial Progenitor Cells and Their Different Contributions to Neovasculogenesis. Arterioscler Thromb Vasc Biol 24: 288–293.
58. Thijssen DHJ, Vos JB, Verseyden C, Van Zonneveld AJ, Smits P, et al. (2006) Haematopoietic stem cells and endothelial progenitor cells in healthy men: effect of aging and training. Aging Cell 5: 495–503.
59. Goto C, Higashi Y, Kimura M, Noma K, Hara K, et al. (2003) Effect of Different Intensities of Exercise on Endothelium-Dependent Vasodilation in Humans: Role of Endothelium-Dependent Nitric Oxide and Oxidative Stress. Circulation 108: 530–535.
60. Zampetaki A, Kirton JP, Xu Q (2008) Vascular repair by endothelial progenitor cells. Cardiovascular Research 78: 413–421.
61. Laufs U, Urhausen A, Werner N, Scharhag J, Heitz A, et al. (2005) Running exercise of different duration and intensity: effect on endothelial progenitor cells in healthy subjects. Journal of Cardiovascular Risk 12: 407–414.
62. Currie KD, Dubberley JB, Mckelvie RS, Macdonald MJ (2013) Low-Volume, High-Intensity Interval Training in Patients with CAD. Medicine & Science in Sports & Exercise 45: 1436–1442 1410.1249/MSS.1430b1013e31828bbbd31824.

Effects of Home-Based Interval Walking Training on Thigh Muscle Strength and Aerobic Capacity in Female Total Hip Arthroplasty Patients: A Randomized, Controlled Pilot Study

Yutaka Morishima[1,2], Takashi Mizushima[2], Katsuya Yamauchi[2], Mayuko Morikawa[1,3], Shizue Masuki[1], Hiroshi Nose[1,3]*

1 Department of Sports Medical Sciences, Shinshu University Graduate School of Medicine, Matsumoto, Japan, **2** Department of Rehabilitation, Hamamatsu University School of Medicine, Hamamatsu, Japan, **3** Jukunen Taiikudaigaku Research Center, Matsumoto, Japan

Abstract

Due to the reduced physical activity of patients who have undergone total hip arthroplasty (THA), there are no home-based exercise training regimens for preventing muscle atrophy and aerobic capacity impairment in these patients. We examined whether interval walking training (IWT) could prevented these issues. Twenty-eight female patients (~60 years of age) who had undergone THA more than 2 months prior were randomly divided into IWT (n = 14) and control (CNT, n = 14) groups. The IWT subjects trained at a target of 60 min of fast walking at >70% peak aerobic capacity for walking (VO_{2peak}) per wk for 12 wk, while those in the CNT maintained their previous sedentary life during the same period. We measured the energy expenditure of the daily physical activity, except during sleeping and bathing, every minute and every day during the intervention. We also measured the isometric knee extension (F_{EXT}) and flexion (F_{FLX}) forces, VO_{2peak}, and anaerobic threshold during the graded cycling exercise (VO_{2AT}) before and after the intervention. All subjects, except for one in IWT, completed the protocol. F_{FLX} increased by 23% on the operated side ($P = 0.003$) and 14% on the non-operated side of IWT ($P = 0.006$), while it only increased on the operated side of CNT ($P = 0.03$). The VO_{2peak} and VO_{2AT} in IWT increased by 8% ($P = 0.08$) and 13% ($P = 0.002$), respectively, and these changes were significantly higher in the IWT than in CNT group (both, $P < 0.05$). In conclusion, IWT might be an effective home-based training regimen for preventing the muscle atrophy from reduced daily physical activity in THA patients.

Trial Registration: UMIN-CTR UMIN000013172

Editor: Naoyuki Hayashi, Tokyo Institute of Technology, Japan

Funding: This study was supported in part by grants from the Ministry of Health, Labor, and Welfare (Comprehensive Research on Aging and Health) and the Japan Society for the Promotion of Science. The funders had no role in study design, data collection and analysis, decision to publish, or preparation of the manuscript.

Competing Interests: The authors have declared that no competing interests exist.

* Email: nosehir@shinshu-u.ac.jp

Introduction

Total hip arthroplasty (THA) is a broadly prescribed surgical treatment for patients with advanced arthritic disorders of the joint. [1] However, THA patients are thought to suffer from muscular atrophy and weakness on the operated limb side more than 2 years after surgery; [2,3] these changes might be accompanied by joint instability, prosthesis loosening, risk of falls, and other complications, [4–7] and they might advance to impaired mobility of the joint, [1,8–11] resulting in reduced daily physical activity and aerobic capacity in a vicious cycle.

To prevent these problems, exercise training for rehabilitation is performed immediately after surgery under the supervision of medical staff while the patient stays in the hospital with financial support from national insurance; however, a maximum period of 2 wk is recommended for hospital management reasons, and this period is too short for recovering muscle strength. Patients are allowed to visit a hospital for rehabilitation up to several months following discharge, and resistance training using machines has also been reported to be effective; [12] however, limited financial support from insurance, impaired mobility, and the inconvenience of the transportation options for travelling to the hospital might discourage patients from continuing exercise training [13–16].

Therefore, the development of a home-based exercise regimen is needed so that THA patients can perform habitual exercise to increase their muscle strength on the side of the treated limb. Recently, we developed an exercise training system for middle-aged and older people featuring 1) interval walking training (IWT), 2) the use of a portable calorimeter, and 3) the e-Health Promotion System. Using the system, we found that middle-aged and older people who performed IWT for 5 months had ~10% increased thigh muscle strength and peak aerobic capacity for walking ($\dot{V}O_{2peak}$) [17,18] with a much higher adherence rate to IWT (94%) than for a standard walking training regimen (~60%); however, there have been no studies on THA patients [19].

Therefore, the purpose of this pilot study was to examine whether the training system is helpful for increasing thigh muscle strength and aerobic capacity as well as improving daily physical activity in THA patients.

Methods

The protocol for this trial and supporting CONSORT checklist are available as supporting information; see Checklist S1 and Protocol S1.

Ethics Statement

This study was approved by the Ethics Committee of Hamamatsu University School of Medicine and was in accordance with the Declaration of Helsinki. All participants provided written informed consent for participation.

Trial registration

The clinical trial was registered after participant recruitment for this study. However, we recruited the first participant for this study after approval by the ethics committee of Hamamatsu University School of Medicine. Additionally, all ongoing and related trials for the exercise training of THA patients are registered.

Participants

The criteria for subjects with total hip arthroplasty were that they were able to walk independently without any assistive devices. The exclusion criteria were suffering from any acetabular and/or femoral prosthesis failure or other comorbidities or the presence of any cardiopulmonary, neurologic, or cognitive diseases.

Figure 1 shows the flow profile of subjects in the present study. Recruitment and screening began on August 1. To recruit subjects for this study, we mailed leaflets to female patients who had undergone THA at Hamamatsu University Hospital and who visited the hospital for rehabilitation before June 2009. As a result, 28 of 98 respondents met the criteria, and all provided written informed consent before participating in the study. They were randomly divided [20] into interval walking training (IWT, n = 14) and control (CNT, n = 14) groups such that there were no significant differences in the medical history, current physical characteristics (**Table 1**), and other measurements before training.

Randomization

Allocation was performed using permuted-block randomization (block of 4). YM generated the random allocation sequence. Each eligible and consenting subject was assigned to one of the groups. Only known one researcher (YM) knew of the exact allocation.

Intervention Protocols

The training experiments were conducted from September 6, 2009 to December 20, 2009. The subjects were instructed to visit the gym at 8:30 am on the assigned day in September after overnight fasting. After interviewing the subjects about their current hip joint pain, their subjective feeling of satisfaction with walking using the visual analogue scale (VAS) and their quality of life with the Medical Outcomes Study 36-item short-form health survey (SF-36), [21,22] we measured their height and body weight. After allowing them to eat a light breakfast and rest for an hour, we measured the thigh muscle strength and $\dot{V}O_{2peak}$. Within a week, the subjects were invited to our laboratory in the hospital an hour or more after breakfast or lunch and were asked to participate in a measurement of the anaerobic threshold by graded cycling exercise ($\dot{V}O_{AT}$). [23] When they left the laboratory after the measurement, we provided them with a portable calorimeter with a tri-axial accelerometer (JD-Mate; Kissei Comtec, Matsumoto, Japan) and instructed them to measure their energy expenditure due to physical activity every minute during the day, except during sleeping and bathing periods, for 7 consecutive days before the start of training.

Before IWT, the subjects visited a gym near the hospital and received instructions about the exercise program. They were told to repeat 5 or more sets of 2- to 3-minute low-intensity walking intervals at ~40% of the pre-training $\dot{V}O_{2peak}$, followed by a 3-minute interval of high-intensity walking at >70% but <85% $\dot{V}O_{2peak}$, ≥4 days/wk; the total fast walking time per week reached ≥60 min. The intensity and steps were monitored with JD-Mate, which was worn on the mid-clavicular line of the right or left waist. A beeping signal alerted subjects when a change of intensity was scheduled, and another sound told them when their walking intensity had reached the target level. Once subjects had learned the program, they were allowed to choose their training time. Additionally, in IWT, the energy expenditure (oxygen consumption rate) due to physical activity other than IWT and steps was measured with JD-Mate during the day, except for during bathing and sleeping periods, while the beeping signal and sounds of the device were switched off. The total energy expenditure due to physical activity is presented in **Table 2**, including that for IWT.

Every 2 weeks, the subjects visited the hospital, and data from the tracking devices were transferred over the internet to a central server in the administrative center for automatic analysis and reporting of the IWT effects from a database of more than 3,000 middle-aged and older people without THA; we call this system the e-Health Promotion System (Kissei Comtec). [24] Physical therapists used these reports to track the daily walking intensity and the other parameters given in **Table 2** to instruct subjects on how best to achieve the target levels. If the targets were not met, they encouraged subjects to increase their efforts to achieve them.

Subjects in CNT were instructed to maintain the same lifestyle as before training. Every 2 weeks during the training period for IWT, they visited the hospital, and the energy expenditure due to daily physical activity and steps during the day, except during sleeping and bathing periods, was transferred over the internet from the tracking devices to the central server in the administrative center, but, unlike in IWT, there was no automatic analysis and reporting.

After the 12-wk training period, we measured the same variables as before training for both groups. After the post-training measurements, we instructed the subjects in both groups to continue measuring their energy expenditure from daily physical activity and steps during the day, except during the sleeping and bathing periods, for 7 consecutive days after the end of training. The data were then transferred to the server after measurements.

Number of subjects for the analyses

In IWT, one subject was excluded from the following analyses because she was absent on one of the measurement days assigned after training. Therefore, we analyzed 13/14 and 14/14 subjects in IWT and CNT, respectively.

Measurements

Thigh muscle strength. Isometric bilateral knee extension (F_{EXT}) and flexion (F_{FLX}) forces were measured with an isometric dynamometer (GT-330; OG Giken, Tokyo, Japan). The higher value from 2 trials each for extension and flexion forces, which were displayed on the screen of the dynamometer, was adopted for

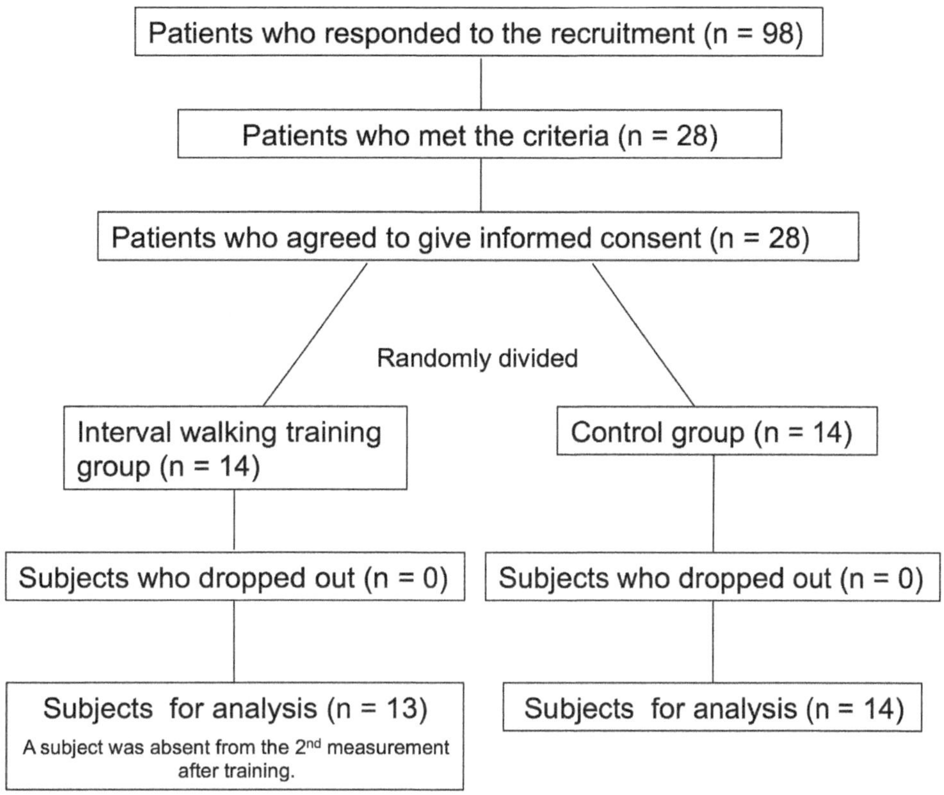

Figure 1. CONSORT flow diagram. Flow profile of the subjects.

analysis. Similarly, we measured the strength of the other knee joint.

Because 3/13 subjects in IWT underwent THA on both hip joints and the remaining 10 subjects underwent THA on one side, we analyzed the effect of IWT on the thigh muscle strength on 16 operated sides and 10 non-operated sides in this group. Similarly, in CNT, 3/14 subjects underwent THA on both hip joints, and the remaining 11 subjects underwent THA on one side. Therefore, we analyzed the thigh muscle strength before and after training for 17 operated sides and 11 non-operated sides in this group.

$\dot{V}O_{2peak}$. Subjects with the accelerometer on their back walked for 3 minutes on a flat floor at 3 graded, subjective velocities (slow, moderate, and fast) with ~25°C room temperature and ~60% relative humidity. At the same time, the heart rate was recorded with an electrocardiogram, and 3-dimensional acceleration was measured at 10-millisecond intervals and recorded as averaged values of the 5-second memories. [25,26] The total impulse from the accelerometer was transferred to a computer and converted to the oxygen consumption rate ($\dot{V}O_2$) using a previously reported equation. [25,26] The $\dot{V}O_{2peak}$ and peak heart rate (HR_{peak}) for walking values are those for the last 30 seconds at the maximal walking speed.

$\dot{V}O_{2AT}$. We determined the $\dot{V}O_{2AT}$ at ~25°C room temperature and ~60% relative humidity with an expired gas analysis system (AE-310S; Minato, Tokyo, Japan). The $\dot{V}O_2$ and carbon dioxide production ($\dot{V}CO_2$) were measured for every breath. The exercise intensity was increased by 10 watts per minute and stopped when the anaerobic threshold was judged to have been

Table 1. Physical characteristics of the subjects.

	CNT (n = 14)	IWT (n = 13)	P (Group)
Age (years)	59.9±5.4 (52–68)	60.3±7.4 (52–74)	NS
Height (cm)	151.9±5.8 (144–166)	153.3±3.4 (146.8–159.4)	NS
Body mass (kg)	57.0±9.6 (48.0–69.8)	54.0±5.3 (43.3–80.6)	NS
BMI (kg/m^2)	24.7±4.1 (20.1–35.4)	23.0±2.6 (19.4–28.5)	NS
Reason for operation	OA: 13; ANFH: 1	OA: 13	NA
Operated side (left/right/bilateral)	7/4/3	5/5/3	NA
Postoperative period (months)	34±46 (2–170)	58±58 (9–181)	NS

Values are given as the means ± SD (range). CNT, control group; IWT, interval walking group; OA, osteoarthritis; ANFH, avascular necrosis of femoral neck head; BMI, body mass index; and NA, not applicable.

Table 2. Total energy expenditure for IWT and physical activity.

	CNT (n = 14)			IWT (n = 13)					
	Before	**During**	**After**	**Before**	**During**	**After**	*P*	*P*	*P*
	(1 wk)	**(12 wk)**	**(1 wk)**	**(1 wk)**	**(12 wk)**	**(1 wk)**	**(Group)**	**(Time)**	**(Group × Time)**
§Total energy expenditure	14614±1496	13616±1361	10258±1827	14032±1133	14744±1012	13824±1495	NS	NS	NS
(O_2 ml/kg/wk)									
Total steps	50537±5411	51636±5411	40159±6749	50693±5845	53016±5845	44619±6105	NS	NS	NS
(steps/wk)									
Fast walking									
§Intensity	10.6±0.6	12.0±1.4	9.7±1.3	9.7±0.6	8.9±0.9	10.2±0.8	NS	NS	NS
(O_2 ml/kg/min)									
Time	76±16	69±15	75±17	100±27	156±15*†	127±18†	<0.0001	<0.0001	<0.0001
(min/wk)									
§Energy expenditure	786±196	805±153	710±176	828±211	1363±157†	1221±169†	.013	NS	NS
(O_2 ml/kg/wk)									

Values are given as the means ± SE. Before, for 1 wk before training; During, for 12 wk during training; and After, for 1 wk after training.
§Resting oxygen consumption is not included.
*Significant difference from the value before training, $P<0.05$;
†Significant difference from the corresponding value in CNT, $P<0.05$. The other abbreviations are the same as in **Table 1**.

reached according to the standard method [23,27,28] by viewing the $\dot{V}O_2$ vs. VCO_2 relationship displayed on the screen of the system during exercise. We also determined the heart rate at $\dot{V}O_{2AT}$ (HR_{AT}).

Total energy expenditure due to IWT and physical activity in daily life. As shown in Table 2, the total energy expenditure due to physical activity was determined by adding the $\dot{V}O_2$ (O_2 ml/kg/min) before (1 wk), during (12 wk), and after (1 wk) the training periods after excluding the energy expenditure at rest, which was assumed to be constant during these periods, and this energy is presented as the O_2 ml/kg/wk. Similarly, the walking steps were determined by summing the steps for the respective periods and are presented as steps/wk. A $\dot{V}O_2$ above 70% $W\dot{V}O_{2peak}$ for individuals was regarded as the intensity for fast walking (O_2 ml/kg/min), and the total energy used for fast walking was determined by summing the $\dot{V}O_2$ for the respective periods, after excluding the rate during rest, and this energy is presented as O_2 ml/kg/wk.

Questionnaires. Hip joint pain was evaluated with the 100-mm VAS scale, where 0 represents "no pain" and 100 represents the "worst pain". Similarly, walking satisfaction was evaluated using 0 as "no satisfaction" and 100 as "full satisfaction". The SF-36 was used to evaluate the quality of daily life [21,22].

Statistical Analysis

The Mann-Whitney *U* test was used to test for differences in the physical characteristics between the IWT and CNT groups (**Table 1**). Two-way analysis of variance (ANOVA) [group (CNT vs IWT)×time (before vs. after training)] for repeated measures was also used to examine any significant differences in the variables before and after training between groups (**Tables 2–4** and the questionnaires). The model was also used to examine any significant changes in the variables after training with an interactive effect of (group×time) on the variables (**Tables 2–4** and the questionnaires). After confirmation of the significance by ANOVA, the Tukey-Kramer method was used as a post-hoc test to examine any significant differences in variables in specific comparisons between groups before and after training (**Tables 2–4** and the questionnaires). We determined significant differences in the changes of the variables after training between groups by ANCOVA after correcting for their pre-training values as covariates (**Figure 2 & 3**). We present the statistical power (1-β) in the text at α= 0.05 in both groups when the variables increased significantly after training or when the increases were significantly greater in IWT than in CNT with the minimum sample sizes to detect the greater increases (**Figures 2 & 3**). All data are reported as the mean±standard error (SE), unless otherwise indicated. The null hypothesis was rejected at $P<0.05$.

Results

The adherence to the program was 100% in IWT (including one subject who was excluded from the analysis). Additionally, there were no adverse events, including musculoskeletal injuries and falling, during the training period.

Table 1 shows the physical characteristics of subjects in the IWT and CNT with no significant differences between groups.

Table 2 shows the total energy expenditure due to physical activity in both groups. We found that the fast walking time was two-fold higher in IWT than in CNT during and after training periods (both, $P = 0.001$). Additionally, the energy expenditure for fast walking was higher in IWT than in CNT during the training periods ($P = 0.018$ and $P = 0.047$, respectively).

The body mass after training was 57.6±2.6 kg in CNT and 54.1±1.5 kg in IWT and it did not significantly differ from the mass before training in either of the two groups ($P = 0.20$ and $P = 0.90$, respectively).

Table 3 shows the thigh muscle strength before and after training in both groups. F_{EXT} and F_{FLX} before and after training in both groups tended to be lower on the operated side than on the non-operated side in each group, but there were no significant differences (all, $P>0.05$). We found that F_{FLX} (Nm/kg) increased on the operated and non-operated sides of IWT ($P = 0.0031$, (1-β) = 0.95, and $P = 0.0063$, (1-β) = 0.95, respectively), while it only increased on the operated side of CNT ($P = 0.028$, (1-β) = 0.62) with an interactive effect of group (CNT and IWT)×time (before and after training) for F_{FLX} on the operated side ($P = 0.023$). This result suggests that the increase in F_{FLX} on the operated side was significantly higher in IWT than in CNT.

Table 4 shows the aerobic capacity before and after training in both groups. $\dot{V}O_{2peak}$ tended to increase in IWT ($P = 0.080$), while it remained unchanged in CNT ($P = 0.13$), with an interactive effect of (group×time) on the change ($P = 0.018$), suggesting that the increase in IWT was significantly higher than that in CNT. Similarly, $\dot{V}O_{2AT}$ increased in IWT ($P = 0.0021$, (1-β) = 0.96), while it remained unchanged in CNT ($P = 0.38$) and there was an interactive effect of (group×time) on the change ($P = 0.0016$), suggesting that the increase was significantly higher in IWT than in CNT. The HR_{peak} remained unchanged after training in both groups, but HR_{AT} increased after the training in IWT ($P = 0.045$, (1-β) = 0.53).

Figure 2 summarizes the changes in the F_{EXT} and F_{FLX} on the operated and non-operated sides after training in both groups and after correcting for the values before training by ANCOVA. Although F_{EXT} on both sides remained unchanged after the training in both groups, F_{FLX} increased by 23% ($P = 0.0031$) and 14% ($P = 0.0063$) on the operated and non-operated sides, respectively, after the training in IWT, while it increased only on the operated side of CNT ($P = 0.028$). The increase on the operated side was significantly higher in IWT than in CNT (ANCOVA, $P = 0.002$, (1-β) = 0.95). The minimum sample size for detecting the difference in the increases in F_{EXT} between group at α= 0.05 and (1-β) = 0.9 was 12 for each group, which is smaller than the size in the present study.

Figure 3 shows the changes in $\dot{V}O_{2peak}$ and $\dot{V}O_{2AT}$ after training in both groups. Although both remained unchanged in CNT (both, $P>0.10$), the increases in the $\dot{V}O_{2peak}$ and $\dot{V}O_{2AT}$ in IWT were 8% ($P = 0.08$) and 13% ($P = 0.0021$), respectively, which were significantly higher in IWT than in CNT (ANCOVA, $P = 0.018$, (1-β) = 0.68 and $P = 0.0016$, (1-β) = 0.94, respectively). The minimum sample size for detecting the differences in the changes in the $\dot{V}O_{2peak}$ and $\dot{V}O_{2AT}$ between groups at α= 0.05 and (1-β) = 0.9 were 23, which is more than in the present study, and 12, which is less than in the present study, for each group, respectively.

The hip pain score was not significantly different between the groups before training ($P>0.55$). After training, the score remained unchanged in both groups on the operated side ($P>0.06$) and on the non-operated side ($P>0.06$).

The walking satisfaction score significantly increased in IWT from 44±9 to 55±8 ($P = 0.047$, (1-β) = 0.53) but not in CNT, whose values changed from 55±10 to 43±10 ($P = 0.24$) with no significant interactive effect of (group×time) ($P = 0.27$).

The "vitality" score in SF-36 significantly increased in IWT from 45±3 to 52±2 ($P = 0.005$, (1-β) = 0.87) but not in CNT, whose values changed from 48±3 to 52±3 ($P = 0.19$). However, there was no significant interactive effect of (group×time)

Table 3. Thigh muscle strength before and after training.

	CNT (n = 14)			IWT (n = 13)			*P*
	Before	**After**	***P* (Time)**	**Before**	**After**	***P* (Time)**	**(Group × time)**
Operated side							
n	17	17		16	16		
F_{EXT} (Nm)	74.6±7.7	74.5±7.5	NS	83.8±5.2	92.5±4.9	NS	NS
(Nm/kg)	1.36±0.15	1.35±0.14	NS	1.56±0.11	1.73±0.12	NS	NS
F_{FLX} (Nm)	36.3±2.3	39.3±2.3*	0.022	37.7±3.3	46.2±2.4**	0.0021	0.036
(Nm/kg)	0.65±0.04	0.70±0.03*	0.028	0.69±0.06	0.85±0.04**	0.0031	0.023
Non-operated side							
n	11	11		10	10		
F_{EXT} (Nm)	96.4±6.5	102.9±11.3	NS	93.3±9.1	88.5±10.1	NS	NS
(Nm/kg)	1.67±0.13	1.72±0.17	NS	1.78±0.19	1.64±0.19	NS	NS
F_{FLX} (Nm)	38.1±4.1	43.4±4.1	NS	40.8±2.1	46.6±2.5**	0.0032	NS
(Nm/kg)	0.64±0.06	0.74±0.07	NS	0.77±0.04	0.87±0.05**	0.0063	NS

Values are given as the means ± SE. F_{EXT}, knee extension force; F_{FLX}, knee flexion force. Significant differences compared to the value before training, *$P<0.05$ and **$P<0.01$.

Table 4. Aerobic capacities before and after training.

	CNT (n = 14)			IWT (n = 13)			*P*
	Before	**After**	***P* (Time)**	**Before**	**After**	***P* (Time)**	**(Group × Time)**
$\dot{V}O_{2peak}$ (ml/kg/min)	16.6±0.8	15.7±0.6	NS	15.8±0.8	17.0±1.1	NS	0.018
HR_{rest}^{1} (beats/min)	81±4	81±3	NS	81±2	79±2	NS	NS
HR_{peak} (beats/min)	141±4	143±4	NS	139±4	138±6	NS	NS
$\dot{V}O_{2AT}$ (ml/kg/min)	13.8±0.6	13.5±0.6	NS	13.7±0.4	15.5±0.5**	0.0021	0.0016
HR_{rest}^{2} (beats/min)	77±2	79±2	NS	77±2	78±2	NS	NS
HR_{AT} (beats/min)	108±2	109±2	NS	110±2	114±2*	0.045	NS

Values are given as the mean ± SE. $\dot{V}O_{2peak}$, peak aerobic capacity for walking; HR_{rest}^{1}, heart rate at rest before starting the exercise for the $\dot{V}O_{2peak}$ measurement; HR_{peak}, peak heart rate at $\dot{V}O_{2peak}$; $\dot{V}O_{2AT}$, anaerobic threshold for cycling; HR_{rest}^{2}, heart rate at rest before starting the exercise for the $\dot{V}O_{2AT}$ measurement; and HR_{AT}, heart rate at $\dot{V}O_{2AT}$. Significant differences compared to the value before training, *$P<0.05$ and **$P<0.01$.

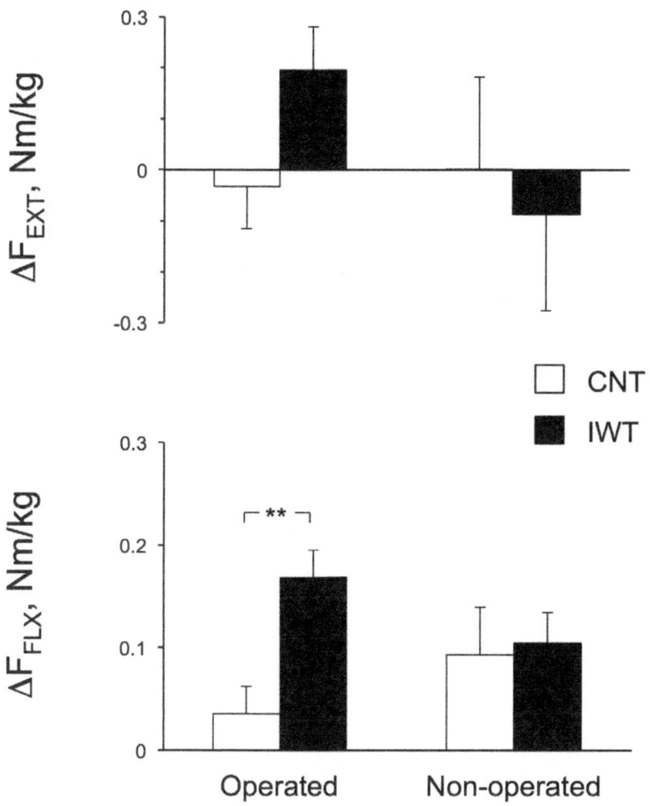

Figure 2. Changes in the thigh muscle strength after training on the operated and non-operated sides. The isometric knee extension (F_{EXT}) and flexion force (F_{FLX}) are shown as the means with SE bars for 17 and 16 measurements on the operated side and 11 and 10 measurements on the non-operated side in 14 and 13 subjects in the control (CNT) and interval walking training (IWT) groups, respectively. Significant difference between the CNT and IWT groups, $^{**}P<0.01$.

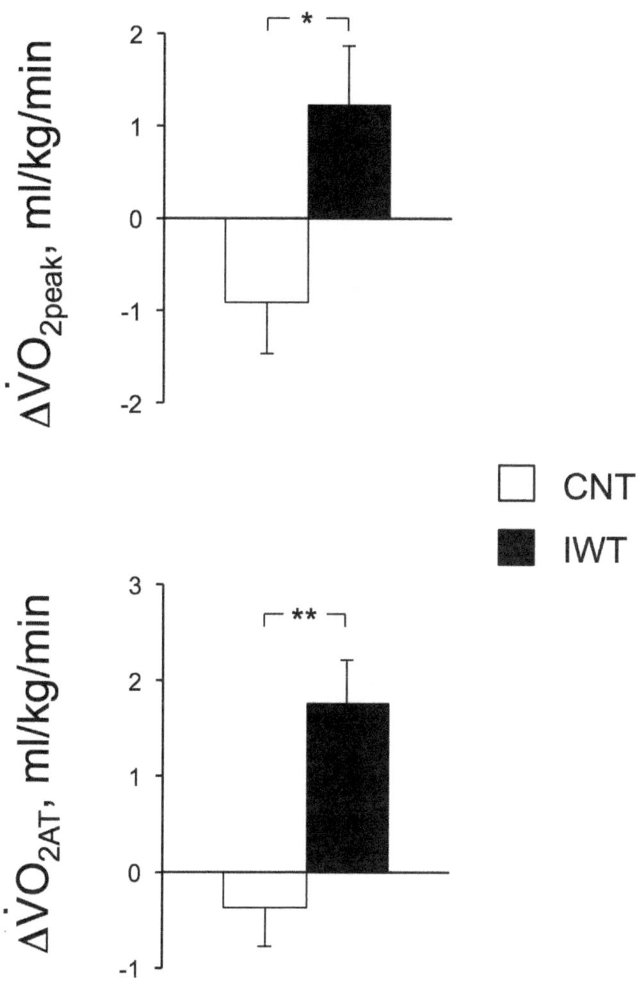

Figure 3. Changes in the aerobic capacities after training. The peak aerobic capacity for walking ($\dot{V}O_{2peak}$) and anaerobic threshold by graded cycling exercise ($\dot{V}O_{2AT}$) are shown as the means with SE bars for 14 and 13 subjects in the CNT and IWT groups, respectively. Significant differences between the CNT and IWT groups, $^{*}P<0.05$ and $^{**}P<0.01$.

($P=0.24$). There were no significant changes in the other items of SF-36 before and after training in either group ($P=0.07$–1.0).

Discussion

In the present study, all THA patients in IWT performed fast walking for more than an average of 60 min per week during the 12-wk training period, leading to increased F_{FLX} on the operated side and increased aerobic capacity, which were accompanied by a lack of hip pain.

We compared the $\dot{V}O_{2peak}$, F_{EXT}, and F_{FLX} before training in CNT and IWT in the present study with those in each of 3 groups that were divided equally according to $\dot{V}O_{2peak}$ (n = 156, each) in the previous study; [18] in that study, we examined the effects of 4-month IWT in 468 middle-aged and older women without THA and with an average age of ~65 years, which was ~5 years older than in the present study. We found that the $\dot{V}O_{2peak}$ and F_{EXT} in the present study were not significantly different from those in the lowest $\dot{V}O_{2peak}$ group ($P>0.05$), while they were significantly lower than those in the middle $\dot{V}O_{2peak}$ group ($P<0.01$). In contrast, the F_{FLX} was significantly lower than that in the lowest $\dot{V}O_{2peak}$ group ($P<0.01$). Therefore, the $\dot{V}O_{2peak}$ and F_{EXT} in the subjects in the present study belong to the bottom 30% group of the age-matched healthy population [20] with a significantly lower F_{FLX} than in that group.

As indicated in **Table 2**, the fast walking time was 87 min/wk higher in IWT than in CNT. Nemoto et al. [17] examined the effects of 5-month IWT on $\dot{V}O_{2peak}$, F_{EXT}, and F_{FLX} in 31 middle-aged women and older women with an average age of ~65 years and no THA, using a target similar to that of the present study, and the researchers reported that the total fast walking time was 32 min/day, the number of walking days was 4.5 days/wk, and the total fast walking time was 144 min/wk. Additionally, Morikawa et al. [18] examined the effects of 4-month IWT on lifestyle-related diseases in 468 middle-aged and older women with an approximate age of ~65 years lacking THA, and the authors reported that the total fast walking time was 22 min/day, the number of walking days was 3.9 day/wk, and the total fast walking time was 85.8 min/wk. Similarly, Okazaki et al. [29] examined the effects of macronutrient supplementation during 5-month IWT on the thigh muscle strength in 35 middle-aged and older women with an approximate age of ~61 years and reported that the total fast walking time was 21.5 min/day, the number of walking days was 4.1 days/wk, and the total fast walking time was

88.2 min/wk. Therefore, the IWT subjects likely accomplished the target of more than 60 min/wk of fast walking at an intensity of more than 70% $\dot{V}O_{2peak}$ as in the previous studies [17,18].

As shown in **Table 3** and **Figure 2**, F_{FLX} in IWT increased significantly by 23% on the operated side and by 14% on the non-operated side, while F_{EXT} remained unchanged after training.

Previous studies have suggested that the response of F_{FLX} to IWT is more sensitive than that of F_{EXT}. [17,18] Nemoto et al. [17] reported that after 5-month IWT, the increase in F_{FLX} was 16% higher than the 12% increase in F_{EXT}. Similar results were also reported in previous studies. [17,27] The precise reasons for the less sensitive response of F_{EXT} remain unclear; however, it might be because the F_{FLX} value is lower than the F_{EXT} value before training. According to the current American College of Sports Medicine guidelines, [30] repetitive contractions above a given percent of maximal force are recommended for increasing muscle strength. In other words, if muscles generate more than a given force in repetitive contractions during training, the strength will increase, but the strength will not otherwise increase. Indeed, Nemoto et al. [17] suggested that the thigh muscle strength remained unchanged after a 5-month moderate-intensity (50% $\dot{V}O_{2peak}$) continuous walking training regimen, while it increased after IWT, which is similar to the results for IWT in the present study. Therefore, the higher sensitivity of F_{FLX} to IWT compared that of F_{EXT} was because the relative exercise intensity was sufficiently high to increase the strength in F_{FLX} but not in F_{EXT}.

As shown in **Table 4** and **Figure 3**, the $\dot{V}O_{2peak}$ and $\dot{V}O_{2AT}$ in IWT increased by 8% and 13%, respectively, while both remained unchanged in CNT.

Nemoto et al. [17] suggested that the $\dot{V}O_{2peak}$ in individual subjects was significantly correlated with their thigh muscle strength and that the increase after 5-month IWT was accompanied by an increase in thigh muscle strength, suggesting that the changes in $\dot{V}O_{2peak}$ and $\dot{V}O_{2AT}$ were caused by the increased oxygen extraction rate in the muscle tissue due to increases in muscle mass, capillary density, and cellular oxidative capacity.

In the present study, the hip pain score remained unchanged in IWT. Generally, THA patients tend to be physically inactive, fearing acetabular cap wear of the implanted joints due to more frequent friction on the surface during walking; [31] however, recent studies have suggested that the wear is not related to the daily physical activity level [32] and, furthermore, the incidence of joint replacement was much higher in patients with less regular exercise, which is most likely due to the reduction in the surrounding muscle mass supporting the joint. [33] We found that the walking satisfaction score, "vitality" in SF-36 in IWT, was improved as the thigh muscle strength increased after training (**Table 3**), which is consistent with the results in the previous study [33].

Limitations

In the present study, we did not measure the hip muscle strength; however, Judd et al. [33] suggested that the hip flexor and abductor forces recovered to those in the age-matched healthy older women within 12 months after surgery in THA patients, while the hip extensor and knee flexor and extensor forces remained ~20% lower than in those in healthy women. In the present study, we confirmed that the F_{EXT} and F_{FLX} before training in both groups were ~20% lower than those in the age-matched total population of healthy women; [18] therefore, the hip and thigh muscle strength likely matched those that were previously reported for THA patients [33].

We only monitored the improvement in daily physical activity for one week after training. Therefore, it is unclear whether the patients would continue IWT afterwards; however, it has been suggested that the adherence rate of 4 months of IWT was 94% in age-matched healthy women, which was due to the instruction service that provided achievement-based feedback over the internet. [18] Therefore, we surmised that most THA patients would continue IWT if the service was provided afterwards.

In the present study, a mild exercise control group was not included; however, Nemoto et al. [17] reported in middle-aged and older people, the F_{EXT} and F_{FLX} significantly increased after high intensity interval walking training for 5 months, while it did not increase after moderate intensity continuous walking training, although the time and steps for training were less in high intensity interval walking training group than in the moderate intensity continuous walking training group. Accordingly, they suggested that high intensity interval walking training increased the thigh muscle strength as resistance training by using machines recommended by the ACSM. [30] We confirmed this in THA patients in the present study.

The subjects in the present study had relatively low BMIs and were middle-aged and older Japanese women. Because this is the first study to evaluate the effects of IWT on THA patients, further studies are needed to assess whether our findings are true for a fatter, Western population.

As mentioned previously, the physical fitness in the subjects in the present study belongs to the bottom 30% group of the age-matched healthy population. [18] Morikawa et al. [18] suggested that the symptoms of life-style related diseases, including hypertension, hyperglycemia, obese, and dyslipidemia, were the worst in the group, but the symptoms improved the most with most increased physical fitness after 5-month interval waling training. Future studies are needed to evaluate the effects of interval walking training on life-style related diseases in THA patients.

Conclusion

IWT might be an effective home-based training regimen for preventing muscle atrophy due to reduced daily physical activity in THA patients.

Supporting Information

Check list S1 CONSORT checklist.

Protocol S1 Trial Protocol.

Protocol S2 Trial Protocol in original language (in Japanese).

Medical Research Ethics Review Application Form S1 Medical Research Ethics Review Application Form.

Medical Research Ethics Review Application Form S2 Medical Research Ethics Review Application Form in original language (in Japanese).

Author Contributions

Conceived and designed the experiments: HN. Performed the experiments: YM TM KY. Analyzed the data: YM SM MM. Contributed reagents/materials/analysis tools: HN. Wrote the paper: YM SM HN.

References

1. Nilsdotter AK, Roos EM, Westerlund JP, Roos HP, Lohmander LS (2001) Comparative responsiveness of measures of pain and function after total hip replacement. Arthritis and rheumatism 45: 258–262.
2. Rasch A, Dalén N, Berg HE (2010) Muscle strength, gait, and balance in 20 patients with hip osteoarthritis followed for 2 years after THA. Acta Orthopaedica 81: 183–188.
3. Rasch A, Byström AH, Dalén N, Martinez-Carranza N, Berg HE (2009) Persisting muscle atrophy two years after replacement of the hip. The Journal of bone and joint surgery British volume 91: 583–588.
4. Long WT, Dorr LD, Healy B, Perry J (1993) Functional recovery of noncemented total hip arthroplasty. Clinical orthopaedics and related research: 73–77.
5. Perrin T, Dorr LD, Perry J, Gronley J, Hull DB (1985) Functional evaluation of total hip arthroplasty with five- to ten-year follow-up evaluation. Clinical orthopaedics and related research: 252–260.
6. Dorr LD, Wan Z (1998) Causes of and treatment protocol for instability of total hip replacement. Clinical orthopaedics and related research: 144–151.
7. Lachiewicz PF, Soileau ES (2002) Stability of total hip arthroplasty in patients 75 years or older. Clinical orthopaedics and related research: 65–69.
8. Murray MP, Gore DR, Brewer BJ, Gardner GM, Sepic SB (1979) A comparison of the funtional performance of patients with Charnley and Müller total hip replacement. A two-year follow-up of eighty-nine cases. Acta orthopaedica Scandinavica 50: 563–569.
9. Victor CR (1987) Rehabilitation after hip replacement: a one year follow up. International journal of rehabilitation research Internationale Zeitschrift für Rehabilitationsforschung Revue internationale de recherches de réadaptation 10: 162–167.
10. Sicard-Rosenbaum L, Light KE, Behrman AL (2002) Gait, lower extremity strength, and self-assessed mobility after hip arthroplasty. The journals of gerontology Series A, Biological sciences and medical sciences 57: M47–51.
11. Madsen MS, Ritter MA, Morris HH, Meding JB, Berend ME, et al. (2004) The effect of total hip arthroplasty surgical approach on gait. Journal of orthopaedic research: official publication of the Orthopaedic Research Society 22: 44–50.
12. Trudelle-Jackson E, Smith SS (2004) Effects of a late-phase exercise program after total hip arthroplasty: a randomized controlled trial. Archives of Physical Medicine and Rehabilitation 85: 1056–1062.
13. Mossey JM, Mutran E, Knott K, Craik R (1989) Determinants of recovery 12 months after hip fracture: the importance of psychosocial factors. American journal of public health 79: 279–286.
14. Magaziner J, Simonsick EM, Kashner TM, Hebel JR, Kenzora JE (1990) Predictors of functional recovery one year following hospital discharge for hip fracture: a prospective study. Journal of gerontology 45: M101–7.
15. Sashika H, Matsuba Y, Watanabe Y (1996) Home program of physical therapy: effect on disabilities of patients with total hip arthroplasty. Archives of physical medicine and rehabilitation 77: 273–277.
16. Jan M-H, Hung J-Y, Lin JC-H, Wang S-F, Liu T-K, et al. (2004) Effects of a home program on strength, walking speed, and function after total hip replacement. Archives of physical medicine and rehabilitation 85: 1943–1951.
17. Nemoto K, Gen-no H, Masuki S, Okazaki K, Nose H (2007) Effects of high-intensity interval walking training on physical fitness and blood pressure in middle-aged and older people. Mayo Clinic proceedings Mayo Clinic 82: 803–811.
18. Morikawa M, Okazaki K, Masuki S, Kamijo Y, Yamazaki T, et al. (2011) Physical fitness and indices of lifestyle-related diseases before and after interval walking training in middle-aged and older males and females. British journal of sports medicine 45: 216–224.
19. Sakai A, Terasawa K, Inaki M (2000) Physical effects of" The Matsumoto physical training program for senior citizens." Shinshu Medical Journal 48: 89–96.
20. Schulz KF, Altman DG, Moher D (2011) CONSORT 2010 statement: updated guidelines for reporting parallel group randomised trials. International journal of surgery (London, England) 9: 672–677.
21. Fukuhara S, Bito S, Green J, Hsiao A, Kurokawa K (1998) Translation, adaptation, and validation of the SF-36 Health Survey for use in Japan. Journal of clinical epidemiology 51: 1037–1044.
22. Fukuhara S, Ware J, Kosinski M (1998) Psychometric and clinical tests of validity of the Japanese SF-36 Health Survey. Journal of clinical epidemiology 51: 1045–1053.
23. Wasserman K, Whipp BJ, Koyl SN, Beaver WL (1973) Anaerobic threshold and respiratory gas exchange during exercise. Journal of applied physiology 35: 236–243.
24. Nose H, Morikawa M, Yamazaki T, Nemoto K-I, Okazaki K, et al. (2009) Beyond epidemiology: field studies and the physiology laboratory as the whole world. The Journal of physiology 587: 5569–5575.
25. Iwashita S, Takeno Y, Okazaki K, Itoh J, Kamijo Y, et al. (2003) Triaxial accelerometry to evaluate walking efficiency in older subjects. Medicine and science in sports and exercise 35: 1766–1772.
26. Yamazaki T, Gen-No H, Kamijo Y-I, Okazaki K, Masuki S, et al. (2009) A new device to estimate VO2 during incline walking by accelerometry and barometry. Medicine and science in sports and exercise 41: 2213–2219.
27. Davis JA, Frank MH, Whipp BJ, Wasserman K (1979) Anaerobic threshold alterations caused by endurance training in middle-aged men. Journal of applied physiology: respiratory, environmental and exercise physiology 46: 1039–1046.
28. Beaver WL, Wasserman K, Whipp BJ (1986) A new method for detecting anaerobic threshold by gas exchange. Journal of applied physiology (Bethesda, Md: 1985) 60: 2020–2027.
29. Okazaki K, Yazawa D, Goto M, Kamijo Y-I, Furihata M, et al. (2013) Effects of macronutrient intake on thigh muscle mass during home-based walking training in middle-aged and older women. Scandinavian journal of medicine & science in sports.
30. Armstrong LE, GJ B, MJ B, SE D, KP D, et al. (2006) General principles of exercise prescription. In: Whayley MH, Brubaker PH, Otto RM, eds. ACSM's guidelines for exercise testing and prescription. 7th ed. Philadelphia: Lippincott Williams & Wilkins.
31. Dowson D (2001) New joints for the Millennium: wear control in total replacement hip joints. Proceedings of the Institution of Mechanical Engineers Part H, Journal of engineering in medicine 215: 335–358.
32. Bennett D, Humphreys L, O'Brien S, Kelly C, Orr J, et al. (2008) Activity levels and polyethylene wear of patients 10 years post hip replacement. Clinical biomechanics (Bristol, Avon) 23: 571–576.
33. Judd DL, Dennis DA, Thomas AC, Wolfe P, Dayton MR, et al. (2013) Muscle Strength and Functional Recovery During the First Year After THA. Clinical orthopaedics and related research.

21

Action Potential-Evoked Calcium Release Is Impaired in Single Skeletal Muscle Fibers from Heart Failure Patients

Marino DiFranco[1], Marbella Quiñonez[1], Perry Shieh[2], Gregg C. Fonarow[3], Daniel Cruz[3], Mario C. Deng[3], Julio L. Vergara[1], Holly R. Middlekauff[1,3]*

1 Department of Physiology, David Geffen School of Medicine, University of California Los Angeles, Los Angeles, California, United States of America, **2** Department of Neurology, David Geffen School of Medicine, University of California Los Angeles, Los Angeles, California, United States of America, **3** Division of Cardiology, Department of Medicine, David Geffen School of Medicine, University of California Los Angeles, Los Angeles, California, United States of America

Abstract

Background: Exercise intolerance in chronic heart failure (HF) has been attributed to abnormalities of the skeletal muscles. Muscle function depends on intact excitation-contraction coupling (ECC), but ECC studies in HF models have been inconclusive, due to deficiencies in the animal models and tools used to measure calcium (Ca^{2+}) release, mandating investigations in skeletal muscle from HF patients. The purpose of this study was to test the hypothesis that Ca^{2+} release is significantly impaired in the skeletal muscle of HF patients in whom exercise capacity is severely diminished compared to age-matched healthy volunteers.

Methods and Findings: Using state-of-the-art electrophysiological and optical techniques in single muscle fibers from biopsies of the locomotive *vastus lateralis* muscle, we measured the action potential (AP)-evoked Ca^{2+} release in 4 HF patients and 4 age-matched healthy controls. The mean peak Ca^{2+} release flux in fibers obtained from HF patients (10 ± 1.2 μM/ms) was markedly (2.6-fold) and significantly ($p<0.05$) smaller than in fibers from healthy volunteers (28 ± 3.3 μM/ms). This impairment in AP-evoked Ca^{2+} release was ubiquitous and was not explained by differences in the excitability mechanisms since single APs were indistinguishable between HF patients and healthy volunteers.

Conclusions: These findings prove the feasibility of performing electrophysiological experiments in single fibers from human skeletal muscle, and offer a new approach for investigations of myopathies due to HF and other diseases. Importantly, we have demonstrated that one step in the ECC process, AP-evoked Ca^{2+} release, is impaired in single muscle fibers in HF patients.

Editor: Nicole Beard, University of Canberra, Australia

Funding: Research reported in this publication was supported by the National Institute of Arthritis and Musculoskeletal and Skin Diseases of the National Institutes of Health under award numbers AR047664, AR54816, and AR041802; the Clinical and Translational Science Institute Grant #UL1TR000124; and funds from the UCLA Department of Medicine and Dean's Office. The funders had no role in study design, data collection and analysis, decision to publish, or preparation of the manuscript.

Competing Interests: The authors have declared that no competing interests exist.

* Email: hmiddlekauff@mednet.ucla.edu

Introduction

Chronic heart failure (HF) patients with systolic dysfunction have benefited from advances in pharmacological and device therapies that have reduced mortality [1]. Nonetheless, residual poor exercise tolerance characterized by skeletal muscle weakness and early fatigue contribute to ongoing suffering and morbidity, leading to 3.5 million hospitalizations per year, 11 million outpatient doctor visits/year, and skyrocketing medical costs [2]. It is a fact that a large proportion of HF patients would trade increased length of life for increased quality of life [3], which in HF patients is directly linked to exercise capacity [4]. Surprisingly, exercise dysfunction in HF patients is not directly related to severity of left ventricular dysfunction, intra-cardiac hemodynamics at rest or during exercise, or inadequate skeletal muscle blood flow [5–8]. Instead, exercise dysfunction is directly related to abnormalities of the skeletal muscles themselves; in fact a skeletal myopathy has been described which includes a fiber shift from type I aerobic fibers to type II anaerobic fibers and decreased mitochondrial volume and metabolic function [8–11].

Skeletal muscle function depends critically on both intact energy metabolism and on the robustness of the sequence of events linking the electrical with the mechanical activation of the muscle fibers (the so-called excitation-contraction coupling [ECC] process). The role of metabolic deficiencies in skeletal muscle function in HF patients on optimal medical therapy has recently been questioned [12–14]. We have recently reported marked abnormalities of several key proteins participating in the ECC process in humans with HF [15]; however, it remains unknown whether these abnormalities in protein content are accompanied by functional abnormalities in calcium (Ca^{2+}) cycling in humans with HF. The integrity of important steps in the ECC chain of events, such as the Ca^{2+} release from the sarcoplasmic reticulum (SR), is a decisive factor for normal exercise ability; ECC impairments are expected to critically contribute to muscle weakness and poor exercise tolerance [8,14–16].

Animal models of HF have been used to investigate ECC abnormalities that may recapitulate the skeletal myopathy seen in HF patients [17–22]. However, these animal studies have intrinsic limitations in that they provide inconsistent information depending on the HF model and they do not fully reproduce the HF phenotype of decreased exercise tolerance [23]. Furthermore, to date, tools capable of measuring the rapid physiological Ca^{2+} release in skeletal muscle fibers have not been utilized in animal models. Altogether, the findings from animal studies are inconclusive and contradictory [18–22]. We chose to bypass the animal models and procure biopsies of the *vastus lateralis* (VL) muscles directly from HF patients and healthy age-matched volunteers, and used state-of-the-art electrophysiological and optical techniques to test our hypothesis that the ECC process is significantly impaired in the locomotive skeletal muscle of HF patients compared to healthy volunteers. Our approach puts special emphasis on the fibers' ability to generate Ca^{2+} transients in response to action potential (AP) stimulation and, by using low affinity Ca^{2+} indicators in conjunction with high internal EGTA concentrations [17–20], allows for a direct comparison of their physiological robustness.

Methods

Ethics Statement

The study was approved by the University of California Los Angeles (UCLA) Human Subjects Protection Committee, and the participants gave their written informed consent.

Study Population

Advanced HF patients, New York Heart Association Class II–III meeting the following eligibility criteria were recruited from the Ahmanson-UCLA Cardiomyopathy Center: 1) age 21–65 years, 2) Left ventricular ejection fraction <35%, 3) HF duration > 1 year, 4) not involved in a formal exercise training program, 5) on stable, guideline appropriate HF medications, and not taking warfarin or non-warfarin oral anticoagulants. Age and gender-matched healthy, non-smoking controls, without chronic illnesses and taking no daily medications, who drank <2 drinks/day, and who did not participate in regular exercise (30 minutes most days), served as controls.

Skeletal muscle biopsy

The procedure was performed at the UCLA Out-Patient Surgery Center under local anesthesia. An incision was made in the lateral aspect of the thigh, at about 20 cm proximal to the patella, and a sample of vastus lateralis (VL) muscle measuring 40 mm in length, 8 mm in width and 5 mm in depth was obtained. The biopsy was transported to the lab in ice-cold oxygenated Tyrode solution, where it was pinned in a Sylgard bottomed Petri dish containing oxygenated Tyrode solution and divided into 10–12 bundles (~2 mm in diameter), as delimited by the perimysium. Bundle pulling was kept at a minimum at all times during dissection. When kept in oxygenated Tyrode solution at room temperature, bundles remained viable for >10 hours. Although not studied systematically, viability was found to be longer the greater the biopsy length. In many cases, bundles 40 mm in length contracted upon stimulation with 10 Hz trains after 1.5 hours from biopsy.

Muscle fiber dissection

A bundle was pinned down at slack length in a dish containing Tyrode, which was subsequently slowly exchanged by relaxing solution (see Solutions). In this solution, fibers became electrically and mechanically inactivated, thus preventing contractures during dissection and increasing the rate of success of intact fiber isolation. A peripheral smaller bundle comprised of ~20 fibers was dissected aside using small Vannas scissors and #5 tweezers. The tissue was divided progressively into smaller bundles until a single fiber of about 20 mm in length was obtained. For this finer dissection, #5 tweezers and retina surgical scissors (gauge 25, Alcon) were used. Fiber stretching was avoided at all times. Only fiber segments crystalline in appearance, devoid of contractured regions, freely flexible, and exhibiting a sharp banding pattern were used for electrophysiological experiments. The degree of difficulty of dissection of fibers from HF biopsies was not significantly different from that of control biopsies.

Fiber mounting and stimulation

Fibers were mounted in an inverted double-gap grease chamber, under stereoscopic microscope observation, as previously described [24,25] but with modifications. Fibers (~8 mm in length) were transferred to the chamber previously flooded with relaxing solution using a heat polished glass capillary connected to a 100 µl pippetor via a Tygon tubing. To avoid adhesion of the fiber to the capillary, it was rinsed in relaxing solution containing 3 mg/ml serum bovine albumin prior to fiber transfer. Using #5 tweezers the fiber was placed across the chamber's gaps, where pre-seals (a shallow layer of grease) had been constructed. Each end of the fiber was secured to the coverslip at the chamber's lateral compartments with grease, and straightened and stretched by ~ 40–50% the slack length by gently pulling the ends embedded in grease. The grease seals were then constructed at the chamber's gaps (Figure 1 in [24]), and the excess solution was removed to render each of the 3 compartments electrically independent. The central pool of the experimental chamber was 300±45 µm (n = 25). The segments of the fiber at the lateral compartments were permeabilized with saponine (10 µg/ml in internal solution, 30 sec). After washing out saponine, internal solution containing the Ca^{2+} sensor was added to the lateral compartments. Finally, the chamber was placed on the stage of the microscope and connected to the perfusion system and the electrical amplifier. Fibers requiring more than −70 nA to be repolarized to −90 mV were discarded. Recordings were started 15–20 min after adding the Ca^{2+} sensor to the lateral pools. The circuit used to stimulate the fibers and to record the membrane potential and currents has been previously described [25]. One cut end of the fiber was connected to a current source, the other was connected to a high impedance amplifier, and the central segment of the fiber was held at virtual ground. APs were elicited by current pulses (0.2 ms, 10–15% above threshold) applied at one cut end. Membrane potential was measured as the difference between the potential at the other cut end (i.e. the myoplasm) and the central pool (i.e. the extracellular milieu).

Ca^{2+} transients

AP evoked Ca^{2+} concentration changes were measured using the low affinity dye OregonGreenBapta488-5N (OGB-5N) [26–29]. OGB5N was added to the internal solution bathing both cut ends of the fibers at a final concentration of 250µM. Large concentrations of EGTA semi-saturated with Ca^{2+} were added to the internal solution with two purposes in mind: a) to prevent fiber movements that would distort optical recordings and potentially dislodge the grease seals; and, b) to allow for the calculation of

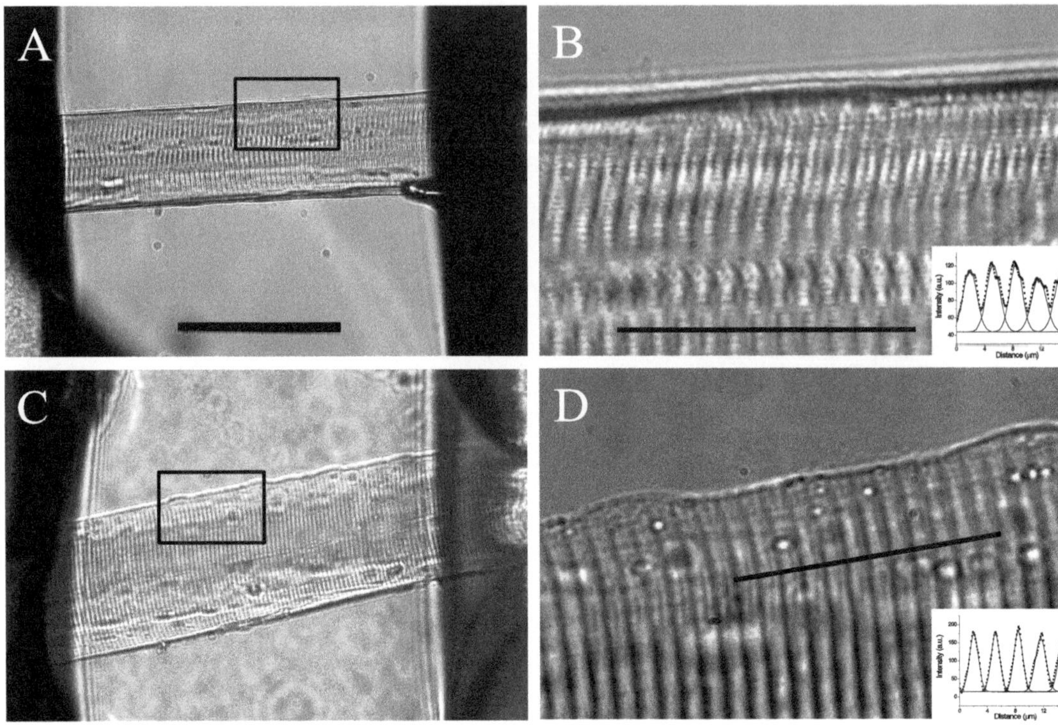

Figure 1. Isolated fibers mounted in the inverted double grease-gap chamber. Panel A: Image of a VL fiber from a healthy volunteer obtained with a 20× objective. The inner part of the grease seals delimiting the experimental pool can be seen at both sides of the image. Panel B: The area delimited by the square in A was imaged with a 100× immersion objective. A sharp banding pattern and smooth border can be seen. Panels C and D shows a VL fiber from a HF patient at the same magnifications as in A and B, respectively. The diameter and sarcomere length were 62.0 and 3.0 μm for the fiber in A, and 80 and 2.8 μm for the fiber in B, respectively. The insets in panels B and D show intensity profiles measured across ~4 sarcomeres. The profiles span ~16 mm along the directions indicated by the lines superimposed in the corresponding images. The dots and lines represent the intensity values and Gaussian fits to the data, respectively. The scale in A corresponds to 100 μm in A and C, and 20 μm in B and D.

peak Ca^{2+} flux from OGB-5N Ca^{2+} transients using a single compartment model that is extensively described elsewhere [27,28,30]. Two mixtures were used: 30:15 and 20:10 EGTA:Ca. The large [EGTA] used are expected to equalize the resting myoplasmic free [Ca] to ~80 nM in all experiments. The Ca^{2+} dependent fluorescence transients (referred to simply as Ca^{2+} transients) are reported as $\Delta F/F$ transients (dimensionless). These transients are used to calculate Ca^{2+} flux transients (μM/ms).

The optical setup was similar to that described elsewhere [28,29]. Briefly, it consisted of an inverted microscope (Olympus IX71) equipped with a standard epifluorescence attachment, a 480-40/510/540-30 nm cube combination, and a 100× 1.4 NA oil immersion objective. The light was focused to a spot with a diameter similar to that of fibers (40–50 μm). In order to reduce stray fluorescence from the grease, the illumination spot was place at the center of the experimental pool. To remove contributions from stray fluorescence to the OGB5N fluorescence, the fluorescence from areas outside the fiber was recorded and subtracted from every Ca^{2+} transient before calculating $\Delta F/F$ transients.

Solutions

The composition of solutions (mM) was:

Tyrode: 150 NaCl, 4KCl, $1MgCl_2$, $2CaCl_2$, 10 glucose, 10 MOPS.

Relaxing solution: 120 K_2SO_4, 10 MOPS, 1 $MgCl_2$, 1 $CaCl_2$, 10 glucose.

Internal solution: 92 K-Aspartate, 20 MOPS, 1 $MgCl_2$, 5 reduced Glutathione, 5 ATP-TRIS, 5 Creatine Phosphate-Na_2, 20 EGTA, 10 $Ca(OH)_2$.

All solutions were adjusted to ph = 7.4 and had 300±5 mOsmol/kg H_2O.

Signal conditioning and statistical analysis

Voltage, current and optical signals were filtered at 10, 5 and 2 kHz (8 pole low-pass-filter; Frequency Devices), respectively, and acquired at 10μs/point. Optical and electrical data from control and HF fibers were compared using the Student's t test. Significance was set at $p<0.05$.

Results

Study population characteristics

Four HF patients at an advanced stage, and four healthy age-matched human volunteers participated in these studies. The major features of the cohorts are presented in Table 1. Importantly, HF patients and healthy volunteers did not differ in age, sex, or body mass index. In addition, HF patients had severe exercise limitation as measured by peak oxygen consumption of 13.1±1.0 ml/kg/min (compared with that of untrained healthy adult values, always >28 ml/kg/min).

Fibers dissected from VL muscle biopsies of healthy volunteers and HF patients appear similarly intact under the light microscope

In contrast to previous reports in rat muscles [19], we found that dissecting single fibers from VL muscle biopsies was not more cumbersome when they were obtained from HF patients

Table 1. Study Population Characteristics.

	Subjects	
	Heart Failure Patients	**Healthy Volunteers**
Number of Subjects	4	4
Age (years)	57.3±2.1	52.8±2.4
BMI[a] (kg/m^2)	29.2±1.6	30.8±2.9
Female	1	1
Druation of HF (years)	8.5±2.2	
Peak VO_2 (ml/kg/min)	13.1±1.0	
LVEF[c](%)	26.0±4.0	
Diabetes mellitus	2	
Hypertension	2	
Etiology of HF		
• CAD[d]	2	
• Idiopathic	2	
• Familial	0	
Medications		
• Beta-blockers	4	
• ACEI[e]	2	
• ARB[f]	1	
• Statin	4	
• Aldosterone antagonist	2	
• Aspirin	3	
• Clopidogrel	0	
• Furosemide	3	
• Digoxin	1	
• Amiodarone	1	

[a]body mass index, [b]peak oxygen consumption, [c]left ventricular ejection fraction, [d]coronary artery disease, [e]angiotensin inhibitor, [f]angiotensin receptor blocker. Values are mean±SEM.

compared to healthy volunteers. Moreover, as illustrated in Figure 1, bright-field images demonstrate that there are no obvious differences in appearance between fibers obtained from healthy volunteers (Figures 1A and B) and HF patients (Figures 1C and D) as they are mounted in the experimental chamber. Specifically, both sets of fibers have comparable diameters. The average diameters (mean±SD) were 75.2±17.2 μm [n = 10; minimum 58.8 μm, maximum = 113.1 μm) for fibers from healthy volunteers, and 75.5±16.4 μm (n = 5; minimum 51.8 μm, maximum = 103.0 μm) for fibers from HF patients. In addition, the fibers exhibited equally sharp sarcomere banding with no indications of contractures or vacuolation suggestive of obvious structural damages. Further, the sets of fibers from HF patients and controls had comparable sarcomere lengths, 3.31±0.34 μm, (range 2.64–3.71 μm) versus 3.21±0.33 μm, (range 2.76–3.69 μm), respectively, confirming that they did not undergo gross contractures. It should be noted that the mean sarcomere length is larger than typical slack sarcomere length (~2.2 μm) because during the mounting process, fibers are slightly stretched (see methods). Even in a more advanced inspection of the structural integrity of the transverse tubular system in live fibers stained with the fluorescence dye di-8-ANEPPS fibers [31], there were no detectable alterations in either set of fibers (see Figure S1).

Fibers dissected from VL muscle biopsies of healthy volunteers and HF patients are comparably healthy in electrical terms

Additional direct evidence for the fibers' intactness was obtained by measuring their spontaneous repolarization after exchanging the high K relaxing solution with Tyrode in the central compartment of the experimental chamber. Isolated fibers from both healthy volunteers and HF patients repolarized spontaneously to a similar membrane potential (−13.6±3.42 mV [n = 8] and −16.5±5.1 mV [n = 10] respectively), and required almost identical holding currents in order to maintain them at a resting potential of −90 mV (−59.2±18.3 nA [n = 8] and −60.8 ±28.5 nA [n = 10] respectively), and V_r changed only slightly throughout the typical 30 min of electrophysiological experimentation. Interestingly, these values are comparable to those previously measured in frog fibers mounted in a similar experimental chamber [24,25], which are known to be resilient to mechanical dissection. We also determined that all fibers responded to pulses of increasing amplitude with a sharp threshold, separating electrotonic from all-or-none responses (i.e. APs). Examples of such responses obtained from a healthy volunteer and a HF patient are shown in Figures 2A and 2B, respectively. When relatively small current pulses (sub-threshold) are applied, similar graded electrotonic responses are elicited in both preparations, which peak at about −50 mV. By increasing the pulse amplitude by 10–15%, comparable all-or-none responses are evoked, which take off from about −40 mV. Threshold potentials were found between these two values. Although the threshold for HF fibers is slightly more depolarized (~3 mV) than healthy fibers, the mean values (±SD) calculated from 10 healthy fibers (−48.3±6.5 mV) and 10 HF fibers (−45.3±4.1 mV) were not significantly different (inset of Figure 2A).

AP-evoked Ca^{2+} release is impaired in isolated fibers from HF patients

Secure that fibers dissected from biopsies of both HF patients and healthy volunteers were equally intact for study in isolation, we proceeded to investigate their respective ability to release Ca^{2+} in response to AP stimulation. A smaller population of fibers was used for this purpose (5 fibers from healthy volunteers and 9 fibers from HF patients). The fibers were allowed to equilibrate with internal solutions containing high [EGTA] and free Ca^{2+} concentration $[Ca^{2+}]$ close to the physiological value ~0.1 μM [26,28]. Figure 3B shows an example of a Ca^{2+} transient recorded in a fiber from a healthy volunteer and equilibrated with internal solution containing 30:15 EGTA:Ca (see Solutions). In response to the AP (Figure 3A), a fast fluorescence transient (Ca^{2+} transient) was elicited that reached a peak ΔF/F of ~0.24. Interestingly, knowing the concentration and Ca^{2+} binding properties of the Ca^{2+} indicator (OGB-5N) and EGTA, we were able to estimate with accuracy the Ca^{2+} release flux (in μM/ms) responsible for this fluorescence transient [26,28–30,32]. The resulting flux record is shown in the inset of Figure 3B; the peak value, representing the maximal rate of Ca^{2+} release, was ~29 μM/ms. In comparison, Ca^{2+} transients recorded from a muscle fiber dissected from a HF patient's VL biopsy under the same conditions as those used for the fiber from the healthy volunteer were ~3-fold smaller amplitude (peak ΔF/F~0.09, Figure 3D). The calculated Ca^{2+} release flux (compare insets of Figures 3B and 3D) was also markedly reduced, ~3-fold (from ~29 to ~10 μM/ms).

This impairment in AP-evoked Ca^{2+} transients was observed in every HF fiber studied, regardless of the EGTA:Ca ratio used to equilibrate control fibers. In order to compare reliably the Ca^{2+} release strength in all fibers studied, we calculated the Ca^{2+} fluxes underlying Ca^{2+} transients recorded at either 30:15 or 20:10 (EGTA:Ca) conditions. As demonstrated in Figure 4A, the mean Ca^{2+} fluxes determined in fibers from healthy volunteers equilibrated with 30:15 (n = 2) and 20:10 (n = 3) EGTA mixtures were comparable to each other. Since the mean flux from fibers was independent of the EGTA:Ca ratio, the data from healthy volunteers was pooled. The results demonstrate that the mean peak Ca^{2+} release flux in fibers obtained from HF patients equilibrated with a 30:15 EGTA:Ca mixture (10±1.2 μM/ms; 4 biopsies, 9 fibers) is substantially (2.6-fold) and significantly ($p < 0.05$) smaller than that in fibers from healthy volunteers (28±3.3 μM/ms; 4 biopsies, 5 fibers). We then compared the frequency distribution of peak Ca^{2+} fluxes from healthy volunteers and HF patients (Figure 4B). The values for AP-evoked Ca^{2+} release fluxes in fibers from healthy volunteers are widely distributed between values as high as ~40 μM/ms to low values of ~18 μM/ms. In contrast, those of fibers from HF patients span a much narrower, left-shifted range of lower values, between ~17 and ~5 μM/ms. AP-evoked Ca^{2+} release fluxes were smaller in all the fibers isolated from HF patients, compared to those from healthy volunteers. Our results demonstrate for the first time that a key step in the ECC process, that is, Ca^{2+} release from the SR, is severely impaired in skeletal muscle fibers of HF patients compared to age-matched healthy volunteers. These findings are consistent with, and expand on, our previous report that the expression of key proteins involved in ECC are reduced in HF fibers [15], to demonstrate that the deficiency in the expression of those proteins has devastating functional implications for HF patients.

Properties of the AP in fibers isolated from biopsies of healthy volunteers and HF patients

Since the AP is the physiological trigger of the ECC process, one potential mechanism underlying the severe reduction in the Ca^{2+} release fluxes observed in fibers from HF patients could be that their AP properties are significantly altered. To our knowledge, there is no published information about the electrical activity of human VL muscle fibers; consequently, we compared the amplitude, full duration at half-maximum (FDHM), time to peak

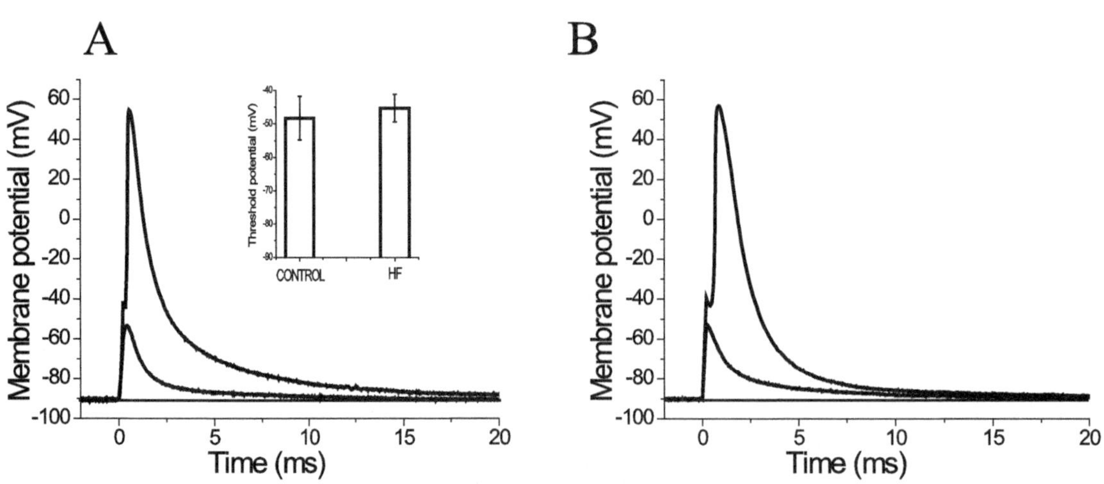

Figure 2. Fibers from healthy volunteers and HF patients have similar thresholds. Panels A and B show electrotonic responses (small depolarizations elicited by sub-threshold current pulses) and actions potentials (large autoregenerative depolarization elicited by suprathreshold current pulses) in a fiber from a healthy volunteer (A) and a HF patient (B). The inset in panel A shows the mean (±SD) threshold potentials for a population of fibers from healthy volunteers (n = 10 fibers) and HF patients (n = 10 fibers).

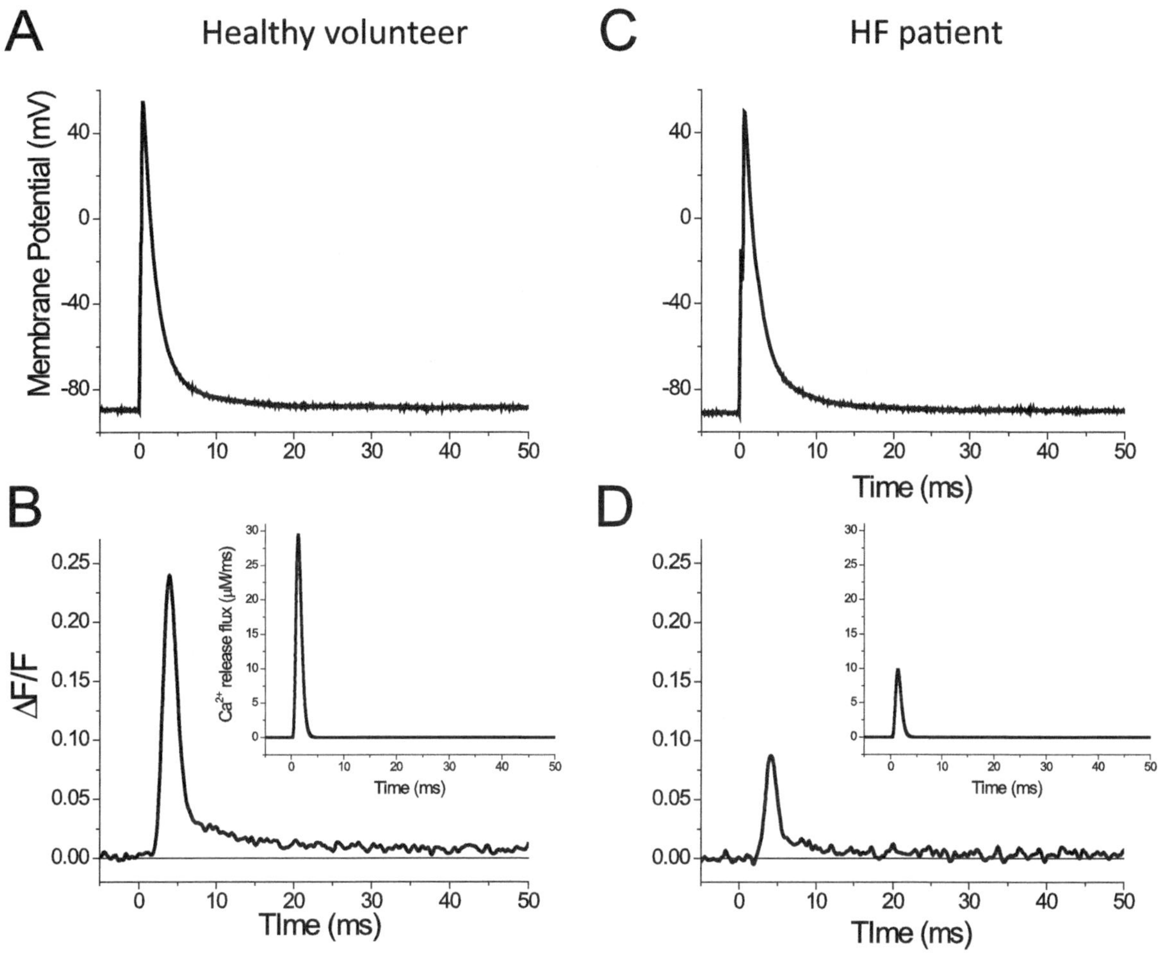

Figure 3. AP evoked Ca^{2+} transients in fibers dissected from a healthy volunteer and a HF patient. Figures A and C are the APs and panels B and D are the corresponding Ca^{2+} transients. The insets in B and D are Ca^{2+} release fluxes (in μM/ms) calculated from the corresponding optical records. The fibers were equilibrated with an internal solution containing 30:15 EGTA:Ca^{2+}.

(TTP), and maximal rate of depolarization ($[dV/dt]_{max}$) of APs recorded in fibers isolated from the skeletal muscle biopsies of HF patients and healthy volunteers (see Table 2). The APs of fibers dissected from biopsies of healthy volunteers and HF patients have almost identical amplitudes and durations. Since the resting potential was kept at −90 mV in both groups of fibers, their APs have similar overshoots (to ~+54 mV). Interestingly, the maximum depolarization rate was significantly faster in fibers from HF patients compared to healthy volunteers ($p<0.05$). Potential implications of this faster depolarization will be addressed in the Discussion.

Discussion

Using state-of-the-art electrophysiological and optical techniques, we have performed studies in single fibers procured from the *vastus lateralis* muscle of advanced HF patients and healthy volunteers, and have demonstrated for the first time that one critical step of the ECC process, specifically, the AP-evoked Ca^{2+} release, is impaired in this locomotive muscle of HF patients. As will be discussed in detail below, these findings are transformative because: 1) they circumvent the inherent limitations of studying ECC in models of HF by utilizing actual tissue obtained directly from patients afflicted with the HF condition; 2) they confirm the feasibility of performing electrophysiological experiments characterizing individual steps of the ECC process in single fibers from human skeletal muscle according to fiber type; and critically, 3) they offer new approaches to investigate other myopathic conditions that may also involve impairments in the ECC process, such as chronic obstructive pulmonary disease and chronic renal disease [33,34].

Inherent limitations in animal models and the need for human studies

Animal models of HF, including the infarct model and the sympathetic hyperactivity-induced model, are critical to our further investigations and improved understanding of human diseases, but have inherent limitations [17–23]. In the rat infarct model, the left coronary artery is ligated, which results in infarction of ~35% of cardiac tissue and elevated left ventricular end-diastolic pressures, mimicking human HF. However, despite significant cardiac damage and dysfunction, HF rats demonstrate no decline in locomotive activity when quantified by the photocell activation technique [23]. That is, the phenotypic expression of decreased exercise tolerance and early fatigue is absent in this model, thereby raising the question of its validity to study exercise dysfunction in patients with HF who suffer from profound exercise limitation. The sympathetic hyperactivity-induced HF model is a

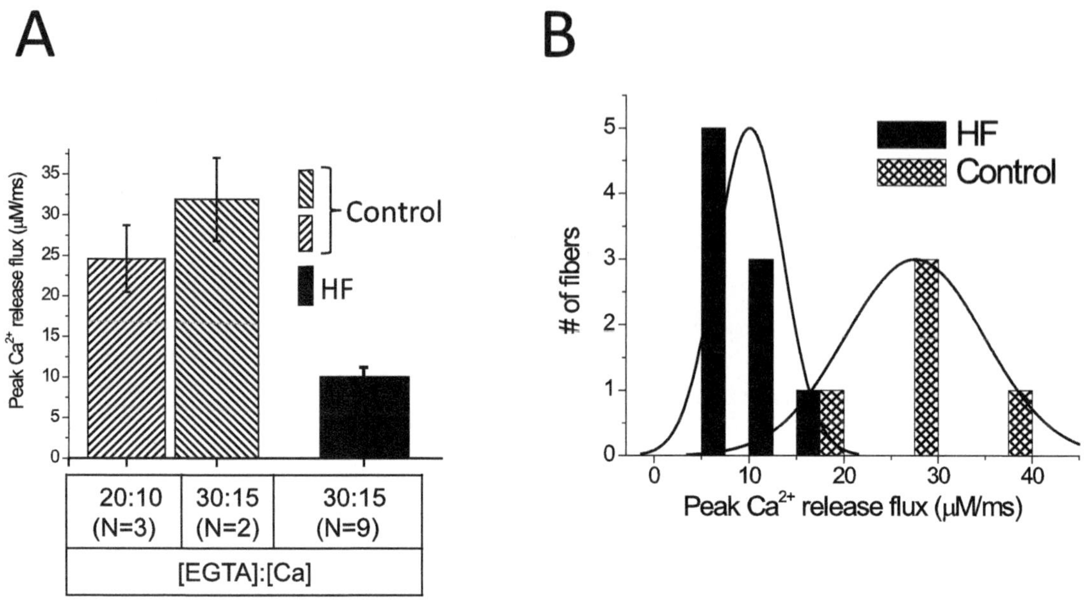

Figure 4. Average values and frequency distribution of peak Ca^{2+} release flux values in fibers from healthy volunteers and HF patients. Panel A shows the mean (±SD) of peak Ca^{2+} flux in fibers of healthy volunteers (hatched) and of HF patients (black) equilibrated with internal solution containing either 30:15 or 20:10 EGTA:Ca. Panel B shows the frequency distribution of peak Ca^{2+} release fluxes from all fibers in panel A. The binning width was 2.5 µM/ms and the lines correspond to fits of the data to standard normal distributions.

congenic α_{2A}/α_{2C} adrenoceptor knockout mouse that leads to sympathetic hyperactivity-induced HF and quantified exercise dysfunction [18]. However, since α_{2A}/α_{2C} adrenoceptors are absent in all tissues, including the skeletal muscle, it is difficult to know whether muscle changes are due to HF, or to the genetic modification. In fact, in this model, the sympathetic hyperactivity leads to early skeletal muscle changes attributable to relatively increased β_2-adrenoceptor activity [17]. These limitations, as well as species' variations in Ca^{2+} cycling proteins and muscle fiber type composition, generally confound data interpretation and detract from these models. As noted earlier, some [18,19,21,35], but not all studies in animal models [20], have uncovered definite, but variable, abnormalities in the ECC process. These intriguing findings in imperfect animal models mandate further investigations in skeletal muscle from HF patients.

Physiological Ca^{2+} release in normal human skeletal fibers

To our knowledge there are no previous studies of the Ca^{2+} release evoked by AP stimulation in human skeletal muscle fibers in health or disease. Two reports of the Ca^{2+} release flux in healthy human fibers performed under voltage-clamp conditions have been published [36,37]. Interestingly, though it would be expected that under these conditions maximal Ca^{2+} fluxes would be recorded, the values calculated in these reports were significantly smaller than ours, by a factor of at least 2-fold. Differences in the fibers' integrity, the use of Ca^{2+} sensors, and calculation methodologies may partially explain these differences. In one study, percutaneous needle biopsies were obtained, yielding only short muscle segments [36]. It is possible that the short length of these fibers adversely affected their functional performance; in our experience electrophysiological integrity of the fibers increases with increasing biopsy length. In the other study [37], a very low

Table 2. Properties of action potentials recorded in fibers from healthy volunteers and HF patients.

	Subjects	
	Heart Failure Patients	Healthy Volunteers
Number of Subjects	4	4
Number of fibers	10	10
AP amplitude (mV)	143.5±3.2	144.1±3.9
FDHM[a] (ms)	2.19±0.16	2.18±0.16
TTP[b] (ms)	0.68±0.16	0.62±0.09
dV/dt (m/s)	791.3±83.0*	647.5±57.7*
Threshold (mV)	−45.3±4.1	−48.3±6.5

For all fibers, the resting potential was maintained at −90 mV. [a]Full-duration-at-half-maximum, [b]time to peak. Values given as Mean±SEM. * HF vs healthy volunteer, $p<0.05$.

rate of success per biopsy was reported, again raising the question of the fibers' integrity. In general, the recording of normal electrical activity and larger Ca^{2+} release fluxes suggests that our fibers were possibly in better physiological condition throughout the experimentation.

Reduced Ca^{2+} release in fibers from HF patients

The most important and novel finding in our study is that the ECC process, specifically AP-evoked Ca^{2+} release, is impaired in fibers from the VL muscle of HF patients compared to those of healthy volunteers. We have previously reported a reduced expression of sarcoplasmic reticulum Ca^{2+}-ATPase (SERCA2a) and dihydropyridine receptor (DHPR) in homogenates of VL muscle from HF patients compared to healthy volunteers, whereas SERCA1a and ryanodine receptor (RyR1) levels were not different [15]. The simplest predictions from those biochemical data would be that SR Ca^{2+} content is reduced in fibers from HF patients compared to those from healthy volunteers, and/or that there are orphaned RyR1s. Either alteration could result in a significant reduction of Ca^{2+} fluxes potentially leading to reduced exercise performance and increased fatigability characteristic of HF patients. Diminished peak Ca^{2+} release was present in response to single APs; a finding that would be expected to result in smaller peak twitch and tetanic tension (i.e. muscle weakness and premature fatigability). Further investigations are necessary to identify the exact step(s) in the ECC process that lead to this marked impairment in AP-evoked Ca^{2+} release in HF patients. Comparisons of the physiological trigger for Ca^{2+} release (the AP which initiates the ECC process) in healthy volunteers and HF patients were performed and essentially eliminated this as a potential cause (see discussion below).

Electrical activity

The amplitude and duration of the transverse tubular system depolarization are key factors in determining the features of Ca^{2+} release. Our measurements demonstrate that the Ca^{2+} release in fibers from HF patients are triggered by unaltered APs. The constancy and similarity of AP amplitude in fibers from both healthy volunteers and HF patients is remarkable; since the "resting" potential is kept close to -90 mV in both fiber groups, this result implies that the AP overshoot was also similar between (i.e. circa +54 mV).

The maximum depolarization rates of the AP in control and HF fibers are similar to that found in frog fibers using a similar method [24]; nevertheless, we found that the rate of depolarization is larger in HF fibers. There may be a number of physiological reasons for this difference, including differences in ionic channel endowment. It has been recently reported that the expression of the adult isoform of the Na^+ channels (NaV1.4) is significantly increased in *soleus muscles* of rat models of muscle disuse, a condition to which HF patients may be prone [38,39]. In fact, an important controversy in the HF literature is whether the skeletal myopathy in HF stems from simple disuse or from the HF condition characterized by neurohumoral activation and inflammation [39]. The increased expression of NaV1.4 might partially explain why paradoxically the weaker fibers of HF patients are electrically more rapid than those of healthy volunteers, lending support to the disuse position. Other possibilities, such as differences in specific capacitance, and/or fine geometry of the transverse tubular system (diameter and luminal resistance of the tubules) may also explain our findings, thus warranting further investigations on this topic.

Ca^{2+} release results may be ubiquitous

Both the kinetics and magnitude of the Ca^{2+} transients have been reported to differ between fast and slow muscle fibers, and to correlate with the myosin heavy chain (MHC) type expressed; specifically, Ca^{2+} release rates are larger in type II than in type I fibers [40]. Exercise fatigue in HF patients has been suggested to result from fiber type transformation [10,13,41]; arguably, a decreased proportion of slow, aerobic, type I fibers with respect to the number of fast, anaerobic, fatigable, type IIx fibers in the locomotion muscles, such as the VL, might explain the fatigability phenotype. However, an increased proportion of type II fibers in which the ECC process is intact in HF patients would be expected to produce more powerful and quicker muscles; of course, this not the case. In our prior report in HF patients [15], we confirmed the previously reported fiber type shift [10,13,41]. We also reported the novel finding that SERCA2a and DHPR protein levels were decreased in homogenates of VL muscle in HF patients compared to healthy volunteers, whereas SERCA1a and ryanodine receptor (RyR1) levels were not different. Although the observed fiber shift could explain the decrease in SERCA2a, which is present only in type I fibers, it cannot explain either the decrease in DHPR level, since DHPR/RyR1 density is greater in type II than type I fibers in rodents [42,43], or the constancy of the SERCA1a and RyR content.

Interestingly, we found a narrow, left-shifted distribution of peak Ca^{2+} fluxes in HF patients, without overlap with the peak Ca^{2+} fluxes in healthy volunteers, consistent with a ubiquitous abnormality affecting the ECC process in every fiber type (I and II) of VL muscles. In other words, the level of Ca^{2+} release from HF fibers with the greatest Ca^{2+} flux, (presumably type II fibers, also expected in larger proportions in the biopsies of HF patients), was even lower than the level of Ca^{2+} release from healthy fibers with the lowest Ca^{2+} flux, presumably type I fibers. A simple fiber-type shift (i.e. from type I to type II) should have resulted in an overall right-shifted distribution of HF fibers, not seen in Figure 4B; that is, a fiber shift would have been expected to produce a larger proportion of the HF fiber population displaying larger Ca^{2+} release.

In summary, our results strongly support the hypothesis that fibers from HF patients have marked and ubiquitous impairments in ECC, specifically AP-evoked Ca^{2+} release that affects all the fibers, independent of their type, in VL muscles.

Limitations

The use of humans, in place of animals, for investigation, has its own limitations, which we acknowledge here: First, patients are on medications including statins, which, for ethical reasons, cannot be interrupted, and these medications may have systemic effects. Nonetheless, it is well established that despite optimal medical therapy HF patients have severe exercise limitations. We would argue that it is precisely these individuals who need to be studied, since despite the best medical therapy, their exercise capacity continues to be impaired. It is worth noting that no patient was diagnosed with a statin myopathy. Secondly, patients have diverse etiologies of HF, however, the severity of exercise dysfunction, and the characteristics of the skeletal myopathy, including the fiber type transformation, are known to be independent of the specific etiology of the HF [44,45]. Finally, since the experiments in fibers from both HF patients and healthy volunteers were performed at room temperature, the absolute values of the Ca^{2+} release fluxes reported here are possibly smaller than those that could be obtained at normal body temperatures. Though future experimentation will take this into account, the observed impairments in Ca^{2+} release of fibers from HF patients are likely to represent a general limitation rather than an experimental peculiarity linked to the choice of temperature.

Conclusion

We report for the first time in single fibers from HF patients compared to healthy volunteers, that AP-evoked Ca^{2+} release is significantly diminished in fibers obtained from the locomotive VL muscle in HF patients. This diminished Ca^{2+} release is not attributable to significant alterations in the AP of fibers from HF patients compared to fibers from healthy volunteers, since the electrical activity in both groups is virtually identical. Our previous findings of diminished DHPR and SERCA2 expression are suggestive of decreased SR Ca^{2+} content, and/or orphaned RyR1; the relative contributions of these abnormalities and others in the ECC process await further investigation. This decrease in Ca^{2+} flux was present in every fiber tested, consistent with a ubiquitous abnormality involving the ECC process in every fiber type in the VL muscle of HF patients, and unlikely to be attributable to a simple fiber type shift. Finally, using this approach, Ca^{2+} fluxes in individual fibers can be compared between muscles of locomotion, vulnerable to disuse, and compared to fibers in non-locomotive muscles, such as the deltoid, to assess if abnormalities of the ECC process are a systemic problem, attributable to systemic neurohumoral activation and inflammation, or a localized problem, more easily explained by disuse. The impact of exercise training on the impairment of ECC and Ca^{2+} release has widespread clinical relevance, both in understanding the role of disuse in this impairment, as well as an important therapeutic approach, and warrants further study.

Supporting Information

Figure S1 The transverse tubular system in live fibers from control and HF individuals. Muscle bundles dissected from biopsies obtained from control individuals (A) and HF patients (B) were stretched to a sarcomere length similar to that in the electrophysiological experiments and pinned down on a Sylgard bottomed dish. The fibers were stained with di-8-ANEPPS and imaged using a two-photon laser scanning microscope (Biorad Radiance 2000). The dye was excited with a 920 nm laser beam, and the emission was collected using a dichroic/band-pass combination of 506 nm/620–650 nm. It can be seen in the optical section in A that, as previously described for other mammalian fibers, di-8-ANEPPS clearly demonstrate the regular double row pattern of the transverse tubular system. The surface membrane can also be seen at the right upper part of the image. The image in B demonstrate that the transverse tubular system of fibers from HF patients is indistinguishable from that of control fibers. The scale represent 15 μm in both images.

Acknowledgments

We thank Dr. Thomas O'Dell (Department of Physiology, UCLA) for the use of his chemiluminescence detection instrument, and Mr. R. Serrano (Staff Research Assistant, Department of Physiology, UCLA) for technical support during the course of the experimentation. We are especially grateful to the generous HF patients of the Ahmanson-UCLA Cardiomyopathy Center, without whom this research would not be possible.

Author Contributions

Conceived and designed the experiments: HRM JLV MD MQ. Performed the experiments: MD MQ. Analyzed the data: HRM MD JLV MQ. Contributed reagents/materials/analysis tools: HRM GCF DC MCD MD MQ JLV PS. Wrote the paper: HRM MD GCF DC MCD JLV MQ PS.

References

1. Yancy CW, Jessup M, Bozkurt B, Butler J, Casey DE Jr, et al. (2013) 2013 ACCF/AHA Guideline for the Management of Heart Failure: Executive Summary: A Report of the American College of Cardiology Foundation/American Heart Association Task Force on Practice Guidelines. Circulation 128: 1810–1852.
2. Go AS, Mozaffarian D, Roger VL, Benjamin EJ, Berry JD, et al. (2013) Heart disease and stroke statistics–2013 update: a report from the American Heart Association. Circulation 127: e6–e245.
3. Stevenson LW, Hellkamp AS, Leier CV, Sopko G, Koelling T, et al. (2008) Changing preferences for survival after hospitalization with advanced heart failure. J Am Coll Cardiol 52: 1702–1708.
4. Dracup K, Walden JA, Stevenson LW, Brecht ML (1992) Quality of life in patients with advanced heart failure. J Heart Lung Transplant 11: 273–279.
5. Franciosa JA, Park M, Barry Levine T (1981) Lack of correlation between exercise capacity and indexes of resting left ventricular performance in heart failure. The American Journal of Cardiology 47: 33–39.
6. Higginbotham MB, Morris KG, Conn EH, Coleman RE, Cobb FR (1983) Determinants of variable exercise performance among patients with severe left ventricular dysfunction. The American Journal of Cardiology 51: 52–60.
7. Maskin CS, Forman R, Sonnenblick EH, Frishman WH, LeJemtel TH (1983) Failure of dobutamine to increase exercise capacity despite hemodynamic improvement in severe chronic heart failure. The American Journal of Cardiology 51: 177–182.
8. Middlekauff HR (2010) Making the Case for Skeletal Myopathy as the Major Limitation of Exercise Capacity in Heart Failure. Circulation: Heart Failure 3: 537–546.
9. Drexler H, Riede U, Munzel T, Konig H, Funke E, et al. (1992) Alterations of skeletal muscle in chronic heart failure. Circulation 85: 1751–1759.
10. Sullivan MJ, Green HJ, Cobb FR (1990) Skeletal muscle biochemistry and histology in ambulatory patients with long-term heart failure. Circulation 81: 518–527.
11. Wilson JR, Rayos G, Yeoh TK, Gothard P (1995) Dissociation between peak exercise oxygen consumption and hemodynamic dysfunction in potential heart transplant candidates. J Am Coll Cardiol 26: 429–435.
12. Mettauer B, Zoll J, Sanchez H, Lampert E, Ribera F, et al. (2001) Oxidative capacity of skeletal muscle in heart failure patients versus sedentary or active control subjects. Journal of the American College of Cardiology 38: 947–954.
13. Williams AD, Selig S, Hare DL, Hayes A, Krum H, et al. (2004) Reduced exercise tolerance in CHF may be related to factors other than impaired skeletal muscle oxidative capacity. J Card Fail 10: 141–148.
14. Middlekauff HR, Verity MA, Horwich TB, Fonarow GC, Hamilton MA, et al. (2013) Intact skeletal muscle mitochondrial enzyme activity but diminished exercise capacity in advanced heart failure patients on optimal medical and device therapy. Clin Res Cardiol 102: 547–554.
15. Middlekauff HR, Vigna C, Verity MA, Fonarow GC, Horwich TB, et al. (2012) Abnormalities of calcium handling proteins in skeletal muscle mirror those of the heart in humans with heart failure: a shared mechanism? J Card Fail 18: 724–733.
16. Rullman E, Andersson DC, Melin M, Reiken S, Mancini DM, et al. (2013) Modifications of skeletal muscle ryanodine receptor type 1 and exercise intolerance in heart failure. J Heart Lung Transplant 32: 925–929.
17. Bacurau AV, Jardim MA, Ferreira JC, Bechara LR, Bueno CR Jr, et al. (2009) Sympathetic hyperactivity differentially affects skeletal muscle mass in developing heart failure: role of exercise training. J Appl Physiol (1985) 106: 1631–1640.
18. Bueno CR Jr, Ferreira JC, Pereira MG, Bacurau AV, Brum PC (2010) Aerobic exercise training improves skeletal muscle function and Ca2+ handling-related protein expression in sympathetic hyperactivity-induced heart failure. J Appl Physiol (1985) 109: 702–709.
19. Lunde PK, Dahlstedt AJ, Bruton JD, Lannergren J, Thoren P, et al. (2001) Contraction and intracellular Ca(2+) handling in isolated skeletal muscle of rats with congestive heart failure. Circ Res 88: 1299–1305.
20. Lunde PK, Sejersted OM, Thorud HM, Tonnessen T, Henriksen UL, et al. (2006) Effects of congestive heart failure on Ca2+ handling in skeletal muscle during fatigue. Circ Res 98: 1514–1519.
21. Perreault CL, Gonzalez-Serratos H, Litwin SE, Sun X, Franzini-Armstrong C, et al. (1993) Alterations in contractility and intracellular Ca2+ transients in isolated bundles of skeletal muscle fibers from rats with chronic heart failure. Circ Res 73: 405–412.

22. Shah KR, Ganguly PK, Netticadan T, Arneja AS, Dhalla NS (2004) Changes in skeletal muscle SR Ca2+ pump in congestive heart failure due to myocardial infarction are prevented by angiotensin II blockade. Can J Physiol Pharmacol 82: 438–447.
23. Simonini A, Long CS, Dudley GA, Yue P, McElhinny J, et al. (1996) Heart failure in rats causes changes in skeletal muscle morphology and gene expression that are not explained by reduced activity. Circ Res 79: 128–136.
24. DiFranco M, Quinonez M, DiGregorio DA, Kim AM, Pacheco R, et al. (1999) Inverted double-gap isolation chamber for high-resolution calcium fluorimetry in skeletal muscle fibers. Pflugers Arch 438: 412–418.
25. Quinonez M, DiFranco M (2000) Novel inverted triple grease-gap isolation chamber for electrophysiological and calcium release studies in skeletal muscle fibers. Jpn J Physiol 50: 457–462.
26. Woods CE, Novo D, DiFranco M, Capote J, Vergara JL (2005) Propagation in the transverse tubular system and voltage dependence of calcium release in normal and mdx mouse muscle fibres. J Physiol 568: 867–880.
27. Woods CE, Novo D, DiFranco M, Vergara JL (2004) The action potential-evoked sarcoplasmic reticulum calcium release is impaired in mdx mouse muscle fibres. J Physiol 557: 59–75.
28. Capote J, DiFranco M, Vergara JL (2010) Excitation-contraction coupling alterations in mdx and utrophin/dystrophin double knockout mice: a comparative study. Am J Physiol Cell Physiol 298: C1077–1086.
29. DiFranco M, Woods CE, Capote J, Vergara JL (2008) Dystrophic skeletal muscle fibers display alterations at the level of calcium microdomains. Proc Natl Acad Sci U S A 105: 14698–14703.
30. Song LS, Sham JS, Stern MD, Lakatta EG, Cheng H (1998) Direct measurement of SR release flux by tracking 'Ca2+ spikes' in rat cardiac myocytes. J Physiol 512 (Pt 3): 677–691.
31. DiFranco M, Capote J, Vergara JL (2005) Optical imaging and functional characterization of the transverse tubular system of mammalian muscle fibers using the potentiometric indicator di-8-ANEPPS. J Membr Biol 208: 141–153.
32. DiFranco M, Novo D, Vergara JL (2002) Characterization of the calcium release domains during excitation-contraction coupling in skeletal muscle fibres. Pflugers Arch 443: 508–519.
33. Troosters T, Gosselink R, Decramer M (2004) Chronic obstructive pulmonary disease and chronic heart failure: two muscle diseases? J Cardiopulm Rehabil 24: 137–145.
34. Adams GR, Vaziri ND (2006) Skeletal muscle dysfunction in chronic renal failure: effects of exercise. Am J Physiol Renal Physiol 290: F753–761.
35. Ward CW, Reiken S, Marks AR, Marty I, Vassort G, et al. (2003) Defects in ryanodine receptor calcium release in skeletal muscle from post-myocardial infarct rats. FASEB J 17: 1517–1519.
36. Delbono O, O'Rourke KS, Ettinger WH (1995) Excitation-calcium release uncoupling in aged single human skeletal muscle fibers. J Membr Biol 148: 211–222.
37. Struk A, Lehmann-Horn F, Melzer W (1998) Voltage-dependent calcium release in human malignant hyperthermia muscle fibers. Biophys J 75: 2402–2410.
38. Desaphy JF, Pierno S, Leoty C, George AL Jr, De Luca A, et al. (2001) Skeletal muscle disuse induces fibre type-dependent enhancement of Na(+) channel expression. Brain 124: 1100–1113.
39. Rehn TA, Munkvik M, Lunde PK, Sjaastad I, Sejersted OM (2012) Intrinsic skeletal muscle alterations in chronic heart failure patients: a disease-specific myopathy or a result of deconditioning? Heart Fail Rev 17: 421–436.
40. Baylor SM, Hollingworth S (2012) Intracellular calcium movements during excitation-contraction coupling in mammalian slow-twitch and fast-twitch muscle fibers. J Gen Physiol 139: 261–272.
41. Schaufelberger M, Eriksson BO, Grimby G, Held P, Swedberg K (1997) Skeletal muscle alterations in patients with chronic heart failure. Eur Heart J 18: 971–980.
42. Ferguson DG, Franzini-Armstrong C (1988) The Ca2+ ATPase content of slow and fast twitch fibers of guinea pig. Muscle Nerve 11: 561–570.
43. Lamb GD, Walsh T (1987) Calcium currents, charge movement and dihydropyridine binding in fast- and slow-twitch muscles of rat and rabbit. J Physiol 393: 595–617.
44. Mancini DM, Coyle E, Coggan A, Beltz J, Ferraro N, et al. (1989) Contribution of intrinsic skeletal muscle changes to 31P NMR skeletal muscle metabolic abnormalities in patients with chronic heart failure. Circulation 80: 1338–1346.
45. Whellan DJ, Nigam A, Arnold M, Starr AZ, Hill J, et al. (2011) Benefit of exercise therapy for systolic heart failure in relation to disease severity and etiology-findings from the Heart Failure and A Controlled Trial Investigating Outcomes of Exercise Training study. Am Heart J 162: 1003–1010.

The Order of Exercise during Concurrent Training for Rehabilitation Does Not Alter Acute Genetic Expression, Mitochondrial Enzyme Activity or Improvements in Muscle Function

Lauren G. MacNeil[1], Elisa Glover[1], T. Graham Bergstra[2], Adeel Safdar[1], Mark A. Tarnopolsky[1,3]*

1 Department of Pediatrics, McMaster University, Hamilton, Ontario, Canada, **2** Department of Health Sciences, McMaster University, Hamilton, Ontario, Canada, **3** Department of Medicine, McMaster University, Hamilton, Ontario, Canada

Abstract

Concurrent exercise combines different modes of exercise (e.g., aerobic and resistance) into one training protocol, providing stimuli meant to increase muscle strength, aerobic capacity and mass. As disuse is associated with decrements in strength, aerobic capacity and muscle size concurrent training is an attractive modality for rehabilitation. However, interference between the signaling pathways may result in preferential improvements for one of the exercise modes. We recruited 18 young adults (10 ♂, 8 ♀) to determine if order of exercise mode during concurrent training would differentially affect gene expression, protein content and measures of strength and aerobic capacity after 2 weeks of knee-brace induced disuse. Concurrent exercise sessions were performed 3x/week for 6 weeks at gradually increasing intensities either with endurance exercise preceding (END>RES) or following (RES>END) resistance exercise. Biopsies were collected from the *vastus lateralis* before, 3 h after the first exercise bout and 48 h after the end of training. Concurrent exercise altered the expression of genes involved in mitochondrial biogenesis (PGC-1α, PRC, PPARγ), hypertrophy (PGC-1α4, REDD2, Rheb) and atrophy (MuRF-1, Runx1), increased electron transport chain complex protein content, citrate synthase and mitochondrial cytochrome *c* oxidase enzyme activity, muscle mass, maximum isometric strength and VO_{2peak}. However, the order in which exercise was completed (END>RES or RES>END) only affected the protein content of mitochondrial complex II subunit. In conclusion, concurrent exercise training is an effective modality for the rehabilitation of the loss of skeletal muscle mass, maximum strength, and peak aerobic capacity resulting from disuse, regardless of the order in which the modes of exercise are performed.

Editor: Guillermo López Lluch, Universidad Pablo de Olavide, Centro Andaluz de Biología del Desarrollo-CSIC, Spain

Funding: Financial support for this study was awarded to MT as a Collaborative Health Research Project from Canadian Institutes of Health Research and Natural Sciences and Engineering Research Council of Canada (CHRP 365655-2009). The funders had no role in study design, data collection and analysis, decision to publish, or preparation of the manuscript.

Competing Interests: The authors have declared that no competing interests exist.

* Email: tarnopol@mcmaster.ca

Introduction

Muscular adaptation to chronic exercise occurs to maintain cellular homeostasis during future bouts. Typically identified as one of two divergent modes, resistance or aerobic, exercise places stresses upon the myofibre that induce phenotypic changes that differ greatly between the modes. Through sets of low-repetition/high-intensity contractions, resistance exercise promotes hypertrophy and improves anaerobic energy supply, thereby increasing strength/short-term force generation [1,2]. Alternately, aerobic exercise is characterized by longer periods of high-repetition/low-intensity contractions that promote an increase in oxidative energy capacity, predominately through mitochondrial biogenesis and increased vascularization [3], improving fatigue resistance. However, these changes are not mutually exclusive as both modes modestly affect characteristics associated with the other [4–6]. It has been suggested that the adaptive processes may interfere with one another [7,8], thereby attenuating the optimal adaptation that could be achieved from either mode individually. As such, training strategies for maximum improvement for a specific physical task, such as sport performance, should be designed with one of these endpoints in mind. However, the desired benefits of exercise may include improvements in both strength and aerobic capacity. For example, rehabilitation of changes that occur in skeletal muscle following disuse atrophy [9–11] and mitigation of the effects of aging [12,13] may require exercise programs utilizing both modes of muscle contraction.

Disuse atrophy is the loss of skeletal muscle mass following a reduction or cessation in physical activity that can be the result of factors such as illness, injury, aging, or lifestyle change. Typically, hypodynamia results in a loss of muscle mass [14–17], muscle function [14–17], and aerobic capacity [17,18]. Incorporating resistance exercise as a clinical recovery strategy is logical to recover lost muscle mass and strength, whilst aerobic exercise may be beneficial to recover aerobic capacity. Combining both modes of exercise into one program is termed concurrent training. Research into the effects of concurrent training as a method of improving both strength and endurance performance are equivocal. Some studies have found that aerobic exercise attenuates the increases in strength [2,19,20], hypertrophy [2,20] and power [2,19] that occur with resistance training alone, potentially by the attenuation of signaling through the Akt-mTOR-S6K cascade by interference from AMPK-PGC-1α signaling [21]. However, others have found equal improvements in strength with concurrent training [22–24]. The effect of concurrent training on improvements in aerobic capacity when compared to aerobic exercise alone seem to indicate that VO_2max is unaffected by competing adaptations [25] and may even be beneficial through increased proportions of type IIa fibres [26].

Concurrent training programs are rarely compared for the effect of the order in which the exercise modes are performed. Results from Coffey et al. suggest that the order in which exercise modes are performed may result in divergent adaption during concurrent training [27]. Following up on these findings, we sought to test whether altering the order of exercise would affect the early gene expression patterns and resulting strength and aerobic capacity changes as part of a rehabilitation strategy.

Materials and Methods

Subjects and anthropometrics

Eighteen young healthy adults (10 men and 8 women) volunteered as participants in this study. All subjects were screened to ensure they had no pre-existing health conditions and they had not regularly participated in resistance or endurance exercise in the preceding 6 months. Menstrual cycle and oral contraceptive use was not controlled in this study; as such all findings represent general responses to disuse in women. Whole body and body compartment composition and were measured using dual energy x-ray absorptiometry (DXA) scans (Lunar Prodigy Advance, GE Healthcare, Madison, WI). The study subject's demographics were (mean ± SD): age −20±2 y; height −171±10 cm; weight −70.2±16.9 kg, BMI −24.0±5.2.

Ethics statement

Each participant was given an information sheet and all of the testing procedures were explained to them before providing written informed consent. The study conformed to the standards outlined in the *Declaration of Helsinki* and was given approval by the Research Ethics Board at McMaster University (REB #09-322).

Study design

Immediately before beginning this study, all participants had completed 2-weeks of single leg knee joint immobilization with the use of a Rehab post-op knee brace (Össur Americas, Foothill Ranch, CA) that was restricted to 90° knee flexion. Participants returned to the lab daily to have the brace removed, at which time the leg was inspected for pain or edema and were allowed to shower without bearing weight on the treatment leg. The brace was replaced, taped and a unique identifier was used to ensure that knee braces were not removed. Walking crutches were provided to assist with mobility. This protocol has been used previously to induce disuse muscle atrophy and loss of strength [15,17,28,29].

Participants were then randomly assigned to one of two concurrent exercise groups: resistance exercise first followed immediately by endurance exercise (RES>END, N = 9) or endurance exercise first followed immediately by resistance exercise (END>RES, N = 9). Peak aerobic capacity (VO_{2peak}), maximum isometric strength and maximum strength (1RM) were tested before immobilization to determine baseline aerobic fitness and strength and to calculate initial rehabilitation exercise values.

VO_{2peak} was measured using a graded incremental cycling test and an Excalibur Sport cycle ergometer (Lode, Groningen, the Netherlands). Following a 5-minute cycling warm up with light resistance, participants began the test at a workload of 50 W and increased by 50 W (men) or 30 W (women) every 2 minutes either until volitional fatigue, defined as the inability to maintain a pedaling frequency above 60 rpm for longer than 5 seconds. Verbal encouragement was provided as participants approached test completion. Heart rate (bpm) and oxygen consumption (L/min) were monitored with a MOXUS modular metabolic system (AEI Technologies, Pittsburg, PA).

Maximum isometric strength of the knee extensors was measured with a System 3 dynamometer (Biodex Medical Systems, Shirley, NY). Participants were seated in the dynamometer, with their knee flexed at 90°, and secured across the thigh, calf, lap and trunk to prevent extraneous movements. All were instructed to maximally contract their knee extensors for 5 seconds. Isometric strength was measured 3 times with a 30 s rest period between each repetition; the highest value (Nm) was recorded for each leg.

1RM was measured as the maximum amount of weight that could be successfully moved through complete range of motion once only for three leg exercises: leg press, knee extension and knee flexion. For each exercise, a brief warm up of 5 repetitions using a submaximal weight and a 1 minute rest was performed before participants attempted 3 repetitions of a weight estimated to be ~80% of maximum. Weights were increased and single repetitions attempted until movement through the complete range of motion was not possible. The heaviest successful repetition was designated as the 1RM.

Acute Exercise protocol

Relative exercise intensities and duration were identical between the END>RES and RES>END groups; the only exception between them was the order in which the exercises were performed. Depending on their assigned group participants began with either 22.5 minutes of stationary cycling at 65% VO_{2peak} or 3×10 repetitions of leg press, knee flexion and knee extension at 65% 1RM and immediately transferred to the opposite protocol. The resistance exercise protocol had a 1 minute rest between sets and exercises and was completed in approximately 22 minutes, resulting in a total exercise time of ~45 minutes.

Rehabilitative Exercise protocol

Participants completed three exercise sessions per week with at least one rest day between sessions. Following the acute exercise protocol, two more identical sessions completed the first training week. Aerobic exercise intensity increased by 5% every two weeks to 70% and 75% of VO_{2peak}; exercise duration remained constant at 22.5 minutes. Resistance exercise intensity increased to 70% 1RM for the second week. Maximum strength was retested every two weeks to ensure the progression over the course of the study matched the participant's rate of strength change. Weeks three and four had intensities of 70% and 75% of the second 1RM test; weeks five and six were 75% and 80% of the third 1RM test (Figure 1).

A muscle biopsy of the *vastus lateralis* was taken under local anesthesia (2% lidocane) using a modified Bergström needle with manual suction from the experimental leg following 2 weeks

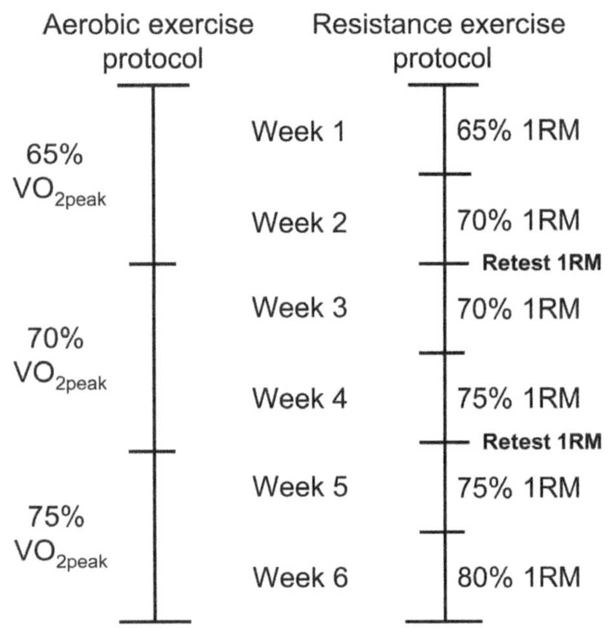

Figure 1. Concurrent exercise program design with weekly intensities for aerobic and resistance exercise protocols.

immobilization (Pre-exercise), 3 hours after the first bout of concurrent exercise (3H) and following 6 weeks of rehabilitative concurrent exercise (Post) (Figure 2). Immediately following excision, the muscle biopsy was dissected free of connective tissue and fat, sectioned into 25–50 mg pieces, placed into 1.5 mL Eppendorff tubes and frozen in liquid nitrogen. Muscle samples were stored at −80°C until processing and analysis. Immediately following each muscle biopsy, blood was collected in BD Vacutainer collection tubes for serum and K_2EDTA plasma from the antecubital vein and treated following manufacturer's specifications. Tubes were centrifuged and the supernatant aliquoted and stored at −20°C for future analyses.

RNA extraction

Total RNA was extracted from skeletal muscle as follows. Muscle tissue (~25 mg) was homogenized using an electric homogenizer (Pro Scientific) in 1 mL of Trizol Reagent (Life Technologies, Cat. No. 15596, Gaithersburg, MD). The homogenate was then incubated for 10 min at room temperature, followed by phase separation using 200 µL of chloroform and precipitation of the total RNA from the aqueous phase using 380 µL of anhydrous ethanol. The RNA was then isolated using Qiagen RNeasy Mini Kits according to manufacturer's instructions, eluted with RNase free water, aliquoted, and stored at −80°C. The concentration and purity of the RNA was determined using a Nanodrop UV-vis spectrophotometer (ND 1000; Thermo Scientific, Wilmington, DE) at 260 and 280 nm. The average purity (OD_{260}/OD_{280}) of the samples was >1.7. Prior to elution, isolated RNA was treated with DNA-free recombinant DNase I (Ambion Inc, Austin, TX) according to the manufacturer's instructions to remove any potential genomic DNA contamination.

qPCR analysis

Changes in gene expression relative to baseline values were measured using quantitative real-time polymerase chain reaction (qPCR). Following confirmation of stable expression at all time points, 18S rRNA was used as the housekeeping gene. The efficiencies of all primers were tested and determined to be greater than 98%. The primer sequences can be found in Table 1.

qPCR was performed using PerfeCta SYBR Green SuperMix, ROX (Quanta BioSciences, Gaithersburg, MD). The primers to each target gene were designed using cDNA sequences in GenBank (http://www.ncbi.nlm.nih.gov/sites/entrez/?db=gene) and primer 3 designer (http://frodo.wi.mit.edu/primer3-0.4.0/input.htm). qPCR was performed on an Applied Biosystems 7300 PCR system (Bio-Rad Laboratories, Hercules, CA). The genes of interest were normalized to the housekeeping gene following the standard method: C_T values of the housekeeping gene were subtracted from the C_T values of the gene of interest (ΔC_T) and normalized to baseline ($\Delta\Delta C_T$). All samples were run in duplicate and C_T was automatically calculated.

Tissue preparation

Total protein was isolated from skeletal muscle tissue samples using an electric homogenizer in 20 µL of 0.05 M KPO_4 buffer (5 mM EDTA, 0.5 mM DTT, 1.15% KCl (w/v)) per milligram of tissue. A protease inhibitor cocktail (Sigma, St. Louis, Missouri) was dissolved in buffer immediately prior to homogenization at a ratio of 1 tablet per 10 mL buffer. Samples were centrifuged at 600 *g* for 10 min at 4°C and the supernatant aliquoted and stored at −80°C. Total protein concentrations were determined using a bicinchoninic acid (BCA) assay (Pierce Biotechnology, Rockford, IL) following manufacturer's instructions and absorbance measured with a plate spectrophotometer (Bio-Rad Laboratories, Hercules, CA).

Western blotting

Proteins were separated on SDS-polyacrylamide gels, transferred to Hybond ECL nitrocellulose membrane (Amersham Biosciences, Piscataway, NJ) and blocked with either 5% BSA (w/v) or 2% milk protein in Tris-buffered saline with 0.1% Tween (vol/vol) (TBST). The following commercially available primary antibodies were used: MitoProfile Total OXPHOS Human Cocktail (abcam, Cambridge, MA; ab110411, 1:1000); Atrogin-1 (abcam; ab67866, 1:1000); MURF1 (abcam; ab96857, 1:1000); total ubiquitin (Santa Cruz Biotechnology, Dallas, TX; sc-8017, 1:1000); NEDD4 (abcam; ab14592, 1:1000). After washing in TBST, membranes were incubated in either HRP-linked anti-

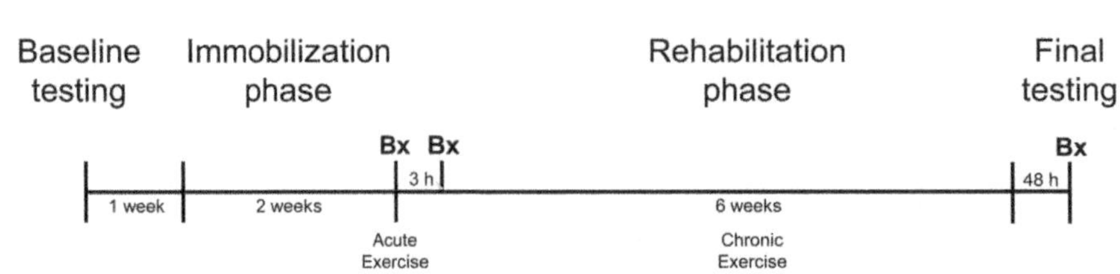

Figure 2. Longitudinal study design. (Bx) - Timing of muscle biopsy.

Table 1. Primer design.

Gene name	Forward primer	Reverse Primer
18S rRNA	CGGTAATTCCAGCTCCAATAG	CGCTCCCAAGATCCAACTAC
PGC-1α	CATCAAAGAAGCCCAGGTACA	GGACTTGCTGAGTTGTGCATAC
PGC-1β	CCTGTTTATGCCTCCCTCAC	GGTGAAGCTGCGATCCTTAC
PGC-1α4	TCACACCAAACCCACAGAGA	CTGGAAGATATGGCACA
PPARγ	AGAAGCTGTTGGCGGAGAT	CAGCGGGAAGGACTTTATGTA
PRC	CCTACCAAGGTGGAGGTCAA	AGCCTTCATCTGGGGACTTT
REDD1	AGTGCCCTCCAAGACAGAGA	TTAGGTGGCTGCCTCAGTTT
REDD2	GTTCCTGAACCCAACCTCAA	AAGGACCTTTGAGCAACCAA
Rheb	TAGCTCGATGTCCGTGTCA	CAGGCAAGGCTGTTCTCAAT
Atrogin-1	AGCTGGATTGGAAGAAGATGTA	TTTGCAGAGCTGAAGGGTATC
MuRF-1	TCCATGTGCAAGGTGTTTG	GCCACCAGCATGGAGATAC
Nedd4	CAAGGATGAGCACCAGGTATAG	ATGAGGGTGGGCATGATTAC
Runx1	TCAGAGTCAGATGCAGGATACA	ATCCCAGGTATTGGTAGGACTG

rabbit or anti-mouse IgG secondary antibody (Amersham Biosciences), washed with TBST and developed using ECL (Amersham Biosciences; model no. RPN2106). Membranes were exposed to x-ray film (Biomax XAR; Kodak, Rochester, New York). Films were then scanned with a Dell 920 scanner (North York, ON, Canada) at 300 DPI and saved in TIFF file format. Using Image J v1.40g software (National Institutes of Health, Bethesda, Maryland), background noise was removed and bands in the region of interest were selected for analysis. Individual profile plots were generated and area under the curve measured in arbitrary units (AU). All proteins were normalized for gel loading using Ponceau S.

Enzyme activity

Maximal enzyme activities were measured with a Cary Bio-300 UV-Vis spectrophotometer (Varian, Inc., Palo Alto, CA). Enzyme activities are expressed as IU · mg of protein^{-1}.

Citrate synthase (CS). Activity was measured by mixing 830 µL Tris buffer (0.1M, pH 8.0, 37°C), 100 µL of DTNB (0.5 mg/mL Tris buffer), 10 µL of Acetyl CoA (6.25 mg/mL Tris Buffer) and 10 µL muscle homogenate in 1.5 mL reference and measurement cuvettes. Cuvettes were placed in spectrophotometer (37°C) and the reaction was started by adding 50 µL of oxaloacetic acid (1.22 mg/mL Tris buffer) to the measurement cuvette only, mixing thoroughly. Absorbance was continuously recorded for 2 minutes at 412 nm and the enzyme activity calculated. Activity was normalized to protein content.

Cytochrome c oxidase (COX). Activity was measured by mixing 970 µL KPO_4 buffer (0.05 M, pH 7.4, 37°C) and 10 µL reduced cytochrome *c* (24 mg/mL KPO_4 buffer) in 1.5 mL reference and measurement cuvettes. Cuvettes were placed in spectrophotometer (37°C) and the reaction was started by adding 20 µL of muscle homogenate to the measurement cuvette only, mixing thoroughly. Absorbance was continuously recorded for 2 minutes at 550 nm and the enzyme activity calculated. Activity was normalized to protein content.

Statistical Analysis

Student's paired t-tests were used to test for differences at baseline for age, height, weight, BMI, body fat percentage, lean body mass, bone mineral content, isometric strength and VO_{2peak} between END>RES and RES>END groups. Two-way repeated measures ANOVAs (group×time) were used to assess if protein levels, enzyme activities, experimental leg mass, isometric strength, aerobic capacity and the linear $2^{-\Delta\Delta CT}$ data sets for gene expression were statistically different. All analyses were completed using STATISTICA for Windows 5.0 (Statsoft, Tulsa, OK); the threshold for significance was set at $P \leq 0.05$. If statistical significance was achieved, Tukey's honestly significant difference (HSD) post-hoc test was used to determine the significance among the means. All data are presented as mean ± SD.

Results

Baseline measurements

There were no differences in average participant age, height, weight, BMI, body fat percentage, lean body mass, bone mineral content, maximum isometric strength (experimental and control leg) or VO_{2peak} between the END>RES and RES>END groups at baseline (BL) (Table 2).

Gene expression changes following acute concurrent exercise

The following genes were measured for their role in aerobic adaptation as regulators of mitochondrial biogenesis: peroxisome proliferative activated receptor (PPAR) gamma coactivator-1α (PGC-1 α), PGC-1β, PPARγ and PGC-1-related coactivator (PRC) (Figure 3A). PGC-1α had the greatest response to acute exercise, increasing its expression level more than 10-fold at 3H. Although not as strongly induced, PRC was increased by almost 570%. Acute PGC-1β expression was not different from pre-exercise level. Only one gene, PPARγ, was expressed at a lower level after acute exercise. The order of exercise did not differentially affect gene expression levels as P values for interactions between group and time ranged between 0.2 and 0.87.

To determine whether concurrent exercise affected mRNA involved in hypertrophy, the following genes were measured as they have been described as regulators of Akt/mTOR pathway signaling (Ras homolog enriched in brain (Rheb), regulated in DNA damage 1 (REDD1) and 2 (REDD2)) and expression of IGF1 and myostatin (PGC-1α, isoform 4 (PGC-1α4)). Acute

Table 2. Subject characteristics before interventions.

	Res-End	End-Res	P value
Age (y)	19±1.3	20±1.6	0.40
Height (cm)	174.2±10.3	168.0±8.6	0.17
Weight (kg)	67.4±16.5	71.4±17.4	0.62
BMI (kg/m^2)	21.9±2.8	25.4±6.2	0.14
Body fat (%)	24.4±11.2	30.8±12.6	0.74
Lean body mass (kg)	45.9±10.8	44.5±10.1	0.77
Bone mineral content (g)	24.4±11.2	24.4±11.2	0.62
Experimental Leg Maximum Isometric Strength (Nm)	212.6±78.9	238.4±76.7	0.49
Control Leg Maximum Isometric Strength (Nm)	229.4±80.9	248.1±76.5	0.62
VO_{2peak} (ml/kg/min)	39.2±7.4	38.7±6.1	0.88
Males (N)	5	5	
Females (N)	4	4	

Mean ± SD.

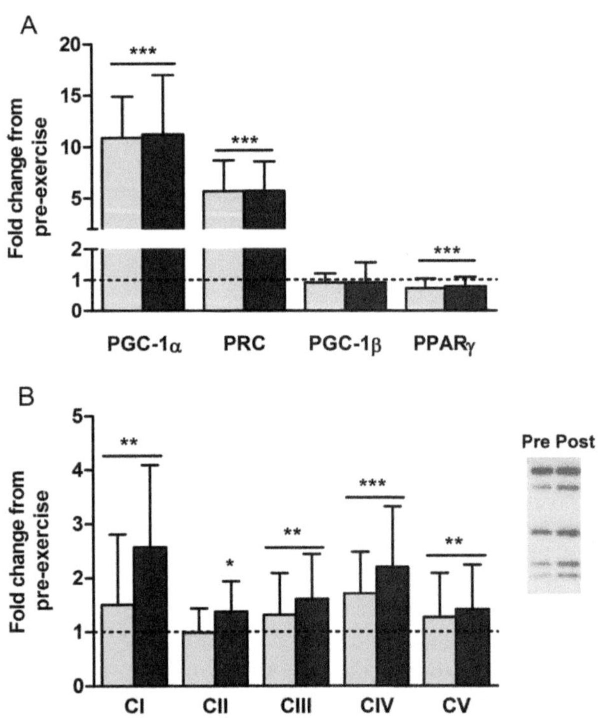

Figure 3. Concurrent exercise alters mRNA content of genes involved in mitochondrial biogenesis and metabolism and increases protein content of subunits of the ETC. A - Gene expression changes in skeletal muscle 3 hours after concurrent rehabilitative exercise for genes involved in aerobic exercise adaption. Peroxisome proliferative activated receptor (PPAR) gamma coactivator-1α (PGC-1α), PGC-1-related coactivator (PRC), PGC-1β, and PPARγ. B - Fold changes in protein content from pre-exercise for subunits of the 5 complexes of the ETC (CI-CV) following 6 weeks of concurrent rehabilitative exercise. Light bars indicate END>RES group, dark bars indicate RES>END group. Representative western blotting image for pre-exercise and post included. *Significant difference from baseline ($P<0.05$). **Significant difference from baseline ($P<0.01$). ***Significant difference from baseline ($P<0.001$). Bar indicates main effect for time and not exercise group. Mean ± SD.

concurrent exercise affected each Akt/mTOR regulator gene differently: REDD1 content was unchanged, REDD2 content was lower, and RheB content was higher. PGC-1α4 had the greatest response to acute exercise, increasing its expression level more than 10-fold at 3H (Figure 4). Order of exercise did not affect gene expression levels as P values for the interaction between group and time for each was greater than 0.77.

The genes selected as regulators of protein degradation either induce (Atrogin-1, muscle-specific RING finger-1 (MuRF-1), neural precursor cell expressed developmentally downregulated protein 4 (Nedd4)) or attenuate (Runt-related transcription factor 1 (Runx1)) skeletal muscle atrophy. There was no difference in the levels of Atrogin-1 and Nedd4 mRNA 3 hours after exercise (Figure 5A). MuRF-1 and Runx1 were both strongly induced by exercise, increasing to more than 500 and 700% of baseline levels

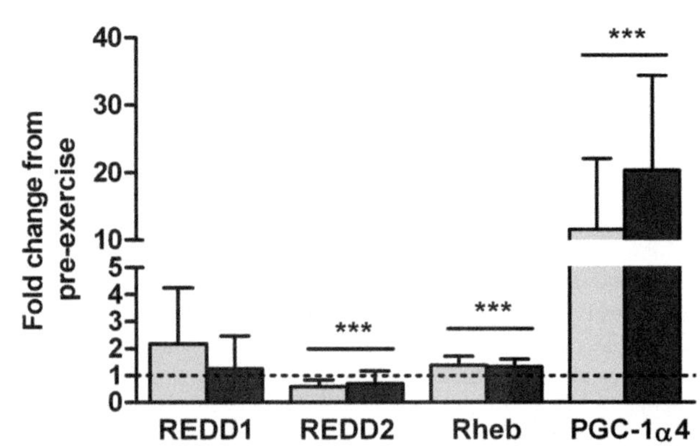

Figure 4. Concurrent exercise alters mRNA content of genes involved in the regulation of mTOR signaling, and proposed IGF-1 and myostatin gene expression. Gene expression changes in skeletal muscle 3 hours after concurrent rehabilitative exercise for genes involved in resistance exercise adaption. Light bars indicate END>RES group, dark bars indicate RES>END group. Regulated in DNA damage 1 (REDD1) and 2 (REDD2), Ras homolog enriched in brain (Rheb), and peroxisome proliferative activated receptor (PPAR) gamma coactivator-1α, isoform 4 (PGC-1α4), ***Significant difference from baseline ($P<0.001$). Bar indicates main effect for time and not exercise group. Mean ± SD.

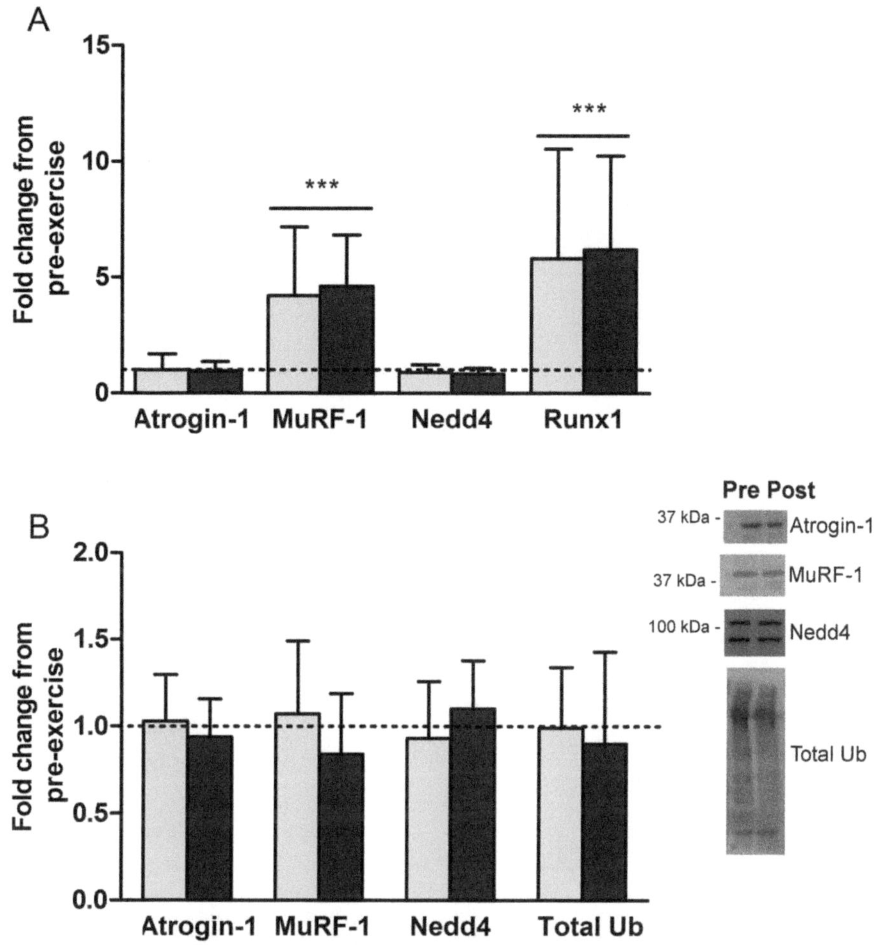

Figure 5. Concurrent exercise acutely increases mRNA content of genes involved in the regulation of muscle atrophy but does not affect chronic protein content of selected E3 ligases or total ubiquitination. A - Gene expression changes in skeletal muscle 3 hours after concurrent rehabilitative exercise for genes involved in regulation of protein breakdown. Atrogin-1, muscle-specific RING finger-1 (MuRF-1), neural precursor cell expressed developmentally downregulated protein 4 (Nedd4), and Runt-related transcription factor 1 (Runx1). B - Fold changes in protein content from pre-exercise levels for muscle specific (Atrogin-1 and MuRF-1) and ubiquitously expressed (Nedd4) E3 ligases, and total ubiquitination (Total Ub) following 6 weeks of concurrent rehabilitative exercise. Light bars indicate END>RES group, dark bars indicate RES>END group. Representative western blotting images for pre-exercise and post included. ***Significant difference from baseline ($P<0.001$). Bar indicates main effect for time and not exercise group. Mean ± SD.

respectively. Again, order of exercise did not affect gene expression levels as the P value for the interaction between group and time was greater than 0.6 for all.

Protein expression changes following 6-weeks of rehabilitative concurrent exercise

Protein content of subunits of complexes I to V (CI –CV) of the electron transport chain (ETC) were measured upon completion of the 6 week rehabilitative exercise program and expressed relative to pre-exercise values. Although there was a main effect for increased protein content with time for all five complexes, CII was the only complex significantly different between the exercise protocols with RES>END higher than END>RES ($P = 0.037$) (Figure 3B).

Protein content of the muscle specific E3 ligases Atrogin-1 and MuRF-1, the ubiquitously expressed E3 ligase Nedd4 and total ubiquitination were measured after rehabilitative exercise. None were different from baseline nor were any differentially affected by order of concurrent exercise (Figure 5B).

Effect of concurrent exercise on mitochondrial enzyme activity

CS and COX maximal activities were 61% ($P<0.001$) and 51% ($P = 0.002$) higher after 6 weeks of concurrent exercise, respectively (Figure 6A and 6B). The COX/CS ratio was unaffected by the exercise protocol (Figure 6C). Order of concurrent exercise did not affect any of the measurements or calculations.

Performance changes after rehabilitative concurrent exercise

Following 6 weeks of rehabilitative exercise, maximum isometric strength of the knee extensors of the immobilized leg increased by 35% from pre-exercise values ($P<0.001$) regaining the strength lost by immobilization (Figure 7A). Maximum isometric strength of the control leg was unchanged over the course of the study (results not shown). Peak aerobic capacity significantly increased by 9% between the baseline measures taken before immobilization and after rehabilitative exercise ($P = 0.006$) (Figure 7B). The order

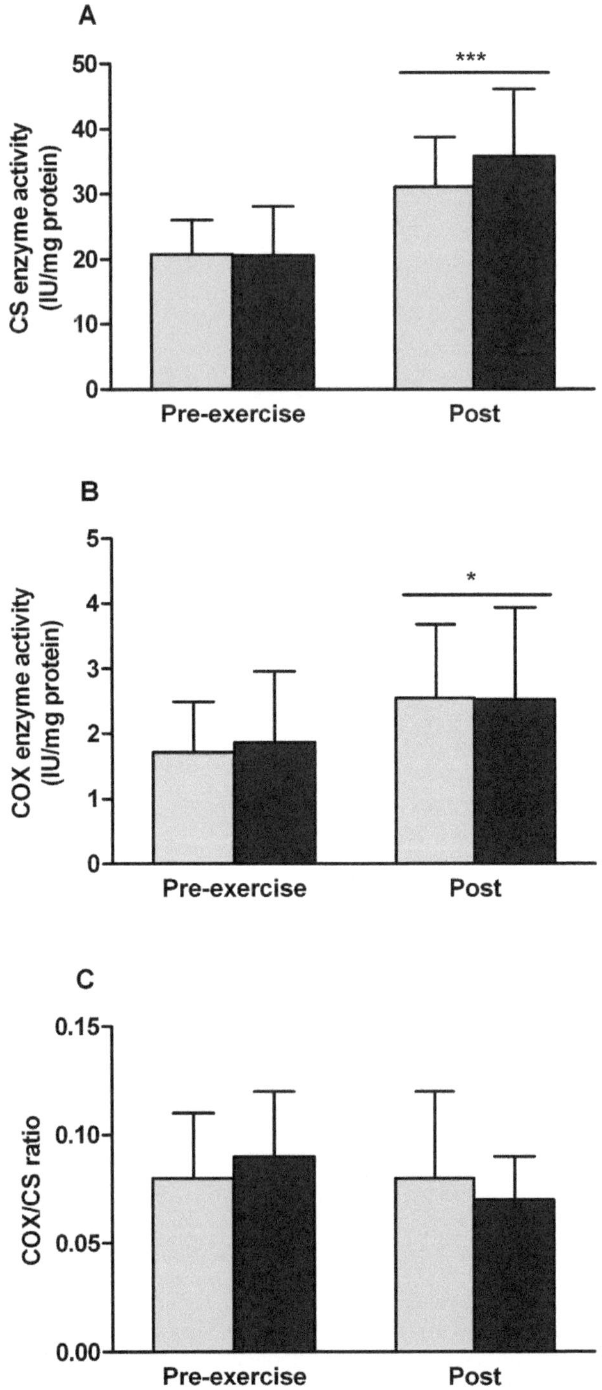

Figure 6. Concurrent exercise increases mitochondrial enzyme activity. Enzyme activities in skeletal muscle before (Pre-exercise) and after 6 weeks of concurrent rehabilitative exercise (Post). A - citrate synthase (CS), B - cytochrome *c* oxidase (COX) and C – COX/CS ratio. Light bars indicate END>RES group, dark bars indicate RES>END group. *Significant difference from baseline ($P<0.05$). ***Significant difference from baseline ($P<0.001$). Bar indicates main effect for time and not exercise group. Mean ± SD.

of concurrent exercise did not affect the increases measured in either maximum isometric strength or VO_{2peak}.

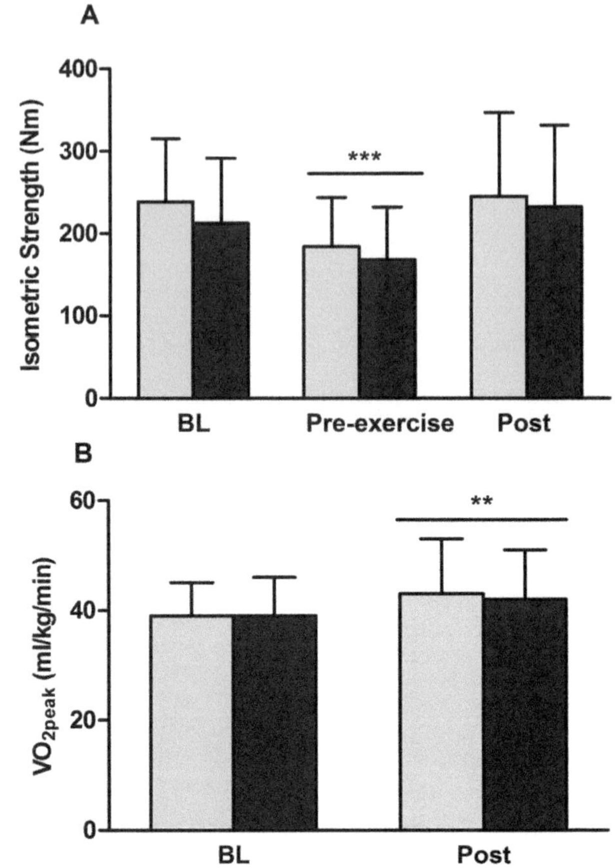

Figure 7. Concurrent exercise recovers maximum isometric strength loss induced by disuse and increases aerobic performance. A - Values for maximum isometric strength of the knee extensors before immobilization (BL), before exercise (pre-exercise) and after 6 weeks of rehabilitative concurrent exercise (Post). B - peak oxygen consumption (VO_{2peak}) before immobilization (BL) and after 6 weeks of concurrent exercise (Post). Light bars indicate END>RES group, dark bars indicate RES>END group. **Significant difference from baseline ($P<0.01$). ***Significant difference from baseline ($P<0.001$). Bar indicates main effect for time and not exercise group. Mean ± SD.

Muscle mass changes after rehabilitative concurrent exercise

Two weeks of immobilization significantly reduced the mass of the experimental leg from 8.6 kg to 8.4 kg ($P = 0.04$). Six weeks of concurrent exercise increased the leg mass, surpassing the amount of tissue lost by disuse by 0.3 kg to reach 8.9 kg ($P<0.001$).

Discussion

Resistance and aerobic exercises are rehabilitation therapies used to regain losses in strength and aerobic capacity that typically occur during injury, illness or chronic disuse of skeletal muscle. Performing these exercises together in the same session as concurrent exercise typically increases both strength and aerobic function; however, some research suggests that interference in the signaling patterns for adaptation favor one phenotypic outcome, depending on the order in which the exercise modes are performed [27,30]. As such, we examined the effects of alternating the order of exercise in concurrent training protocols as a rehabilitation strategy for preferentially improving strength or aerobic capacity following 2 weeks of induced hypodynamia.

Contrary to our hypothesis we did not find differences in the gene expression patterns, most protein content changes, and the increases in isometric strength or peak aerobic capacity between groups that completed concurrent exercise protocols in which the first mode was either endurance exercise or resistance exercise.

Concurrent exercise is an effective and efficient method of reversing losses in strength and aerobic capacity that may result from prolonged skeletal muscle disuse. Regardless of the order in which the exercise modes are performed, we observed almost identical improvements in both maximum isometric strength and VO_{2peak} after 6 weeks of rehabilitative concurrent exercise. A meta-analysis of 21 studies examining concurrent training and the interferences between aerobic and resistance exercise concluded that concurrent training provides similar respective increases in strength and VO_{2max} as those found with resistance and aerobic exercise alone [25]. They reported that the mean overall effect size (ES) for increasing strength using resistance training alone (ES = 1.76, 95% CI: 1.34, 2.18) was not significantly different from concurrent exercise (ES = 1.44, 95% CI: 1.03, 1.84) [25]. Similarly, the improvements in VO_{2max} following either endurance only or as part of a concurrent training model were almost identical; 1.37 (95% CI: 0.85, 1.88) and 1.41 (95% CI: 0.93, 2.95) respectively [25]. Although it we do not know whether greater gains in either metric could have been achieved by focusing on one exercise mode only for rehabilitation, we did not observe preferential adaptation based on the order of the exercises performed.

As highlighted by the above meta-analysis, many studies have compared the outcome metrics and signaling patterns following concurrent and single mode exercise protocol. However, none have tested the benefits of concurrent exercise as a mechanism for muscle rehabilitation following disuse atrophy. Additionally, studies examining if outcome measures are affected by the order in which the modes of exercise are performed during a concurrent exercise session are limited. Two studies that were found used trained males in 2 week crossover study designs to compare acute gene expression and protein signaling after single mode and concurrent exercise [27,30]; the primary difference between them being that one used maximum sprint intervals (10×6 s) [30] and the other submaximal cycling (30 min @ 70% VO_{2max}) [27]. They reported a greater increase in MuRF-1 mRNA content when resistance exercise was performed before both endurance or sprint exercise [27,30], a greater increase in insulin-like growth factor-1 (IGF-1) and hexokinase II (HKII) mRNA when resistance exercise preceded endurance exercise [27] and attenuated expression of a regulator of mitochondrial biogenesis (PGC-1α) when resistance exercise preceded sprint but not endurance exercise [27,30]. These results led the authors to conclude that the acute response to concurrent exercise is affected by the order in which the exercises are performed [27,30]. We, however, did not find differential expression patterns in any of the genes we selected, including MuRF-1 or PGC-1α, although both were induced by concurrent exercise. Reasons for the different results may be due to differences in exercise protocols, timing of exercise and biopsies, or training status (detrained vs. well-trained) of the individuals at the time of testing. However, our conclusion that order of exercise did not affect mRNA content of any of the genes we measured agrees with the similar improvements in outcome performance metrics between RES>END and END>RES groups.

We also sought to determine whether altering the order of exercise had an effect on other genes involved in mitochondrial biogenesis. Originally identified for its role in oxidative metabolism in brown adipose tissue, PGC-1α translocates to the nucleus and mitochondria of skeletal muscle following exercise to induce the transcription of nuclear and mitochondrial DNA-encoded mitochondrial genes [31,32]. Two additional coactivators of mitochondrial biogenesis are PRC [33] and PGC-1β [34]. Acting in a similar manner to PGC-1α, PRC expression is increased with endurance exercise [35,36] and enhanced when performed concurrently with resistance exercise [37]. To the contrary, chronic endurance exercise appears to attenuate resting PGC-1β protein content [38] though acute exercise does not affect mRNA values [39]. PPARγ, although not abundantly expressed in skeletal muscle, is a regulator of insulin signaling and metabolism as it promotes molecular storage of energy [40,41]. Elevated muscle PPARγ mRNA expression has been measured with obesity and type II diabetes and is thought to negatively affect insulin resistance [42]. Taken together, the expression changes of PGC-1α, PRC, and PPARγ all support a modification to the transcriptome to increase mitochondrial content and function after concurrent exercise. In support of this, we measured higher protein content of all five complexes of the electron transport chain, higher CS and COX enzyme activity and higher VO_{2peak} at the end of training. Although statistical analyses reported similar increases in VO_{2peak}, CS enzyme activity, COX enzyme activity, and 4 of the 5 ETC complexes between RES>END and END>RES groups, there may be trend for greater protein content of the ETC complexes and CS enzyme activity when resistance exercise followed endurance. Further work is needed to determine if this would become significant at different time points or using different exercise intensities and modes.

A major regulator of the protein synthesis associated with hypertrophy is the protein kinase, mammalian target of rapamycin (mTOR) [43–45]. Once activated, mTOR phosphorylates substrates involved in the translation of mRNA for protein accretion [45,46]. Activation and regulation of mTOR occurs in response to many stimuli that include but are not limited to growth factors, nutrients, cellular stress and a number of small proteins [45]. Rheb is a small GTPase that positively regulates mTOR [43,45,47] while REDD1 and REDD2 negatively regulate mTOR [45,47–49]. The lack of change in REDD1 mRNA expression, reduced REDD2 expression and increased Rheb expression suggest a coordinate response for positive regulation of mTOR signaling by concurrent exercise, that was unaffected by order in which the modes of exercise were performed. The specific actions of PGC-1α4, a recently identified isoform of PGC-1α, remain to be well-defined. This splice variant was first described as important in the adaptation to strengthening exercise rather than aerobic exercise as its target genes were important for hypertrophy (IGF-1 and myostatin), and was stimulated by resistance not endurance exercise [32]. However, subsequent work has not supported this unique response as both PGC1α and PGC1α4 can be induced by either resistance or endurance exercise separately [50,51]. Our data suggests that PGC-1α4 can be highly upregulated immediately following concurrent exercise and unaffected by order of exercise mode. Together, these early gene responses are supported by the increased strength and lean tissue mass following rehabilitation that was not different between RES>END and END>RES groups.

The ubiquitin proteasome pathway is the primary cellular mechanism for protein breakdown [52]. Targeting of specific proteins for degradation by the proteasome is achieved through binding of the chains of the regulatory protein ubiquitin (polyubiquitination) by E3 ligases [53]. Muscle contains two specific E3 ligases, Atrogin-1 and MuRF-1, whose gene expression levels are higher following unweighting and immobilization in humans [53–55]. Additionally, as part of the breakdown initiated as part of the remodeling process [56,57], expression of both of these genes may be increased following unaccustomed resistance exercise [58,59]. Unlike the muscle specific expression of Atrogin-1 and MuRF-1, Nedd4 is a ubiquitously expressed E3 ligase that is also upregulated in muscle following unloading and denervation in rodents [60,61] and human patients with severe COPD [62]. Negative regulation of skeletal muscle atrophy is also necessary to conserve muscle mass in times of disuse [63,64]. One of the first autophagy suppressors described was Runx1 [63]. Although the exact mechanism for its suppression is unclear, it may be through the modulation of FoxO3 [65], a mediator of Atrogin-1 and MuRF-1 mRNA expression [66]. Our results indicate that MuRF-1 and Runx1 were highly induced by concurrent exercise following immobilization. As positive and negative regulators of autophagy, the ultimate outcome of their signaling is unknown, although the increase in muscle mass suggests that they may have regulated muscle remodeling. The lack of change in Atrogin-1 and Nedd4 content at 3H may have been a result of the time selected for measurement, or induction following immobilization may not have been possible. Protein levels of Atrogin-1, MuRF-1, Nedd4 and total ubiquitination were not different when measured after 6 weeks of rehabilitative exercise, likely because the muscle had habituated to the exercise regime and muscle protein synthesis superseded breakdown to aid in hypertrophy. None of our measurements of markers of autophagy were affected by the order of exercises performed, suggesting that alternating concurrent exercises may affect autophagy similarly when used as a modality for rehabilitation.

Conclusion

Concurrent exercise is an effective and efficient rehabilitation protocol for regaining lost strength and muscle mass associated with prolonged disuse. When performed immediately after one another, the order of exercise does not differentially influence the chronic mitochondrial enzyme activities changes or increases in maximum strength or aerobic capacity. Although the genes and most proteins we selected were not different between groups, adaptation to multimode exercise involves coordination of a myriad of unmeasured signaling pathways that may have been different. However, in the absence of an effect on performance any single difference may be acute or opposed by another. As a result, we have shown for the first time that concurrent exercise sessions provide a reproducible intervention for the clinical treatment of short term muscle atrophy. This is important as the translation of the adaptations following exercise interventions in health people to those in need of rehabilitation is questionable.

Author Contributions

Conceived and designed the experiments: LM EG MT. Performed the experiments: LM EG TB AS. Analyzed the data: LM TB AS. Contributed reagents/materials/analysis tools: MT. Contributed to the writing of the manuscript: LM MT.

References

1. D'Antona G, Pellegrino MA, Adami R, Rossi R, Carlizzi CN, et al. (2003) The effect of ageing and immobilization on structure and function of human skeletal muscle fibres. J Physiol 552: 499–511.
2. Kraemer WJ, Patton JF, Gordon SE, Harman EA, Deschenes MR, et al. (1995) Compatibility of high-intensity strength and endurance training on hormonal and skeletal muscle adaptations. J Appl Physiol (1985) 78: 976–989.
3. Yan Z, Lira VA, Greene NP (2012) Exercise training-induced regulation of mitochondrial quality. Exerc Sport Sci Rev 40: 159–164.
4. Di Donato DM, West DW, Churchward-Venne TA, Breen L, Baker SK, et al. (2014) Influence of aerobic exercise intensity on myofibrillar and mitochondrial protein synthesis in young men during early and late postexercise recovery. Am J Physiol Endocrinol Metab 306: E1025–1032.
5. Harber MP, Konopka AR, Douglass MD, Minchev K, Kaminsky LA, et al. (2009) Aerobic exercise training improves whole muscle and single myofiber size and function in older women. Am J Physiol Regul Integr Comp Physiol 297: R1452–1459.
6. Lundberg TR, Fernandez-Gonzalo R, Gustafsson T, Tesch PA (2012) Aerobic exercise alters skeletal muscle molecular responses to resistance exercise. Med Sci Sports Exerc 44: 1680–1688.
7. Creer A, Gallagher P, Slivka D, Jemiolo B, Fink W, et al. (2005) Influence of muscle glycogen availability on ERK1/2 and Akt signaling after resistance exercise in human skeletal muscle. J Appl Physiol (1985) 99: 950–956.
8. Hawley JA (2009) Molecular responses to strength and endurance training: are they incompatible? Appl Physiol Nutr Metab 34: 355–361.
9. Alkner BA, Tesch PA (2004) Knee extensor and plantar flexor muscle size and function following 90 days of bed rest with or without resistance exercise. Eur J Appl Physiol 93: 294–305.
10. Campbell EL, Seynnes OR, Bottinelli R, McPhee JS, Atherton PJ, et al. (2013) Skeletal muscle adaptations to physical inactivity and subsequent retraining in young men. Biogerontology 14: 247–259.
11. Berg HE, Tesch PA (1996) Changes in muscle function in response to 10 days of lower limb unloading in humans. Acta Physiol Scand 157: 63–70.
12. Allen J, Morelli V (2011) Aging and exercise. Clin Geriatr Med 27: 661–671.
13. Baumgartner RN, Wayne SJ, Waters DL, Janssen I, Gallagher D, et al. (2004) Sarcopenic obesity predicts instrumental activities of daily living disability in the elderly. Obes Res 12: 1995–2004.
14. Hvid L, Aagaard P, Justesen L, Bayer ML, Andersen JL, et al. (2010) Effects of aging on muscle mechanical function and muscle fiber morphology during short-term immobilization and subsequent retraining. J Appl Physiol (1985) 109: 1628–1634.
15. Yasuda N, Glover EI, Phillips SM, Isfort RJ, Tarnopolsky MA (2005) Sex-based differences in skeletal muscle function and morphology with short-term limb immobilization. J Appl Physiol 99: 1085–1092.
16. de Boer MD, Selby A, Atherton P, Smith K, Seynnes OR, et al. (2007) The temporal responses of protein synthesis, gene expression and cell signalling in human quadriceps muscle and patellar tendon to disuse. J Physiol 585: 241–251.
17. Abadi A, Glover EI, Isfort RJ, Raha S, Safdar A, et al. (2009) Limb immobilization induces a coordinate down-regulation of mitochondrial and other metabolic pathways in men and women. PLoS One 4: e6518.
18. Adhihetty PJ, O'Leary MF, Chabi B, Wicks KL, Hood DA (2007) Effect of denervation on mitochondrially mediated apoptosis in skeletal muscle. J Appl Physiol (1985) 102: 1143–1151.
19. Hakkinen K, Alen M, Kraemer WJ, Gorostiaga E, Izquierdo M, et al. (2003) Neuromuscular adaptations during concurrent strength and endurance training versus strength training. Eur J Appl Physiol 89: 42–52.
20. Hickson RC (1980) Interference of strength development by simultaneously training for strength and endurance. Eur J Appl Physiol Occup Physiol 45: 255–263.
21. Atherton PJ, Babraj J, Smith K, Singh J, Rennie MJ, et al. (2005) Selective activation of AMPK-PGC-1alpha or PKB-TSC2-mTOR signaling can explain specific adaptive responses to endurance or resistance training-like electrical muscle stimulation. FASEB J 19: 786–788.
22. Balabinis CP, Psarakis CH, Moukas M, Vassiliou MP, Behrakis PK (2003) Early phase changes by concurrent endurance and strength training. J Strength Cond Res 17: 393–401.
23. McCarthy JP, Pozniak MA, Agre JC (2002) Neuromuscular adaptations to concurrent strength and endurance training. Med Sci Sports Exerc 34: 511–519.
24. McCarthy JP, Agre JC, Graf BK, Pozniak MA, Vailas AC (1995) Compatibility of adaptive responses with combining strength and endurance training. Med Sci Sports Exerc 27: 429–436.
25. Wilson JM, Marin PJ, Rhea MR, Wilson SM, Loenneke JP, et al. (2012) Concurrent training: a meta-analysis examining interference of aerobic and resistance exercises. J Strength Cond Res 26: 2293–2307.
26. Aagaard P, Andersen JL (2010) Effects of strength training on endurance capacity in top-level endurance athletes. Scand J Med Sci Sports 20 Suppl 2: 39–47.
27. Coffey VG, Pilegaard H, Garnham AP, O'Brien BJ, Hawley JA (2009) Consecutive bouts of diverse contractile activity alter acute responses in human skeletal muscle. J Appl Physiol 106: 1187–1197.
28. Glover EI, Yasuda N, Tarnopolsky MA, Abadi A, Phillips SM (2010) Little change in markers of protein breakdown and oxidative stress in humans in immobilization-induced skeletal muscle atrophy. Appl Physiol Nutr Metab 35: 125–133.
29. Oates BR, Glover EI, West DW, Fry JL, Tarnopolsky MA, et al. (2010) Low-volume resistance exercise attenuates the decline in strength and muscle mass associated with immobilization. Muscle Nerve 42: 539–546.
30. Coffey VG, Jemiolo B, Edge J, Garnham AP, Trappe SW, et al. (2009) Effect of consecutive repeated sprint and resistance exercise bouts on acute adaptive

responses in human skeletal muscle. Am J Physiol Regul Integr Comp Physiol 297: R1441–1451.
31. Safdar A, Little JP, Stokl AJ, Hettinga BP, Akhtar M, et al. (2011) Exercise increases mitochondrial PGC-1alpha content and promotes nuclear-mitochondrial cross-talk to coordinate mitochondrial biogenesis. J Biol Chem 286: 10605–10617.
32. Ruas JL, White JP, Rao RR, Kleiner S, Brannan KT, et al. (2012) A PGC-1alpha isoform induced by resistance training regulates skeletal muscle hypertrophy. Cell 151: 1319–1331.
33. Andersson U, Scarpulla RC (2001) Pgc-1-related coactivator, a novel, serum-inducible coactivator of nuclear respiratory factor 1-dependent transcription in mammalian cells. Mol Cell Biol 21: 3738–3749.
34. Scarpulla RC (2002) Nuclear activators and coactivators in mammalian mitochondrial biogenesis. Biochim Biophys Acta 1576: 1–14.
35. Psilander N, Wang L, Westergren J, Tonkonogi M, Sahlin K (2010) Mitochondrial gene expression in elite cyclists: effects of high-intensity interval exercise. Eur J Appl Physiol 110: 597–606.
36. Wang L, Psilander N, Tonkonogi M, Ding S, Sahlin K (2009) Similar expression of oxidative genes after interval and continuous exercise. Med Sci Sports Exerc 41: 2136–2144.
37. Wang L, Mascher H, Psilander N, Blomstrand E, Sahlin K (2011) Resistance exercise enhances the molecular signaling of mitochondrial biogenesis induced by endurance exercise in human skeletal muscle. J Appl Physiol (1985) 111: 1335–1344.
38. Mathai AS, Bonen A, Benton CR, Robinson DL, Graham TE (2008) Rapid exercise-induced changes in PGC-1alpha mRNA and protein in human skeletal muscle. J Appl Physiol (1985) 105: 1098–1105.
39. Mortensen OH, Plomgaard P, Fischer CP, Hansen AK, Pilegaard H, et al. (2007) PGC-1beta is downregulated by training in human skeletal muscle: no effect of training twice every second day vs. once daily on expression of the PGC-1 family. J Appl Physiol (1985) 103: 1536–1542.
40. Hu S, Yao J, Howe AA, Menke BM, Sivitz WI, et al. (2012) Peroxisome proliferator-activated receptor gamma decouples fatty acid uptake from lipid inhibition of insulin signaling in skeletal muscle. Mol Endocrinol 26: 977–988.
41. Loviscach M, Rehman N, Carter L, Mudaliar S, Mohadeen P, et al. (2000) Distribution of peroxisome proliferator-activated receptors (PPARs) in human skeletal muscle and adipose tissue: relation to insulin action. Diabetologia 43: 304–311.
42. Park KS, Ciaraldi TP, Abrams-Carter L, Mudaliar S, Nikoulina SE, et al. (1997) PPAR-gamma gene expression is elevated in skeletal muscle of obese and type II diabetic subjects. Diabetes 46: 1230–1234.
43. Sofer A, Lei K, Johannessen CM, Ellisen LW (2005) Regulation of mTOR and cell growth in response to energy stress by REDD1. Mol Cell Biol 25: 5834–5845.
44. Fingar DC, Salama S, Tsou C, Harlow E, Blenis J (2002) Mammalian cell size is controlled by mTOR and its downstream targets S6K1 and 4EBP1/eIF4E. Genes Dev 16: 1472–1487.
45. Corradetti MN, Guan KL (2006) Upstream of the mammalian target of rapamycin: do all roads pass through mTOR? Oncogene 25: 6347–6360.
46. Gingras AC, Raught B, Sonenberg N (2001) Regulation of translation initiation by FRAP/mTOR. Genes Dev 15: 807–826.
47. Kimball SR, Do AN, Kutzler L, Cavener DR, Jefferson LS (2008) Rapid turnover of the mTOR complex 1 (mTORC1) repressor REDD1 and activation of mTORC1 signaling following inhibition of protein synthesis. J Biol Chem 283: 3465–3475.
48. Murakami T, Hasegawa K, Yoshinaga M (2011) Rapid induction of REDD1 expression by endurance exercise in rat skeletal muscle. Biochem Biophys Res Commun 405: 615–619.
49. Brugarolas J, Lei K, Hurley RL, Manning BD, Reiling JH, et al. (2004) Regulation of mTOR function in response to hypoxia by REDD1 and the TSC1/TSC2 tumor suppressor complex. Genes Dev 18: 2893–2904.
50. Ydfors M, Fischer H, Mascher H, Blomstrand E, Norrbom J, et al. (2013) The truncated splice variants, NT-PGC-1alpha and PGC-1alpha4, increase with both endurance and resistance exercise in human skeletal muscle. Physiol Rep 1: e00140.
51. Lundberg TR, Fernandez-Gonzalo R, Norrbom J, Fischer H, Tesch PA, et al. (2014) Truncated splice variant PGC-1alpha4 is not associated with exercise-induced human muscle hypertrophy. Acta Physiol (Oxf).
52. Rock KL, Gramm C, Rothstein L, Clark K, Stein R, et al. (1994) Inhibitors of the proteasome block the degradation of most cell proteins and the generation of peptides presented on MHC class I molecules. Cell 78: 761–771.
53. Favier FB, Benoit H, Freyssenet D (2008) Cellular and molecular events controlling skeletal muscle mass in response to altered use. Pflugers Arch 456: 587–600.
54. Chen YW, Gregory CM, Scarborough MT, Shi R, Walter GA, et al. (2007) Transcriptional pathways associated with skeletal muscle disuse atrophy in humans. Physiol Genomics 31: 510–520.
55. Gustafsson T, Osterlund T, Flanagan JN, von Walden F, Trappe TA, et al. (2010) Effects of 3 days unloading on molecular regulators of muscle size in humans. J Appl Physiol (1985) 109: 721–727.
56. Cunha TF, Moreira JBN, Paixao NA, Campos JC, Monteiro AWA, et al. (2012) Aerobic exercise training upregulates skeletal muscle calpain and ubiquitin-proteasome systems in healthy mice. Journal of Applied Physiology 112: 1839–1846.
57. Leger B, Cartoni R, Praz M, Lamon S, Deriaz O, et al. (2006) Akt signalling through GSK-3beta, mTOR and Foxo1 is involved in human skeletal muscle hypertrophy and atrophy. J Physiol 576: 923–933.
58. Stefanetti RJ, Zacharewicz E, Della Gatta P, Garnham A, Russell AP, et al. (2014) Ageing has no effect on the regulation of the ubiquitin proteasome-related genes and proteins following resistance exercise. Front Physiol 5: 30.
59. Stefanetti RJ, Lamon S, Rahbek SK, Farup J, Zacharewicz E, et al. (2014) Influence of divergent exercise contraction mode and whey protein supplementation on atrogin-1, MuRF1 and FOXO1/3A in human skeletal muscle. J Appl Physiol (1985).
60. Koncarevic A, Jackman RW, Kandarian SC (2007) The ubiquitin-protein ligase Nedd4 targets Notch1 in skeletal muscle and distinguishes the subset of atrophies caused by reduced muscle tension. FASEB J 21: 427–437.
61. Batt J, Bain J, Goncalves J, Michalski B, Plant P, et al. (2006) Differential gene expression profiling of short and long term denervated muscle. FASEB J 20: 115–117.
62. Plant PJ, Brooks D, Faughnan M, Bayley T, Bain J, et al. (2010) Cellular markers of muscle atrophy in chronic obstructive pulmonary disease. Am J Respir Cell Mol Biol 42: 461–471.
63. Wang X, Blagden C, Fan J, Nowak SJ, Taniuchi I, et al. (2005) Runx1 prevents wasting, myofibrillar disorganization, and autophagy of skeletal muscle. Genes Dev 19: 1715–1722.
64. Sandri M (2010) Autophagy in skeletal muscle. FEBS Lett 584: 1411–1416.
65. Wildey GM, Howe PH (2009) Runx1 is a co-activator with FOXO3 to mediate transforming growth factor beta (TGFbeta)-induced Bim transcription in hepatic cells. J Biol Chem 284: 20227–20239.
66. Suzuki N, Motohashi N, Uezumi A, Fukada S, Yoshimura T, et al. (2007) NO production results in suspension-induced muscle atrophy through dislocation of neuronal NOS. J Clin Invest 117: 2468–2476.

Clinical Effectiveness of Protein and Amino Acid Supplementation on Building Muscle Mass in Elderly People

Zhe-rong Xu[1], Zhong-ju Tan[1], Qin Zhang[1], Qi-feng Gui[1], Yun-mei Yang[2]*

1 Department of Geriatrics, First Affiliated Hospital, School of Medicine, Zhejiang University, Hangzhou, China, **2** State Key Laboratory for Diagnosis and Treatment of Infectious Diseases, Department of Geriatrics, First Affiliated Hospital, School of Medicine, Zhejiang University, Hangzhou, China

Abstract

Objective: A major reason for the loss of mobility in elderly people is the gradual loss of lean body mass known as sarcopenia. Sarcopenia is associated with a lower quality of life and higher healthcare costs. The benefit of strategies that include nutritional intervention, timing of intervention, and physical exercise to improve muscle loss unclear as finding from studies investigating this issue have been inconsistent. We have performed a systematic review and meta-analysis to assess the ability of protein or amino acid supplementation to augment lean body mass or strength of leg muscles in elderly patients.

Methods: Nine studies met the inclusion criteria of being a prospective comparative study or randomized controlled trial (RCT) that compared the efficacy of an amino acid or protein supplement intervention with that of a placebo in elderly people (≥65 years) for the improvement of lean body mass (LBM), leg muscle strength or reduction associated with sarcopenia.

Results: The overall difference in mean change from baseline to the end of study in LBM between the treatment and placebo groups was 0.34 kg which was not significant (P = 0.386). The overall differences in mean change from baseline in double leg press and leg extension were 2.14 kg (P = 0.748) and 2.28 kg (P = 0.265), respectively, between the treatment group and the placebo group.

Conclusions: These results indicate that amino acid/protein supplements did not increase lean body mass gain and muscle strength significantly more than placebo in a diverse elderly population.

Editor: Conrad P. Earnest, Texas A&M University, United States of America

Funding: The authors have no support or funding to report.

Competing Interests: The authors have declared that no competing interests exist.

* Email: gbbf2000@sina.com

Introduction

Sarcopenia is an age related loss of muscle mass and strength, and is associated with a lower quality of life resulting from a reduced ability to perform daily living tasks [1]. Sarcopenia results in increased healthcare costs of approximately $900 per elderly adult which in the USA is approximately $18.5 billion per year [2]. Prevalence of sarcopenia differs by gender, living circumstances, and continent: 13.2% of Chinese men and 4.8% of Chinese women who are ≥70 years of age have sarcopenia, while 45–70% and 7–17.5% of American men and 2%–59% and 4–10% of American women have sarcopenia, respectively [3]. Age-related muscle loss is highly prevalent in nursing homes, with rates being as high as 68% in elderly men and 21% in elderly females [4], whereas community dwelling elderly have lower prevalence rates in males (10%) but higher rates in women (33%) [5].

Inadequate nutrition, oxidative stress, low physical activity levels, inflammation, and reduced hormone concentrations contribute to age related muscle loss [6]. Possible strategies that reliably increase muscle mass and strength in the elderly have been actively investigated, but conclusions on the benefits of different nutritional interventions, timing of administration, and physical exercise from studies have been conflicting [7–20].

Several nutritional interventions such as creatine monohydrate, whey protein, caseinate, and essential amino acids appear to augment protein synthesis in muscles [1,21,22]. Numerous studies have found that these nutritional supplements enhance the magnitude of gain in lean body mass and muscle strength in older adults undergoing exercise training [1,6,15]. Essential amino acid and leucine supplementation have increased protein synthesis in muscles and are thought to be better strategies for offsetting muscle loss than intact protein [7,16,22–24], due in part to their higher absorption [22]. However, several studies that compared the effect of whey protein or amino acid supplementation on skeletal muscle mass, lean body mass, or strength in healthy elderly to that of placebos have not detected a significant difference between the two groups [8,17].

Many of the studies evaluating the impact of protein or amino acid supplementation on sarcopenia have been small and

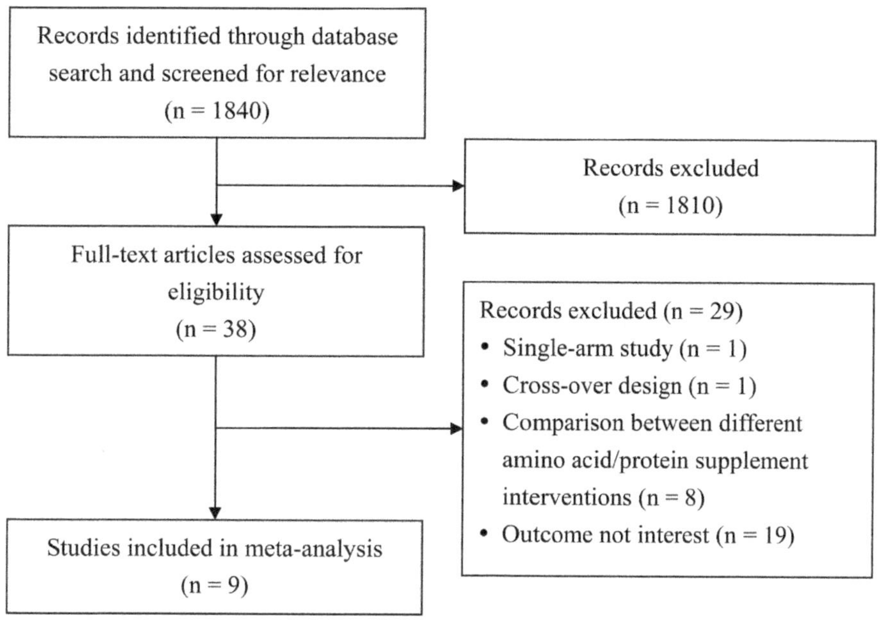

Figure 1. Flow diagram of study selection.

evaluated different supplements. In order to maximize the biostatical power of placebo controlled clinical trials, we have performed a meta-analysis to assess the ability of protein or amino acid supplementation to augment lean body mass or strength of leg muscles in elderly patients.

Experimental Methods

PubMed, Google Scholar, The Cochrane Library, EMBASE, and ClinicalTrials.gov were searched from inception to 13 Jun 2014 using combinations of the following terms: aging, elder, older, muscle loss or muscular atrophy, protein, amino acid. Inclusion criteria for the meta-analysis required that an article be published in a peer-reviewed reviewed journal that described a prospective study or randomized controlled trial (RCT) which compared the efficacy of an amino acid or protein supplement with placebo in improving lean body mass, leg muscle strength in elderly people (≥65 years of age). Single group uncontrolled studies, cross sectional studies, or retrospective studies were excluded. Studies published as letters, comments, editorials, or case reports were also excluded, as well as studies that included people <65 years of age. We utilized the Delphi list to assess the quality of the included studies [25].

Data extraction

Full text articles for the relevant titles were assessed for eligibility which included studies that measured changes in lean body mass (LBM), and may have included evaluation of muscle strength of leg extension and double leg press. Two independent reviewers (coders) extracted the following information from each eligible study: cited reference, type of study, type and duration of interventions, participant number in the intervention and placebo groups, demographics of participants (age, sex, mean body mass index [BMI]), and mean values of the outcome measures (LBM, muscle strength in double leg press, muscle strength in leg extension) at baseline and post intervention. In case of a disagreement, a third reviewer resolved the issue.

To assess coder drift, agreement between coders was calculated by dividing the number of variables coded the same by the total number of variables. Mean agreement of ≥0.90 was considered to be acceptable.

Biostatistics

Treatment effectiveness was evaluated by comparison of LBM (primary outcome) and muscle strength of double leg press and leg extension (secondary outcomes) in elderly subjects at baseline and after nutritional intervention for 6 months (24 weeks). For treatment consistency, only studies providing protein supplementation were considered for meta-analysis. The means with standard deviations (SD) for the LBM, mean muscle strength (leg press and leg extension) were calculated for each group at baseline and post study completion. The difference in mean change (from baseline to end of study) with 95% confidence interval (95% CI) was calculated as the mean change of the protein intervention (treatment group) minus mean change of the placebo or non-nutritious supplements (control group) for each outcome.

Heterogeneity was determined by calculating Cochran Q and the I^2 statistic. The Q statistic indicated statistically significant heterogeneity at $P<0.10$. The I^2 statistic reflected the percentage of the observed between-study variability and provided a scale of heterogeneity: 0 to 24% = no heterogeneity; 25 to 49% = moderate heterogeneity; 50 to 74% = large heterogeneity; and 75 to 100% = extreme heterogeneity. If heterogeneity existed between studies (a Q statistic with $P<0.1$ or an I^2 statistic >50%), we performed the random-effects model (DerSimonian-Laird method). Otherwise, the fixed-effects model was recommended (Mantel-Haenszel method). Combined difference in mean change from baseline to end of study was calculated and a 2-sided P value <0.05 was considered to indicate statistical significance. Sensitivity analysis was performed using the leave-one-out approach. Publication bias was only assessed for lean body mass by constructing funnel plots and exacerbations rate by Egger's test. The absence of publication bias is indicated by the data points forming a symmetric funnel-shaped distribution and one-tailed significance level $P>0.05$ in Egger's test. All statistical analyses

Table 1. Quality assessment of the 9 studies included in the systematic review and meta-analysis as determined using the Delphi List.

Author (Year)	Was a method of randomization used?	Were the groups similar at baseline regarding the most important prognostic indicators?	Were the eligibility criteria specified?	Was the outcome assessor blinded?	Was the care provider blinded?	Was the patient blinded?	Were point estimate and measures of variability presented for the primary outcome measures?	Did the analysis include an intention-to-treat analysis?
Daly et al [27]	Yes	Yes	Yes	No	No	Yes	Yes	Yes
Vermeeren et al [28]	Yes	Yes	Yes	Yes	Yes	Yes	Yes	No
Chale et al [8]	Yes	Yes	Yes	Yes	Yes	Yes	Yes	Yes
Alemán-Mateo et al [29]	Yes	Yes	Yes	Yes	No	No	Yes	Yes
Tieland et al [20]	Yes	Yes	Yes	Yes	Yes	Yes	Yes	Yes
Tieland et al [26]	Yes	Yes	Yes	Yes	Yes	Yes	Yes	Yes
Leenders et al [19]	Yes	Yes	Yes	Yes	Yes	Yes	Yes	No
Ferrando et al [18]	Yes	Gender different, others similar	Yes	No	No	Yes	Yes	No
Verhoeven et al [17]	Yes	Yes	Yes	Yes	ND	Yes	Yes	No

ND, not described.

Study name	Comparison	Difference in means	Lower limit	Upper limit	Z-Value	P-Value	Relative Weight
Daly et al (2014)	Protein vs. Control	0.50	-0.46	1.46	1.02	0.310	62.32
Vermeeren et al (2014)	Protein vs. Control	-0.10	-1.62	1.42	-0.13	0.897	25.22
Chale et al (2013)	Protein vs. Control	0.30	-3.55	4.15	0.15	0.879	3.91
Aleman-Mateo et al (2012)	Protein vs. Control	0.00	-3.97	3.97	0.00	1.000	3.69
Tieland et al (2012)a	Protein vs. Control	0.10	-4.63	4.83	0.04	0.967	2.60
Tieland et al (2012)b	Protein vs. Control	1.60	-3.46	6.66	0.62	0.535	2.27
		0.34	-0.42	1.10	0.87	0.386	

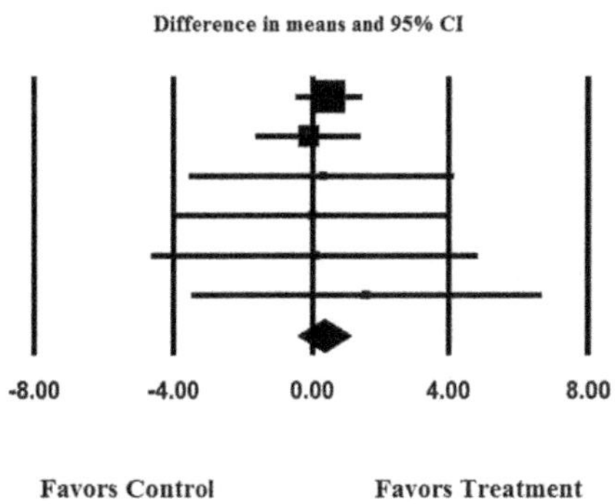

Heterogeneity test: Q=0.71, df = 5, P = 0.982, I-square =0.00%

Figure 2. Forest plot showing results for the meta-analysis of difference in mean change from baseline in lean-body-mass after intervention: treatment vs. control. Abbreviation: CI, confidence interval.

were performed using the statistical software Comprehensive Meta-Analysis, version 2.0 (Biostat, Englewood, NJ, USA).

Results

Out of 1840 studies identified by the data base searches, 38 were screened for eligibility, and 29 were excluded for one of the following reasons: no comparison group (n = 1), no placebo (n = 8), cross over design (n = 1) or no value for mean muscle mass or leg muscle strength (n = 19) (Figure 1). Nine prospective studies met the inclusion criteria (Figure 1) [8,17–20,26–29].

All but one of the studies [18] were at least 75% compliant with the Delphi list (Table 1). Eight of the 9 studies were randomized, placebo-controlled clinical trials [8,17,19,20,26–29]. Five of the trials included an intention-to-treat analysis [8,20,26,27,29]. The 75%–100% compliance levels of 8 of the 9 studies to the Delphi criteria suggest that the studies provided high quality evidence. Coder drift was calculated to be 0.93, indicating satisfactory reliability between coders.

The number of total participants in all 9 studies who had taken the intervention was 267 (range, 10 to 53) and who had received placebo were 244 (range, 11 to 47). Six of the 9 studies provided a protein supplement (whey) to 203 elderly participants and placebo to 191 elderly subjects (controls) [8,20,26–29], 2 studies supplied leucine supplementation to 54 elderly participants and placebo to 42 controls [17,19], and one provided essential amino acids (EAA) to 10 elderly participants and 11 controls [18] (Table 2). The duration of intervention ranged from 10 days to 6 months (Table 2).

Lean Body Mass

Among the 6 studies with protein supplementation [8,20,26–29], three reported that nutritional supplementation significantly increased LBM in the elderly compared to placebo [8,26,27]. Two studies observed a significantly greater LBM in both the placebo and nutritional intervention groups [829]. Pooling of data from the 6 studies revealed no heterogeneity (Q = 0.71, df = 5, P = 0.982; $I^2 = 0.0\%$); therefore, a fixed-effects model was used to assess the difference in mean change in LBM from baseline to end of study between the placebo and protein supplementation groups. The difference in mean change of LBM from baseline to end of study between the placebo and protein supplementation groups ranged from −0.1 to 1.60 kg. The overall difference in mean change in LBM between treatment intervention and placebo was 0.34 kg which was not significant (95% CI = −0.42 to 1.10 kg, P = 0.386, Figure 2).

We compared the health status of the participants in the 9 studies to determine whether the health status of the elderly correlated with the greater gain in LBM. No significant gains in LBM compared to the controls were observed in subjects with diabetes [19], chronic obstructive pulmonary disease [29], limited mobility, who were sedentary [8], moderately active [18], or healthy and independent [17] (Table 3).

Muscle strength: double leg press

Five of the 9 studies assessed the effect of nutritional intervention on muscle strength be double leg press [8,17,19,20,26]. Three of 5 studies reported that the strength of the leg press significantly increased in both placebo and intervention groups during the duration of the study and the mean change was similar in both groups [8]. Two studies reported no significant change in the strength of the leg press with respect to treatment time or group [17,20].

Three studies were included in the analysis of the influence of protein supplements on leg strength [8,20,26]. No heterogeneity was found among 3 studies (Q = 0.147, df = 2, $P = 0.929$; $I^2 = 0.0\%$); and the fixed-effects model revealed no significant difference in mean change in muscle strength by double leg press between the placebo and treatment groups. The difference in mean change from baseline to end of study ranged from −1.00 to 5 kg, with the overall difference in mean change being 2.14 kg (95% CI = −10.92 to 15.20 kg, P = 0.748, Figure 3A).

Muscle strength: leg extension

Six studies evaluated the effect of nutritional intervention on muscle strength by comparing leg extension muscle strength between the intervention and placebo groups [17,19,20,26–28]. Five of the 6 studies reported that the strength of the leg extension significantly increased in both groups during the duration of the study [8,19,26–28]. Two studies reported no significant change in the strength of the leg extension versus treatment time or group [17,20].

Among the 6 studies with protein supplementation, 2 did not provide the mean muscle strength of leg extension for both groups at baseline and at completion of study [8,17], hence the meta-analysis included 4 studies [20,26,28]. Since moderate heterogeneity was found among the studies (Q = 4.52, df = 3, $P = 0.210$; $I^2 = 33.66\%$), a fixed-effects model was used for the meta-analysis.

Table 2. Characteristics of studies included in the systematic review and meta-analysis.

Author (Year)	Study type	Comparison	Duration of Intervention	Number of cases	Mean Age (year)	Sex (Male %)	Mean BMI (kg/m^2)	Lean body mass (kg)		Muscle strength (kg), double leg press		Muscle strength (kg), leg extension	
								Before	After	Before	After	Before	After
Daly et al [27]	RCT	Protein vs Control	4 months	53 vs 47	72 vs 74	0 v. 0	28 vs 28	0.6 (0.3, 0.8)* vs 0.1 (−0.4, 1.1)*		NA	NA	28 (18, 39)* vs 10 (−1, 21)*	
Vermeeren et al [28]	RCT	Protein vs Control	mean 9 days	23 vs 24	66 vs 65	61 vs 75	20 vs 21	Mean change from baseline: –0.5±2.6 vs -0.4±2.7		NA	NA	Mean change from baseline: 3±8 vs 2±9	
Chale et al [8]	RCT	Protein vs Control	6 months	42 vs 38	78 vs 77.3	40 vs 42	27 vs 26.9	46.7±8.6 vs 46.4±8.4	47.3±8.6 vs 46.7±8.4	125±39 vs 128±47	151±58 vs 149±54	NA	NA
Alemán-Mateo et al [29]	RCT	Protein vs Control	3 months	20 vs 20	75 vs 77	40 vs 45	27 vs 26	37.1±6.3 vs 36.8±6.4	37.9±6.5 vs 37.6±6.4	NA	NA	NA	NA
Tieland et al [20]	RCT	Protein vs Control	24 weeks	34 vs 31	78 vs 81	41.2 vs 48.9	27 vs 26.2	45.8±9.9 vs 46.7±9.5	45.8±9.9 vs 46.6±9.5	118±47 vs 124±50	136±47 vs 139±50	57±29 vs 57±28	68±29 vs 63±28
Tieland et al [26]	RCT	Protein vs Control	24 weeks	31 vs 31	78 vs 79	35 vs 32	28.7 vs 28.2	47.2±9.6 vs 45.7±8.9	48.5±9.4 vs 45.4±8.9	124±39 vs 116±36	169±39 vs 162±41	56±17 vs 58±17	77±18 vs 79±18
Leenders et al [19]	RCT	Leucine vs Control	24 weeks	39 vs 28	71 vs 71	100 vs 100	27.4 vs 27.2	61.9±6.9 vs 62.2±6.9	62.0±6.2 vs 62.2±6.9	202±44 vs 205±37	217±50 vs 218±42	80±12 vs 88±16	84±19 vs 94±21
Ferrando et al [18]	RCT	Amino acid vs Control	10 days	10 vs 11	71 vs 68	10 vs 50	NA	43.0±0.6 vs 46.8±1.0	42.1±0.6 vs 45.3±1.0	NA	NA	NA	NA
Verhoeven et al [17]	RCT	Leucine vs Control	12 weeks	15 vs 14	NA	100 vs 100	25.9 vs 26.3	54.6±5.8 vs 55.8±3.4	55.0±5.8 vs 56.2±4.1	170±8 vs 172±6	NA	85±3 vs 85±3	NA

NA, not available; RCT: randomized controlled trial.
*values are within-group mean absolutes of the change from baseline with 95% confidence intervals in parentheses.

Table 3. Summary of 9 trials included in the systematic review and meta-analysis.

Author (Year)	Condition of elderly	Supplement given	Significant increased LBM to baseline	Significant increased Leg press to baseline	Significant increased Leg extension to baseline	Significant increased Physical performance
Daly et al [27]	Healthy	Max.45 g protein/twice daily	Significant increased in protein group, different between groups	ND	Significant increased in protein group, different between groups	Significant increased in both group, similar between groups
Vermeeren et al [28]	COPD	125 ml/three times daily	Neither group	ND	Neither group	ND
Chale et al [8]	Mobility limited	20 g protein/day twice daily	Both groups improved, and also significant different between groups	Both groups to baseline	Both groups to baseline	Significant for whey group
Alemán-Mateo et al [29]	Healthy	15 g protein/day	Both groups improved, but no significant different between groups	ND	ND	ND
Tieland et al [20]	Pre-frail and frail	15 g protein twice daily	Neither group	Both groups to baseline	Both groups to baseline	Both groups
Tieland et al [26]	Pre-frail and frail	15 g protein twice daily	Significant increased in protein group, different between groups	Neither group	Trend toward significant improvement in protein group vs control.	Significant improvement in protein group vs control.
Leenders et al [19]	Type 2 diabetes	2.5 g leucine three times daily	None	Increased vs time in both groups, similar between groups	Increased vs time in both groups, similar between groups	ND
Ferrando et al [18]	Moderately active	15 g EAA three times daily	None	ND	ND	Increased vs time in both groups, similar between groups
Verhoeven et al [17]	Healthy	2.5 g leucine three times daily	None vs time or groups	None vs time or groups	None vs time or groups	ND

COPD, chronic obstructive pulmonary disease; EAA, essential amino acids; LBM, lean body mass; ND, not described.

The difference in mean change from baseline to end of study in the 4 studies ranged from 0 to 18 kg with the overall difference in mean change from baseline to end of study being 2.28 kg (95% CI = −1.73 to 6.29 kg, P = 0.265, Figure 3B). The combined difference in mean change of muscle strength by leg extension from baseline to end of study revealed no significant difference between the control and treatment groups.

Sensitivity analysis

To assess the effect of a single study on the results of the meta-analysis, we removed each study in turn for LBM (Figure 4A), muscle strength by double leg press (Figure 4B), and muscle strength by leg extension (Figure 4C). The removal of any study did not alter the magnitude and direction; taken together, these results indicated that the meta-analysis showed good reliability.

Publication Bias

Publication bias (Figure 5) was assessed using the LBM results only as more than 5 studies reported results for this outcome (note: more than five studies are required to detect funnel plot asymmetry [30]). Egger's test results showed that there was no publication bias in LBM results among studies (Figure 5, t = 0.046, one-tailed P = 0.483).

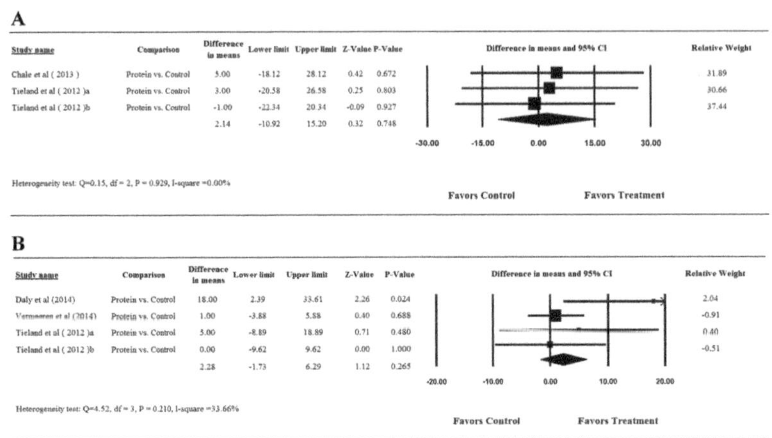

Figure 3. Forest plot showing results for the meta-analysis of difference in mean change from baseline in (A) muscle strength of double leg press and (B) muscle strength of leg extension after intervention: treatment vs. control. Abbreviation: CI, confidence interval.

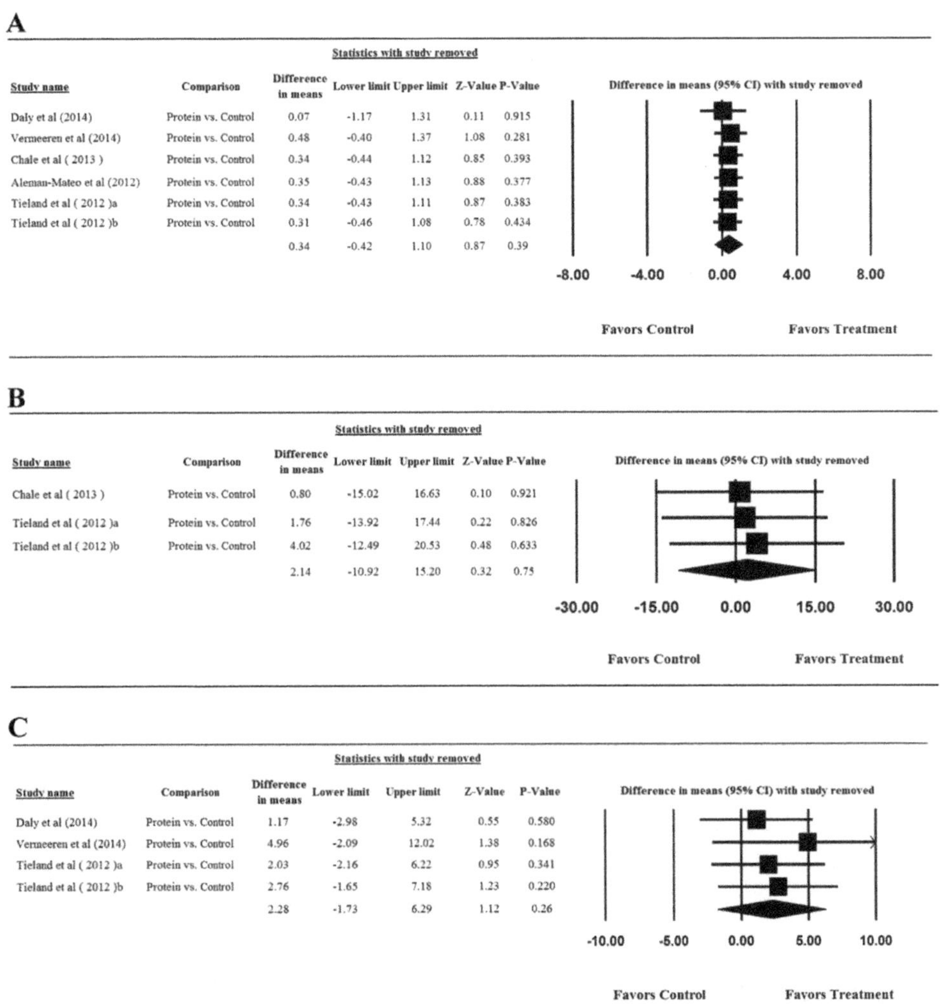

Figure 4. Results of sensitivity analysis to examine the influence of individual studies on pooled estimates as determined using the leave-one-out approach: (A) lean-body-mass; (B) muscle strength of double leg press. Abbreviation: CI, confidence interval.

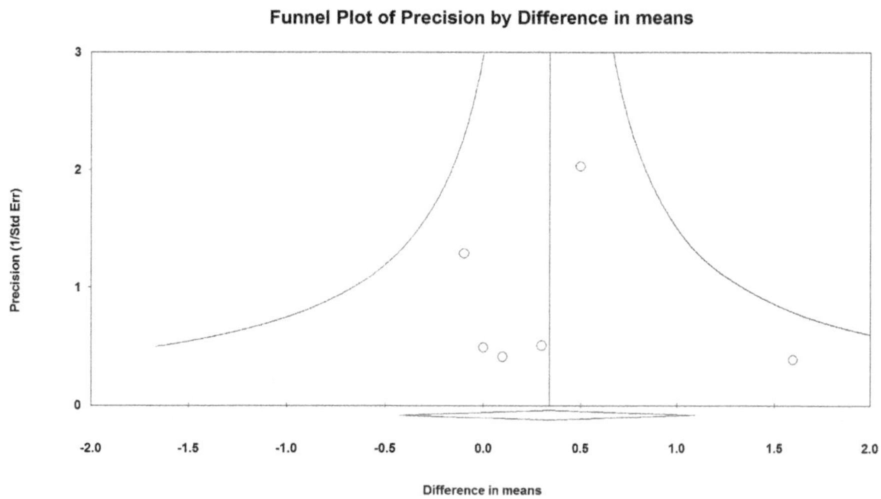

Figure 5. Funnel plot for the assessment of publication bias for studies included in the meta-analysis of the assessment of the mean change from baseline in lean body mass after intervention.

Discussion

This meta-analysis of 9 placebo-controlled studies assessed protein and amino acid supplementation on improving LBM in elderly subjects. Our analysis detected no significant differences between placebo and treatment groups in mean change from baseline to the end of the studies of LBM or muscle strength as measured by double leg press or leg extension in a mixed elderly population.

Multiple studies, several of which were included in our meta-analysis, found no significant benefit of protein supplementation compared to placebo in improving LBM [8,20,26–29,31]. However, protein supplementation has increased LBM and strength in some studies [32]. This inconsistency raises questions of whether it may be due to differences in study design, difference in efficacy of the supplements tested, or differences among the populations analyzed. Identification of the variables that influence the outcome of high protein intake towards a significant increase in LBM or leg strength would provide important guidance for physicians and for cost effective usage of protein supplementation.

The health and physical status of the patient may influence outcomes. Physical condition may affect response to protein or amino acid supplementation. One study showed that whey supplementation augmented LBM significantly more than placebo in pre-frail and frail elderly subjects receiving resistance training [20] but not in another study of elderly subjects with limited mobility that also received protein supplements and resistance training [8]. These findings suggest that the physical condition of the elderly is not solely responsible for the divergent results. Undernourishment may be another condition that significantly affects the outcome [33]. An earlier meta-analysis showed that protein supplementation induced significant weight gain in undernourished elderly subjects and may reduce mortality [33]. In addition, some elderly subjects may have reduced sensitivity to the amino acid induced anabolic signals and thus have a higher propensity to muscle wasting [21]. Addition of leucine appeared to normalize these anabolic signals [14,32]. The health status or stage of the skeletal muscle (whether the person does or does not have sarcopenia) may also affect their ability to respond to protein or amino acid supplementation.

The provided supplement or its dosage also may impact treatment outcomes since supplementation with essential amino acid was not as efficacious in increasing LBM in elderly subjects as whey protein in a direct comparison [32]. Both whey and caseinate supplementation induced a similar increase in protein synthesis after heavy resistance training in healthy elderly participants [12]. Interestingly, a fortified, hydrolyzed collagen protein supplement added to a relatively low-protein diet maintained LBM to a greater extent than whey protein [34]. In some studies [7,11,13], supplementation with essential amino acids improved LBM or muscle protein synthesis rate in elderly subjects; however, another study did not find any benefit of supplementing with amino acids [14].

Loss of muscle tissue or development of sarcopenia is accelerated by bed rest and lack of physical activity [23]. The elderly in the Tieland et al study [26] performed resistance-type exercise 2 times per week for 24 weeks and had a significant increase in LBM in the supplement group, whereas 5 of the included studies involved participants on bed rest [18], no exercise program [17,20,29], or patients who were hospitalized [28]. All participants in the study reported by Daly et al [27] performed resistance training. Consistent with the findings of Tieland et al [26], Daly et al [27] found that participants in supplement group had a significant increase in LBM compared with participants in the control group. The participants of the Chale et al study [8] also performed resistance training and both treatment and placebo groups had similar increases in LBM and leg muscle strength; although, the whey group showed a significant improvement in physical performance [8]. Similarly, in the study by Leenders et al [19] both treatment and control groups reported a mean of 1.55 h physical exercise daily and both groups had similar but significant increases in mean leg strength (both leg press and extension). The resistance training regimen in the study by Tieland et al [26] included several more types of exercises than that of Chale et al [8], while the training regimen in the study of Daly et al [27] involved progressive resistance training. Hence, the beneficial interaction between resistance training and whey protein supplementation on muscle mass and strength gain may depend to some extent on the type of resistance training regimen used. In support for the benefits of concurrent resistance training, a meta-analysis of six studies of older participants reported that protein supplementation augmented loss of fat free mass [35].

There are several limitations to this analysis that should be considered when interpreting the findings. There are a number of outcomes that this analysis did not assess primarily due to limitations of the included studies. These outcomes included (but are not limited to) gender, physical performance and activity, and muscle stage. We also included only RCT. Some non-RCT trials have been done that indicate protein or amino acid supplementation may improve LMB [36]. The relatively small number of included studies, the small subject populations, diverse supplements administered, different outcomes measured and study designs used in the 9 included studies further confounds the analysis. In particular, several studies incorporated exercise (for both intervention and control participants) as part of the study [8,26,27], while the others did not. Although our meta-analysis suggests that exercise had little effect on the change in LBM in the individual studies, this possibility clearly warrants examination in appropriately designed studies. In addition, it is not clear whether our findings will be applicable to elderly subjects who receive other types of supplements, had different exercise regimens, or health status than those used in the 9 included studies. The small number of RCTs that address the question of the use of protein or amino acid supplements to reduce muscle loss in elderly subjects highlights the need for more controlled studies to address this medically important question.

In conclusion, these results indicate that amino acid or protein supplements did not increase lean body mass gain and muscle strength significantly more than placebo in a diverse elderly population. The ability of protein or amino acid supplementation to augment muscle mass and strength may depend on the nutritional physical status of the participants, or their ability to digest protein and absorb the amino acids, the sensitivity of the anabolic pathways in muscles, and the resistance training regimen itself.

Author Contributions

Conceived and designed the experiments: ZRX YMY. Performed the experiments: QZ. Analyzed the data: QZ. Wrote the paper: QFG. Definition of intellectual content, literature research, data acquisition: ZJT. Manuscript preparation, literature research, guarantor of integrity of the entire study: ZRX.

References

1. Forbes SC, Little JP, Candow DG (2012) Exercise and nutritional interventions for improving aging muscle health. Endocrine 42: 29–38.
2. Janssen I, Shepard DS, Katzmarzyk PT, Roubenoff R (2004) The healthcare costs of sarcopenia in the United States. J Am Geriatr Soc 52: 80–85.
3. Cheng Q, Zhu X, Zhang X, Li H, Du Y, et al. (2014) A cross-sectional study of loss of muscle mass corresponding to sarcopenia in healthy Chinese men and women: reference values, prevalence, and association with bone mass. J Bone Miner Metab 32: 78–88.
4. Landi F, Liperoti R, Fusco D, Mastropaolo S, Quattrociocchi D, et al. (2012) Prevalence and risk factors of sarcopenia among nursing home older residents. J Gerontol A Biol Sci Med Sci 67: 48–55.
5. Masanes F, Culla A, Navarro-Gonzalez M, Navarro-Lopez M, Sacanella E, et al. (2012) Prevalence of sarcopenia in healthy community-dwelling elderly in an urban area of Barcelona (Spain). J Nutr Health Aging 16: 184–187.
6. Candow DG, Forbes SC, Little JP, Cornish SM, Pinkoski C, et al. (2012) Effect of nutritional interventions and resistance exercise on aging muscle mass and strength. Biogerontology 13: 345–358.
7. Dillon EL, Sheffield-Moore M, Paddon-Jones D, Gilkison C, Sanford AP, et al. (2009) Amino acid supplementation increases lean body mass, basal muscle protein synthesis, and insulin-like growth factor-I expression in older women. J Clin Endocrinol Metab 94: 1630–1637.
8. Chale A, Cloutier GJ, Hau C, Phillips EM, Dallal GE, et al. (2013) Efficacy of whey protein supplementation on resistance exercise-induced changes in lean mass, muscle strength, and physical function in mobility-limited older adults. J Gerontol A Biol Sci Med Sci 68: 682–690.
9. Fiatarone MA, O'Neill EF, Ryan ND, Clements KM, Solares GR, et al. (1994) Exercise training and nutritional supplementation for physical frailty in very elderly people. N Engl J Med 330: 1769–1775.
10. Groen BB, Res PT, Pennings B, Hertle E, Senden JM, et al. (2012) Intragastric protein administration stimulates overnight muscle protein synthesis in elderly men. Am J Physiol Endocrinol Metab 302: E52–60.
11. Baier S, Johannsen D, Abumrad N, Rathmacher JA, Nissen S, et al. (2009) Year-long changes in protein metabolism in elderly men and women supplemented with a nutrition cocktail of beta-hydroxy-beta-methylbutyrate (HMB), L-arginine, and L-lysine. JPEN J Parenter Enteral Nutr 33: 71–82.
12. Dideriksen KJ, Reitelseder S, Petersen SG, Hjort M, Helmark IC, et al. (2011) Stimulation of muscle protein synthesis by whey and caseinate ingestion after resistance exercise in elderly individuals. Scand J Med Sci Sports 21: e372–383.
13. Koopman R, Verdijk LB, Beelen M, Gorselink M, Kruseman AN, et al. (2008) Co-ingestion of leucine with protein does not further augment post-exercise muscle protein synthesis rates in elderly men. Br J Nutr 99: 571–580.
14. Koopman R, Verdijk L, Manders RJ, Gijsen AP, Gorselink M, et al. (2006) Co-ingestion of protein and leucine stimulates muscle protein synthesis rates to the same extent in young and elderly lean men. Am J Clin Nutr 84: 623–632.
15. Kim HK, Suzuki T, Saito K, Yoshida H, Kobayashi H, et al. (2012) Effects of exercise and amino acid supplementation on body composition and physical function in community-dwelling elderly Japanese sarcopenic women: a randomized controlled trial. J Am Geriatr Soc 60: 16–23.
16. Solerte SB, Gazzaruso C, Bonacasa R, Rondanelli M, Zamboni M, et al. (2008) Nutritional supplements with oral amino acid mixtures increases whole-body lean mass and insulin sensitivity in elderly subjects with sarcopenia. Am J Cardiol 101: 69E–77E.
17. Verhoeven S, Vanschoonbeek K, Verdijk LB, Koopman R, Wodzig WK, et al. (2009) Long-term leucine supplementation does not increase muscle mass or strength in healthy elderly men. Am J Clin Nutr 89: 1468–1475.
18. Ferrando AA, Paddon-Jones D, Hays NP, Kortebein P, Ronsen O, et al. (2010) EAA supplementation to increase nitrogen intake improves muscle function during bed rest in the elderly. Clin Nutr 29: 18–23.
19. Leenders M, Verdijk LB, van der Hoeven L, van Kranenburg J, Hartgens F, et al. (2011) Prolonged leucine supplementation does not augment muscle mass or affect glycemic control in elderly type 2 diabetic men. J Nutr 141: 1070–1076.
20. Tieland M, van de Rest O, Dirks ML, van der Zwaluw N, Mensink M, et al. (2012) Protein supplementation improves physical performance in frail elderly people: a randomized, double-blind, placebo-controlled trial. J Am Med Dir Assoc 13: 720–726.
21. Cuthbertson D, Smith K, Babraj J, Leese G, Waddell T, et al. (2005) Anabolic signaling deficits underlie amino acid resistance of wasting, aging muscle. FASEB J 19: 422–424.
22. Paddon-Jones D, Sheffield-Moore M, Katsanos CS, Zhang XJ, Wolfe RR (2006) Differential stimulation of muscle protein synthesis in elderly humans following isocaloric ingestion of amino acids or whey protein. Exp Gerontol 41: 215–219.
23. Phillips SM (2012) Nutrient-rich meat proteins in offsetting age-related muscle loss. Meat Sci 92: 174–178.
24. Leenders M, van Loon LJ (2011) Leucine as a pharmaconutrient to prevent and treat sarcopenia and type 2 diabetes. Nutr Rev 69: 675–689.
25. Verhagen AP, de Vet HC, de Bie RA, Kessels AG, Boers M, et al. (1998) The Delphi list: a criteria list for quality assessment of randomized clinical trials for conducting systematic reviews developed by Delphi consensus. J Clin Epidemiol 51: 1235–1241.
26. Tieland M, Dirks ML, van der Zwaluw N, Verdijk LB, van de Rest O, et al. (2012) Protein supplementation increases muscle mass gain during prolonged resistance-type exercise training in frail elderly people: a randomized, double-blind, placebo-controlled trial. J Am Med Dir Assoc 13: 713–719.
27. Daly RM, O'Connell SL, Mundell NL, Grimes CA, Dunstan DW, et al. (2014) Protein-enriched diet, with the use of lean red meat, combined with progressive resistance training enhances lean tissue mass and muscle strength and reduces circulating IL-6 concentrations in elderly women: a cluster randomized controlled trial. Am J Clin Nutr 99: 899–910.
28. Vermeeren MA, Wouters EF, Geraerts-Keeris AJ, Schols AM (2004) Nutritional support in patients with chronic obstructive pulmonary disease during hospitalization for an acute exacerbation; a randomized controlled feasibility trial. Clin Nutr 23: 1184–1192.
29. Aleman-Mateo H, Macias L, Esparza-Romero J, Astiazaran-Garcia H, Blancas AL (2012) Physiological effects beyond the significant gain in muscle mass in sarcopenic elderly men: evidence from a randomized clinical trial using a protein-rich food. Clin Interv Aging 7: 225–234.

30. Sutton AJ, Duval SJ, Tweedie RL, Abrams KR, Jones DR (2000) Empirical assessment of effect of publication bias on meta-analyses. BMJ 320: 1574–1577.
31. Nissen SL, Sharp RL (2003) Effect of dietary supplements on lean mass and strength gains with resistance exercise: a meta-analysis. J Appl Physiol (1985) 94: 651–659.
32. Katsanos CS, Chinkes DL, Paddon-Jones D, Zhang XJ, Aarsland A, et al. (2008) Whey protein ingestion in elderly persons results in greater muscle protein accrual than ingestion of its constituent essential amino acid content. Nutr Res 28: 651–658.
33. Milne AC, Potter J, Avenell A (2005) Protein and energy supplementation in elderly people at risk from malnutrition. Cochrane Database Syst Rev: CD003288.
34. Hays NP, Kim H, Wells AM, Kajkenova O, Evans WJ (2009) Effects of whey and fortified collagen hydrolysate protein supplements on nitrogen balance and body composition in older women. J Am Diet Assoc 109: 1082–1087.
35. Cermak NM, Res PT, de Groot LC, Saris WH, van Loon LJ (2012) Protein supplementation augments the adaptive response of skeletal muscle to resistance-type exercise training: a meta-analysis. Am J Clin Nutr 96: 1454–1464.
36. Borsheim E, Bui QU, Tissier S, Kobayashi H, Ferrando AA, et al. (2008) Effect of amino acid supplementation on muscle mass, strength and physical function in elderly. Clin Nutr 27: 189–195.

Voluntary Exercise Prevents Cisplatin-Induced Muscle Wasting during Chemotherapy in Mice

Pernille Hojman[1]*, Jonas Fjelbye[1], Bo Zerahn[2], Jesper F. Christensen[3], Christine Dethlefsen[1], Camilla K. Lonkvist[4], Claus Brandt[1], Hanne Gissel[5†], Bente Klarlund Pedersen[1], Julie Gehl[4]*

1 The Centre of Inflammation and Metabolism and the Centre for Physical Activity Research, Department of Infectious Diseases, Rigshospitalet, University of Copenhagen, Copenhagen, Denmark, **2** Department of Clinical Physiology and Nuclear Medicine, Copenhagen University Hospital Herlev, Herlev, Denmark, **3** Copenhagen University Hospital, The University Hospitals Centre for Health Care Research (UCSF), Copenhagen, Denmark, **4** Department of Oncology, Copenhagen University Hospital Herlev, Herlev, Denmark, **5** Institute of Biomedicine, University of Aarhus, Aarhus C, Denmark

Abstract

Loss of muscle mass related to anti-cancer therapy is a major concern in cancer patients, being associated with important clinical endpoints including survival, treatment toxicity and patient-related outcomes. We investigated effects of voluntary exercise during cisplatin treatment on body weight, food intake as well as muscle mass, strength and signalling. Mice were treated weekly with 4 mg/kg cisplatin or saline for 6 weeks, and randomized to voluntary wheel running or not. Cisplatin treatment induced loss of body weight (29.8%, $P<0.001$), lean body mass (20.6%, $P=0.001$), as well as anorexia, impaired muscle strength (22.5% decrease, $P<0.001$) and decreased glucose tolerance. In addition, cisplatin impaired Akt-signalling, induced genes related to protein degradation and inflammation, and reduced muscle glycogen content. Voluntary wheel running during treatment attenuated body weight loss by 50% ($P<0.001$), maintained lean body mass ($P<0.001$) and muscle strength ($P<0.001$), reversed anorexia and impairments in Akt and protein degradation signalling. Cisplatin-induced muscular inflammation was not prevented by voluntary wheel running, nor was glucose tolerance improved. Exercise training may preserve muscle mass in cancer patients receiving cisplatin treatment, potentially improving physical capacity, quality of life and overall survival.

Editor: Antonio Musaro, University of Rome La Sapienza, Italy

Funding: CIM is supported by a grant from the Danish National Research Foundation (DNRF55). CFAS is supported by a grant from Trygfonden. This study was further supported by grants from the Danish Council for Independent Research and by grants from the Novo Nordic Foundation, Lundbeck Foundation, and Fabrikant Einar Willumsens legat. JG is a Royal Swedish Academy of Sciences Research Fellow supported by a grant from the Acta Oncologica Foundation. The funders had no role in study design, data collection and analysis, decision to publish, or preparation of the manuscript.

Competing Interests: The authors have declared that no competing interests exist.

* Email: phojman@inflammation-metabolism.dk (PH); Julie.Gehl@regionh.dk (JG)

† Deceased.

Background

Loss of muscle mass is a common clinical finding across cancer diagnoses and stages attributable to a range of factors related to both anti-cancer treatment, patient lifestyle and the cancer disease itself [1]. In both patients with early and advanced stage disease, muscle mass significantly impacts patient-reported and clinical outcomes, including survival and disease progression.

Cisplatin is a cornerstone in curative and adjuvant treatment of several solid tumours including testicular-, head and neck-, uterine cervix and lung cancer [2–4]. Cisplatin is highly effective but also associated with plethora of adverse reactions including nausea, anorexia, dysphagia, pain, and fatigue, all of which may be associated with muscular dysfunction. Studies in muscle cell culture suggest that cisplatin can induce atrophy-related genes, proteosomal proteolysis and inflammation in muscle cells [5,6].

Currently, there is emerging enthusiasm for exercise interventions in cancer patients due to accumulating evidence of beneficial effects on fitness, body composition, muscle strength, functional performance and patient reported quality of life [7–9]. Structured exercise training induces a wide range of biochemical alterations, which, under normal circumstances, improve the contractile, metabolic and endocrine properties of skeletal muscle [10]. However, these exercise-induced adaptations may be affected by concomitant influence of cisplatin. For the anthracycline, doxorubicin, exercise has been shown to reverse doxorubicin-induced oxidative stress by induction of muscular antioxidant enzymes and heat shock protein 72 [11]. Evidence of such direct protective mechanisms of exercise remains to be determined for other chemotherapeutics including cisplatin.

Thus, we propose that voluntary wheel running during cisplatin treatment may ameliorate cisplatin-induced adverse effects on muscle mass and function in mice. Specifically, we investigated the effect of voluntary exercise during cisplatin treatment on body weight, food intake as well as muscle mass, strength and signalling. Moreover, we tested if there was an influence on results of anti-emetic treatment, and if exercise during recovery from cisplatin treatment could augment muscle mass restoration.

Materials and Methods

Animals and ethical considerations

All animal experiments were conducted in accordance with the recommendations of the European Convention for the Protection of Vertebrate Animals used for Experimentation and after approval of the experimental protocol by the Danish Animal Experiments Inspectorate. All animal experiments were performed according to the ARRIVE guidelines (Checklist S1). To ensure animal welfare, cisplatin treatment was discontinued if body weight fell below 20 g, for completion rates, please see Table 1. Eight-to-twelve week old female NMRI mice (own breed, FELASA tested) were housed in a temperature- and humidity-controlled room and maintained on a 12:12-h light-dark cycle with food and water *ad libitum*, with 3 mice per cage.

Cisplatin treatment and voluntary exercise

Mice were randomised to receive weekly cisplatin 4 mg/kg (Hospira Nordic, Sweden) or to saline-control for a duration of 6 weeks. Following the initial group allocation, the mice were further randomized to cages with running wheels or not. Average running distances for experiment 3 are reported in Fig S1.

Experiment 1: Effect of cisplatin and exercise. Sixty-eight mice were randomly assigned to one of four groups: control sedentary (CON, n = 16), control exercise (CON+EX, n = 16), cisplatin sedentary (CIS, n = 18) and cisplatin exercise (CIS+EX, n = 18). All mice were weekly evaluated for body weight and food intake, and upon completion of the six-week period were measured as follows: body weight, weight of organs and blood sampling at termination. In addition, half of the mice were DXA scanned, performed hang tests and had a glucose tolerance test made, before they were euthanized at rest. The other half of each study group performed an acute swimming bout in 35°C water prior to euthanization.

Experiment 2: effect of antiemetic drugs. Fifty-eight mice were randomized to one of six groups, three of which were identical to groups in experiment one: control sedentary (CON, n = 9), cisplatin sedentary (CIS, n = 10), cisplatin exercise (CIS+EX, n = 10) and three groups given antiemetic drugs by i.p. injection for 3 days concomitant with each of the 6 weekly cisplatin treatments: cisplatin sedentary+ondansetron 1 mg/kg (Fresenius Kabi) (CIS+ondansetron, n = 10), cisplatin+sedentary+dexamethasone 5 mg/kg (Galen) (CIS+DEXA, n = 9) or cisplatin + dexametasone+exercise (CIS +DEXA+EX, n = 10). Three days before the first and 7 days after the last cisplatin treatment, all mice were DXA scanned. In addition, body weight and food intake were monitored weekly, and blood samples were collected at termination, 7 days after last cisplatin administration.

Experiment 3: effect of exercise on muscular recovery from cisplatin treatment. To evaluate recovery, we followed mice for a 6-wk pretreatment period (pre-CIS), a 6-wk treatment period (CIS) and a 6-wk follow-up period (recovery). Twenty-seven mice were randomized to one of three groups: saline-control sedentary (CON, n = 9), cisplatin sedentary (CIS, n = 9) or cisplatin exercise in the recovery period (CIS+Ex, n = 9). All mice were evaluated weekly for body mass and food intake, and further evaluated for body composition (DXA scan) prior to the treatment period, immediately after cisplatin-treatment and after the follow-up period.

DXA scanning

Assessment of lean body mass (LBM) and fat mass (FM) were performed using a LUNAR Prodigy dual-energy X-ray absorptiometry (DXA) scanner (GE Healthcare Systems, LUNAR, Madison WI) with the "small animal" software application (software version 8.10). Mice were anaesthetized and placed side-by-side on the scan table and scanned en bloc five consecutive times. Regions of interest (ROIs) for analysis of whole-body composition were manually adjusted once around each mouse and then copied to the four subsequent scans. Mean LBM and FM for each mouse in a group was then calculated from the 5 consecutive scans.

Hang test

The mouse was placed on a suspended wire for a 3 minute-period. When the mouse fell off the wire time was paused, and the mouse put back on the wire. Deliberate and accidental falls were not included. From an initial score of 10, each fall decreased the score by 1, and the total number of falls over the 3 minute-period was noted as test result [12].

Glucose tolerance test

Mice were fasted for 3 hours and given an i.p. injection of glucose (2 g/kg body weight) in order to test glucose tolerance (n = 8–9). Blood samples were taken from the tail at 0, 15, 30, 60 and 120 min after glucose injection.

PCR

Total RNA was isolated from frozen muscle tissue samples (n = 8) by tissue homogenization and RNA extraction using the TRIzol method (Invitrogen). Purity and quantity of the isolated RNA were determined by a Nanodrop spectrophotometer (Thermo Scientific). Total RNA (500 ng) was reversely transcribed into complementary DNA (cDNA) using the High Capacity cDNA Reverse Transcription kit with random hexamer primers (Applied Biosystems). PCR amplification was monitored in real time using the WiiA7 real-time PCR machine (Applied Biosystems) and SYBR green as a fluorescence marker (SYBRGreen PCR Master Mix, Applied Biosystem). Quantification was performed by normalizing to standard curves for each gene. The target genes presented as their ratio to ribosomal 18S RNA.

Western blotting

Muscle tissue samples were homogenized in a Tris lysis buffer with the use of Qiagen Tissuelyser. Proteins were separated on a 4–15% Criterion TGX Precast Gel (Bio-Rad) by electrophoresis and transferred to a polyvinylidene difluoride membrane (Bio-Rad), using the Trans-Blot Turbo Transfer system at 2.5A–25V for 10 min (Bio-Rad). After blocking with 1% Fish Skin Gelatin (Sigma-Aldrich), the membrane was incubated overnight at 4°C with either anti-Akt (Cell Signalling), anti-phospho-Akt (Ser473, Cell Signalling), anti-mTOR (Cell Signalling) or anti-phospho-mTOR (Ser2448, Cell Signalling) antibodies in 1% Fish Skin Gelatin. Secondary anti-bodies used were HRP-conjugated Polyclonal Goat Anti-Rabbit Immunoglobulins (DAKO) in 1% Fish Skin Gelatin, and proteins were visualised with super signal west femto luminol/enhancer solution (Thermo Scientific). Proteins were analysed by the ChemiDoc XRS system (Bio-Rad) and the Quantity One software (Bio-Rad). Unspecific staining of proteins with Reactive Brown (Sigma-Aldrich) was used as loading and transfer control.

ELISA

Serum interleukin 6 (IL-6) concentrations were measured by a sandwich ELISA (R&D Systems). The sensitivity was 6.27 pg/ml and the intra-assay coefficient of variation was below 15%. Serum ghrelin concentrations were measured by the Luminex ghrelin

Table 1. Treatment completion rates.

Group	Treatment	Week 1	Week 2	Week 3	Week 4	Week 5	Week 6
Study 1							
1	CON	100% (16/16)	100% (16/16)	100% (16/16)	100% (16/16)	100% (16/16)	100% (16/16)
2	CIS	100% (16/16)	100% (16/16)	100% (16/16)	100% (16/16)	87% (14/16)	87% (14/16)
3	CON + EX	100% (18/18)	100% (18/18)	100% (18/18)	100% (18/18)	100% (18/18)	100% (18/18)
4	CIS + EX	100% (18/18)	100% (18/18)	100% (18/18)	100% (18/18)	100% (18/18)	100% (18/18)
Study 2							
1	CON	100% (9/9)	100% (9/9)	100% (9/9)	100% (9/9)	100% (9/9)	100% (9/9)
2	CIS	100% (10/10)	100% (10/10)	100% (10/10)	90% (9/10)	80% (8/10)	80% (8/10)
3	CIS + ONS	100% (10/10)	100% (10/10)	100% (10/10)	90% (9/10)	90% (9/10)	80% (9/10)
4	CIS + STER	100% (9/9)	100% (9/9)	100% (9/9)	88% (8/9)	88% (8/9)	78% (7/9)
5	CIS + STER + EX	100% (10/10)	100% (10/10)	100% (10/10)	100% (10/10)	100% (10/10)	90% (9/10)
6	CIS + EX	100% (10/10)	100% (10/10)	100% (10/10)	100% (10/10)	100% (10/10)	100% (10/10)
Study 3							
1	CON	100% (9/9)	100% (9/9)	100% (9/9)	100% (9/9)	100% (9/9)	100% (9/9)
2	CIS	100% (9/9)	100% (9/9)	100% (9/9)	100% (9/9)	100% (9/9)	100% (9/9)
3	CIS + EX in recovery	100% (9/9)	100% (9/9)	100% (9/9)	100% (9/9)	100% (9/9)	100% (9/9)

Percentage and number of mice completing cisplatin treatment. CON: Saline treated mice, CIS: cisplatin treated mice, ONS: Onsedansetron, STER: steroids, dexamethasone, EX: access to running wheels, and CIS + EX in recovery: access to running wheels in the 6 weeks recovery phase.

In study 1 in each group, the mice were divided between termination at rest or after 1 hour of acute exercise (swimming). Both groups had the following measurements made: body weight, food intake, weight of organs at termination and blood sampling at termination. In addition, the rest group were DXA scanned, performed the hang tests and had a glucose tolerance test made.

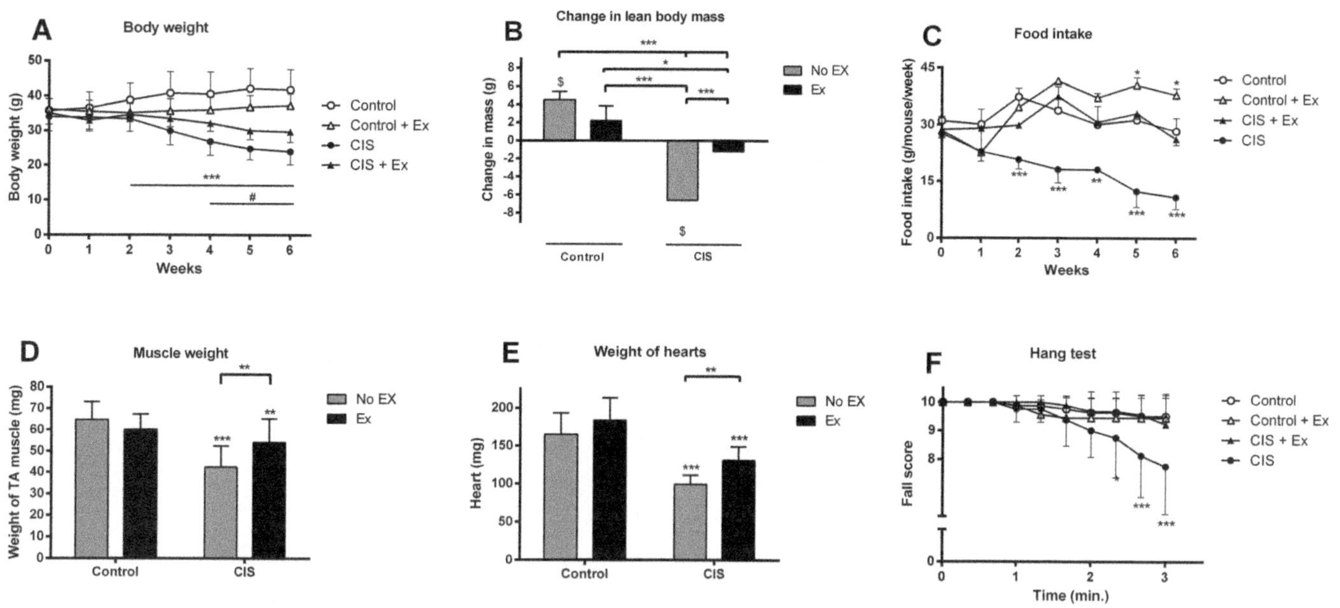

Figure 1. The effect of cisplatin and voluntary wheel running on muscle mass, strength, food intake and body weight. Mice (n = 16–18) were treated with 4 mg/kg cisplatin (CIS) or saline (Control) once weekly for 6 weeks. During treatment mice were assigned to running wheels in their home cages (Ex) or not. A) Body weight was recorded weekly during the intervention. *** Indicates a significant effect of time (change from baseline, $P<0.001$), # indicates significant different from the control group ($P<0.001$)(No Ex = 16, Ex = 18). B) Change in lean body mass (LBM) by DXA scanning before and after the 6 weeks intervention (No Ex = 8, Ex = 9). C) Food intake was recorded per cage with 3 mice. A significant effect of time ($P<0.001$), cisplatin treatment ($P<0.001$) and the interaction ($P<0.001$) between the two was observed (n = 6). D) Weight of TA muscle (No Ex = 16, Ex = 18). E) Weight of heart (No Ex = 16, Ex = 18). F) Fall score from hang test performed 3 days after last cisplatin treatment (No Ex = 8, Ex = 9). Results are presented as means ± SEM. Statistical analysis was performed by 2-way ANOVA with repeated measurements and post hoc test (A, C, D) or post hoc paired T-tests (B) with Bonferroni corrections. * $P<0.05$, ** $P<0.01$, ***$P<0.001$ indicates statistical significance compared to non-exercising control or as indicated by the lines except in A) or $^{\$}P<0.05$ compared to pre-treatment levels (B).

singleplex kit (Millipore) in serum samples from the second study. The sensitivity was 5.18 pg/ml and the intra-assay coefficient of variation was below 10%.

Intramuscular ion and glycogen content

For ion content, total Na^+, K^+ and Mg^{2+} were extracted by trichloroacetic acid, and Mg^{2+} content was determined by atomic absorption spectrophotometry (Solaar AAS, Thermo), while Na^+ and K^+ were determined with a Radiometer FLM3 flame photometer, as previously described [13]. For glycogen content, quadriceps femoris (QF) muscles (n = 8) were acid hydrolyzed in 1 N HCl for 2 hours at boiling point and subsequent neutralized in 1 N NaOH. The liberated free-glycosyl units were determined spectrophotometrically by using FluoroSkan (Ascent, Labsystems) at 355 nm excitation wavelength and 460 nm emission wavelength using software Ascent version 2.4.

Statistics

For multiple comparisons, statistical analysis was performed using two-way analysis of variance (2-way ANOVA) followed by post hoc tests with Bonferroni corrections. A 2-way ANOVA with repeated measures was used when the effects of experimental factors was analyzed at different time-points. The statistical significance of the difference between measurements (pre- vs. post-treatment) was obtained from a two-tailed paired T-test. Data analysis was performed using the GraphPad Prism version 5.0 software. Results are expressed as means ± standard error of mean (SEM). The criterion for significance was set at a probability of less than 0.05.

Results

Exercise ameliorates effects of cisplatin on body weight, lean mass, food intake and strength

Six weeks of cisplatin treatment induced a 29.8% loss of body weight ($P<0.001$, n = 16) compared to pre-treatment levels in sedentary mice (FIG. 1A), and these mice weighed 43% less than control mice. Evaluations of DXA scans showed that the sedentary cisplatin-treated mice lost 6.6+/−3.6 g of LBM from pre-treatment levels ($P<0.001$, n = 8 mice, FIG. 1B), which was on average 8.4 g lower in comparison to saline treated mice after treatment. Sedentary cisplatin-treated mice became anorexic, eating less than 50% than saline control mice ($P<0.001$, n = 6 cages per group, FIG. 1C). Weight reductions of 22.3±2.4 mg tibialis anterior (TA) muscle and 65.4±7.0 mg heart was found in sedentary cisplatin-treated mice compared with controls (FIG. 1D–E), and sedentary cisplatin-treated mice had an average of two falls during the 3 min hang test, compared to no falls in saline control mice ($P<0.001$, CON: n = 8, EX: n = 9) (FIG. 1F).

Voluntary exercise, by access to running wheels, attenuated weight loss to 15% compared to pre-treatment level in cisplatin-treated mice ($P<0.001$, n = 18, FIG. 1A), halving the weight loss compared to non-exercising cisplatin-treated mice ($P<0.001$), but still causing a significant drop in body weight compared to saline-treated exercising mice ($P<0.001$). Wheel running prevented loss of LBM by maintaining muscle mass in cisplatin-treated mice, while exercising control mice gained 2.2+/−0.5 g LBM during the treatment period ($P<0.05$, n = 9)(FIG. 1B). Food intake was normalized, as exercising cisplatin-treated mice ate the same amount of fodder as saline treated mice and 58.8% more than the sedentary cisplatin-treated mice ($P<0.001$, n = 6 cages per group)

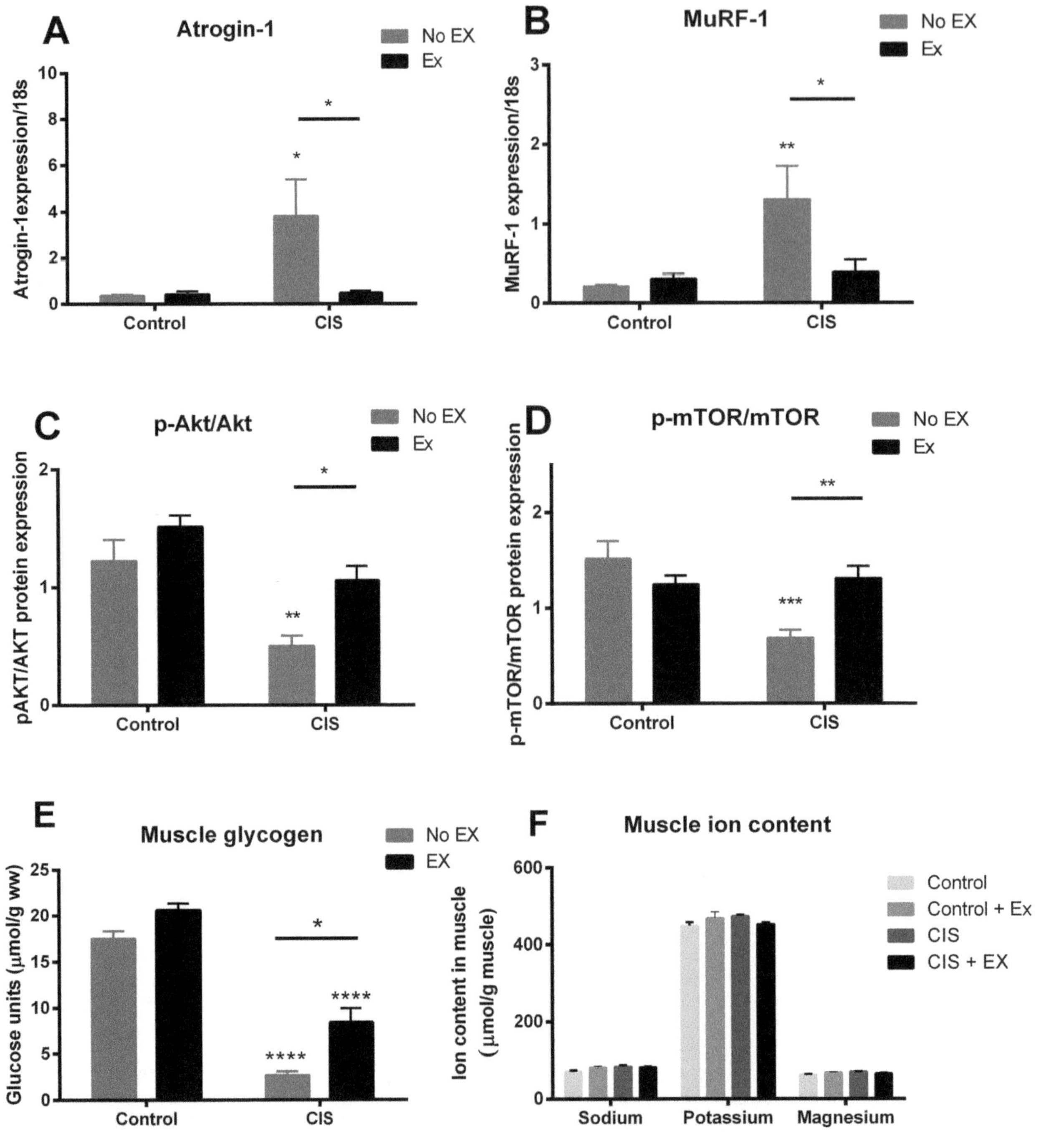

Figure 2. Changes in muscular signalling after cisplatin treatment. Gene expression of A) Atrogin-1 and B) MuRF-1 was determined in muscles from cisplatin-treated (CIS) or saline-treated mice (Control), randomized to exercise training during treatment (Ex). Ratio between phosphorylated and total C) Akt (Ser473) and D) mTOR (Ser2448) was measured by Western blotting. Total-Akt and total-mTOR protein abundance did not differ significantly between groups (data not shown). For pAkt/Akt, a significant effect of exercise ($P<0.001$) and cisplatin treatment ($P<0.0001$) was observed in the 2-way ANOVA, while for p-mTOR/mTOR, a significant effect of cisplatin treatment ($P<0.001$) was observed, (No Ex = 8, Ex = 9). E) Muscle glycogen content, and F) muscular ion content. Results are presented as means ± SEM (n = 8). Statistical analysis was performed by 2-way ANOVA with Bonferroni's post hoc test. *$P<0.05$, **$P<0.01$, ****$P<0.0001$ indicates statistical significance compared to non-exercising control or as indicated by the lines.

(FIG. 1C). The weight reductions of TA muscle and heart was attenuated in the exercising cisplatin-treated mice (FIG. 1D–E). Muscle strength was also maintained, as defined by no falls in the hang test (FIG. 1F).

Cisplatin-induced signalling events in muscle

In line with the cisplatin-induced loss of muscle mass, we found a 6 and 10-fold up regulation of the two muscle atrophy-related genes, *MuRF-1 and atrogin-1* in the sedentary cisplatin group ($P<0.01$, FIG. 2A–B). Voluntary wheel running during cisplatin

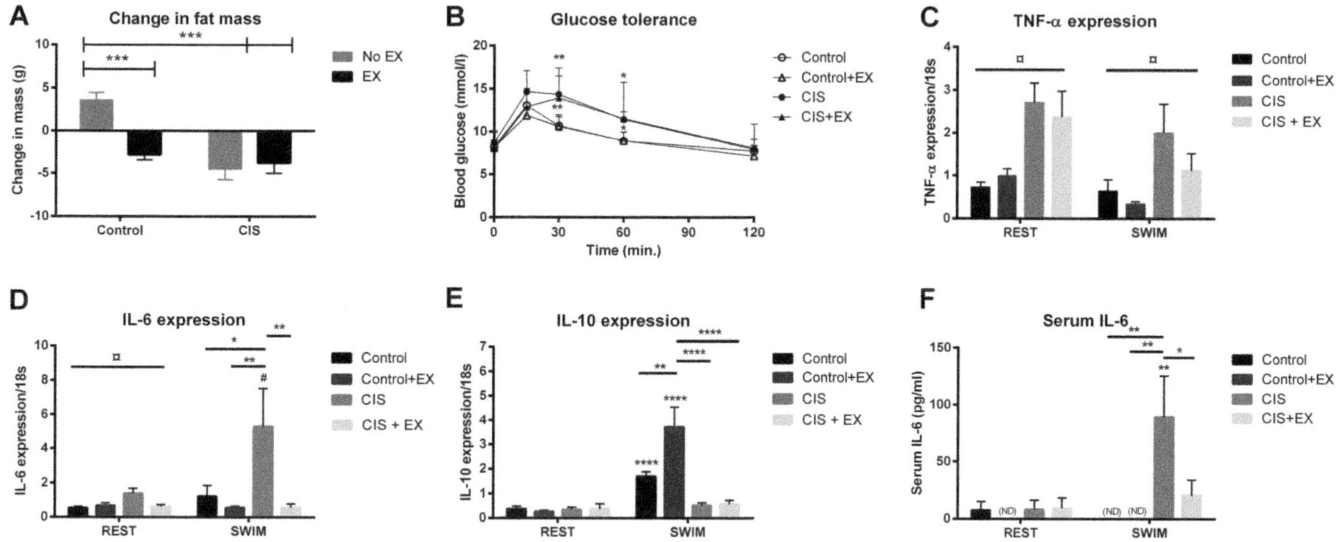

Figure 3. Exercise does not reverse cisplatin induced inflammation and glucose intolerance. After 6 weeks of cisplatin treatment, A) change in fat mass (FM) by DXA scanning, and B) blood glucose levels during a glucose tolerance test, were determined. Before euthanasia, half of the mice performed a single bout of acute exercise (60 min swimming). Gene expression of C) TNF-α, D) IL-6 and E) IL-10 and F) serum IL-6 in mice euthanized before swimming (REST) or immediately after the swimming exercise (SWIM). ND: Values below detection rate. Results are presented as means ± SEM (n = 8). Statistical analysis was performed by 2-way ANOVA with Bonferroni's post hoc test and post hoc T-test for the CIS group. ¤ indicates cisplatin treatment effect (P<0.05) by 2-way ANOVA. *P<0.05, **P<0.01, ***P<0.001, ****P<0.0001 indicates significance in post hoc tests indicates compared to non-exercising control or as indicated by the lines.

treatment abolished this cisplatin-induced expression of *MuRF-1* and *atrogin-1* mRNA (P<0.05, FIG. 2A–B). By western blotting, we showed reduced phosphorylation of the hypertrophy-related proteins Akt and mTOR in muscles of cisplatin-treated mice (P< 0.01) (FIG. 2C–D, FIG. S2). This repression of Akt and mTOR was reversed in the exercising cisplatin-treated mice.

Muscular energy and ion status

Glycogen content in the cisplatin-treated muscles were 14.8% of the glycogen content in the control muscles (P<0.001). Access to running wheels increased glycogen content in cisplatin-treated mice to 47.8% of the control muscles (P<0.001 compared to control muscles; P<0.01 compared to CIS muscle, FIG. 2E). Cisplatin did not alter muscular water and ion content (FIG. 2F).

Whole body metabolism and control of inflammation during acute exercise

Both cisplatin-treated groups lost fat mass (FM) (P<0.01, CON: n = 8, EX: n = 9) (FIG. 3A), and showed significant impairment in glucose tolerance (FIG. 3B). These effects were unaffected by voluntary wheel running during cisplatin treatment. Glucose tolerance can be impaired by local muscular inflammation. In line with this, we found that cisplatin treatment induced TNF-α and IL-6 mRNA expression (P<0.01, n = 8) (FIG. 3C+D). Exercise during cisplatin attenuated the cisplatin-dependent induction of IL-6, but this could not prevent induction of TNF-α.

Acute exercise is known to have direct anti-inflammatory effects. To test this response after cisplatin treatment, half of the mice performed a 60 min swimming bout. The acute exercise induction of IL-10 mRNA expression observed in control mice was completely blunted in cisplatin-treated mice (P<0.05, n = 8). Voluntary wheel running during the cisplatin treatment did not rescue the acute exercise induction of IL-10 (FIG. 3E, n = 9), potentially explaining why exercise did not prevent muscular inflammation. We found a 4-fold induction of IL-6 mRNA expression and 12-fold increase in serum IL-6 in cisplatin-treated mice following swimming (P<0.01 and P<0.001 respectively, n = 8, FIG. 3D+F), while wheel running tended to attenuate this induction (P = 0.102, n = 9, FIG. 3D+F). The induction of IL-6 is highly dependent on glycogen depots in the muscles, and correlates with the reductions in these during the 1 hour of swimming.

No effect of antiemetic drugs on food intake

As exercise was shown to normalise food intake in the cisplatin-treated groups, we investigated if anti-emetic drugs would influence food intake. I.p. administration of the antiemetic drugs (ondansetron or dexamethasone) was not able to normalize food intake or prevent loss of body weight in this model (FIG. 4A–B). In addition, we found a significant correlation between decreased food intake and loss of body weight ($R^2 = 0.53$, P = 0.025, FIG. 4C), as well as loss of LBM ($R^2 = 0.47$, P = 0.041, FIG. 4E) in the non-exercising groups. These correlations dissipated in the exercising groups (FIG. 4D+F). Stressing the effect of exercise on food intake, we found that the appetite hormone ghrelin was up-regulated in the exercising cisplatin-treated groups (7491+/−948 pg/ml, n = 18) compared to non-exercising cisplatin-treated mice (5333+/−622 pg/ml, n = 24) and saline-injected controls (3664+/−777, n = 9, P<0.05) (FIG. 5).

No observable effect of exercise on muscular mass restoration after cisplatin treatment

In order to evaluate muscle mass restoration, mice were followed for a 6 week recovery period after the initial 6 weeks of cisplatin treatment. During the recovery period, mice returned to pre-treatment levels of body weight and food intake (FIG. 6A–B), and regained all lost LBM and fat mass as determined by DXA scanning (FIG. 6C+D). Exercise during the recovery phase had no additional effect on muscle mass restoration after cisplatin

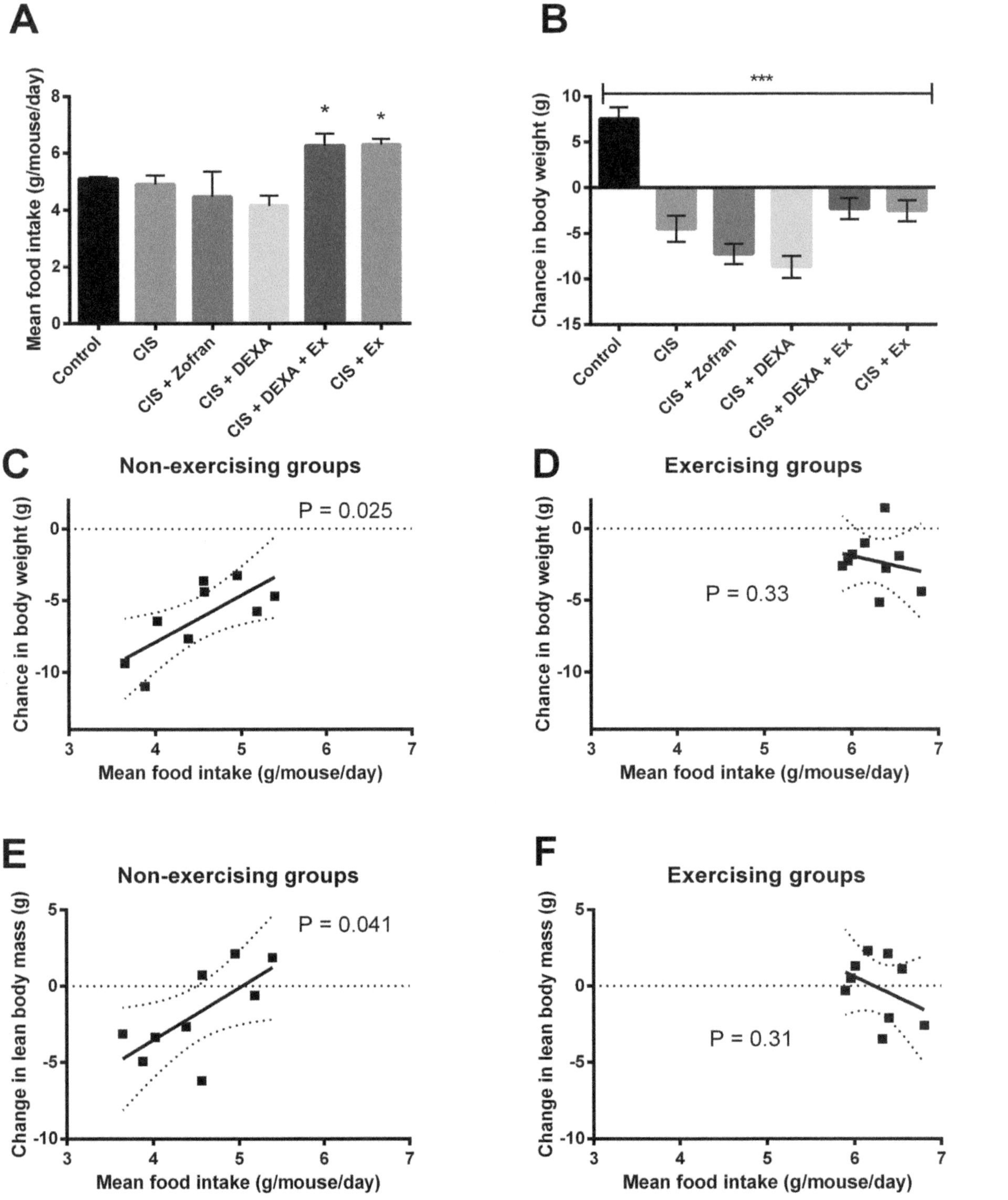

Figure 4. Effect of anti-emetic medication on body weight and mean food intake. Mice were treated with 4 mg/kg cisplatin (CIS) or saline (Control) once weekly for 6 weeks and received concomitant ondansetron (Zofran) or dexamethasone (DEXA) for 3 consecutive days after each cisplatin treatment. A) Mean food intake, and B) change in body weight. Statistical analysis was performed by oneway ANOVA with Bonferroni's post hoc test (Mean $\pm$ SEM, N = 10). *$P<0.05$, ***$P<0.001$ compared with Control mice. Linear regression analyses between mean food intake (calculated from 3–5 cages per group) and change in body weight (C+D) (mean of mice in each cage), or change in lean body mass (E+F) (mean of mice in each cage) in non-exercising cisplatin-treated groups (CIS, CIS+Zofran and CIS+DEXA) and exercising cisplatin-treated groups (CIS+DEXA+EX and CIS+EX) were performed.

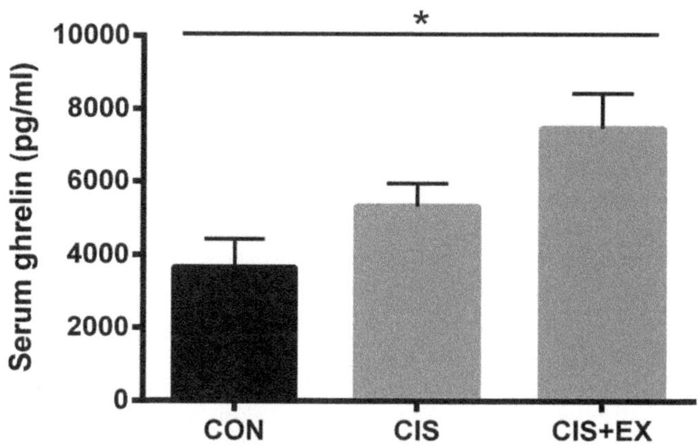

Figure 5. Exercise during cisplatin treatment stimulates the appetite hormone ghrelin. In the control, non-exercising cisplatin-treated (CIS) and exercising cisplatin-treated (CIS+EX) groups from fig. 2, serum ghrelin was determined by ELISA. Statistical analysis was performed by 1-way ANOVA with Bonferroni's post hoc test. *P<0.05 indicates significance in post hoc tests as indicated by the line.

treatment (FIG. 6A–C). In addition, cisplatin no effect on satellite cell proliferation (data not shown), nor was myoD gene expression affected by cisplatin treatment or exercise (data not shown).

Discussion

The present study explores the capacity of exercise to counteract cisplatin-induced adverse effects in skeletal muscle. There were two principal findings: 1) cisplatin treatment induced muscular dysfunction as defined by reductions in muscle mass and strength, and impairments in insulin resistance and inflammation. 2) Voluntary wheel running could effectively abrogate cisplatin-induced loss of muscle mass and strength, as well as attenuate intramuscular signalling events, in parallel with normalization of body weight and food intake. Yet, voluntary wheel running had no protective effect on impaired glucose tolerance or inflammatory status. In concert, these findings provide novel evidence for both direct and indirect effects of cisplatin on muscular function, as well as elucidating the capacity and limitations of exercise as therapeutic countermeasure for cisplatin-induced muscle dysfunction.

Protective mechanisms of voluntary exercise in mice

In our cisplatin-treated mice, we found severe reductions in lean mass, which mostly likely was driven by reduced food intake, given the close correlation between reduction in food intake and the level muscle wasting during the treatment period. Importantly, voluntary wheel running normalized food intake, preserving muscle mass and function. Exercise is generally recognized for increasing appetite, explaining why exercise interventions in overweight individuals do not always result in the expected weight

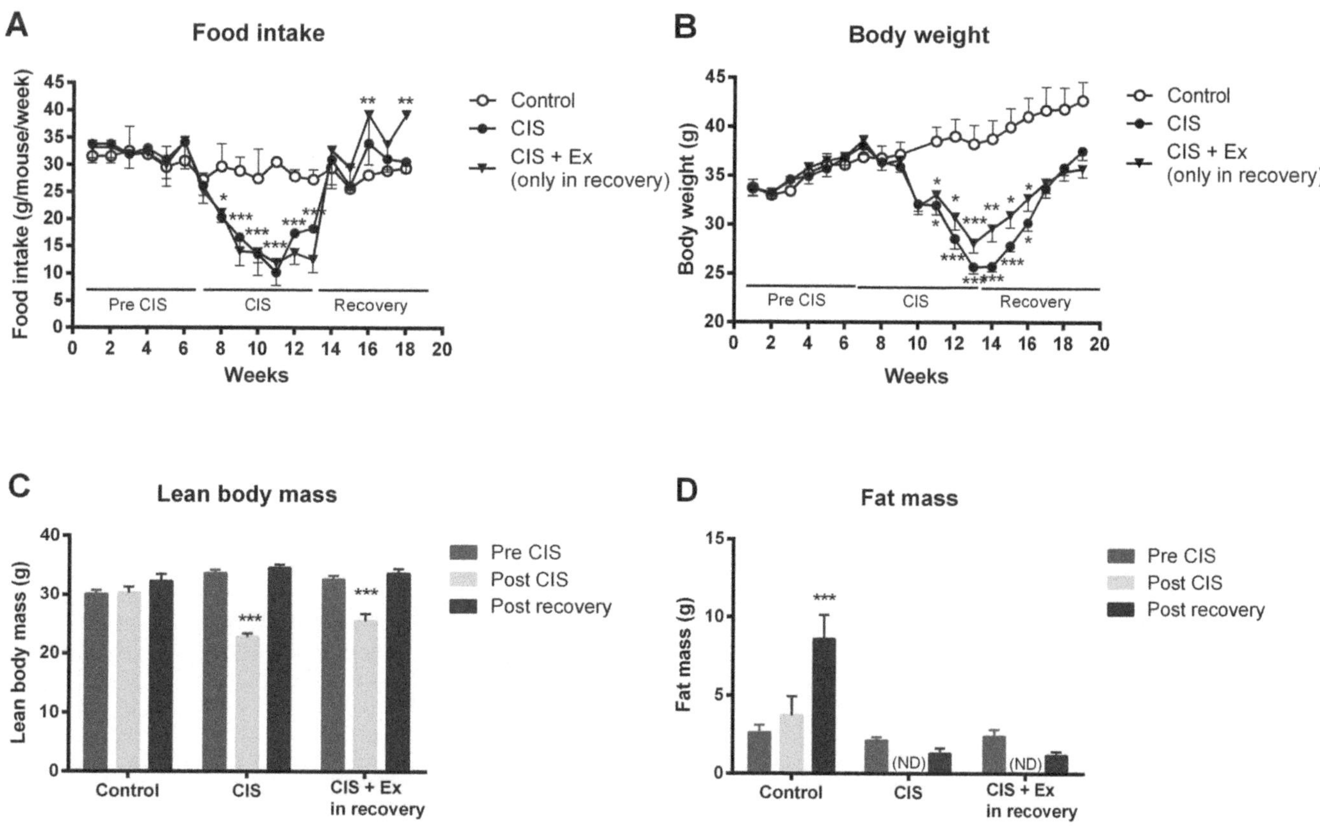

Figure 6. Muscle restoration in cisplatin treated mice. To evaluate the regenerative response, mice were treated weekly for 6 weeks with cisplatin (4 mg/kg), and then followed for additional 6 weeks. A) Body weight and B) food intake was recorded weekly. C) Lean body mass (LBM) and D) fat mass (FM) was determined by DXA scanning before cisplatin treatment (pre CIS), immediately after the 6 weeks cisplatin treatment (post CIS) and after 6 weeks recovery (post recovery). ND: values below detection limit. Results are presented as means ± SEM. *P<0.05, **P<0.01, ***P<0.001 indicates significant difference compared to baseline control.

loss. Conversely, limited information is available on regulation of appetite by exercise in anorexic or undernourished states. In our mouse model, we found that exercise increased the systemic levels of the appetite hormone, ghrelin, indicating that exercise induces direct hormonal effects on food intake in these anorexic mice. In an attempt to control the energy intake, we investigated the concurrent effect of anti-emetic drugs. Neither i.p. dexamethasone nor ondansetron, two agents commonly administered as supportive care medication, improved food intake in our mouse model. Thus we cannot in the present study separate the effects of exercise from the derived effect of increased food intake.

Irreversible muscular inflammation and insulin resistance

Cisplatin treatment has been associated with substantial systemic and nephritic inflammation [14]. After 6 weeks of cisplatin treatment, we observed a marked induction of TNF-α expression in the muscles, which was not reversed by exercise. This discrepancy between TNF-α expression and loss of LBM indicates that inflammation-driven muscle wasting is not an important pathway in cisplatin-induced muscle wasting in our model. TNF-α can impair glucose uptake by altering insulin signal transduction in skeletal muscle, as shown through infusions of TNF-α at physiological relevant systemic concentrations in healthy humans [15]. These findings may explain the impaired glucose tolerance in both the sedentary and exercising cisplatin-treated groups.

Training comprises of repeated bouts of acute exercise, during which the systemic concentration of anti-inflammatory cytokines i.e. IL-1ra and IL-10 increases, driving the anti-inflammatory response of exercise [16]. During an acute bout of exercise, we observed that the induction of IL-10 mRNA was completely blunted in both cisplatin-treated groups. This lack of release of anti-inflammatory cytokines during acute exercise, may explain why TNF-α could not be controlled by voluntary wheel running in the exercising cisplatin-treated group.

In contrast, IL-6 expression increased during an acute bout of swimming in both the sedentary groups, yet most pronounced in the cisplatin-treated group. This response was completely blunted in both exercising groups. IL-6 expression in the muscle is highly dependent on the glycogen content of the muscle, and the induction of IL-6 during acute exercise is a sensor of carbohydrate availability. Thus exercise-induced release of IL-6 can signal from the contracting muscle to other organs, increasing hepatic glucose output and gluconeogenesis, as well as lipolysis in the adipose tissue [17]. In line with this, we found that induction of IL-6 expression correlated with glycogen depletion in the muscles of cisplatin treated mice.

Exercise as muscle preserving intervention in cancer patients

Exercise intervention is increasingly being promoted in cancer patients, as numerous trials have proven safe, feasible and efficient in improving functional capacity, fitness, lean mass and strength, as well as psychosocial parameters [7,18,19]. Most studies have been performed in patients with breast and prostate cancer, yet studies in patient groups receiving cisplatin-based therapy are emerging [20,21,21–23].

Traditionally exercise is divided into endurance training with focus on improving cardiovascular output, fitness levels and energy expenditure, and strength training concentrating on building muscle mass [10]. Both modalities have been tested in cancer patients undergoing chemotherapy, showing that they can improve functional capacity and muscle mass [7]. For patients receiving cisplatin treatment, the urgent concern for restoring muscle mass implies that strength training would be an effective intervention in this group. Yet for the sedentary cancer patient any engagement in physical activity would stimulate muscular hypertrophy signals and based on the results here stimulate food consumption.

In this study, we chose to use the voluntary wheel running model of exercise. This model, in contrast to other rodent exercise regimens, is entirely unforced as the mice run at night at their own pace and will. This model has the benefit of inducing minimal stress, or no stress at all, with high exercise performance.

This study supports a general recommendation for exercise in patients receiving cisplatin-based treatments. Our results show that even under anorexia and energy-depleted states, exercise not only prevents muscle wasting, but normalizes energy intake possibly through a direct effect on the appetite hormone ghrelin. In addition, both the numerous exercise trials in cancer patients and controlled exercise trials in mice clearly demonstrate that exercise does not have any tumour promoting effects, if anything exercise seems to decrease tumour growth through yet unidentified mechanisms [24–26]. These findings can have relevance for daily clinical practice since weekly administration of cisplatin is used routinely, e.g. during radiotherapy of head- and neck, and cervical cancer [27,28]. There has been considerable focus on treatment of nausea and emesis. Yet maintenance of appetite is an equally important factor, and this study points out that exercise may independently improve appetite.

Conclusion

In summary, we found that exercise during treatment could alleviate cisplatin-induced muscle wasting and signalling impairments in protein degradation and hypertrophic pathways in healthy mice. Thus exercise training might be a promising strategy for preservation of muscle mass in cancer patients receiving treatment with cisplatin, and holds the potential for improving physical capacity, quality of life and overall survival.

Acknowledgments

Anne Boye, Lone Christensen, Henriette Pilegaard and Vibeke Uhre are acknowledged for their technical assistance. Our dear colleague Hanne Gissel unfortunately passed away in the final phases of the preparation of this article.

Supporting Information

Figure S1 Running distance was evaluated weekly in the groups of experiment 3 (N = 3 cages). Statistical analysis was performed by 2-way ANOVA with Bonferroni's post hoc test. *$P<0.05$, ***$P<0.001$ indicates significance in post hoc tests from the control group.

Figure S2 Representative western blotting bands of the data presented in FIG. 2C-D of phospho-Akt (p-Akt), total Akt, phospho-mTOR (p-mTOR), and total mTOR, as well as the whole gel stained with reactive brown as loading control.

Checklist S1 ARRIVE guideline checklist.

Author Contributions

Conceived and designed the experiments: PH JFC HG BKP JG. Performed the experiments: PH JF BZ CD CB HG. Analyzed the data: PH JF BZ JG. Contributed reagents/materials/analysis tools: BZ CB HG. Wrote the paper: PH JFC CKL JG.

References

1. Christensen JF, Jones LW, Andersen JL, Daugaard G, Rorth M, et al. (2014) Muscle dysfunction in cancer patients. Ann Oncol, 25(5):947–58.
2. Scatchard K, Forrest JL, Flubacher M, Cornes P, Williams C (2012) Chemotherapy for metastatic and recurrent cervical cancer. Cochrane Database Syst Rev 10, CD006469.
3. Reveiz L, Rueda JR, Cardona AF (2012) Chemotherapy for brain metastases from small cell lung cancer. Cochrane Database Syst Rev 6, CD007464.
4. Feldman DR, Bosl GJ, Sheinfeld J, Motzer RJ (2008) Medical treatment of advanced testicular cancer. JAMA 299: 672–684.
5. Damrauer JS, Stadler ME, Acharyya S, Baldwin AS, Couch ME, et al. (2008) Chemotherapy-induced muscle wasting: assocation with NF-kappabeta and cancer cachexia. Basic Applied Myology 18: 139–148.
6. Fanzani A, Zanola A, Rovetta F, Rossi S, Aleo MF (2010) Cisplatin triggers atrophy of skeletal C2C12 myotubes via impairment of Akt signalling pathway and subsequent increment activity of proteasome and autophagy systems. Toxicol Appl Pharmacol 250: 312–321.
7. Brown JC, Winters-Stone K, Lee A, Schmitz KH (2012) Cancer, physical activity, and exercise. Compr Physiol 2: 2775–2809.
8. Ballard-Barbash R, Friedenreich CM, Courneya KS, Siddiqi SM, McTiernan A, et al. (2012) Physical activity, biomarkers, and disease outcomes in cancer survivors: a systematic review. J Nat Cancer Inst 104: 815–840.
9. Kushi LH, Doyle C, McCullough M, Rock CL, Demark-Wahnefried W, et al. (2012) American Cancer Society Guidelines on nutrition and physical activity for cancer prevention: reducing the risk of cancer with healthy food choices and physical activity. CA Cancer J Clin 62: 30–67.
10. Egan B, Zierath JR (2013) Exercise metabolism and the molecular regulation of skeletal muscle adaptation. Cell Metab 17: 162–184.
11. Smuder AJ, Kavazis AN, Min K, Powers SK. (2011) Exercise protects against doxorubicin-induced oxidative stress and proteolysis in skeletal muscle. J Appl Physiol 110: 935–942.
12. van Putten M (2011) The use of hanging wire tests to monitor muscle strength and condition over time. TREAT-NMD Neuromscular Network/Wellstone Muscular Dystrophy Center, Washington, DC.
13. Gissel H (2010) Effects of varying pulse parameters on ion homeostasis, cellular integrity, and force following electroporation of rat muscle in vivo. Am J Physiol Regul Integr Comp Physiol 298: R918–R929.
14. dos Santos NA, Carvalho-Rodrigues MA, Martins NM, dos Santos AC (2012) Cisplatin-induced nephrotoxicity and targets of nephroprotection: an update. Arch Toxicol 86: 1233–1250.
15. Plomgaard P, Fischer CP, Ibfelt T, Pedersen BK, van Hall G (2008) Tumor necrosis factor-alpha modulates human in vivo lipolysis. J Clin Endocrinol Metab 93: 543–549.
16. Pedersen BK (2013) Muscle as a secretory organ. Compr Physiol 3: 1337–1362.
17. Pedersen BK, Febbraio MA (2012) Muscles, exercise and obesity: skeletal muscle as a secretory organ. Nat Rev Endocrinol 8: 457–465.
18. Segal RJ, Reid RD, Courneya KS, Malone SC, Parliament MB, et al. (2003) Resistance exercise in men receiving androgen deprivation therapy for prostate cancer. J Clin Oncol 21: 1653–1659.
19. Courneya KS, Segal RJ, Mackey JR, Gelmon K, Reid RD, et al. (2007) Effects of aerobic and resistance exercise in breast cancer patients receiving adjuvant chemotherapy: a multicenter randomized controlled trial. J Clin Oncol 25: 4396–4404.
20. Quist M, Rørth M, Langer S, Jones LW, Laursen JH, et al. (2012) Safety and feasibility of a combined exercise intervention for inoperable lung cancer patients undergoing chemotherapy: a pilot study. Lung Cancer 75: 203–208.
21. Samuel SR, Maiya GA, Babu AS, Vidyasagar MS (2013) Effect of exercise training on functional capacity and quality of life in head and neck cancer patients receiving chemoradiotherapy. Indian J Med Res 137: 515–520.
22. Christensen JF, Andersen JL, Adamsen L, Lindegaard B, Mackey AL, et al. (2011) Progressive resistance training and cancer testis (PROTRACT) - efficacy of resistance training on muscle function, morphology and inflammatory profile in testicular cancer patients undergoing chemotherapy: design of a randomized controlled trial. BMC Cancer 11.
23. Quist M, Langer S, Rørth M, Christensen KB, Adamsen L (2013) "EXHALE": exercise as a strategy for rehabilitation in advanced stage lung cancer patients: a randomized clinical trial comparing the effects of 12 weeks supervised exercise intervention versus usual care for advanced stage lung cancer patients. BMC Cancer 13: 477.
24. Jones LW, Viglianti BL, Tashjian JA, Kothadia SM, Keir ST, et al. (2010) Effect of aerobic exercise on tumor physiology in an animal model of human breast cancer. J Appl Physiol 108: 343–348.
25. Jones LW, Antonelli J, Masko EM, Broadwater G, Lascola CD, et al. (2012) Exercise modulation of the host-tumor interaction in an orthotopic model of murine prostate cancer. J Appl Physiol 113: 263–272.
26. Hojman P, Dethlefsen C, Brandt C, Hansen J, Pedersen L, et al. (2011) Exercise-induced muscle-derived cytokines inhibit mammary cancer cell growth. Am J Physiol Endocrinol Metab 301: E504–E510.
27. Green JA, Kirwan JM, Tierney JF, Symonds P, Fresco L, et al. (2001) Survival and recurrence after concomitant chemotherapy and radiotherapy for cancer of the uterine cervix: a systematic review and meta-analysis. Lancet 358: 781–786.
28. Pignon JP, le Maitre A, Maillard E, Bourhuis J, MACH-NC Collaborative Group (2009) Meta-analysis of chemotherapy in head and neck cancer (MACH-NC): an update on 93 randomised trials and 17,346 patients. Radiother Oncol 92: 4–14.

Physical Activity Level of Urban Pregnant Women in Tianjin, China

Yan Zhang[1], Shengwen Dong[1], Jianhua Zuo[2], Xiangqin Hu[3], Hua Zhang[1], Yue Zhao[1]*

1 School of Nursing, Tianjin Medical University, Tianjin, China, **2** Obstetrics and Gynecology Department, Wangdingdi Hospital, Tianjin, China, **3** Tianjin Central Hospital of Gynecology and Obstetrics, Tianjin, China

Abstract

Objective: To determine the physical activity level and factors influencing physical activity among pregnant urban Chinese women.

Methods: This prospective cross-sectional study enrolled 1056 pregnant women (18–44 years of age) in Tianjin, China. Their socio-demographic characteristics were recorded, and the Pregnancy Physical Activity Questionnaire was used to assess their physical activity during pregnancy. The data were analyzed by multinomial logistic regression with adjustment for potential confounders.

Results: Median total energy expenditure of pregnant women in each of the three trimesters ranged from 18.50 to 21.90 metabolic equivalents of task (METs) h/day. They expended 1.76–1.85 MET h/day on moderate and vigorous activities and 0.11 MET h/day on exercise. Only 117 of the women (11.1%) met the international guideline for physical activity in pregnancy (≥150 min moderate intensity exercise per week). The most frequent reason given for not being more physically active was the fear of miscarriage. Higher education level (OR: 4.11, 95% CI: 1.59–10.62), habitual exercise before pregnancy (OR: 2.14, 95% CI: 1.39–3.28), and husbands who exercised regularly (OR: 2.21, 95% CI: 1.33–3.67) significantly increased the odds of meeting the guideline ($p<0.001$). A low pre gravid body mass index (OR: 0.42, 95% CI: 0.20–0.87) significantly decreased the odds ($p<0.001$).

Conclusions: Few urban Chinese pregnant women met the recommended physical activity guideline. They also expended little energy exercising. Future interventions should be based on the clinic environment and targeting family members as well as the subjects. All pregnant women should be targeted, not just those in high-risk groups.

Editor: Noel Christopher Barengo, University of Tolima, Colombia

Funding: This study was supported by the Scientific Research Program of the Health Department of Tianjin, China (grant No. 2013KZ085). The funder had no role in study design, data collection and analysis, decision to publish, or preparation of the manuscript.

Competing Interests: The authors have declared that no competing interests exist.

* Email: yuezhao35@hotmail.com

Introduction

Pregnancy is an important period for both women and their children, and excessive gestational weight gain (GWG) is a common phenomenon globally because many women decrease their physical activity during pregnancy [1]. Excessive GWG can lead to pregnancy complications such as gestational diabetes, and may also promote negative health outcomes for the child such as excess weight or obesity [2]. Physical activity during pregnancy may reduce the risk of prenatal complications and prevent excessive GWG [3,4]; however, the incidence of low levels of physical activity during pregnancy is increasing globally because many women stop exercising and choose to rest and relax instead [5].

In 2002, the American College of Obstetricians and Gynecologists (ACOG) updated their guidelines on exercise for pregnant women and recommended moderate intensity exercise for at least 30 min per day on most days of the week [6]. However, the findings of studies on the levels of physical activity in pregnant women in Western countries are inconsistent. In 2012, a survey of 3482 pregnant women in Norway showed that only 14.6% followed the recommended guideline (≥3 times a week, 20 min per session, moderate intensity) at 17–21 weeks gestation [7], but in 1991 and 1992, a British study of 9889 pregnant women reported that approximately 50% participated in vigorous activity for at least 3 h per week at 18 and 32 weeks of gestation [8]. In 2004, a report from the UK showed that 39% of pregnant women who exercised regularly before pregnancy stopped exercising after becoming pregnant [9]. Another study showed that 21.5% healthy pregnant women in Ireland met the recommended guideline [10]. A cohort study of 1280 pregnant American women 1999–2006 revealed that only 22.9% met the ACOG recommended guidelines [11]; however, another study, conducted in the United States in 2013, found that 94.5% of women (52/55) at 18 weeks of pregnancy accumulated ≥150 min of moderate-to-vigorous activity weekly [12]. Various factors have been shown to influence the amount of physical activity or exercise taken by pregnant women, including educational level [13], pre gravid body mass index (BMI) [4], discomfort symptoms [4,7], age [14], unemployment [14], and their husband's exercise habits [14]. Studies conducted in Brazil and Australia found that the main reasons given by pregnant women for not being more physically active were incontinence, discomfort, lack of time, and feeling tired [15,16].

Most previous studies included mainly Caucasian women [7,8,9,10,11,12] and only a few were carried out in Asian populations including Chinese populations [17]. China is the most populous country in the world. At the present time, excessive GWG is a public health problem in China [3]. A cohort study of 862 pregnant Chinese women found that more than 50% of participants experienced excessive weight gain during pregnancy [3]. Most pregnant women decreased their physical activity, reduced house-work or even quit their jobs as soon as they became pregnant. At the same time they increased their sedentary activities [17]. The prevalence of adherence to appropriate levels of physical activity, as defined by the international recommended guideline, by pregnant women in China remains unknown. Moreover, the factors that influence physical activity in this population have not yet been explored. Tianjin, the third largest city in China, is located in the eastern coastal area in China. In recent years, Tianjin has experienced rapid economic development and urbanization in line with overall national development. These transitions maybe influence physical activity behavior and related perceptions [18]. This population-based cross-sectional study conducted in Tianjin, evaluated physical activity level during pregnancy and factors that influence physical activity during pregnancy. The objective was to identify barriers that prevent pregnant Chinese women from exercising.

Material and Methods

Ethics

The study was approved by the Ethics Committee of the Tianjin Medical University (TMUhMEC 2012010). All participants were informed of the purposes and procedures of the study and all provided both verbal and written consent.

Study design

For this population-based cross-sectional study, 1100 pregnant women in any of the three trimesters were recruited consecutively between February 2012 and February 2013 at two community hospitals, one obstetrics and gynecology hospital, and one general hospital during prenatal care visits. All study centers were located in urban districts of Tianjin, China. Pregnant women who had medical or obstetric complications that limited their physical activity or who were unwilling to take part in the study were excluded. A total of 40 subjects were excluded due to missing exercise-related information, and another four subjects who suffered discomfort while filling out the questionnaires were also excluded; thus 1056 pregnant women were included in the current analysis.

At the time of recruitment, just after their prenatal check, the women were informed about the purposes and procedures of this study. They were then informed about the questionnaires that would be administered by the investigators if they consented to participate. All subjects were assured that the questionnaires would be anonymous, therefore ensuring their privacy. After this introduction, the women were invited to participate in the study and after giving oral and written consent, the participants completed two questionnaires over a period of 15 min in a quiet place in the clinic. The questionnaires were then placed in a sealed box that could only be opened by the researchers.

Questionnaires and measurements

The socio-demographic information was divided into two sections. The first included questions about the subject's socio-demographic characteristics (e.g., age, education level, pre gravid and current work status). The second section collected general information on exercise characteristics including whether the subject had ever received exercise advice from a health professional during pregnancy, what the subject's prepregnancy exercise habits were, and what the husband's exercise habits were. A baseline BMI was calculated from pre gravid weight and height, which were recorded in the medical records.

In 2004, Chasan-Taber *et al.* [19] developed the Pregnancy Physical Activity Questionnaire (PPAQ) to assess physical activity during pregnancy. This questionnaire includes 32 activities: household/caregiving activities (thirteen activities), occupational activities (five activities), sports/exercise activities (eight activities), transportation activities (three activities), and inactivity (three activities). The PPAQ measures the frequency and duration of activities, and gives an intensity value to each activity. The activities can be analyzed by type, by intensity or for the total energy expenditure. The PPAQ was validated by 7 days of testing with accelerometer measurements in a group of 54 pregnant women. The PPAQ was found to be a reliable measure of the physical activity of pregnant women in Australia [19], France [20], Japan [21] and Vietnam [22].

Few structured and validated questionnaires that can measure the physical activity of pregnant women have been developed in China [23]. Most available questionnaires do not include household or childcare activities, which make up a large part of physical activity during pregnancy [19]. The existing questionnaires cannot calculate the energy consumption of physical activity in pregnant women [23].

Regarding the accuracy and validity of PPAQ, with the approval of Chasan-Taber *et al.*, we translated the PPAQ into Chinese, adapted it to culture conditions in China, and then translated it back into English. Five experts (including two chief physicians and one chief nurse majoring in obstetrics, one professor specializing in physical activity and sports, and one nursing educational specialist) were then invited to analyze the face and content validity of the Chinese version of the PPAQ. The resulting questionnaire lacked three items that were present in the Western version. These were, "holding children", "mowing the lawn by riding a mower", and "mowing the lawn by using a walking mower, raking, and gardening". Two items were added, namely, "riding a bicycle" and "going up and down the stairs". The modified Chinese version of the PPAQ thus included 31 items for measuring physical activity during pregnancy. They comprise household/caregiving activities (ten activities), occupational activities (five activities), sports/exercise activities (eight activities), transportation activities (five activities), and inactivity (three activities).

Following its development, 30 pregnant Chinese women were surveyed using the revised questionnaire. They were then asked to wear Live Pod-02 human motion energy consumption meters to monitor their energy consumption for 7 days. At the end of the 7 days, the correlation between the questionnaire results and the meter results was analyzed. The content validity and test-retest reliability of the questionnaire were 0.940 and 0.944, respectively, while the correlation coefficient between meter and questionnaire results was 0.768 [23].

The energy expenditure for each activity was then calculated by multiplying the self-reported time spent in each activity per day by the activity intensity. The total activity expenditure was expressed as metabolic equivalents of task (METs) h per day, obtained by

Table 1. Socio-demographic of pregnant women n (%).

Characteristic		Overall	1st trimester	2nd trimester	3rd trimester
N		1056 (100.0)	172 (16.3)	512 (48.5)	372 (35.2)
Age		27.89±3.53	28.28±2.65	28.28±3.14	27.18±4.23
Race	Han Chinese	1002 (95.0)	160 (93.0)	482 (94.1)	360 (96.8)
	Others	54 (5.0)	12 (7.0)	30 (5.9)	12 (3.2)
Currently employed		590 (55.9)	132 (76.7)	318 (62.1)	140 (37.6)
Education	Lower than high school	180 (17.0)	8 (4.7)	89 (17.4)	83 (22.3)
	High school graduate	424 (40.2)	64 (37.2)	206 (40.2)	154 (41.4)
	College or higher degree	452 (42.8)	100 (58.1)	217 (42.4)	135 (36.3)
Monthly household income (RMB)	≤3500	368 (34.9)	28 (16.3)	144 (28.2)	196 (52.7)
	~3501	274 (25.9)	64 (37.2)	136 (26.6)	74 (19.9)
	~5001	338 (32.0)	70 (40.7)	192 (37.5)	76 (20.4)
	≥10,000	76 (7.2)	10 (5.8)	40 (7.9)	26 (7.0)
Pre-gravid health status	Very healthy	422 (40.0)	68 (39.5)	212 (41.4)	144 (38.7)
	Healthy	500 (47.3)	90 (52.3)	244 (47.7)	166 (44.6)
	General	134 (12.7)	14 (8.1)	56 (10.9)	62 (16.7)
Pre-gravid work status (employed)		750 (71.0)	136 (79.1)	361 (70.5)	253 (68.0)
Pre-gravid BMI (kg/m^2)	Low (≤18.4)	164 (15.5)	24 (14.0)	72 (14.1)	68 (18.3)
	Normal (~18.5)	764 (72.4)	122 (70.9)	386 (75.4)	356 (95.7)
	Overweight (~25.0)	128 (12.1)	26 (15.1)	54 (10.5)	48 (12.9)
Previous live births	0	946 (89.6)	168 (97.7)	470 (91.8)	306 (82.2)
	1	100 (9.5)	2 (1.2)	36 (7.0)	62 (16.7)
	2	10 (0.9)	2 (1.2)	4 (0.8)	4 (1.1)
Discomfort symptoms (yes)		792 (75.0)	132 (76.7)	348 (68.0)	312 (83.9)

summing all activities. Each activity was classified according to intensity (sedentary, <1.5 METs; light, ~1.5 METs; moderate, ~3.0 METs]; and vigorous, ~6.0 METs) and type (i.e., household/caregiving, occupational, and sports/exercise). The average number of METs h per day for each intensity level and activity type was calculated [19]. The total time spent in sports/exercise activities per week was calculated by multiplying the self-reported time spent on each sports/exercise activity per day by the activity intensity based the on PPAQ. Pregnant women who reported more than 2 h moderate intensity sports/exercise activity per week were deemed to meet the international guideline [6,7,12].

Statistical analysis

The subjects who met the guideline, socio-demographic characteristics, exercise-related information, and energy expenditure were expressed as numbers, percentages, and means. The significance of differences in the results for continuous and categorical variables among the women within each trimester group were determined by one-way ANOVA and the chi-square test, respectively. Multinomial logistic regression analysis was used to estimate the odds ratios (ORs) and 95% confidence intervals (CIs) of meeting the activity guideline. The results were presented as crude and adjusted ORs with 95% CIs. p-values of <0.05 were considered to indicate statistical significance. All data were analyzed using SPSS 17.0 (SPSS, Chicago, IL).

Results

Of these participants, 172 (16.3%), 512 (48.5%), and 372 (35.2%) were in the first, second, and third trimester, respectively. The mean age of the participants was 27.89±3.53 years. The other socio-demographic characteristics of the subjects are presented in Table1.

Of the 1056 participants, 87 (8.2%) had received advice about physical activity from a medical professional, and 786 (74.4%) women reported that they had become progressively less active during their pregnancy. In general, the participants considered their husband to be the most important person influencing their decision about exercise. Walking slowly was the most popular exercise. The most common reason given for not engaging in more physical activity during pregnancy was the fear of miscarriage (Table 2).

Based on the PPAQ, 117 (11.1%) women met the guideline. The rates of meeting the guideline did not differ significantly among the three trimesters (Table 3). Women in the first trimester had significantly higher median total energy expenditure (21.90 MET h/day) than women in the second and third trimesters (19.44 and 18.50 MET h/day, respectively; p<0.001). The median, moderate, and vigorous intensity expenditures during the three trimesters ranged from 1.75 to 1.86 MET h/day, and the median energy expenditure on sports/exercise for all subjects was 0.11 MET h/day. As shown in Table 4, sedentary activities accounted for more than half of the energy expenditure of all

Table 2. Exercise-related characteristics of pregnant women (N = 1056) n (%).

Characteristic		Overall	1st trimester	2nd trimester	3rd trimester
Exercise advices from medical professional		87 (8.2)	17(9.9)	34 (6.6)	36(9.7)
Habitually exercise before pregnancy		376 (35.6)	70 (40.7)	174 (34.0)	132 (35.5)
Self-evaluation of physical activity level	Low	448 (42.4)	66 (38.4)	217 (42.4)	165 (44.4)
	Moderate	600 (56.8)	103 (59.9)	291 (56.8)	206 (55.4)
	High	8 (0.8)	3 (1.7)	4 (0.8)	1 (0.3)
Self-evaluation of physical activity changes after pregnancy	Less active	786 (74.4)	129 (75.0)	381 (74.4)	276 (74.2)
	Increased activity	28 (2.7)	2 (1.2)	14 (2.7)	12 (3.2)
	No change	242 (22.9)	41 (23.8)	117 (22.9)	84 (22.6)
Having to go with husband who habitually exercises		820 (77.7)	139 (80.8)	398 (77.7)	283 (76.1)
		698 (66.1)	111 (64.5)	343 (67.0)	244 (65.6)
Sources of information about exercise	Books and newspapers	662 (62.7)	120 (69.7)	298 (58.3)	244 (65.6)
	Friends or relatives	346 (32.8)	68 (39.5)	178 (34.8)	100 (26.9)
	Multi-media	512 (48.4)	100 (58.2)	262 (51.2)	150 (40.3)
	Medical institutions	102 (9.7)	0 (0.0)	56 (10.9)	46 (12.4)
	Public announcement	142 (13.4)	52 (30.2)	58 (11.3)	32 (8.6)
Desirable sources of information about exercise	Medical institutions	554 (52.5)	90 (52.3)	278 (54.3)	186 (50.0)
	Public announcement	274 (25.9)	68 (39.6)	100 (19.5)	106 (28.5)
	Multi-media	192 (18.1)	22 (12.8)	102 (20.0)	68 (18.3)
	Books and newspapers	118 (11.2)	16 (9.3)	60 (11.7)	42 (11.3)
	Friends or relatives	126 (11.9)	12 (7.0)	74 (14.5)	40 (10.7)
The person deciding about the exercise	Husband or partner	848 (80.3)	156 (90.7)	436 (85.2)	256 (68.8)
	Medical staff	334 (31.6)	50 (29.1)	240 (46.9)	44 (11.8)
	Other family members or friends	300 (28.6)	60 (34.9)	116 (22.7)	124 (33.3)
The preferred exercise	Walking slowly	1032 (98.0)	172 (100.0)	506 (98.8)	354 (95.2)
	Prenatal exercise class	324 (30.7)	60 (34.9)	180 (35.2)	84 (22.6)
	Swimming	30 (2.8)	6 (3.5)	16 (3.1)	8 (2.2)
	Climb hill	18 (1.7)	4 (2.3)	8 (1.6)	6 (1.6)
	Dancing	10 (0.9)	2 (1.2)	2 (0.4)	6 (1.6)
	Walking quickly	8 (0.8)	0 (0.0)	4 (0.8)	4 (1.1)
	Running slowly	6 (0.5)	2 (1.2)	2 (0.4)	2 (0.5)
	Running quickly	3 (0.3)	0 (0.0)	3 (0.6)	0 (0.0)
Reasons hindering exercise activities	Fear of miscarriage	704 (66.7)	138 (80.2)	390 (76.2)	176 (47.3)
	Discomfort	370 (35.0)	68 (39.5)	216 (42.2)	86 (23.1)
	Lacking exercise knowledge	264 (25.0)	38 (22.1)	170 (33.2)	56 (15.1)
	Too tired	244 (23.1)	48 (27.9)	82 (16.0)	114 (30.6)
	Having no exercise habits	150 (14.2)	14 (8.1)	82 (16.0)	54 (14.5)
	Lack of venues or equipment	120 (11.4)	10 (5.8)	92 (18.0)	18 (4.8)
	Having no time	102 (9.7)	24 (14.0)	50 (9.8)	28 (7.5)
	Having no one to go with	90 (8.5)	4 (2.3)	52 (10.2)	34 (9.1)
	Dislikes exercise	56 (5.3)	10 (5.8)	24 (4.7)	22 (5.9)
	Weight gain	54 (5.1)	2 (11.6)	30 (5.9)	22 (5.9)

subjects (52.7–57.6%). By contrast, exercise accounted for only 1.7–2.4% of the energy expenditure for all subjects (Table 4).

As shown in Table 5, after adjusting for a number of factors, several variables strongly influenced the ORs of meeting the guideline. Pregnant women who had college degrees or higher education were more likely to meet the guideline (OR: 4.11, 95% CI: 1.59–10.62). However, having a low pre gravid BMI decreased the ORs of meeting the guideline (OR: 0.42, 95% CI: 0.20–0.87). Women who exercised regularly before pregnancy had an increased likelihood of meeting the guideline (OR: 2.14, 95%

Table 3. Physical activities during pregnancy.

Characteristic	1st trimester (≤13 weeks)			2nd trimester (14–27 weeks)			3rd trimester (≥28 weeks)				
	Mean[a]	Median[a]	25th, 75th percentile	Mean[a]	Media[a]	25th, 75th percentile	Mean[a]	Median[a]	25th, 75th percentile	*H*	*P value*[b]
Meet the guideline *n* (%)	20 (11.6)			58 (11.3)			39 (10.5)			0.219	0.896
Total energy expenditure per day	23.98	21.90	14.78, 28.04	20.41	19.44	12.31, 27.29	20.11	18.50	12.21, 26.71	22.000	0.000
By activity intensity											
Sedentary	13.82	11.74	7.70, 16.71	11.74	9.85	7.08, 16.4	10.59	9.58	6.63, 16.55	31.256	0.000
Light	5.76	5.29	2.61, 9.31	5.85	4.68	2.50, 7.93	6.03	4.53	2.53, 7.20	2.677	0.262
Moderate	4.28	1.86	0.86, 4.58	2.78	1.75	0.75, 4.19	3.45	1.75	0.75, 3.86	22.787	0.000
Vigorous	0.11	0.00	0.00, 0.00	0.02	0.00	0.00, 0.00	0.04	0.00	0.00, 0.00	10.611	0.005
By type of activity											
Household/caregiving	3.09	3.03	1.21, 5.33	3.75	3.03	1.25, 5.74	5.34	3.03	1.28, 5.74	41.139	0.000
Occupational	8.23	6.00	0.00, 10.15	5.49	2.06	0.00, 10.15	4.02	0.20	0.00, 10.15	73.347	0.000
Sports/exercise	0.57	0.11	0.00, 0.51	0.34	0.11	0.00, 0.36	0.43	0.11	0.00, 0.35	41.326	0.000
Transportation	3.89	2.75	0.38, 4.09	3.02	2.25	1.03, 4.00	2.35	2.00	1.12, 3.63	42.519	0.000

[a] MET-hours/day.
[b] Kruskal–Wallis test of differences in ranks.

Table 4. Contribution of each type of activity to the total expenditure across different trimesters.

Characteristics	1st trimester (≤13 weeks) (%)	2nd trimester (14–27 weeks) (%)	3rd trimester (≥28 weeks) (%)
Total energy expenditure	100.0	100.0	100.0
Sedentary	57.7	57.6	52.7
Light	24.0	28.7	30.0
Moderate	17.8	13.6	17.1
Vigorous	0.5	0.1	0.2
Total energy expenditure[a]			
Household/caregiving	12.9	18.4	26.6
Occupational	34.3	26.9	20.0
Sports/exercise	2.4	1.7	2.1
Transportation	16.2	14.8	11.7

[a] Sitting accounted for 34% to 40% of total energy expenditure in the three trimesters.

CI: 1.39–3.28). The odds of meeting the guideline were higher in women with a self-evaluation of current physical activity as moderate (OR: 2.43, 95% CI: 1.53–3.86) or high (OR: 9.49, 95% CI: 1.77–50.88), and those having a husband who exercised habitually (OR: 2.21, 95% CI: 1.33–3.67). Receiving advice from medical professionals did not increase the odds (OR: 0.74, 95% CI: 0.19–2.83) (Table 5).

Discussion

Only 11.1% of the pregnant women who participated in this study met the international recommended guideline for physical activity during pregnancy. This rate is lower than the rates recorded in Ireland (21.5%) [10] and the United States (22.9% and 94.5%) [11,12]. In addition, the subjects in this study expended less total energy during pregnancy (approximately 20 MET h/day) than pregnant women in the United States (25.4 MET h/day) [12], Australia (30.0 MET h/day) [13], and France (29.0 MET h/day) [20]. However, the contributions of specific activities to the total energy expenditure found in this study population were similar to the Australian and French study populations [13,20].

The women in this study expressed concern about the safety of exercise, reporting that the primary reason for not exercising during pregnancy was fear of miscarriage. By contrast, women who participated in studies conducted in Brazil and Australia stated that their primary reasons for lack of exercise in pregnancy were feeling tired, lack of time, and incontinence [15,16]. This difference may be related to traditional Chinese culture, which defines pregnancy as a vulnerable period that requires rest and protection. Therefore, to avoid spontaneous miscarriage and reduce pressure from family and friends, pregnant Chinese women tend to obey traditional taboos such as "no jumping", "no moving heavy objects", "no fast walking", and "not too much walking" [24]. This may partly explain why the pregnant Chinese women reported that their most common form of exercise was slow walking, which is very different from pregnant British women, who report that fast walking, swimming, and prenatal exercise classes are their most popular forms of exercise [14]. The cultural taboos against exercise in pregnancy in China are exacerbated by the Family Planning Policy, which has greatly increased the focus of family members on the fetus and the pregnant woman [25]. As a result, it is believed that cutting back on exercise and even household/caregiving activities aids the growth of the fetus [24]. These cultural factors may explain why 74.4% of these study subjects become less physically active during pregnancy and why exercise contributed little to total energy expenditure. The fact that a large number of women in China stop exercising after becoming pregnant had been observed previously; moreover, more than half of Chinese women become overweight during pregnancy [3]. Evenson *et al.* have previously noted that the influence of different cultural beliefs on physical activity during pregnancy needs further exploration [26].

The present study showed that only 8.2% of the pregnant Chinese participants were given advice by medical professionals about physical activity. By contrast, an American study showed that 63% of pregnant women in the United States were given advice about physical activity during pregnancy and that more than half believed that such advice from doctors could improve their exercise behavior in pregnancy [27]. A recent systematic review of nine randomized controlled trials of behavioral interventions for improving physical activity among pregnant women suggests that medical providers play a key role in such interventions [28]. However, in this study, receiving advice from health professionals did not increase the rate at which the participants met the international guideline. A study in Taiwan found that individual counseling on diet and physical activity provided during routine clinic visits made the pregnant women healthier and more active and thus assisted with weight management during pregnancy [29]. Therefore, because nonsystematic medical advice may not be adequate for changing the exercise behaviors of pregnant women in China, a systematic clinic-based intervention protocol may be warranted.

Consistent with previous studies, the pregnant women who had higher educational levels were more active during their pregnancy than women with lower educational levels [4,13]. This correlation may be related to the possibility that women with higher educational levels have more access to knowledge about physical activity during pregnancy and thus are more likely to exercise [13]. Moreover, the present study showed that women who exercised regularly and evaluated their current level of physical activity as moderate or high were more likely to meet the guideline. This finding suggests that this self-evaluation is relatively objective, and that habitual exercise before pregnancy can influence women to

Table 5. Association between participants' characteristics and the odds of meeting the guideline.

Characteristics		*n (%)*	*OR (95% CI)*	
			Unadjusted	**Adjusted**
Age		27.89±3.53	1.04 (0.99, 1.10)	1.02 (0.95, 1.10)
Race	Minority	54 (5.0)	0.30 (0.07, 1.23)	0.26 (0.06, 1.16)
Currently employed	Working	590 (55.9)	1.82 (1.21, 2.74)	1.10 (0.65, 1.87)
Education	Lower than high school	180 (17.0)	1.0 (Ref)	1.0 (Ref)
	High school graduate	424 (40.2)	1.93 (0.92, 4.06)	2.24 (0.95, 5.25)
	College or higher degree	452 (42.8)	3.42 (1.67, 7.02)	4.11 (1.59, 10.62)
Monthly household income	≤3500	368 (34.9)	0.41 (0.20, 0.85)	0.71 (0.31, 1.63)
(RMB)	~3501	274 (25.9)	0.91 (0.45, 1.84)	1.30 (0.60, 2.83)
	~5001	338 (32.0)	0.70 (0.35, 1.40)	0.70 (0.33, 1.51)
	≥10000	76 (7.2)	1.0 (Ref)	1.0 (Ref)
Previous live births	0	946 (89.6)	0.52 (0.11, 2.46)	0.64 (0.11, 3.68)
	1	100 (9.5)	0.30 (0.05, 1.70)	0.51 (0.08, 3.39)
	2	10 (0.9)	1.0 (Ref)	1.0 (Ref)
Pre-pregnancy work status	Working	750 (71.0)	1.41 (0.90, 2.22)	0.76 (0.42,1.36)
Pre-pregnancy health status	Very healthy	422 (40.0)	1.0 (Ref)	1.0 (Ref)
	Healthy	500 (47.3)	0.83 (0.55, 1.25)	1.04 (0.66, 1.63)
	General	134 (12.7)	0.92 (0.50, 1.69)	1.03 (0.52, 2.04)
Pre-gravid BMI (kg/m^2)	Low (≤18.4)	164 (15.5)	0.39 (0.19, 0.78)	0.42 (0.20, 0.87)
	Normal (~18.5)	764 (72.4)	1.0 (Ref)	1.0 (Ref)
	Overweight (~25.0)	128 (12.1)	0.44 (0.21, 0.93)	0.64 (0.16, 2.58)
Discomfort symptoms	Yes	792 (75.0)	0.83 (0.54, 1.28)	0.75 (0.49, 1.85)
Stage of pregnancy	First trimester	172 (16.3)	1.12 (0.63, 1.99)	0.95 (0.55, 2.09)
	Second trimester	512 (48.5)	1.09 (0.71, 1.68)	0.86 (0.52, 1.41)
	Third trimester	372 (35.2)	1.0 (Ref)	1.0 (Ref)
Exercise before pregnancy	Yes	376 (35.6)	2.33 (1.58, 3.44)	2.14 (1.39, 3.28)
Self-evaluation of current physical activity level	Low	448 (42.4)	1.0 (Ref)	1.0 (Ref)
	Moderate	600 (56.8)	1.94 (1.26, 2.96)	2.43 (1.53, 3.86)
	High	8 (0.8)	12.58 (3.00,52.58)	9.49 (1.77,50.88)
Having to go with husband who habitually exercises	Yes	820 (77.7)	1.20 (0.74, 1.94)	1.14 (0.69, 1.90)
	Yes	698 (66.1)	1.72 (1.10, 2.69)	2.21 (1.33, 3.67)
Exercise advice from medical professional	Yes	87(8.2)	0.51(0.24, 1.07)	0.74(0.19, 2.83)

continue exercising during pregnancy. The latter observation has also been made previously [4].

A previous study in Australia showed that women with high pre gravid BMIs were less active during pregnancy than women with lower pre gravid BMIs [4]. By contrast, the present study showed that Chinese women with low pre gravid BMIs were less likely to meet the guideline than those with higher BMIs. Huang *et al.* [30] observed that a low weight before pregnancy also increased the risk of excessive GWG in women in Taiwan, which may reflect several cultural beliefs in China. First, traditional Chinese medicine holds that one is healthy when the *yin* and the *yang* are balanced, and that pregnancy can cause a harmful imbalance in the pregnant women's body [31]. To prevent this imbalance, Chinese women are encouraged to greatly increase their consumption of food and to decrease their physical activity [25]. This is exacerbated by the belief of the older women in Chinese families that it is necessary to gain weight during pregnancy. This belief reflects the experiences of these women with food shortages experienced in previous decades [29]. Notably, previous interventions for improving the physical activity of pregnant women mainly focused on high-risk groups such as obese women [28], but our observation that women with low pre gravid BMI were more likely not to meet the guideline than women with higher BMI indicates that future interventions should target all women, not just the high-risk women.

The present study also showed that pregnant women with husbands who exercised habitually were more likely to meet the guideline than women with less active husbands. The exercise levels of pregnant women correlated positively with their partner's physical activity levels. The observation that women living with an active partner may be more active during pregnancy than women without an active partner has been reported previously [14].

Thornton *et al.* [32] also posited that the husband is the most important influence on decisions about exercise in pregnancy because the husband provides the pregnant women with the most social support. In Chinese culture, antenatal taboos are mainly imparted by family members [25]. Further studies are required to determine whether maximizing the positive role of family members such as husbands will encourage Chinese women to increase their physical activity during pregnancy.

There were several limitations in present study. First, only one city was included, and all of the participants were urban residents. The study results may thus not be generalizable to all Chinese populations, including rural pregnant women. Studies examining the residents in multiple Chinese cities and in rural areas are warranted. Second, the reliability of self-reported measurements is lower than that of data obtained by accelerometry. However, the PPAQ is a validated tool for assessing the duration and intensity of exercise, and defining the types of physical activity that pregnant women engage in, and it is better than unstructured questions [19]. In addition, the questionnaire can collect data on some activities that could not be detected with accelerometry [33]. Third, data from this cross-sectional study do not illustrate exercise conditions throughout pregnancy. Therefore, longitudinal follow-up is warranted in future studies. Finally, although we explored a considerable number of factors influencing physical activity during pregnancy, we could not measure the influence of other factors such as social and cultural factors [26]. In the future, multicenter studies are needed for measuring additional factors influencing physical activity during pregnancy in China.

Conclusions

Few urban Chinese pregnant women met the recommended physical activity guideline. They also expended little energy on exercise. Physical activity interventions that are conducted in the clinic environment and that target family members and social networks in addition to the pregnant woman herself, may improve the physical activity and health of pregnant Chinese women and should be explored. Moreover, pregnant women with low pre gravid BMIs should also be given as much attention in future interventions as women who are deemed to be at high risk.

Author Contributions

Conceived and designed the experiments: Y. Zhang HZ Y. Zhao. Performed the experiments: Y. Zhang SD JZ HZ XH. Analyzed the data: Y. Zhang HZ. Wrote the paper: Y. Zhang.

References

1. Fell DB, Joseph KS, Armson BA, Dodds L, Nelson ME, et al. (2009) The impact of pregnancy on physical activity level. Matern Child Health J 13: 597–603.
2. Hedderson MM, Gunderson EP, Ferrara A (2010) Gestational weight gain and risk of gestational diabetes mellitus. Obstet Gynecol 115: 597–604.
3. Jiang H, Qian X, Li M, Lynn H, Fan Y, et al. (2012) Can physical activity reduce excessive gestational weight gain? Findings from a Chinese urban pregnant women cohort study. Int J Behav Nutr Phys Act 9: 12.
4. Foxcroft KF, Rowlands IJ, Byrne NM, McIntyre HD, Callaway LK (2011) Exercise in obese pregnant women: the role of social factors, lifestyle and pregnancy symptoms. BMC Pregnancy Childbirth 11: 4.
5. Pivarnik J, Chambliss H, Clapp JI (2006) Impact of physical activity during pregnancy and postpartum on chronic disease risk. Med Sci Sports Exerc 38: 989–1006.
6. ACOG (2002) ACOG Committee opinion. Number 267, January 2002: exercise during pregnancy and the postpartum period. Obstet Gynecol 99: 171–173.
7. Gjestland K, Bo K, Owe KM, Eberhard-Gran M (2012) Do pregnant women follow exercise guidelines? Prevalence data among 3482 women, and prediction of low-back pain, pelvic girdle pain and depression. Br J Sports Med 47: 515–520.
8. Liu J, Blair SN, Teng Y, Ness AR, Lawlor DA, et al. (2011) Physical activity during pregnancy in a prospective cohort of British women: results from the Avon longitudinal study of parents and children. Eur J Epidemiol 26: 237–247.
9. Clarke PE, Gross H (2004) Women's behaviour, beliefs and information sources about physical exercise in pregnancy. Midwifery 20: 133–141.
10. Walsh JM, McGowan C, Byrne J, McAuliffe FM (2011) Prevalence of physical activity among healthy pregnant women in Ireland. Int J Gynaecol Obstet 114: 154–155.
11. Evenson KR, Wen F (2010) National trends in self-reported physical activity and sedentary behaviors among pregnant women: NHANES 1999–2006. Prev Med 50: 123–128.
12. Smith KM, Campbell CG (2013) Physical activity during pregnancy: impact of applying different physical activity guidelines. J Pregnancy 2013: 165617.
13. Schmidt MD, Pekow P, Freedson PS, Markenson G, Chasan-Taber L (2006) Physical activity patterns during pregnancy in a diverse population of women. J Womens Health (Larchmt) 15: 909–918.
14. Liu J, Blair SN, Teng Y, Ness AR, Lawlor DA, et al. (2011) Physical activity during pregnancy in a prospective cohort of British women: results from the Avon longitudinal study of parents and children. Eur J Epidemiol 26: 237–247.
15. Ribeiro CP, Milanez H (2011) Knowledge, attitude and practice of women in Campinas, Sao Paulo, Brazil with respect to physical exercise in pregnancy: A descriptive study. Reprod Health 8: 31.
16. Duncombe D, Wertheim EH, Skouteris H, Paxton SJ, Kelly L (2009) Factors related to exercise over the course of pregnancy including women's beliefs about the safety of exercise during pregnancy. Midwifery 25: 430–438.
17. Li Q, Xiong R, Wang L, Cui J, Shi L, et al. (2014) Associations of dietary habits, physical activity and cognitive views with gestational diabetes mellitus amongChinese women. Public Health Nutr 17: 1850–1857.
18. Ding D, Sallis JF, Hovell MF, Du J, Zheng M, et al. (2011) Physical activity and sedentary behaviours among rural adults in Suixi, China: a cross-sectional study. Int J Behav Nutr Phys Act 8: 37.
19. Chasan-Taber L, Schmidt MD, Roberts DE, Hosmer D, Markenson G, et al. (2004) Development and validation of a Pregnancy Physical ActivityQuestion-naire. Med Sci Sports Exerc 36: 1750–1760.
20. Chandonnet N, Saey D, Almeras N, Marc I (2012) French Pregnancy Physical Activity Questionnaire compared with an accelerometer cut point to classify physical activity among pregnant obese women. PLOS One 7: e38818.
21. Matsuzaki M, Haruna M, Ota E, Yeo S, Murayama R, et al. (2010) Translation and cross-cultural adaptation of the Pregnancy Physical Activity Questionnaire (PPAQ) to Japanese. Biosci Trends 4: 170–177.
22. Ota E, Haruna M, Yanai H, Suzuki M, Anh DD, et al. (2008) Reliability and validity of the Vietnamese version of the Pregnancy Physical Activity Questionnaire (PPAQ). Southeast Asian J Trop Med Public Health 39: 562–570.
23. Zhang Y, Zhao Y, Dong SW, Xiong Y, XQ H (2013) Reliability and validity of the Chinese version of the Pregnancy Physical Activity Questionnaire(PPAQ). Chinese Journal Of Nursing 48: 825–827.
24. Lee DT, Ngai IS, Ng MM, Lok IH, Yip AS, et al. (2009) Antenatal taboos among Chinese women in Hong Kong. Midwifery 25: 104–113.
25. Gao H, Stiller CK, Scherbaum V, Biesalski HK, Wang Q, et al. (2013) Dietary intake and food habits of pregnant women residing in urban and rural areas of Deyang City, Sichuan Province, China. Nutrients 5: 2933–2954.
26. Evenson KR, Bradley CB (2010) Beliefs about exercise and physical activity among Pregnant women. Patient Educ Couns, 79(1):124–129.
27. Krans EE, Gearhart JG, Dubbert PM, Klar PM, Miller AL, et al. (2005) Pregnant women's beliefs and influences regarding exercise during pregnancy. J Miss State Med Assoc 46: 67–73.
28. Pearce EE, Evenson KR, Downs DS, Steckler A (2013) Strategies to Promote Physical Activity During Pregnancy: A Systematic Review of Intervention Evidence. Am J Lifestyle Med 7.
29. Huang TT, Yeh CY, Tsai YC (2011) A diet and physical activity intervention for preventing weight retention among Taiwanese childbearing women: a randomised controlled trial. Midwifery 27: 257–264.
30. Huang TT, Dai FT (2007) Weight retention predictors for Taiwanese women at six-month postpartum. J Nurs Res 15: 11–20.
31. Raven JH CQ, Tolhurst RJ, Garner P (2007) Traditional beliefs and practices in the postpartum period in Fujian Province, China: a qualitative study. BMC Pregnancy Childbirth 21: 8.
32. Thornton PL, Kieffer EC, Salabarria-Pena Y, Odoms-Young A, Willis SK, et al. (2006) Weight, diet, and physical activity-related beliefs and practices among pregnant and postpartum Latino women: the role of social support. Matern Child Health J 10: 95–104.
33. Bell R, Tennant PW, McParlin C, Pearce MS, Adamson AJ, et al. (2013) Measuring physical activity in pregnancy: a comparison of accelerometry and self-completion questionnaires in overweight and obese women. Eur J Obstet Gynecol Reprod Biol 1: 90–95.

26

The Acute Satellite Cell Response and Skeletal Muscle Hypertrophy following Resistance Training

Leeann M. Bellamy[1,◑], Sophie Joanisse[1,◑], Amanda Grubb[1,◑], Cameron J. Mitchell[1], Bryon R. McKay[1], Stuart M. Phillips[1], Steven Baker[3], Gianni Parise[1,2*]

1 Department of Kinesiology, McMaster University, Hamilton, Ontario, Canada, **2** Department of Medical Physics and Applied Radiation Sciences, McMaster University, Hamilton, Ontario, Canada, **3** Department of Medicine, McMaster University, Hamilton, Ontario, Canada

Abstract

The extent of skeletal muscle hypertrophy in response to resistance training is highly variable in humans. The main objective of this study was to explain the nature of this variability. More specifically, we focused on the myogenic stem cell population, the satellite cell (SC) as a potential mediator of hypertrophy. Twenty-three males (aged 18–35 yrs) participated in 16 wk of progressive, whole body resistance training, resulting in changes of 7.9±1.6% (range of −1.9–24.7%) and 21.0±4.0% (range of −7.0 to 51.7%) in quadriceps volume and myofibre cross-sectional area (CSA), respectively. The SC response to a single bout of resistance exercise (80% 1RM), analyzed via immunofluorescent staining resulted in an expansion of type II fibre associated SC 72 h following exercise (pre: 11.3±0.9; 72 h: 14.8±1.4 SC/type II fibre; $p<0.05$). Training resulted in an expansion of the SC pool associated with type I (pre: 10.7±1.1; post: 12.1±1.2 SC/type I fibre; $p<0.05$) and type II fibres (pre: 11.3±0.9; post: 13.0±1.2 SC/type II fibre; $p<0.05$). Analysis of individual SC responses revealed a correlation between the relative change in type I associated SC 24 to 72 hours following an acute bout of resistance exercise and the percentage increase in quadriceps lean tissue mass assessed by MRI ($r^2=0.566$, $p=0.012$) and the relative change in type II associated SC following 16 weeks of resistance training and the percentage increase in quadriceps lean tissue mass assessed by MRI ($r^2=0.493$, $p=0.027$). Our results suggest that the SC response to resistance exercise is related to the extent of muscular hypertrophy induced by training.

Editor: Atsushi Asakura, University of Minnesota Medical School, United States of America

Funding: This study was funded by a Natural Science and Engineering Research Council Discovery grant awarded to GP. The funders had no role in study design, data collection and analysis, decision to publish, or preparation of the manuscript.

Competing Interests: The authors have declared that no competing interests exist.

* Email: pariseg@mcmaster.ca

◑ These authors contributed equally to this work.

Introduction

There is a high degree of inter-individual variation in skeletal muscle hypertrophy following resistance exercise training despite exposure to exercise of the same relative intensity [1,2]. Individuals response to hypertrophic stimuli like resistance exercise leads to a highly variable response with respect to the accretion of lean tissue [1]. The basis for the variability in hypertrophic responses to training is poorly understood; however factors such as genetic variation [3], genetic polymorphisms [4,5], transcriptomic profiles [6] the ability to activate specific signaling proteins known to be important in muscle protein synthesis [7], and microRNA expression [8] have been identified as potential control points in regulating the hypertrophic response.

Skeletal muscle possesses a functional population of resident stem cells commonly referred to as satellite cells (SC) [9]. SC are activated, proliferate and fuse giving rise to nascent myotubes or fuse to existing muscle fibres in response to various stressors such as mechanical loading or injury [10]. The progression of SC from activation, proliferation through to terminal differentiation is governed by a network of transcription factors referred to as myogenic regulatory factors (MRF) [11–13]. Although the essential role that SC play in the maintenance of healthy skeletal muscle function is widely accepted their role in mediating exercise induced skeletal muscle hypertrophy is debatable. Various findings from studies of resistance exercise training-induced hypertrophy in humans highlight the association of SC with muscle hypertrophy [2,14]. However based on results from rodent models others propose that SC are dispensable in mediating muscle hypertrophy [15,16]. We propose, however, that because hypertrophy can occur in SC-depleted rodent models does not necessarily render their contribution unimportant in contributing to hypertrophy in humans under physiological conditions. Instead, models of selective SC depletion that demonstrate hypertrophy, under conditions of extreme overload, merely establish the capacity of redundant mechanisms to compensate and result in hypertrophy.

In humans a growing body of evidence has characterized the response of SC to resistance exercise and implied a role for nuclear addition during muscle fibre adaptation [9,17–21]. Only one previous study in humans has, however, attempted to correlate the variability in the myogenic response to acute resistance exercise or following resistance training [2,14].

Myostatin (MSTN, or growth-differentiation factor 8, GDF-8), a transforming growth factor-beta (TGF-β) family member, is a negative regulator of muscle growth [22]. Knockouts of MSTN in multiple species (including a human case study) resulted in gross muscle hypertrophy and an overall increase in body mass of 2–3 fold as compared to wild-type counterparts [22]. Importantly, there appears to be a conserved role for MSTN in humans, which we demonstrated by showing an acute reduction in the co-localization of MSTN to SC in human skeletal muscle *in vivo* following a single exercise bout. Furthermore, aging was found to be associated with an impaired ability to decrease the proportion of SC co-localized with MSTN following exercise [9]. Collectively, these results imply a role for MSTN in the regulation of human SC function and suggest that MSTN may regulate hypertrophy [23].

The purpose of this investigation was to determine whether either the acute SC response to a bout of resistance exercise or the expansion of the SC pool was related to muscle hypertrophy following training. We hypothesized that individuals with an elevated acute SC response, based on expansion of the SC pool and progression of SCs through the myogenic program, would also demonstrate the greatest increase in lean tissue mass.

Methods

Subjects

Twenty-three previously untrained healthy males (age 18–35 years) completed 16 weeks of whole body resistance training. Participants were recreationally active but had no formal weight training experience within the past year. This study was approved by the McMaster University Research Ethics Board and adhered to the principles expressed in the Declaration of Helsinki. Informed written consent was obtained from all participants prior to commencement of the study. Complete subject characteristics have been previously published [24].

Exercise Training

The training program has been previously described elsewhere [24]. In brief, however, training consisted of four supervised sessions per week, divided into two upper and two lower body sessions. The upper body sessions consisted of chest press, shoulder press, lat pull down, row, bicep curl and triceps extension exercise. The lower body sessions consisted of leg press, leg extension, leg curl, calf press, and abdominal exercise. Training progressed from two sets performed at 70% of 1 repetition maximum (RM) to four sets performed at 85% of 1RM, with all sets performed to the point of momentary muscle exhaustion. At the conclusion of each workout, participants consumed a beverage containing 30 g of whey protein, 25.9 g of carbohydrates and 3.4 g of fat (Musashi p30, Notting Hill Victoria, Australia).

Acute Exercise Protocol

Prior to the onset of the resistance training program subjects completed an intensity matched (80% 1RM) acute bout of resistance exercise. The acute exercise consisted of four sets and eight reps each of leg press, leg extension, calf press and leg curl. The final set was performed to volitional failure. All exercises (with the exception of leg press) were performed using HUR circuit training-type exercise equipment (HUR, Kokkola Finland).

Magnetic Resonance Imaging and Dual-Energy X-ray Absorptiometry

Magnetic resonance imaging (MRI) scans of the quadriceps were completed by all participants prior to and following the training program. Prior to scanning, participants rested in the supine position for 1 h to prevent the influence of fluid shift on muscle volume. Imaging was performed in a 3T HD scanner (Signa MRI System, GE Medical, Milwaukee, WI). Image acquisition in the axial plane was performed with the following parameters: repetition time/echo time = 2100 ms/23.58 ms; field of view = 28 cm; matrix size = 320/320 reconstructed to 512/512 phase/frequency; slice thickness = 5 mm. Thigh image acquisition utilized an eight-channel torso coil with two excitations. There was a 10 mm gap between slices. Quadriceps volume was measured from the first slice where the rectus femoris was visible to the first slice where the gluteus maximus was visible, and calculated by multiplying the slice area by the distance between slices. The area of each slice was determined with Image J software (U. S. National Institutes of Health, Bethesda, Maryland, USA). Time of day, joint angle and leg compression were matched in all pre- and post-training scans.

Body composition was assessed using whole body dual-energy X-ray absorptiometry (DEXA) scan (QDR-4500A, software version 12.31; Hologic, Bedford, MA). Subjects were fasted and had not completed any exercise prior to the scan. All scans were performed and analyzed by a trained technician. All scans were completed according to the AIS whole-body DEXA protocol [24,25]. Prior to the measurement the DEXA was calibrated as per manufacture guidelines. All subjects were centrally aligned prior to the scan, hands and feet were secured for consistency.

Sample Collection

Muscle biopsies were obtained from the *vastus lateralis* before, 24 h and 72 h after an acute exercise bout prior to (Pre-1, 24-1, 72-1) and following (Pre-2, 24-2, 72-2) 16 weeks of exercise training using a modified 5 mm Bergström needle with manual suction under local anaesthesia (2% xylocaine). Subjects had not participated in any physical activity at least 96 hours before the collection of the baseline biopsy (Pre). Upon excision, the muscle samples were immediately dissected into pieces that were snap frozen in liquid nitrogen (gene expression analysis), embedded in optimal cutting temperature (OCT) compound for immunofluorescence analysis, or maintained as fresh tissue in growth media (Dulbecco's modified eagle medium - DMEM containing 20% fetal bovine serum - FBS) for flow cytometry analysis.

Flow Cytometry

Approximately 65 mg of muscle obtained from biopsies prior to training (Pre-1, 24-1, 72-1) were prepared for flow cytometry analysis. Briefly, muscle samples were weighed prior to mulching with sterile surgical scissors in 35 mm tissue culture plates. Single cell suspensions were achieved using enzymatic digestion. 400 μl of Collagenase/dispase solution (10 mg/ml Collagenase B, Roche Diagnotsics, Mannheim, Germany; 2.4 U/ml dispase, Life Technologies, Garlsbad, CA, USA; containing 5 μl/ml of 0.5 M $CaCl_2$) was added to each plate, triturated for ~2 min, and incubated at 37°C for 9 min, this step was then repeated with an incubation time of 5 min. The sample was then filtered using a 70 μm mesh filter and centrifuged at 800 g for 5 min to obtain a pellet of mononuclear cells. Cells were fixed in ice cold 70% ethanol and stored at −20°C. Samples were prepared as previously described [26] by incubation in Pax7 primary antibody (neat, Developmental Studies Hybridoma Bank, Iowa City, IA, USA), Alexa Fluor 488 goat anti-mouse secondary antibody (1:500, Invitrogen, Carlsbad, CA, USA), and propidium iodide. Flow cytometry analysis was completed on a Beckman-Coulter Epics XL (Beckman-Coulter Inc., Brea, CA, USA) instrument operated by a trained technician.

Immunofluorescence

Muscle cryosections, 7 μm in thickness, were prepared from OCT embedded samples, allowed to air dry for 15–45 minutes and stored at −80°C. Tissue sections were fixed in 4% paraformaldehyde (PFA) for 10 min, washed 3×5 min in PBST, blocked for 60 min at RT (in PBS containing 2% bovine serum albumin, 5% FBS, 0.2% Triton x-100, 0.1% NaAzide, and 2% goat serum), and subsequently incubated in primary antibodies Pax7 (neat, DSHB), Laminin (1:250 or 1:750, Abcam, Cambridge, MA, USA), MHCI (neat, DSHB, Iowa City, IA, USA), MHCII (1:1000, Abcam, Cambride, MA, USA), and Myostatin (1:150, Millipore, Etobicoke, ON, Canada) for 2 hr at RT or overnight at 4°C. Secondary antibody detection included Pax7 (Alexa Fluor 594 goat anti-mouse, 1:500), Laminin (Alexa Fluor 488 goat anti-rabbit, 1:500), MHCI (Alexa Fluor 488 goat anti-mouse, 1:500), MHCII and Myostatin (Alexa Fluor goat anti-rabbit, 1:500), all from Invitrogen, Carlsbad, CA, USA, for 2 hr at RT. Nuclei were labelled with DAPI (4′,6-diamidino-2-phenylindole) (1:20000, Sigma-Aldrich, Oakville, ON, Canada), prior to cover slipping slides with fluorescent mounting media (DAKO, Burlington, ON, Canada). Images were taken with a Nikon Eclipse 90i microscope at 20× magnification and captured with a high-resolution QImaging fluorescent camera (Nikon Instruments, Melville, NY, USA). SC quantity and myostatin positive cells were quantified using the Nikon NIS Elements AR 3.0 software (Nikon Instruments, Melville, NY, USA) on large scale images consisting of ≥ 100 fibres/subject/timepoint in a blinded fashion.

RNA Isolation

RNA was isolated from 15–25 mg of muscle using the Trizol/RNeasy method. All samples were homogenized with 1 mL of Trizol Reagent (Life Technologies, Burlington, ON, Canada), in Lysing Maxtrix D tubes (MP Biomedicals, Solon, OH, USA), with the FastPrep-24 Tissue and Cell Homogenizer (MP Biomedicals, Solon, OH, USA) for a duration of 40 sec at a setting of 6 m/sec. Following a five minute room temperature incubation, homogenized samples were stored at −80°C for one month (samples may be stored up to one year), until further processing. After thawing on ice, 200 μl of cholorform reagent (Sigma-Aldrich, Oakville, ON, Canada) was added to each sample, mixed vigorously for 15 sec, incubated at RT for 5 min, and spun at 12000 g for 10 min at 4°C. The RNA (aqueous) phase was purified using the commercially available E.Z.N.A. Total RNA Kit 1 (Omega Bio-Tek, Norcross, GA, USA) as per manufacturer's instructions. RNA concentration (ng/μl) and purity (260/280) was determined with the Nano-Drop 1000 Spectorophotometer (Thermo Fisher Scientific, Rockville, MD, USA). RNA integrity reported via RNA integrity numbers (RIN scale of 0–10) were determined with the Agilent 2100 Bioanalyzer (Agilent Technologies, Toronto, ON, Canada). Samples were reverse transcribed using the commercially available high capacity cDNA reverse transcription kit (Applied Biosystems, Foster City, CA, USA) in 20 μl reaction volumes, as per manufacturer's instructions, using an Eppendorf Mastercycler epgradient thermal cycler (Eppendorf, Mississauga, ON, Canada) to obtain cDNA for gene expression analysis.

Quantitative real time RT-PCR

All QPCR reactions were run in duplicate in 25 μl volumes containing RT Sybr Green qPCR Master Mix (Qiagen Sciences, Valencia, CA, USA), prepared with the epMotion 5075 Eppendorf automated pipetting system (Eppendorf, Mississauga, ON, Canada), and carried out using an Eppendorf realplex^2 Master Cycler epgradientS (Eppendorf, Mississauga, ON, Canada). Expression levels of Pax7 (fwd: 5′-GCTCCGGGGCAGAAC-TACC-3′; rev: 5′-GCACGCGGCTAATCGAACTC-3′), myostatin (fwd: 5′-TGGTCATGATCTTGCT GTAACCTT-3′; rev: 5′-TGTCTGTTACCTTGACCTCTAAAA-3′), follistatin (fwd: 5′-AGTC CAGTACCAAGGCAGATGT-3′; rev: 5′-GGTCA-CACAGTAGGCA TTATTGG-3′) and FSTL-1 (fwd: 5′-AGAG-GAGGAGATGACCAGATATG-3′; rev: 5′-CGCTGAAGTG-GAGAA GATGC-3′) were normalized to the housekeeping gene Beta-2-microglobulin (fwd: 5′-ATGAG TATGCCTGC-CGTGTGA-3′; rev: 5′-GGCATCTTCAAACCTCCATG-3′).

Statistical Analysis

Statistical analysis was performed using Sigma Stat 3.1.0 analysis software (Systat Software, Chicago, IL, USA). One-way repeated measures ANOVA tests, paired two-tailed t-tests and Pearson's correlations were performed where appropriate. Statistical significance was considered to be $p \leq 0.05$ with data reported as mean ± standard error of the mean (SEM).

Results

Skeletal muscle hypertrophy and nuclear content

Sixteen weeks of whole body resistance training resulted in skeletal muscle hypertrophy as assessed by DEXA, MRI and immunofluorescence (Fig 1). DEXA and MRI scans revealed a significant increase in total lean mass (pre: 62.6±2.0 kg; post: 64.8±2.1 kg; $p<0.001$) (Fig 1A), and in quadriceps volume (pre: 1837±82 cm^3; post: 1970±53 cm^3; $p<0.001$) (Fig 1B), respectively following training. Fibre CSA was assesed via immunofluorescent staining of muscle cross sections for type I (MHCI) and type II (MHCII); 16 weeks of training increased CSA for both type I (pre: 5355±324 μm^2; post: 6099±310 μm^2) and type II fibres (pre: 6284±390 μm^2; post: 7543±362 μm^2; $p<0.001$), as previously reported [24]. Myonuclear domain size, defined as the fiber CSA per nuclei, was maintained in type I (pre: 1409.6±72.5 μm^2/nuclei; post: 1341.1±61.5 μm^2/nuclei) and in type II fibres (pre: 1799.6±96.7 μm^2/nuclei; post: 1987.1±111.8 μm^2/nuclei), with an increase in the number of nuclei per muscle cross section of type I fibres (pre: 3.9±0.2; post: 4.6±0.2; $p<0.05$) and a strong trend for an increase in type II fibres (pre: 3.6±0.2; post: 3.9±0.2; $p=0.07$) observed with training (Fig 2A and B).

SC response following acute resistance exercise and training

The fibre type-specific SC response was quantified via immunofluorescence of muscle cross sections (Fig 3A). 72 hours following an acute bout of resistance exercise the number of SC associated with type II muscle fibres increased (pre: 11.3±0.9; 72 h: 14.8±1.4 SC/100 type II fibres; $p<0.05$) (Fig 3B). Following 16 weeks of resistance exercise training there was an expansion of the SC pool associated with both type I (pre: 10.7±1.1; post: 12.1±1.2 SC/100 type I fibres; $p<0.05$) and type II fibres (pre: 11.3±0.9; post: 13.0±1.2 SC/100 type II fibres; $p<0.05$, Fig 3C).

Gene expression analysis of Pax7 was conducted on whole muscle homogenates. In accordance with the fibre type-specific SC response Pax7 gene expression was increased 2.1-fold and 1.9-fold above baseline at 24 and 72 hours, respectively, following the acute bout of whole body resistance exercise that was completed before the onset of training ($p<0.05$, Fig 3D). In addition 16 weeks of training led to a 2.1-fold increase in basal Pax7 mRNA expression ($p<0.05$, Fig 3E).

There was an increase in the number of Pax7$^+$ cells progressing through the cell cycle as determined by flow cytometry analysis following the bout of acute exercise completed before training.

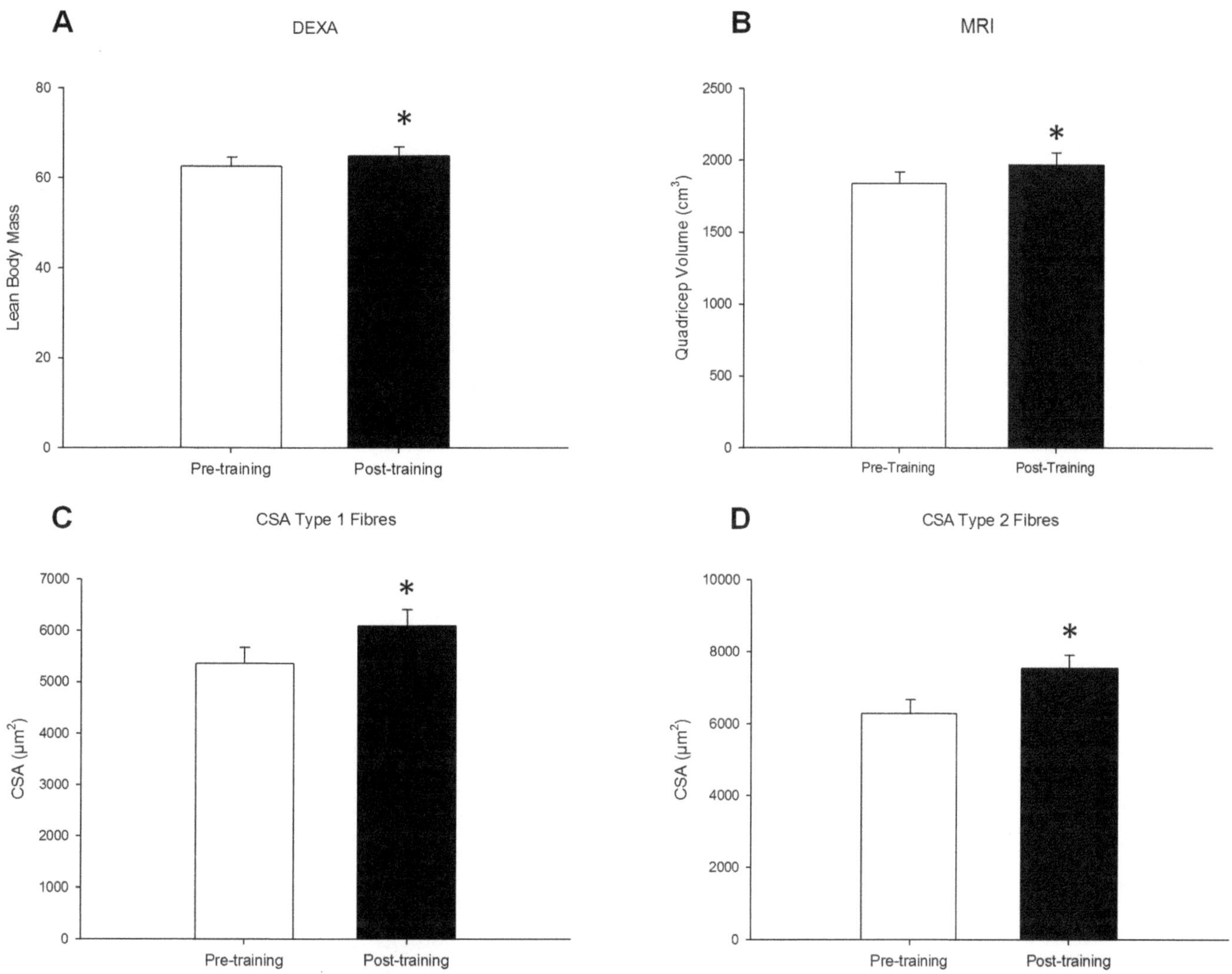

Figure 1. Skeletal muscle hypertrophy following training. Skeletal muscle hypertrophy was assessed by taking measures pre- and post-training using (A) DEXA, (B) MRI, and (C and D) cross-sectional area specific to both type 1 and type 2 fibers respectively. Significant increases were seen in all measures. * denotes a significant difference from pre-training ($p<0.001$).

Specifically, the percentage of SC in S-phase progressively increased by 33.9%±14.9 and 50.2%±23.5 24 and 72 hours respectively following exercise (Fig 4). This coincides with the increase in Pax7 mRNA expression 24 and 72 hours post-acute exercise (Fig 3D, E).

SC response and its relation to muscle hypertrophy

To determine the relationship between the acute exercise-mediated SC responses and the changes in baseline SC content following resistance training the relative changes in these variables were individually compared to relative gains in lean tissue mass. Acute exercise completed before training resulted in a highly variable SC response across individuals; however examination of individual responses revealed a significant correlation between the relative changes in SC associated with type I fibres between 24 and 72 hours following acute exercise completed before the onset of training and the relative change in quadriceps volume as assessed by MRI following 16 weeks of training ($r^2=0.566$; $p=0.012$, Fig 5A). There was no correlation in SC associated with type II fibres with the relative change in quadriceps volume following training ($r^2=0.248$; $p=0.307$, Fig 5B). There was a correlation between the change in SC associated with type II fibres following training and the change in quadriceps volume ($r^2=0.49$; $p=0.027$, Fig 5C). However, there was no correlation with the change in SC associated with type I fibres and the change in quadriceps volume following training ($r^2=0.110$; $p=0.653$).

MSTN co-localization with SC following acute resistance exercise and training

To further describe the SC response following acute resistance exercise and following a resistance training program the relation of MSTN, a known negative regulator of myogenesis, specific to the SC was assessed via immunofluorescence of muscle cross sections (Fig 6A). The proportion of MSTN positive SC associated with type I (pre: 66±4%; 24 hrs: 51±3%; 72 hrs: 33±5% type I SC positive for MSTN) and type II fibres (pre: 65±3%; 24 hrs: 49±2%; 72 hrs: 29±2% type II SC positive for MSTN) decreased 24 and 72 hours following acute resistance exercise completed before training (Fig 6B). Resistance training did not affect the proportion of SC positive for MSTN associated with either fibre type (Fig 6C).

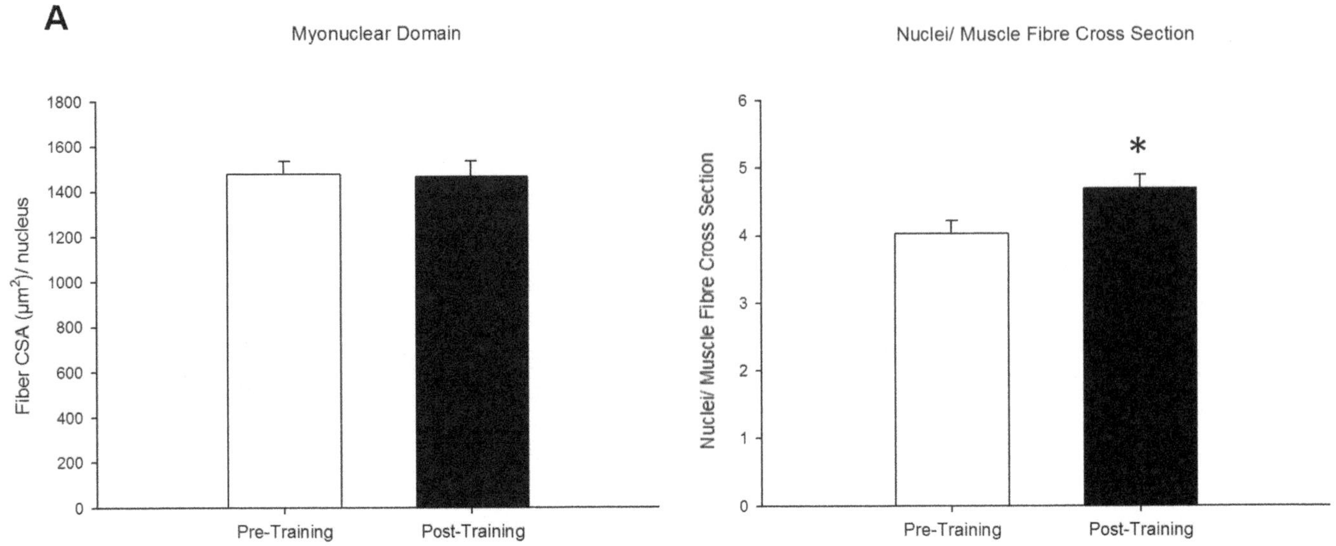

Figure 2. Myonuclear contribution to muscle hypertrophy. Myonuclear content and fibre size were quantified by visualization of nuclei (Pax7/DAPI) and myofibre borders (laminin) on muscle cross sections. Calculations of (A) myonuclear domain (fibre area (μm2) per nucleus) and (B) nuclei per muscle fibre cross section are reported. * denotes a significant difference from pre-training ($p<0.05$).

Discussion

For the first time, we report a relationship between the acute temporal SC response to exercise and the accretion of lean mass as a result of exercise training. Together this suggests that the acute SC response is important in the hypertrophic response to resistance training. Additionally, we demonstrated that an expansion of the SC pool following exercise training is also related to muscle hypertrophy. Finally we showed that basal MSTN co-localization to SC following resistance training was not affected with resistance training indicating that basal expression of MSTN within the SC appears to be independent of training status. In agreement with previous, work we also reported an increase in the number of SC associated with type II fibres following acute resistance exercise [9]. This increase in the SC pool following acute exercise was supported by cell cycle analysis demonstrating an increase in the number of SC entering S-phase indicative of SC proliferation to support remodeling. Whether SC are a contributor to muscle hypertrophy has been hotly debated but the question remains unresolved. While ours is not the first investigation to correlate myonuclear content of skeletal muscle cross sections and muscle fibre CSA [1,27] or demonstrate an increase in SC number in conjunction with hypertrophy [14,28,29], we are the first to demonstrate an association between the acute SC response associated with type I fibres following a single bout of resistance exercise with the degree of hypertrophy observed following a resistance training program.

To date, numerous factors have been identified for their role in regulating skeletal muscle hypertrophy yet these factors can only account for a small degree of the variation in muscle growth [30]. During hypertrophy in humans the addition of new nuclei via the SC is necessary in order to support myofiber growth and maintain the myonuclear domain [31]. Consistent with others [1] we observed a great degree of individual variability in muscle growth assessed using various measures. The observation of unaltered myonuclear domain size in both type I and II fibres in addition to an increase in the average number of nuclei per muscle fibre cross section of type I myofibre and a strong trend for an increase per type II myofibre ($p = .07$) following training strongly suggests a role for nuclear addition in the process of hypertrophy. CSA of type I and II fibres increased following training with a concomitant increase in the number of myonuclei and of SC per fibre suggesting that SC contribute to hypertrophy. Consistent with previous work [27,32,33] our data suggests that as myofibre size increases there is a concomitant increase in the progenitor pool to maintain and support growth of the myofibre.

Following acute exercise we demonstrated that the acute response of type I associated SC was associated with skeletal muscle hypertrophy. In line with other reports we observed a significant increase in the number of SC associated with both type II [34] and type I [27] fibres following training, consistent with the increase in CSA observed in both fibre types. Previous work has demonstrated an increase in the basal SC pool following resistance training in individuals who had the greatest gains in muscle mass when 'clusters' of responders were examined [35]. Here we extend previous findings showing that the expansion of the SC pool associated with type II, but not type I, fibres was associated with the greatest degree of hypertrophy with training. Collectively, our results along with previous investigations [27,34] suggest a role for myonuclear contribution in the process of muscle adaptation and growth.

Further analysis of the acute SC response suggests that individuals who saw the greatest gains in muscle mass following training were also the ones with a progressive increase in SC associated, with both type I and II fibres, 24 to 72 hours following acute exercise in all individuals except for one (Figure S2 B, D). While individuals who had the smallest or no gains in muscle mass following training all had a decrease in the number of SC associated with type I and II fibres between 24 and 72 hours except for one individual (Figure S2 A,C). It seems likely that the ability to sustain an increase in the SC response beyond 24 hours following acute resistance exercise is an important factor in determining the degree of muscle hypertrophy. The positive correlation between the number of SC associated with type I fibres from 24 to 72 hours following exercise and the degree of muscle hypertrophy following training suggests that the variability in the response of type I associated SC coincides with gains in muscle

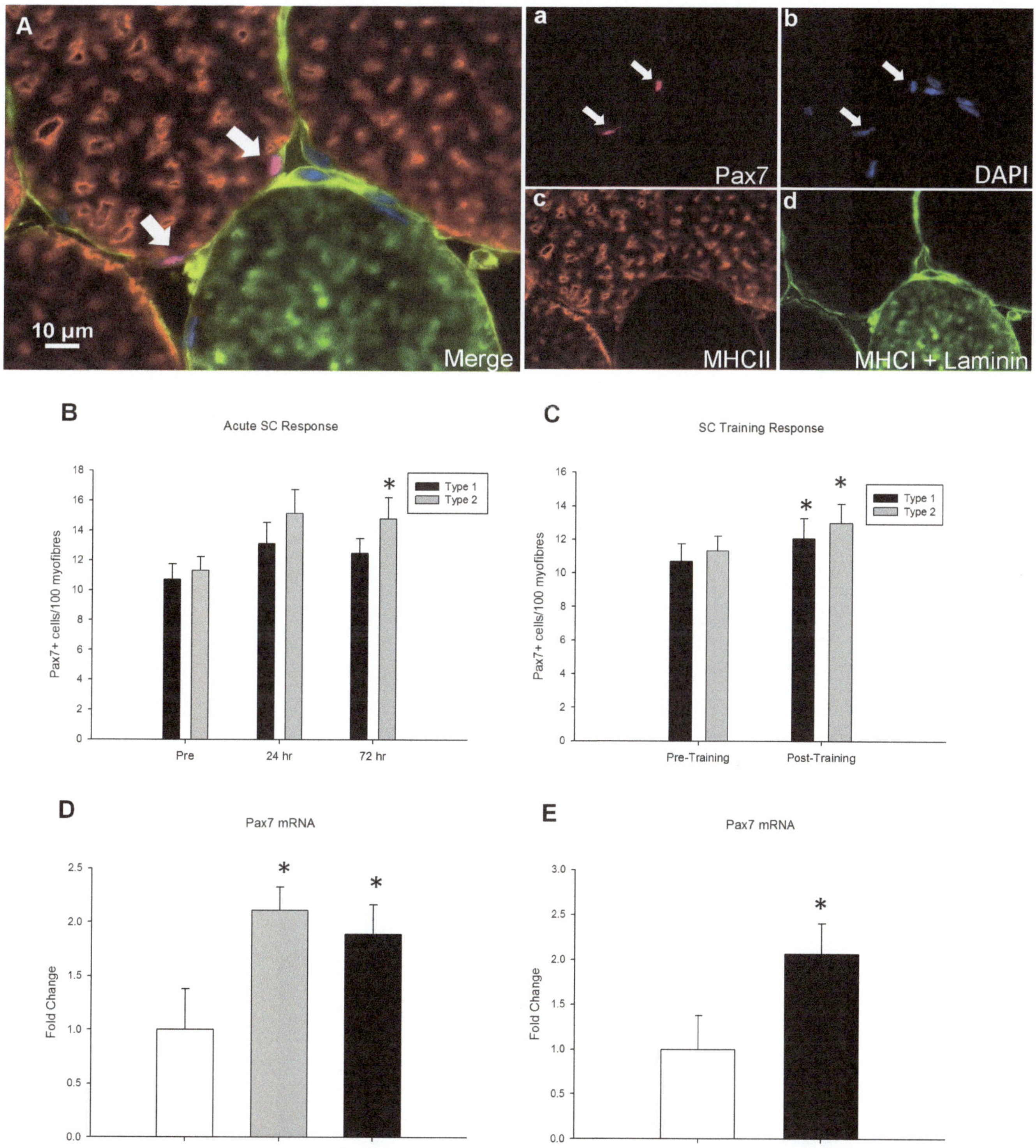

Figure 3. The SC response to an acute bout of resistance exercise and to 16 wks of resistance training. (A), representative image (merge) of a Pax7/Laminin/MHCI/MCHII immunofluorescent stain. Arrow denotes a Pax7+ cell associated with a type 2 fibre. Single channel views of (a) Pax7 (pink), (b) DAPI (blue), (c) MHCII (red), (d) MHCI and laminin (green)are provided. Scale bar measures 10 µm. SC response to (B) an acute bout of resistance exercise and (C) 16 weeks of training are expressed as satellite cell number per 100 myofibres and are specific to fiber type. Changes in SC number correspond to increases in whole muscle Pax7 mRNA in both (C) the acute time course and (D) the training response of Pax7 mRNA. * denotes significant differences from pre- time point ($p \leq 0.05$).

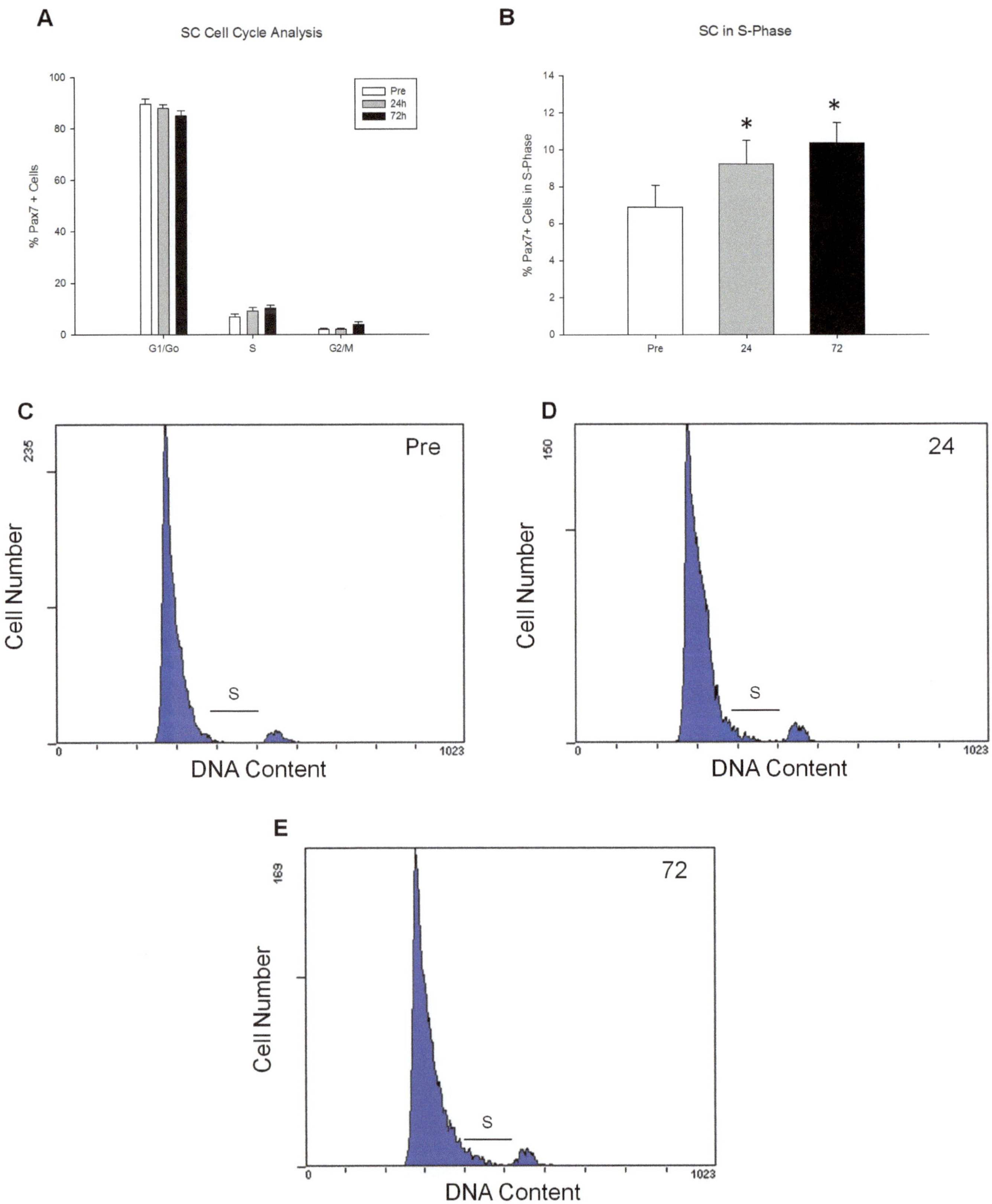

Figure 4. Cell cycle kinetics following an acute bout of resistance exercise. SC cell cycle kinetics in response to a bout of resistance exercise was analyzed through flow cytometry analysis of Pax7/PI staining in the acute time-course pre-training. Percentage of SC ($Pax7^+$) in (A) all cell cycle phases (G_o/G_I, S, G_2/M), and (B) S-phase are demonstrated. Representative FACS plots of cell cycle of Pax7+ cells pre (C), 24 h (D) and 72 h (E) following an acute bout of exercise. S phase is highlighted in each representative plot. Pax7+ cells in S phase represent 8.2% (C), 9.2% (D), and 12.3% (E) of total cells pre, 24 h and 72 h respectively. * denotes a significant difference from respective Pre timepoint ($p<0.01$).

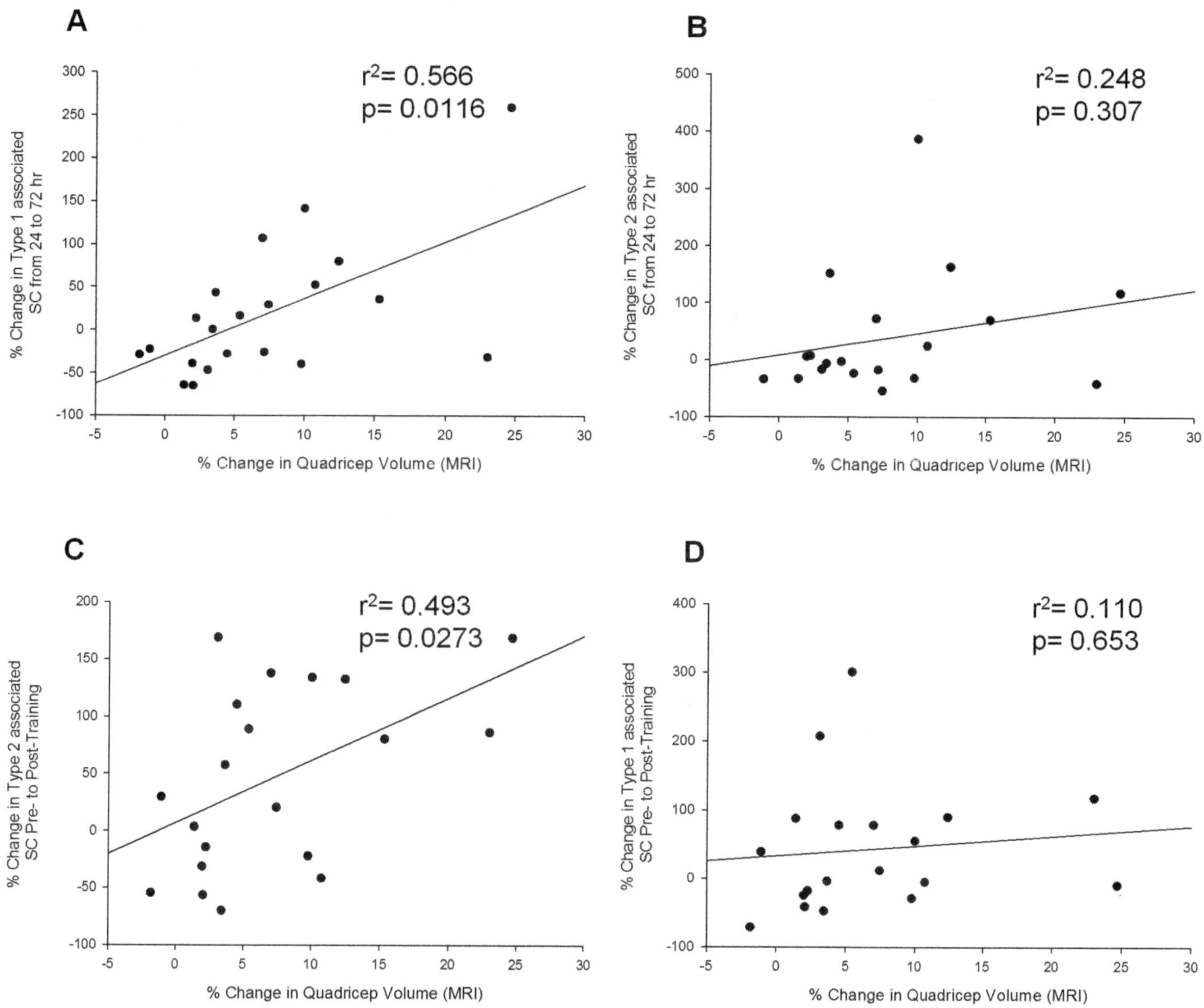

Figure 5. The relationship between the acute SC and teh expansion of the SC pool to skeletal muscle hypertrophy. (A) displays a significant correlation between the increases in quadricep volume as measured by MRI as a result of training and type 1 fibre associated SC pool expansion from 24 to 72 hours after exercise. No such correlation is seen in (B) the type 2 fibre associated SC at that time point. However, a significant correlation (C) was seen between the MRI measured increase in quadricep volume and type 2 fibre associated SC pool expansion as a result of training. No correlation (D) associated with the increase in type 1 fibre associated SC as a result of training was seen with hypertrophy.

mass. All but one of the individuals with the greatest gains in muscle mass had an increase in the number of SC associated with type II fibres following training; while individuals with the smallest/no gains in muscle mass, with the exception of one subject, experienced a decrease or no change in the number of SC associated with type II fibres following training. These data reinforce that although a relationship exists between the acute response of SC associated with type I fibres following acute exercise and muscle growth it is the expansion of the SC pool associated with type II fibres following a period of resistance training that is associated with the greatest gains in muscle mass.

MSTN has been recognized as one of the most potent regulators of muscle mass. Some reports suggest that MSTN gene expression is down-regulated in response to a resistance exercise bout [9], and 24 hours following remobilization after two weeks of immobilization [36]. Furthermore, MSTN has been implicated in the regulation of SC function by impairing activation and differentiation in animals [37] and cell culture models [38]. Recent work from our lab demonstrated an acute down-regulation of the proportion of SC co-localizing with MSTN in response to an acute exercise bout in young and older men [9]. In the current investigation we demonstrate a reduction in the proportion of SC co-localizing with MSTN in both type I and II fibres 24 and 72 hours following acute resistance exercise (Fig 6B); however, following 16 weeks of resistance training with significant hypertrophy, there was no difference in the extent of MSTN co-localization with the SC. This finding is in accordance with some reports which suggest that the inhibition of MSTN resulting in hypertrophy may be associated with changes in MSTN at the myofibre level and not the SC [39,40]. Although not significant, whole muscle mRNA expression analysis revealed a trend ($p = 0.103$) for a decrease in MSTN expression following training

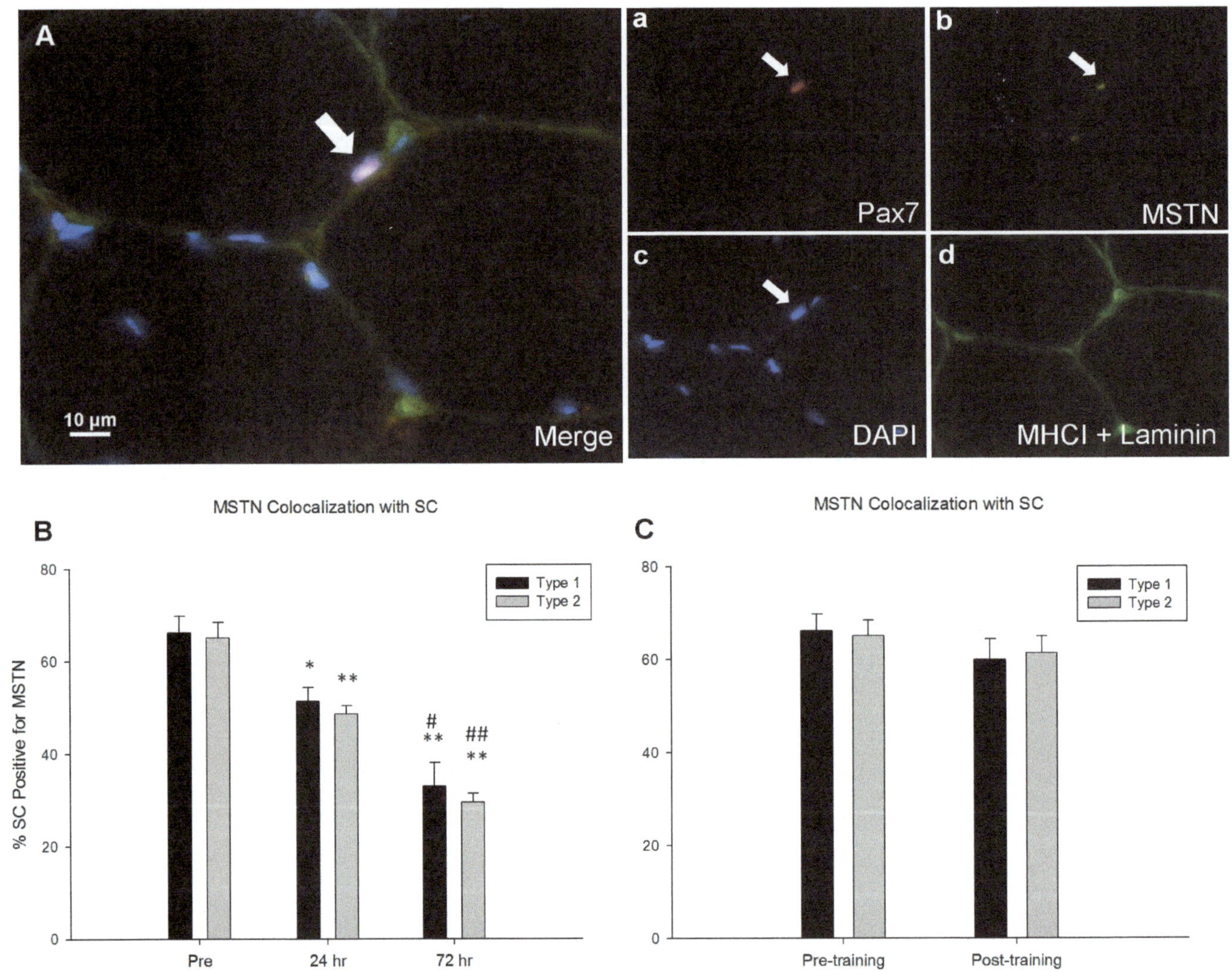

Figure 6. The association of MSTN with SC following an acute bout of resistance exercise and 16 wks of resistance training. (A), representative image (merge) of a MSTN/Pax7/Laminin/MHCI immunofluorescent stain. The arrow denotes a MSTN+/Pax7+ cell associated to a type 2 fibre. Single channel views of (a) Pax7 (red), (b) MSTN (yellow), (c) DAPI (blue), and (d) MHCI and Laminin (green) are provided, scale bar measures 10 µm. Quantification of MSTN colocalization to SCs was done in a fiber type specific manner. The changes in colocalization as a result of (B) an acute bout of resistance exercise and (C) 16 weeks of training is displayed. * and ** denote significant differences from the pre timepoint ($p<0.05$ and $p<0.001$ respectively). # and ## denote significant differences from the 24 hour timepoint ($p<0.05$ and $p<0.001$ respectively).

and a significant increase in follistatin like 1 (FSTL1) expression (Figure S1). FSTL1 is an antagonist of MSTN and its up-regulation may in part mediate the gains in muscle mass following training. Our results suggest that myostatin may play a role in acute SC regulation following exercise but that MSTN-induced training adaptation appear to be mediated at the whole muscle level rather than the SC.

In summary, the results presented in this investigation confirm previous findings demonstrating an acute expansion of the SC pool associated with type II fibres following exercise [9]. Additionally, an expansion of the basal SC pool associated with both fibre types occurred following 16 weeks of resistance training. Although an acute expansion of the SC pool associated with type I fibres was not observed, our study is the first to demonstrate a relationship between the acute response of SC associated with type I fibres and the extent of muscle hypertrophy following training. This highlights that the variability within individuals of the acute type I associated SC response is associated with hypertrophy following training. We also demonstrate a relationship with the expansion of the SC pool associated with type II fibres and the extent of muscle hypertrophy following training. Although MSTN co-localization with SC is down-regulated following acute exercise there is no difference in the proportion of SC expressing MSTN following training. Together these data suggest that under physiological conditions the contribution of nuclei to myofibres by SC is an important event in the regulation of muscle hypertrophy.

Supporting Information

Figure S1 Gene expression following 16 wks of resistance training. The training effect on whole muscle (A) MSTN, (B) follistatin and (C) FSTL1 mRNA. Pre and post- 16 week training measures are shown. * denotes significant differences from p<0.05.

Figure S2 The acute SC response in the top and bottom 5 gainers. The type I associated SC response 24 to 72 hours following resistance exercise of the bottom 5 (A) and the top 5 (B) gainers. The type II associated SC response Pre- and Post-training of the bottom 5 (C) and the top 5 (D) gainers.

Acknowledgments

We would like to thank Dr. Dan Moore and Mr. Josh Nederveen for their technical expertise during tissue analysis.

Author Contributions

Conceived and designed the experiments: LMB SMP SKB GP. Performed the experiments: LMB SJ AG BRM. Analyzed the data: LMB SJ AG CJM BRM. Contributed reagents/materials/analysis tools: GP. Wrote the paper: LMB SJ CJM BRM GP.

References

1. Hubal MJ, Gordish-Dressman H, Thompson PD, Price TB, Hoffman EP, et al. (2005) Variability in muscle size and strength gain after unilateral resistance training. Med Sci Sports Exerc 37: 964–972.
2. Petrella JK, Kim J-S, Mayhew DL, Cross JM, Bamman MM (2008) Potent myofiber hypertrophy during resistance training in humans is associated with satellite cell-mediated myonuclear addition: a cluster analysis. J Appl Physiol 104: 1736–1742.
3. Pescatello LS, Kostek MA, Gordish-Dressman H, Thompson PD, Seip RL, et al. (2006) ACE ID genotype and the muscle strength and size response to unilateral resistance training. Med Sci Sports Exerc 38(6): 1074–81.
4. Clarkson PM, Devaney JM, Gordish-Dressman H, Thompson PD, Hubal MJ, et al. (2005) ACTN3 genotype is associated with increases in muscle strength in response to resistance training in women. J Appl Physiol 99(1): 154–63.
5. Riechman SE, Balasekaran G, Roth SM, Ferrell RE (2004) Association of interleukin-15 protein and interleukin-15 receptor genetic variation with resistance exercise training responses. J Appl Physiol 97: 2214–2219.
6. Phillips BE, Williams JP, Gustafsson T, Bouchard C, Rankinen T, et al. (2013) Molecular Networks of Human Muscle Adaptation to Exercise and Age. PLoS Genet 9.
7. Terzis G, Georgiadis G, Stratakos G, Vogiatzis I, Kavouras S, et al. (2008) Resistance exercise-induced increase in muscle mass correlates with p70S6 kinase phosphorylation in human subjects. Eur J Appl Physiol 102: 145–152.
8. Davidsen PK, Gallagher IJ, Hartman JW, Tarnopolsky MA, Dela F, et al. (2011) High responders to resistance exercise training demonstrate differential regulation of skeletal muscle microRNA expression. J Appl Physiol 110: 309–317.
9. McKay BR, Ogborn DI, Bellamy LM, Tarnopolsky MA, Parise G (2012) Myostatin is associated with age-related human muscle stem cell dysfunction. FASEB J 26: 2509–2521.
10. Yin H, Price F, Rudnicki M (2013) Satellite cells and the muscle stem cell niche. Physiol Rev 93: 23–67.
11. Arnold H, Winter B (1998) Muscle differentiation: more complexity to the network of myogenic regulators. Curr Opin Genet Dev: 539–544.
12. Rudnicki MA, Le Grand F, McKinnell I, Kuang S (2008) The molecular regulation of muscle stem cell function. Cold Spring Harb Symp Quant Biol 73: 323–331.
13. Ten Broek RW, Grefte S, Von den Hoff JW (2010) Regulatory factors and cell populations involved in skeletal muscle regeneration. J Cell Physiol 224: 7–16.
14. Petrella JK, Kim J, Cross JM, Kosek DJ, Bamman MM (2006) Efficacy of myonuclear addition may explain differential myofiber growth among resistance-trained young and older men and women. Am J Physiol Endocrinol Metab 291: E937–E946.
15. Jackson JR, Mula J, Kirby TJ, Fry CS, Lee JD, et al. (2012) Satellite cell depletion does not inhibit adult skeletal muscle regrowth following unloading-induced atrophy. AJP Cell Physiol 303: C854–C861.
16. McCarthy JJ, Mula J, Miyazaki M, Erfani R, Garrison K, et al. (2011) Effective fiber hypertrophy in satellite cell-depleted skeletal muscle. Development 138: 3657–3666.
17. Crameri RM, Langberg H, Magnusson P, Jensen CH, Schrøder HD, et al. (2004) Changes in satellite cells in human skeletal muscle after a single bout of high intensity exercise. J Physiol 558: 333–340.
18. Dreyer HC, Blanco CE, Sattler FR, Schroeder ET, Wiswell RA (2006) Satellite cell numbers in young and older men 24 hours after eccentric exercise. Muscle Nerve 33: 242–253.
19. McKay BR, De Lisio M, Johnston APW, Reilly CE, Phillips SM, et al. (2009) Association of interleukin-6 signalling with the muscle stem cell response following muscle-lengthening contractions in humans. PLOS One 4.
20. McKay BR, O'Reilly CE, Phillips SM, Tarnopolsky MA, Parise G (2008) Co-expression of IGF-1 family members with myogenic regulatory factors following acute damaging muscle-lengthening contractions in humans. J Physiol 586: 5549–5560.
21. Toth KG, McKay BR, de Lisio M, Little JP, Tarnopolsky MA, et al. (2011) IL-6 induced STAT3 signalling is associated with the proliferation of human muscle satellite cells following acute muscle damage. PLOS One 6.
22. McPherron AC, Lee SJ (1997) Double muscling in cattle due to mutations in the myostatin gene. Proc Natl Acad Sci U S A 94: 12457–12461.
23. Kim J, Cross JM, Bamman MM (2005) Impact of resistance loading on myostatin expression and cell cycle regulation in young and older men and women. Am J Physiol Endocrinol Metab 288: E1110–E1119.
24. Mitchell CJ, Churchward-Venne TA, Bellamy L, Parise G, Baker SK, et al. (2013) Muscular and Systemic Correlates of Resistance Training-Induced Muscle Hypertrophy. PLOS One 8.
25. Nana A, Slater GJ, Hopkins WG, Burke LM (2012) Effects of daily activities on dual-energy X-ray absorptiometry measurements of body composition in active people. Med Sci Sports Exerc 44: 180–189.
26. McKay BR, Toth KG, Tarnopolsky MA, Parise G (2010) Satellite cell number and cell cycle kinetics in response to acute myotrauma in humans: immunohistochemistry versus flow cytometry. J Physiol 588: 3307–3320.
27. Mackey AL, Andersen LL, Frandsen U, Sjøgaard G (2011) Strength training increases the size of the satellite cell pool in type I and II fibres of chronically painful trapezius muscle in females. J Physiol 589: 5503–5515.
28. Kadi F, Eriksson A, Holmner S, Butler-Browne GS, Thornell LE (1999) Cellular adaptation of the trapezius muscle in strength-trained athletes. Histochem Cell Biol 111: 189–195.
29. Sinha-Hikim I, Roth SM, Lee MI, Bhasin S (2003) Testosterone-induced muscle hypertrophy is associated with an increase in satellite cell number in healthy, young men. Am J Physiol Endocrinol Metab 285: E197–205.
30. Timmons JA (2011) Variability in training-induced skeletal muscle adaptation. J Appl Physiol 110: 846–853.
31. Allen DL, Roy RR, Edgerton VR (1999) Myonuclear domains in muscle adaptation and disease. Muscle Nerve 22: 1350–1360.
32. Eriksson A, Kadi F, Malm C, Thornell L-E (2005) Skeletal muscle morphology in power-lifters with and without anabolic steroids. Histochem Cell Biol 124: 167–175.
33. O'Connor RS, Pavlath GK (2007) Point: Counterpoint: Satellite cell addition is/is not obligatory for skeletal muscle hypertrophy. J Appl Physiol 103: 1099–1100.
34. Verdijk LB, Gleeson BG, Jonkers RAM, Meijer K, Savelberg HHCM, et al. (2009) Skeletal muscle hypertrophy following resistance training is accompanied by a fiber type-specific increase in satellite cell content in elderly men. J Gerontol A Biol Sci Med Sci 64: 332–339.
35. Raue U, Slivka D, Jemiolo B, Hollon C, Trappe S (2006) Myogenic gene expression at rest and after a bout of resistance exercise in young (18–30 yr) and old (80–89 yr) women. J Appl Physiol 101: 53–59.
36. Jones SW, Hill RJ, Krasney PA, O'Conner B, Peirce N, et al. (2004) Disuse atrophy and exercise rehabilitation in humans profoundly affects the expression of genes associated with the regulation of skeletal muscle mass. FASEB J 18: 1025–1027.
37. Langley B, Thomas M, Bishop A, Sharma M, Gilmour S, et al. (2002) Myostatin inhibits myoblast differentiation by down-regulating MyoD expression. J Biol Chem 277: 49831–49840.
38. McCroskery S, Thomas M, Maxwell L, Sharma M, Kambadur R (2003) Myostatin negatively regulates satellite cell activation and self-renewal. J Cell Biol 162: 1135–1147.
39. Wang Q, McPherron AC (2012) Myostatin inhibition induces muscle fibre hypertrophy prior to satellite cell activation. J Physiol 590: 2151–2165.
40. Lee S-J, Huynh T V, Lee Y-S, Sebald SM, Wilcox-Adelman SA, et al. (2012) Role of satellite cells versus myofibers in muscle hypertrophy induced by inhibition of the myostatin/activin signaling pathway. Proc Natl Acad Sci U S A 109: E2353–60.

Association between Combined Lifestyle Factors and Non-Restorative Sleep in Japan

Minako Wakasugi[1]*, Junichiro James Kazama[2], Ichiei Narita[3], Kunitoshi Iseki[3], Toshiki Moriyama[3], Kunihiro Yamagata[3], Shouichi Fujimoto[3], Kazuhiko Tsuruya[3], Koichi Asahi[3], Tsuneo Konta[3], Kenjiro Kimura[3], Masahide Kondo[3], Issei Kurahashi[4], Yasuo Ohashi[5], Tsuyoshi Watanabe[3]

1 Center for Inter-organ Communication Research, Niigata University Graduate School of Medical and Dental Sciences, Niigata, Japan, **2** Department of Clinical Nephrology and Rheumatology, Niigata University Graduate School of Medical and Dental Sciences, Niigata, Japan, **3** Steering Committee for "Design of the comprehensive health care system for chronic kidney disease (CKD) based on the individual risk assessment by Specific Health Checkups," Fukushima, Japan, **4** iAnalysis LLC, Tokyo, Japan, **5** Department of Integrated Science and Engineering for Sustainable Society, Chuo University, Tokyo, Japan

Abstract

Background: Although lifestyle factors such as cigarette smoking, excessive drinking, obesity, low or no exercise, and unhealthy dietary habits have each been associated with inadequate sleep, little is known about their combined effect. The aim of this study was to quantify the overall impact of lifestyle-related factors on non-restorative sleep in the general Japanese population.

Methods and Findings: A cross-sectional study of 243,767 participants (men, 39.8%) was performed using the Specific Health Check and Guidance System in Japan. A healthy lifestyle score was calculated by adding up the number of low-risk lifestyle factors for each participant. Low risk was defined as (1) not smoking, (2) body mass index<25 kg/m^2, (3) moderate or less alcohol consumption, (4) regular exercise, and (5) better eating patterns. Logistic regression analysis was used to examine the relationship between the score and the prevalence of non-restorative sleep, which was determined from questionnaire responses. Among 97,062 men (mean age, 63.9 years) and 146,705 women (mean age, 63.7 years), 18,678 (19.2%) and 38,539 (26.3%) reported non-restorative sleep, respectively. The prevalence of non-restorative sleep decreased with age for both sexes. Compared to participants with a healthy lifestyle score of 5 (most healthy), those with a score of 0 (least healthy) had a higher prevalence of non-restorative sleep (odds ratio, 1.59 [95% confidence interval, 1.29–1.97] for men and 2.88 [1.74–4.76] for women), independently of hypertension, hypercholesterolemia, diabetes, and chronic kidney disease. The main limitation of the study was the cross-sectional design, which limited causal inferences for the identified associations.

Conclusions: A combination of several unhealthy lifestyle factors was associated with non-restorative sleep among the general Japanese population. Further studies are needed to establish whether general lifestyle modification improves restorative sleep.

Editor: Mathias Basner, University of Pennsylvania Perelman School of Medicine, United States of America

Funding: This study was supported by a Health and Labor Sciences Research Grant for "Design of a comprehensive health care system for chronic kidney disease (CKD) based on individual risk assessment by Specific Health Checkups" (H24-intractible(renal)-ippan-006) from the Ministry of Health, Labor, and Welfare of Japan. The funders had no role in study design, data collection and analysis, decision to publish, or preparation of the manuscript.

Competing Interests: The authors have declared that no competing interests exist.

* Email: minakowa@med.niigata-u.ac.jp

Introduction

A combination of healthy lifestyle factors, such as abstaining from smoking, maintaining a body mass index (BMI) of less than 25 kg/m^2, consuming alcohol moderately, exercising regularly, and having a healthy diet, is reportedly associated with a significantly reduced risk of developing several diseases, such as coronary heart disease [1–2], type 2 diabetes mellitus [3], stroke [4], sudden cardiac death [5], chronic kidney disease [6], cancer [7–9], and total mortality [10]. A clear linear relationship was observed in these studies between risk reduction and the number of healthy lifestyle factors, suggesting that an analysis of combined lifestyle factors may demonstrate their influence better than analyses based on single factors due to the complexity and multiple dimensions of habitual health behaviors. In addition, maintaining an overall healthy lifestyle throughout young adulthood was strongly associated with a low cardiovascular disease risk profile in middle age regardless of sex, race, or a parental history of myocardial infarction, suggesting that genetic factors may not be very important in determining a low risk profile [11]. Most of these studies were conducted in non-Japanese populations except for a few studies [6,9]; however, a combination of healthy lifestyle factors may play a prominent role regardless of sex, race, or genetics.

Little is known about the impact of combined lifestyle factors on inadequate sleep. There is growing evidence that inadequate sleep, which includes short sleep duration and poor sleep quality, is associated with lifestyle factors that include obesity, insufficient physical exercise, and consumption of substances such as caffeine, alcohol, and nicotine [12]. Inadequate sleep may also modify eating patterns, thereby mediating or contributing to the observed relationship between sleep disturbance and obesity [13].

Inadequate sleep is associated with several chronic diseases. Epidemiological studies have shown that short sleep duration is associated with a higher risk of lifestyle-related diseases such as obesity [14–17], type 2 diabetes mellitus [18–19], hypertension [20], dyslipidemia [21], coronary heart disease [22], and chronic kidney disease [23]. Sleep quality is important in modifying the association between sleep duration and these diseases [24–26].

We hypothesized that a combination of unhealthy lifestyle factors is associated with inadequate sleep. Evidence of a relationship could have important clinical and public health implications. If a combination of unhealthy behaviors is associated with inadequate sleep, lifestyle interventions have the potential to reduce its occurrence. We present the results of a large cross-sectional study on the prevalence of non-restorative sleep (NRS), typically defined as subjectively feeling unrefreshed upon waking [27], and its association with a combination of lifestyle factors in the general Japanese population.

Methods

Study population and design

This cross-sectional study used baseline data from a prospective cohort study of 667,218 participants, aged 40 to 74 years, obtained from the Japanese Specific Health Check and Guidance System (SHC) created in 2008. Twenty-four of the prefectures participating in this nationwide project (Hokkaido, Miyagi, Yamagata, Fukushima, Ibaraki, Tochigi, Tokyo, Saitama, Kanagawa, Niigata, Nagano, Ishikawa, Gifu, Osaka, Okayama, Tokushima, Kochi, Fukuoka, Saga, Nagasaki, Oita, Kumamoto, Miyazaki, and Okinawa) agreed to participate in our study and were included in the present analysis. Data were sent to and verified by an independent data center, the NPO Japan Clinical Research Support Unit (Tokyo, Japan). All participants remained anonymous, and the study was conducted according to Japanese privacy protection laws and ethical guidelines for epidemiological studies published by the Ministry of Education, Science, and Culture and the Ministry of Health, Labor, and Welfare. The study protocol was approved by the ethics committee in Fukushima Medical University (No. 1485).

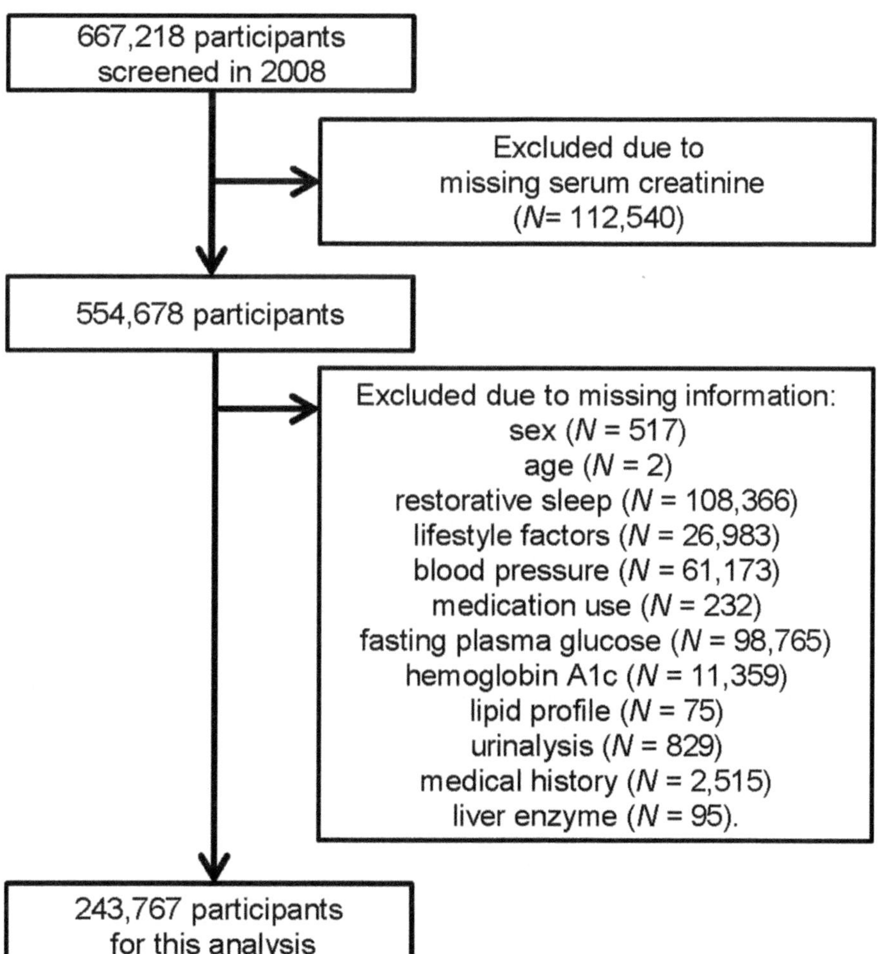

Figure 1. Flow chart of participant selection. Of the 667,218 SHC participants screened in 2008, we excluded anyone with missing information, resulting in a final sample size of 243,767.

Table 1. Clinical characteristics of male participants by restorative sleep achievement.

Characteristics	Total (N=97,062)	Restorative sleep (N=78,384 [80.8%])	Non-restorative sleep (N=18,678 [19.2%])	P value
Age, years	63.9 (8.5)	64.4 (8.2)	61.7 (9.5)	<0.0001
Healthy lifestyle score, *n* (%)				<0.0001
0	484 (0.5)	360 (0.5)	124 (0.7)	
1	5,049 (5.2)	3,715 (4.7)	1,334 (7.1)	
2	16,986 (17.5)	13,140 (16.8)	3,846 (20.6)	
3	30,331 (31.3)	24,326 (31.0)	6,005 (32.2)	
4	31,355 (32.3)	25,735 (32.8)	5,620 (30.1)	
5	12,857 (13.3)	11,108 (14.2)	1,749 (9.4)	
Components of the healthy lifestyle score				
Current smoker, *n* (%)	25,359 (26.1)	20,214 (25.8)	5,145 (27.5)	<0.0001
Body mass index, kg/m^2	23.6 (3.0)	23.6 (2.9)	23.7 (3.2)	0.05
Alcohol<20 g/day, *n* (%)	67,556 (69.6)	53,924 (68.8)	13,632 (73.0)	<0.0001
Regular exercise				
Exercise to sweat lightly, *n* (%)	46,069 (47.5)	39,055 (49.8)	7,014 (37.6)	<0.0001
Walking>1 hour/day, *n* (%)	53,950 (55.6)	45,253 (57.7)	8,697 (46.6)	<0.0001
Eating pattern				
Snacks after supper, *n* (%)	12,000 (12.4)	8,775 (11.2)	3,225 (17.3)	<0.0001
Skipping breakfast, *n* (%)	11,060 (11.4)	7,818 (10.0)	3,242 (17.4)	<0.0001
Past history, *n* (%)				
Stroke	4.938 (5.1)	4,003 (5.1)	935 (5.0)	0.59
Heart disease	7,964 (8.2)	6,285 (8.0)	1,679 (9.0)	<0.0001
Renal disease	552 (0.6)	417 (0.5)	135 (0.7)	0.002
Comorbidities, *n* (%)				
Hypertension	49,135 (50.6)	40,406 (51.5)	8,729 (46.7)	<0.0001
Diabetes	14,596 (15.0)	11,965 (15.3)	2,631 (14.1)	<0.0001
Hypercholesterolemia	33, 258 (34.3)	26,878 (34.3)	6,380 (34.2)	0.74
Chronic kidney disease	22,570 (23.3)	18,481 (23.6)	4,089 (21.9)	<0.0001
Medication, *n* (%)				
Antihypertensive drugs	30,756 (31.7)	25,382 (32.4)	5,374 (28.8)	<0.0001
Antidiabetic medication	6,649 (6.9)	5,457 (7.0)	1,192 (6.4)	0.005
Cholesterol-lowering drugs	10,779 (11.1)	8,856 (11.3)	1,923 (10.3)	<0.0001
Systolic pressure, mmHg	131 (17)	132 (17)	130 (17)	<0.0001
Diastolic pressure, mmHg	78 (11)	78 (11)	78 (11)	0.001
Fasting plasma glucose, mg per 100 mL	102 (25)	102 (24)	102 (26)	0.66
Hemoglobin A_{1c}, %	5.79 (0.79)	5.79 (0.77)	5.78 (0.85)	0.02
LDL cholesterol, mg per 100 mL	120.9 (30.0)	120.8 (29.9)	121.1 (30.4)	0.21
Triglycerides, mg per 100 mL	107 (77, 154)	107 (77, 153)	107 (76, 155)	0.58
HDL cholesterol, mg per 100 mL	57 (15)	57 (15)	57 (15)	0.96
Creatinine, mg per 100 mL	0.85 (0.23)	0.85 (0.23)	0.84 (0.23)	0.03
eGFR, mL min^{-1} per 1.73 m^2	74.4 (16.4)	74.2 (16.3)	75.6 (16.9)	<0.0001
Proteinuria, *n* (%)	7,670 (7.9)	6,157 (7.9)	1,513 (8.1)	0.26

Numbers in the table are means (standard deviation) for continuous variables except triglycerides (median and interquartile range) or numbers (percentages) for categorical variables.
LDL, low-density lipoprotein; HDL, high-density lipoprotein; eGFR, estimated glomerular filtration rate.

The SHC has been previously described [6,28]. Briefly, it is a new healthcare strategy initiated by the Japanese Government in 2008 for the early diagnosis and intervention of metabolic syndrome. The proportion of men to women in the SHC does not necessarily reflect the national population. This is because the SHC is designed for people who have National Health Insurance, or dependents (e.g., spouse) of salaried workers who have health insurance. In this system, participants answer a self-administered questionnaire that covers medical history, smoking habits, alcohol intake, exercise habits, and eating patterns. Trained staff then

Table 2. Clinical characteristics of female participants by restorative sleep achievement.

Characteristics	Total (*N*= 146,705)	Restorative sleep (*N*= 108,166 [73.7%])	Non-restorative Sleep (*N*= 38,539 [26.3%])	*P* value
Age, years	63.7 (7.9)	64.2 (7.7)	62.6 (8.5)	<0.0001
Healthy lifestyle score, *n* (%)				<0.0001
0	63 (0.0)	35 (0.0)	28 (0.1)	
1	1,283 (0.9)	765 (0.7)	518 (1.3)	
2	9,909 (6.8)	6,502 (6.0)	3,407 (8.8)	
3	35,999 (24.5)	25,208 (23.3)	10,791 (28.0)	
4	71,637 (48.8)	53,100 (49.1)	18,537 (48.1)	
5	27,814 (19.0)	22,556 (20.9)	5,258 (13.6)	
Components of the healthy lifestyle score				
Current smoker, *n* (%)	9,763 (6.7)	6,655 (6.2)	3,108 (8.1)	<0.0001
Body mass index, kg/m^2	22.7 (3.4)	22.7 (3.3)	22.6 (3.5)	<0.0001
Alcohol<20 g/day, *n* (%)	142,216 (96.9)	105,038 (97.1)	37,178 (96.5)	<0.0001
Regular exercise				
Exercise to sweat lightly, *n* (%)	58,932 (40.2)	46,404 (42.9)	12,528 (32.5)	<0.0001
Walking>1 hour/day, *n* (%)	76,043 (51.8)	58,492 (54.1)	17,551 (45.5)	<0.0001
Eating pattern				
Snacks after supper, *n* (%)	20,361 (13.9)	13,630 (12.6)	6,731 (17.5)	<0.0001
Skipping breakfast, *n* (%)	11,791 (8.0)	7,429 (6.9)	4,362 (11.3)	<0.0001
Past history, *n* (%)				
Stroke	3.902 (2.7)	2,813 (2.6)	1,089 (2.8)	0.02
Heart disease	7,606 (5.2)	5,271 (4.9)	2,335 (6.1)	<0.0001
Renal disease	632 (0.4)	436 (0.4)	196 (0.5)	0.007
Comorbidities, *n* (%)				
Hypertension	62,034 (42.3)	46,822 (43.3)	15,212 (39.5)	<0.0001
Diabetes	11,623 (7.9)	8,625 (8.0)	2,998 (7.8)	<0.0001
Hypercholesterolemia	74,371 (50.7)	55,682 (51.5)	18,689 (48.5)	<0.0001
Chronic kidney disease	21,762 (14.8)	16,146 (14.9)	5,616 (14.6)	<0.0001
Medication, *n* (%)				
Antihypertensive drugs	39,592 (27.0)	29,884 (27.6)	9,708 (25.2)	<0.0001
Antidiabetic medication	5,373 (3.7)	3,960 (3.7)	1,413 (3.7)	0.96
Cholesterol-lowering drugs	28,802 (19.6)	21,771 (20.1)	7,031 (18.2)	<0.0001
Systolic pressure, mmHg	128 (18)	129 (18)	130 (18)	<0.0001
Diastolic pressure, mmHg	75 (11)	75 (11)	75 (11)	<0.0001
Fasting plasma glucose, mg per 100 mL	95 (18)	95 (17)	95 (19)	0.03
Hemoglobin A_{1c}, %	5.71 (0.59)	5.72 (0.58)	5.70 (0.60)	<0.0001
LDL cholesterol, mg per 100 mL	130.0 (30.3)	130.2 (30.2)	129.2 (30.8)	<0.0001
Triglycerides, mg per 100 mL	92 (68, 127)	92 (69, 127)	91 (67, 126)	<0.0001
HDL cholesterol, mg per 100 mL	65.7 (16.0)	65.5 (16.0)	66.3 (16.2)	<0.0001
Creatinine, mg per 100 mL	0.63 (0.15)	0.63 (0.15)	0.63 (0.16)	0.005
eGFR, mL min^{-1} per 1.73 m^2	75.6 (15.9)	75.4 (15.9)	76.3 (16.1)	<0.0001
Proteinuria, *n* (%)	5,777 (3.9)	4,169 (3.9)	1,608 (4.2)	0.006

Numbers in the table are means (standard deviation) for continuous variables except triglycerides (median and interquartile range) or numbers (percentages) for categorical variables.
LDL, low-density lipoprotein; HDL, high-density lipoprotein; eGFR, estimated glomerular filtration rate.

measure the height, weight, blood pressure, and waist circumference of each participant, after which serum and spot urine samples are collected. BMI is calculated by dividing body weight in kilograms by the square of height in meters. Blood samples are analyzed using an automated clinical chemical analyzer within 24 h of sampling. All blood analyses are conducted at a local, rather than a central, laboratory. Although the methods used for blood analyses are not calibrated between laboratories, analyses

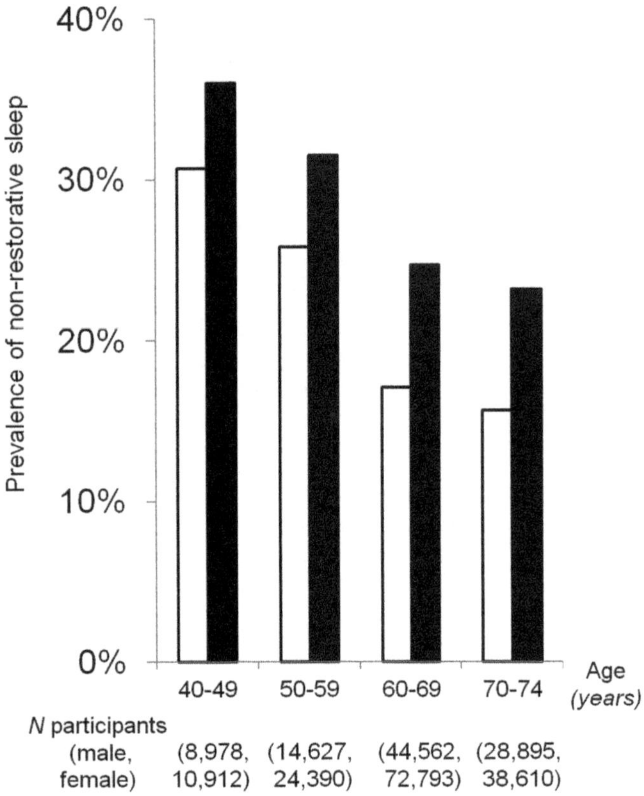

Figure 2. Prevalence of non-restorative sleep by sex and age. Trends were significant for both males (□; *P*<0.0001) and females (■; *P*<0.0001).

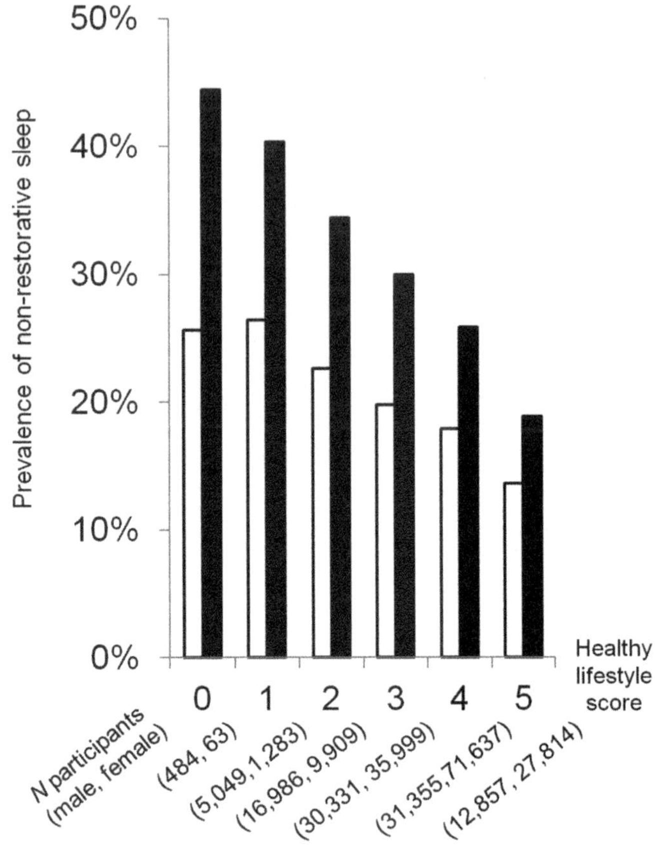

Figure 3. Prevalence of non-restorative sleep by healthy lifestyle score. Trends were significant for both males (□; *P*< 0.0001) and females (■; *P*<0.0001).

are performed according to the Japan Society of Clinical Chemistry-recommended methods for laboratory tests, which have been widely adopted by laboratories across Japan [29]. Participants diagnosed with metabolic syndrome are obligated to receive repeated lifestyle guidance over a six-month period after an annual health examination.

Participants from 40 to 74 years of age without missing information were included in this study. The complete selection process is presented in Figure 1.

Primary outcome

The primary outcome was NRS, which was assessed using this question from the self-administered questionnaire: 'Do you feel refreshed after a night's sleep?' Participants answered either yes or no. NRS was considered present when the answer was 'no'.

Lifestyle factors and covariates

For each lifestyle factor (smoking, BMI, alcohol intake, exercise habits, and eating patterns), we created a binary low-risk variable in which participants were given a score of 1 if they met the criteria for low risk or a score of 0 if otherwise, based on previous research [6]. The a priori definition of low risk was based on current literature, recommended guidelines, and realistically obtainable levels within the general population. We calculated a healthy lifestyle score by adding the total number of lifestyle factors for which each participant was at low risk. The score ranged from 0 (least healthy) to 5 (most healthy).

For smoking, we defined low risk as currently not smoking. Optimal body weight was defined as a BMI of <25 kg/m^2, the standard World Health Organization cutoff for healthy weight. For alcohol, average daily consumption over 20 g was considered high risk. Alcohol consumption was assessed by the following questions: "How often do you drink alcohol (sake, shochu [distilled spirits], beer, liquor, etc.)?" to which participants responded by selecting (1) every day, (2) sometimes, or (3) rarely (can't drink); and "How much do you drink a day, in terms of glasses of refined sake? (A glass [180 mL] of refined sake is equivalent to a medium bottle [500 mL] of beer, 80 mL of shochu (alcohol content 35 percent), a glass [double, 60 mL] of whiskey, and 2 glasses [240 mL] of wine)," to which participants responded by selecting (1) <1 drink per day, (2) 1–2 drinks per day, (3) 2–3 drinks per day, or (4) ≥3 drinks per day'. The ethanol content per drink was calculated to be equivalent to 20 g. For exercise habits, two questions were asked: 'Are you in the habit of exercising to sweat lightly for over 30 minutes each time, two times weekly, for over a year?' and 'In your daily life, do you walk or do any equivalent amount of physical activity for more than one hour a day?' Low risk patients were defined as those who answered 'yes' to both questions on the basis of a current Japanese guideline [30]. For eating patterns, two questions were asked: 'Do you skip breakfast more than three times a week?' and 'Do you eat snacks after supper more than three times a week?' Low risk patients were defined as those who answered 'no' to both questions.

Hemoglobin A1c (HbA1c) was estimated as a National Glycohemoglobin Standardization Program equivalent value using the following equation [31]: HbA1c (%) = HbA1c (Japan Diabetes Society) (%)+0.4%. Diabetes was defined in accordance with American Diabetes Association guidelines [32] as a fasting plasma glucose concentration of 126 mg/dL or higher, HbA1c of

Table 3. Multivariate analysis of the relationship between categories from the healthy lifestyle score and prevalence of non-restorative sleep ($N = 243{,}767$).

Variable	Male ($N = 97{,}062$)		Female ($N = 146{,}705$)	
	Age-adjusted odds ratio (95%CI)	Multivariate odds ratio[a] (95%CI)	Age-adjusted odds ratio (95%CI)	Multivariate odds ratio[a] (95%CI)
Categories				
Current smoker				
No (ref)	1.00	1.00	1.00	1.00
Yes	0.90 (0.87–0.93)****	0.90 (0.87–0.93)****	1.09 (1.04–1.14)****	1.09 (1.04–1.14)****
Body mass index				
<25 m/kg^2 (ref)	1.00	1.00	1.00	1.00
≥25 m/kg^2	0.97 (0.93–1.00)	0.97 (0.94–1.01)	0.98 (0.95–1.00)	0.99 (0.96–1.02)
Alcohol consumption				
<20 g/day (ref)	1.00	1.00	1.00	1.00
≥20 g/day	0.83 (0.80–0.86)****	0.83 (0.80–0.86)****	1.03 (0.96–1.10)	1.03 (0.96–1.10)
Regular exercise				
Yes (ref)	1.00	1.00	1.00	1.00
No	1.57 (1.51–1.62)****	1.57 (1.51–1.63)****	1.52 (1.47–1.58)****	1.52 (1.48–1.56)****
Eating pattern				
Healthy (ref)	1.00	1.00	1.00	1.00
Less healthy	1.54 (1.48–1.60)****	1.54 (1.48–1.60)****	1.44 (1.40–1.48)****	1.44 (1.40–1.48)****
Age				
40–49 years	1.96 (1.85–2.08)****	1.95 (1.84–2.07)****	1.56 (1.48–1.63)****	1.50 (1.43–1.57)****
50–59 years	1.63 (1.55–1.71)****	1.62 (1.54–1.71)****	1.35 (1.30–1.40)****	1.32 (1.27–1.37)****
60–69 years	1.09 (1.04–1.13)****	1.09 (1.04–1.13)****	1.06 (1.03–1.09)****	1.05 (1.02–1.09)**
70–74 years (ref)	1.00	1.00	1.00	1.00
Hypertension		0.96 (0.93–1.00)*		0.94 (0.91–0.96)****
Diabetes mellitus		0.99 (0.95–1.04)		1.06 (1.02–1.11)**
Hypercholesterolemia		0.97 (0.93–1.00)		0.95 (0.92–0.97)****
Chronic kidney disease		1.04 (1.00–1.08)		1.04 (1.00–1.08)*

[a] Adjusted for age (years), sex, hypertension, diabetes, hypercholesterolemia, and chronic kidney disease.
Definitions of these factors are described in the text.
*$P<0.05$,
**$P<0.01$,
***$P<0.001$,
****$P<0.0001$.

6.5% or higher, or self-reported use of anti-hyperglycemic drugs. Hypertension was defined as using antihypertensive medications, a systolic blood pressure ≥140 mmHg, a diastolic blood pressure ≥ 90 mmHg, or both. Hypercholesterolemia was defined as using cholesterol-lowering medications, a low-density lipoprotein (LDL) cholesterol level ≥140 mg/dL, or both. Chronic kidney disease was defined as proteinuria in urinalysis, a glomerular filtration rate (GFR) less than 60 mL/min/1.73 m^2, or both [33]. Proteinuria was defined as a dipstick urinalysis score of 1+ or greater (equivalent to ≥30 mg/dL) because of poor discrimination between negative and trace positive dipstick readings [34]. Estimated GFR was calculated using the Japanese equation [35].

Statistical analysis

Data were analyzed separately by sex. First, we calculated the prevalence of NRS stratified by age categories. Age was categorized as 40–49, 50–59, 60–69, and 70–74 years. Second, we analyzed clinical and laboratory parameters stratified by the presence or absence of NRS. The chi-square test, Student's t-test, and Mann-Whitney U test were used to assess differences among participant characteristics in relation to NRS. Spearman and Pearson correlation coefficients were calculated to evaluate the relationship among each independent variable. To evaluate the association between prevalent NRS and each variable of the healthy lifestyle score, multivariable-adjusted odds ratios (ORs) and their corresponding 95% confidence intervals (CIs) were calculated using the category conventionally believed to be most healthy as the reference group. Data were initially adjusted for age. Next, we added age, hypertension, diabetes, hypercholesterolemia, and chronic kidney disease to multivariate models (Model 1). Finally, we added history of stroke, heart disease, and renal failure to Model 1 (Model 2).

To assess the robustness of the main results, we conducted several subsidiary analyses. First, subgroup analyses were stratified by age categories because age is associated with NRS. Healthy lifestyle scores from 0 (least healthy) to 1 (second-least healthy) were combined into one category because there were few cases. Age was also added as a continuous variable. Second, subgroup analyses were conducted among nonusers of medications to avoid variations in results due to medications. Nonusers of medications were defined as individuals who took no medications for diabetes, hypertension, and hypercholesterolemia. Finally, the analyses were repeated after excluding participants with obesity (BMI≥25 kg/m^2) to enhance the association between healthy lifestyle and NRS, as obese participants could modify their lifestyle to lose weight. Because increased BMI may be a consequence rather than a component of an unhealthy lifestyle, another healthy lifestyle score was created to incorporate all variables except BMI. This score ranged from 0 to 4 points.

$P<0.05$ was considered statistically significant, and all tests were two-tailed. All analyses were performed with the SPSS for Windows statistical package (Version 18.0; SPSS, Chicago, IL, USA) and Stata/MP software (Version 12.1; Stata Corp, College Station, TX, USA).

Results

Participant flow

Of the 667,218 SHC participants screened in 2008, we excluded those who did not have serum creatinine levels measured ($n = 112{,}540$) because it is not mandatory for the SHC but is included independently in some areas. We also excluded anyone with missing information ($n = 310{,}911$), resulting in a final sample size of 243,767 (Figure 1). There were no substantial differences between included and excluded participants for characteristics such as prevalence of NRS, sex, age, and healthy lifestyle score (Table S1).

Demographic characteristics of participants

Among 97,062 men and 146,705 women, 18,678 (19.2%) and 38,539 (26.3%) were identified as having NRS, respectively. Tables 1 and 2 present the associations between various clinical characteristics and NRS. Both male and female participants with NRS were younger, had higher prevalence of current smokers, higher BMI, lower prevalence of exercise habits, and higher prevalence of less healthy eating patterns. They were also more likely to have a history of heart or renal disease and less likely to have hypertension, diabetes, and chronic kidney disease. Some differences were observed between sexes. Women with NRS were less likely to have an adequate intake of daily alcohol, while this was more likely in men with NRS compared to those without NRS. In addition, the proportion of those with a history of stroke was significantly higher in women with NRS, but not in men with NRS.

Associations between the healthy lifestyle score and NRS

The prevalence of NRS decreased with increasing age for both men and women (*P* for trend <0.0001, Figure 2), and was lower among men than women for all age groups. An inverse, dose-response relationship was observed between healthy lifestyle scores and prevalence of NRS for both male and female participants (*P* for trend <0.0001, Figure 3).

When each variable of the healthy lifestyle score was considered individually, less healthy eating patterns and no regular exercise were associated with a higher prevalence of NRS (Table 3), but there were no apparent associations between BMI and the prevalence of NRS. Some differences were observed between men and women. Current smokers were associated with a higher prevalence of NRS in women and a lower prevalence in men. In addition, alcohol consumption was not associated with NRS in women but was associated with a lower prevalence in men.

Tables 4 and 5 show that participants with a score of 0 (least healthy) had an age-adjusted OR of 1.56 (95% CI, 1.26–1.93) for men and 2.76 (95% CI, 1.68–4.56) for women, compared to those with a score of 5 (most healthy). Additional adjustments for potential consequences of an unhealthy lifestyle (i.e., hypertension, diabetes mellitus, hypercholesterolemia, and chronic kidney disease) only partially changed risk (OR for men: 1.59, 95% CI, 1.29–1.97; OR for women: 2.88, 95% CI, 1.74–4.76). This association was not changed by additional adjustments for history of stroke, heart disease, and renal failure (Model 2).

When stratified by age categories, the association between a healthy lifestyle score and prevalence of NRS was similar when compared with the entire study population for both men and women (Figure 4). Among participants who currently took no medications for diabetes, hypertension, or hypercholesterolemia, a similar association was also observed for both sexes. Furthermore, the associations were consistent among obese and non-obese participants.

Discussion

Our findings support the hypothesis that a combination of unhealthy lifestyle factors is associated with inadequate sleep. A

Table 4. Odds ratios for the association between the healthy lifestyle score and prevalent non-restorative sleep in men ($N = 97{,}062$).

Healthy lifestyle score	Unadjusted	Age-adjusted	Model 1	Model 2
0	2.19 (1.77–2.70)****	1.56 (1.26–1.93)****	1.59 (1.29–1.97)****	1.60 (1.29–1.98)****
1	2.28 (2.10–2.47)****	1.73 (1.59–1.88)****	1.76 (1.62–1.91)****	1.77 (1.63–1.92)****
2	1.86 (1.75–1.98)****	1.54 (1.44–1.64)****	1.56 (1.46–1.66)****	1.56 (1.46–1.66)****
3	1.57 (1.48–1.66)****	1.40 (1.32–1.48)****	1.41 (1.33–1.49)****	1.41 (1.33–1.50)****
4	1.39 (1.31–1.47)****	1.31 (1.24–1.39)****	1.32 (1.24–1.40)****	1.32 (1.24–1.40)****
5 (ref)	1.00	1.00	1.00	1.00

Model 1: adjusted for age (years), hypertension, diabetes, hypercholesterolemia, and chronic kidney disease.
Model 2: adjusted Model 1 plus history of stroke, heart disease, and renal failure.
*$P<0.05$,
**$P<0.01$,
***$P<0.001$,
****$P<0.0001$.

Table 5. Odds ratios for the association between the healthy lifestyle score and prevalent non-restorative sleep in women ($N = 146,705$).

Healthy lifestyle score	Unadjusted	Age-adjusted	Model 1	Model 2
0	3.43 (2.09–5.65)****	2.76 (1.68–4.56)****	2.88 (1.74–4.76)****	2.88 (1.74–4.75)****
1	2.91 (2.59–2.26)****	2.43 (2.16–2.73)****	2.48 (2.21–2.79)****	2.47 (2.20–2.78)****
2	2.25 (2.14–2.37)****	2.00 (1.90–2.11)****	2.04 (1.94–2.15)****	2.03 (1.93–2.14)****
3	1.84 (1.77–1.91)****	1.71 (1.65–1.78)****	1.74 (1.67–1.81)****	1.73 (1.67–1.80)****
4	1.50 (1.45–1.55)****	1.44 (1.39–1.49)****	1.45 (1.40–1.50)****	1.44 (1.39–1.49)****
5 (ref)	1.00	1.00	1.00	1.00

Model 1: adjusted for age (years), hypertension, diabetes, hypercholesterolemia, and chronic kidney disease.
Model 2: adjusted Model 1 plus history of stroke, heart disease, and renal failure.
*$P<0.05$,
**$P<0.01$,
***$P<0.001$,
****$P<0.0001$.

combination of healthy lifestyle factors was associated with a decreased prevalence of NRS in both men and women of any age, even after adjusting for comorbidities such as hypertension, diabetes mellitus, hypercholesterolemia, chronic kidney disease, and history of stroke, heart disease, and renal failure. Although further study is needed to strengthen the association between the combined lifestyle factors and inadequate sleep, these findings raise the possibility that a healthy lifestyle could not only reduce the risk of developing several diseases but also improve sleep quality. If healthy lifestyle factors can provide restorative sleep, gaining satisfying rest would be a strong motivator for lifestyle modification.

Insomnia is an important public health issue [36] characterized by nighttime sleep problems. These may be manifest as difficulties in initiating or maintaining sleep, NRS, a combination of these complaints, or daytime symptoms [37]. Although there is a lack of consistency in the definition of NRS, and reports on NRS have been less extensive compared with other symptoms of primary insomnia (i.e., sleep latency and total sleep time), mounting evidence suggests that NRS is a frequent symptom observed in the general population. NRS prevalence was reported to be 10.8% in the non-institutionalized general population in seven European countries (France, the United Kingdom, Germany, Italy, Portugal, Spain, and Finland) [38], 35% in the participants of the Atherosclerosis Risk in Community Study in the United States [39], and 14.8% in the general South Korean population [40]. Although our methodology and questionnaire were not the same as those used in these studies, our findings were consistent in that NRS is frequently observed in the general Japanese population. The prevalence of NRS was higher in women than in men and decreased with age in our study. These results are in line with previous studies from Europe [38], the United States [36,39], South Korea [40], as well as an international survey conducted in Finland, Greece, Jordan and Lebanon, Morocco, Mexico, the Philippines, Portugal, Sweden, and Switzerland [41]. Although the prevalence of insomnia differs from one country to another [40], a decrease in NRS prevalence with age is commonly observed. This suggests that some common risk factors may be shared among young people with different racial, ethnic, cultural, and environmental background.

With regard to individual lifestyle factors, we found associations between NRS and physical inactivity or unhealthy eating patterns. Both physical activity and a healthy diet are known to be associated with sleep quality. A high level of exercise is related to better sleep patterns such as higher sleep quality, shortened sleep latency, and fewer awakenings during the night [42], while lack of habitual exercise is associated with more reported sleep complaints [43–44]. Meanwhile, skipping breakfast and a regular habit of snacking are more common in individuals with short sleep duration than in those with normal sleep duration [45]. A randomized crossover study showed that skipping breakfast in a nocturnal lifestyle, i.e., sleeping at 1:30 a.m. and waking at 8:30 a.m., was associated with decreased secretion of melatonin and leptin [46], suggesting that those lifestyle factors might be both a cause and a consequence of inadequate sleep. Although information is limited about NRS and physical inactivity or eating patterns, our findings are in line with these studies.

We found no association between NRS and BMI. Although obesity is associated with sleep apnea, little is known about its connection to NRS. Previous literature has shown that BMI is not associated with the prevalence of NRS, except in underweight individuals (BMI$<$20 kg/m^2) who had a higher prevalence of NRS than those with normal BMI (20–24 kg/m^2) [40]. A possible reason for this discrepancy is that use of a binary variable in our analysis did not detect an association between being underweight and having NRS that might only be observed when analyzed quantitatively.

Notably, sex differences were observed for smoking and alcohol consumption. Although smoking was associated with increases in NRS in women, the opposite relationship was observed in men, and adequate alcohol consumption was associated with increases in NRS among only male participants. It has generally been found that both alcohol consumption and smoking are associated with increases in sleep disorders [47–49], but associations between NRS and alcohol consumption or smoking are still controversial. Smoking has been associated with NRS in some studies [40,48] but not in another [39]. While alcohol consumption is not associated with NRS [39], some studies have found that alcohol abuse [50] and alcohol dependence [40] are connected to NRS. These inconsistencies may be primarily due to the different definitions of NRS, which only represents a single dimension or item of sleep symptoms [36]. It is also possible that using the binary variable in our study influenced results. Although associations between NRS and alcohol or smoking differed between men and women, the combined effect of healthy lifestyle factors on NRS were similar for both, suggesting that lifestyle factors cooperate with one another and are important for restorative sleep. Furthermore, a comprehensive analysis of

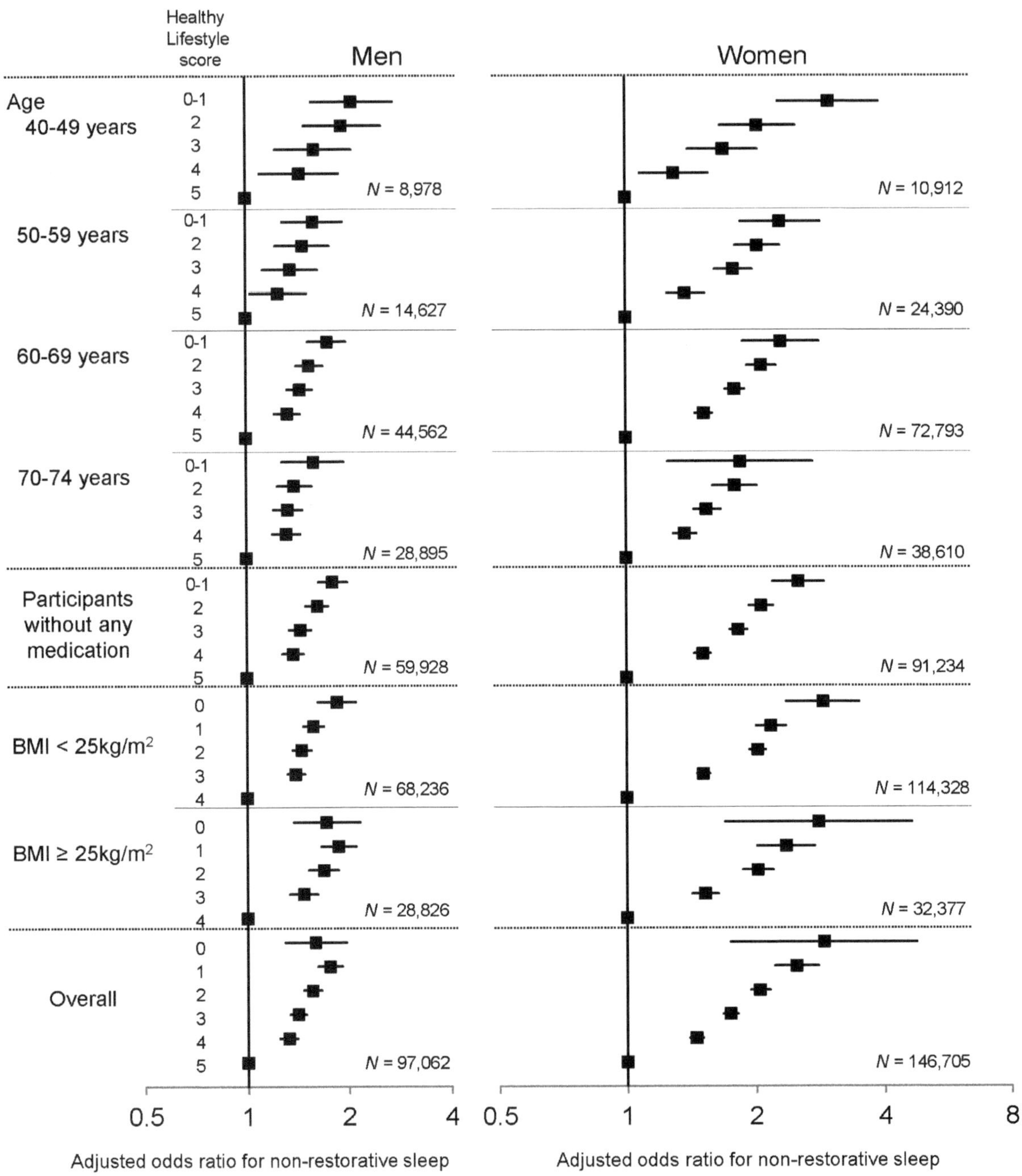

Figure 4. Subgroup analysis. Forest plot shows odds ratio with 95% confidence interval for the association between a healthy lifestyle score and prevalent non-restorative sleep in subgroups and in the entire study population. All analyses were adjusted for the following covariates: age (in years), hypertension, diabetes, hypercholesterolemia, and chronic kidney disease.

healthy lifestyle may capture influence of individual factors better than analyses based on a single factor, given the complexity and multiple dimensions of habitual health behaviors. Further investigation is needed to determine whether critical thresholds exist for each lifestyle factor and to establish combined effects and interaction effects as well as individual effects.

Patients with NRS were recently reported to have higher C-reactive protein (CRP) levels, a marker for systemic inflammation, than those without NRS [51]. Elevated CRP has also been associated with lifestyle risk factors such as obesity [52], physical inactivity [53], cigarette smoking [54], and alcohol consumption [55,56]. These findings together suggest that participants with NRS have higher CRP levels due to unhealthy lifestyle behaviors, although no information about CRP was available in our study. It is possible that sleep deprivation [57,58] or stress [59] leads to increased CRP levels. Further investigation is warranted to clarify these aspects of the relationship between NRS and lifestyle factors.

Our study has several limitations. First, a selection bias of subjects might exist. Because participants in this cohort received annual physical checkups, they might be more health-conscious than the average Japanese population. Second, NRS was determined solely based on self-reported information and may not be accurate. A single retrospective item has limitations that need to be addressed, such as recall bias and demand characteristics. In addition, frequency (i.e., more than three times per week) and sleep duration were not included in the questionnaire used to assess NRS. However, there is no reliable and well-validated patient-reported outcome instrument currently available for evaluating NRS [27]. Third, we cannot exclude the possibility that residual confounding factors exist, which were not measured in the present study, such as marital status [38], educational level [36,50], employment status [38], work schedule [50], level of stress [50], psychiatric disorders [38], and use of sleep medications. Whether these factors affect the relationship between lifestyle factors and NRS should be assessed in the future. Fourth, we gave equal weight to each lifestyle factor to achieve the main purpose of the study. That may have resulted in conservative estimates for multiple lifestyle factors. Fifth, the nutritive content in diet could not be evaluated due to lack of information. Evidence regarding the associations between diet and NRS is scarce, although a cross-sectional study using data from the National Health and Nutrition Examination Survey (NHANES) from the United States has shown that NRS is positively associated with butanoic acid, moisture, cholesterol, and negatively associated with calcium, vitamin C, and water [60]. Sixth, odds ratios do not approximate well to the relative risk when the effect sizes are large and the prevalence of the outcome of interest is high [61]. In our study, the prevalence of NRS was relatively high, whereas the effect sizes were not large. In addition, qualitative judgments based on interpreting odds ratios as though they were relative risks are unlikely to be seriously in error [61]. Therefore, we consider that our results demonstrate important effects. Finally, the cross-sectional study design limited our ability to determine the direction of the association or causality. NRS might be the cause, rather than the consequence, of one or more unhealthy lifestyle factors.

Our study also has several strengths. First, it was a large-scale cross-sectional study with participants from all over Japan. Second, this is the first report, to the best of our knowledge, to demonstrate the prevalence of NRS in the general Japanese population and assess the association between combined lifestyle factors and NRS.

In conclusion, a combination of healthy lifestyle factors was associated with an increase in restorative sleep independently of age, sex, and comorbidities in the general Japanese population. Further studies are needed to establish whether general lifestyle modification improves restorative sleep.

Supporting Information

Table S1 Clinical characteristics of participants included and excluded in the analysis. Numbers in the table are means (standard deviation) for continuous variables except triglycerides (median and interquartile range) or numbers (percentages) for categorical variables. Note that the percentages are computed based only on the total number of non-missing cases. LDL, low-density lipoprotein; HDL, high-density lipoprotein; eGFR, estimated glomerular filtration rate.

Author Contributions

Conceived and designed the experiments: MW IN. Performed the experiments: MW JJK IN. Analyzed the data: MW. Wrote the first draft of the manuscript: MW. Contributed to drafting the manuscript: MW JJK IN. ICMJE criteria for authorship read and met: MW JJK IN KI TM KY SF KT KA TK KK MK IK YO TW. Agree with manuscript results and conclusions: MW JJK IN KI TM KY SF KT KA TK KK MK IK YO TW.

References

1. Stampfer MJ, Hu FB, Manson JE, Rimm EB, Willett WC (2000) Primary prevention of coronary heart disease in women through diet and lifestyle. N Engl J Med 343: 16–22.
2. Chiuve SE, McCullough ML, Sacks FM, Rimm EB (2006) Healthy lifestyle factors in the primary prevention of coronary heart disease among men: benefits among users and nonusers of lipid-lowering and antihypertensive medications. Circulation 114: 160–167.
3. Hu FB, Manson JE, Stampfer MJ, Colditz G, Liu S, et al. (2001) Diet, lifestyle, and the risk of type 2 diabetes mellitus in women. N Engl J Med 345: 790–797.
4. Kurth T, Moore SC, Gaziano JM, Kase CS, Stampfer MJ, et al. (2006) Healthy lifestyle and the risk of stroke in women. Arch Intern Med 166: 1403–1409.
5. Chiuve SE, Fung TT, Rexrode KM, Spiegelman D, Manson JE, et al. (2011) Adherence to a low-risk, healthy lifestyle and risk of sudden cardiac death among women. JAMA 306: 62–69.
6. Wakasugi M, Kazama JJ, Yamamoto S, Kawamura K, Narita I (2013) A combination of healthy lifestyle factors is associated with a decreased incidence of chronic kidney disease: a population-based cohort study. Hypertens Res 36: 328–333.
7. Platz EA, Willett WC, Colditz GA, Rimm EB, Spiegelman D, et al. (2000) Proportion of colon cancer risk that might be preventable in a cohort of middle-aged US men. Cancer Causes Control 11: 579–588.
8. Jiao L, Mitrou PN, Reedy J, Graubard BI, Hollenbeck AR, et al. (2009) A combined healthy lifestyle score and risk of pancreatic cancer in a large cohort study. Arch Intern Med 169: 764–770.
9. Sasazuki S, Inoue M, Iwasaki M, Sawada N, Shimazu T, et al. (2012) Combined impact of five lifestyle factors and subsequent risk of cancer: the Japan Public Health Center Study. Prev Med 54: 112–116.
10. van Dam RM, Li T, Spiegelman D, Franco OH, Hu FB (2008) Combined impact of lifestyle factors on mortality: prospective cohort study in US women. BMJ 337: a1440.
11. Liu K, Daviglus ML, Loria CM, Colangelo LA, Spring B, et al. (2012) Healthy lifestyle through young adulthood and the presence of low cardiovascular disease risk profile in middle age: the Coronary Artery Risk Development in (Young) Adults (CARDIA) study. Circulation 125: 996–1004.
12. Shochat T (2012) Impact of lifestyle and technology developments on sleep. Nature Science Sleep 4: 19–31.
13. Peuhkuri K, Sihvola N, Korpela R (2012) Diet promotes sleep duration and quality. Nutrition Research 32: 309–319.
14. Hasler G, Buysse DJ, Klaghofer R, Gamma A, Ajdacic V, et al. (2004) The association between short sleep duration and obesity in young adults: a 13-year prospective study. Sleep 27: 661–666.
15. Gangwisch JE, Malaspina D, Boden-Albala B, Heymsfield SB (2005) Inadequate sleep as a risk factor for obesity: analyses of the NHANES I. Sleep 28: 1289–1296.
16. Patel SR, Malhotra A, White DP, Gottlieb DJ, Hu FB (2006) Association between reduced sleep and weight gain in women. Am J Epidemiol 164: 947–954.
17. Chaput JP, Després JP, Bouchard C, Tremblay A (2008) The association between sleep duration and weight gain in adults: a 6-year prospective study from the Quebec Family Study. Sleep 31: 517–523.
18. Ayas NT, White DP, Al-Delaimy WK, Manson JE, Stampfer MJ, et al. (2003) A prospective study of self-reported sleep duration and incident diabetes in women. Diabetes Care 26: 380–384.
19. Gangwisch JE, Heymsfield SB, Boden-Albala B, Buijs RM, Kreier F, et al. (2007) Sleep duration as a risk factor for diabetes incidence in a large U.S. sample. Sleep 30: 1667–1673.
20. Gangwisch JE, Heymsfield SB, Boden-Albala B, Buijs RM, Kreier F, et al. (2006) Short sleep duration as a risk factor for hypertension: analyses of the first National Health and Nutrition Examination Survey. Hypertension 47: 833–839.
21. Kaneita Y, Uchiyama M, Yoshiike N, Ohida T (2008) Associations of usual sleep duration with serum lipid and lipoprotein levels. Sleep 31: 645–652.
22. Ayas NT, White DP, Manson JE, Stampfer MJ, Speizer FE, et al. (2003) A prospective study of sleep duration and coronary heart disease in women. Arch Intern Med 163: 205–209.
23. Yamamoto R, Nagasawa Y, Iwatani H, Shinzawa M, Obi Y, et al. (2012) Self-reported sleep duration and prediction of proteinuria: a retrospective cohort study. Am J Kidney Dis 59: 343–355.
24. Chang ET (2009) The impact of daytime naps on the relation between sleep duration and cardiovascular events. Arch Intern Med 169: 717. doi:10.1001/archinternmed.2009.29.
25. Chandola T, Ferrie JE, Perski A, Akbaraly T, Marmot MG (2010) The effect of short sleep duration on coronary heart disease risk is greatest among those with

sleep disturbance: a prospective study from the Whitehall II cohort. Sleep 33: 739–744.
26. Hoevenaar-Blom MP, Spijkerman AM, Kromhout D, van den Berg JF, Verschuren WM (2011) Sleep duration and sleep quality in relation to 12-year cardiovascular disease incidence: the MORGEN study. Sleep 34: 1487–1492.
27. Vernon MK, Dugar A, Revicki D, Treglia M, Buysse D (2010) Measurement of non-restorative sleep in insomnia: A review of the literature. Sleep Med Rev 14: 205–212.
28. Kohro T, Furui Y, Mitsutake N, Fujii R, Morita H, et al. (2008) The Japanese national health screening and intervention program aimed at preventing worsening of the metabolic syndrome. Int Heart J 49: 193–203.
29. Tsuruya K, Yoshida H, Nagata M, Kitazono T, Hirakata H, et al. (2014) Association of the triglycerides to high-density lipoprotein cholesterol ratio with the risk of chronic kidney disease: analysis in a large Japanese population. Atherosclerosis. 233: 260–267.
30. The Office for Lifestyle-Related Diseases Control, General Affairs Division, Health Service Bureau, Ministry of Health, Labour and Welfare of Japan (2006) Exercise and Physical Activity Guide for Health Promotion 2006 - To Prevent Lifestyle-related Diseases - <Exercise Guide 2006>Prepared in August, 2006. Available: http://www.nih.go.jp/eiken/programs/pdf/exercise_guide.pdf. Accessed 13 September 2011.
31. The Committee of Japan Diabetes Society on the diagnostic criteria of diabetes mellitus (2010) Report of the Committee on the classification and diagnostic criteria of diabetes mellitus. J Jpn Diabetes Soc 53: 450–467.
32. American Diabetes Association (2011) Diagnosis and classification of diabetes mellitus. Diabetes Care (Suppl 1): S62–S69.
33. National Kidney Foundation (2002) K/DOQI clinical practice guidelines for chronic kidney disease: evaluation, classification, and stratification. Am J Kidney Dis 39 (Suppl 1): S1–S266.
34. Harrison NA, Rainford DJ, White GA, Cullen SA, Strike PW (1989) Proteinuria: What value is the dipstick? Br J Urol 63: 202–208.
35. Matsuo S, Imai E, Horio M, Yasuda Y, Tomita K, et al. (2009) Revised equations for estimated GFR from serum creatinine in Japan. Am J Kidney Dis 53: 982–992.
36. Grandner MA, Petrov ME, Rattanaumpawan P, Jackson N, Platt A, et al. (2013) Sleep symptoms, race/ethnicity, and socioeconomic position. J Clin Sleep Med. 9: 897–905; 905A–905D.
37. Roth T, Zammit G, Lankford A, Mayleben D, Stern T, et al. (2010) Nonrestorative sleep as a distinct component of insomnia. Sleep 33: 449–458.
38. Ohayon MM (2005) Prevalence and correlates of nonrestorative sleep complaints. Arch Intern Med 165: 35–41.
39. Phillips B, Mannino D (2005) Correlates of sleep complaints in adults: the ARIC study. J Clin Sleep Med 1: 277–283.
40. Kim BS, Jeon HJ, Hong JP, Bae JN, Lee JY, et al. (2012) DSM-IV psychiatric comorbidity according to symptoms of insomnia: a nationwide sample of Korean adults. Soc Psychiatry Psychiatr Epidemiol 47: 2019–2033.
41. Léger D, Partinen M, Hirshkowitz M, Chokroverty S, EQUINOX (Evaluation of daytime QUality Impairment by Nocturnal awakenings in Outpatient's eXperience) Survey Investigators, et al. (2010) Characteristics of insomnia in a primary care setting: EQUINOX survey of 5293 insomniacs from 10 countries. Sleep Med. 11: 987–998.
42. Brand S, Gerber M, Beck J, Hatzinger M, Pühse U, et al. (2010) High exercise levels are related to favorable sleep patterns and psychological functioning in adolescents: a comparison of athletes and controls. J Adolesc Health 46: 133–141.
43. Kim K, Uchiyama M, Okawa M, Liu X, Ogihara R (2000) An epidemiological study of insomnia among the Japanese general population. Sleep 23: 41–47.
44. Morgan K (2003) Daytime activity and risk factors for late-life insomnia. J Sleep Res 12: 231–238.
45. Kim S, DeRoo LA, Sandler DP (2011) Eating patterns and nutritional characteristics associated with sleep duration. Public Health Nutr 14: 889–895.
46. Qin LQ, Li J, Wang Y, Wang J, Xu JY, et al. (2003) The effects of nocturnal life on endocrine circadian patterns in healthy adults. Life Sci 73: 2467–2475.
47. Phillips BA, Danner FJ (1995) Cigarette smoking and sleep disturbance. Arch Intern Med 155: 734–737.
48. Wetter DW, Young TB (1994) The relation between cigarette smoking and sleep disturbance. Prev Med 23: 328–334.
49. Brower KJ (2003) Insomnia, alcoholism and relapse. Sleep Med Rev 7: 523–539.
50. Ohayon MM, Hong SC (2002) Prevalence of insomnia and associated factors in South Korea. J Psychosom Res 53: 593–600.
51. Zhang J, Lamers F, Hickie IB, He JP, Feig E, et al. (2013) Differentiating nonrestorative sleep from nocturnal insomnia symptoms: demographic, clinical, inflammatory, and functional correlates. Sleep 36: 671–679.
52. Choi J, Joseph L, Pilote L (2013) Obesity and C-reactive protein in various populations: a systematic review and meta-analysis. Obes Rev 14: 232–244.
53. Kasapis C, Thompson PD (2005) The effects of physical activity on serum C-reactive protein and inflammatory markers: A systematic review. J Am Coll Cardiol 45: 1563–1569.
54. Bazzano LA, He J, Muntner P, Vupputuri S, Whelton PK (2003) Relationship between cigarette smoking and novel risk factors for cardiovascular disease in the United States. Ann Intern Med 138: 891–897.
55. Albert MA, Glynn RJ, Ridker PM (2003) Alcohol consumption and plasma concentration of C-reactive protein. Circulation 107: 443e7.
56. Averina M, Nilssen O, Arkhipovsky VL, Kalinin AG, Brox J (2006) C-reactive protein and alcohol consumption: Is there a U-shaped association? Results from a population-based study in Russia. The Arkhangelsk study. Atherosclerosis 188: 309–315.
57. van Leeuwen WM, Lehto M, Karisola P, Lindholm H, Luukkonen R, et al. (2009) Sleep restriction increases the risk of developing cardiovascular diseases by augmenting proinflammatory responses through IL-17 and CRP. PLoS One. 4: e4589.
58. Meier-Ewert HK, Ridker PM, Rifai N, Regan MM, Price NJ, et al. (2004) Effect of sleep loss on C-reactive protein, an inflammatory marker of cardiovascular risk. J Am Coll Cardiol. 43: 678–683.
59. Johnson TV, Abbasi A, Master VA (2013) Systematic review of the evidence of a relationship between chronic psychosocial stress and C-reactive protein. Mol Diagn Ther. 17: 147–164.
60. Grandner MA, Jackson N, Gerstner JR, Knutson KL (2014) Sleep symptoms associated with intake of specific dietary nutrients. J Sleep Res. 23: 22–34.
61. Davies HT, Crombie IK, Tavakoli M (1998) When can odds ratios mislead? BMJ. 316: 989–991.

Permissions

All chapters in this book were first published in PLOS ONE, by The Public Library of Science; hereby published with permission under the Creative Commons Attribution License or equivalent. Every chapter published in this book has been scrutinized by our experts. Their significance has been extensively debated. The topics covered herein carry significant findings which will fuel the growth of the discipline. They may even be implemented as practical applications or may be referred to as a beginning point for another development.

The contributors of this book come from diverse backgrounds, making this book a truly international effort. This book will bring forth new frontiers with its revolutionizing research information and detailed analysis of the nascent developments around the world.

We would like to thank all the contributing authors for lending their expertise to make the book truly unique. They have played a crucial role in the development of this book. Without their invaluable contributions this book wouldn't have been possible. They have made vital efforts to compile up to date information on the varied aspects of this subject to make this book a valuable addition to the collection of many professionals and students.

This book was conceptualized with the vision of imparting up-to-date information and advanced data in this field. To ensure the same, a matchless editorial board was set up. Every individual on the board went through rigorous rounds of assessment to prove their worth. After which they invested a large part of their time researching and compiling the most relevant data for our readers.

The editorial board has been involved in producing this book since its inception. They have spent rigorous hours researching and exploring the diverse topics which have resulted in the successful publishing of this book. They have passed on their knowledge of decades through this book. To expedite this challenging task, the publisher supported the team at every step. A small team of assistant editors was also appointed to further simplify the editing procedure and attain best results for the readers.

Apart from the editorial board, the designing team has also invested a significant amount of their time in understanding the subject and creating the most relevant covers. They scrutinized every image to scout for the most suitable representation of the subject and create an appropriate cover for the book.

The publishing team has been an ardent support to the editorial, designing and production team. Their endless efforts to recruit the best for this project, has resulted in the accomplishment of this book. They are a veteran in the field of academics and their pool of knowledge is as vast as their experience in printing. Their expertise and guidance has proved useful at every step. Their uncompromising quality standards have made this book an exceptional effort. Their encouragement from time to time has been an inspiration for everyone.

The publisher and the editorial board hope that this book will prove to be a valuable piece of knowledge for researchers, students, practitioners and scholars across the globe.

List of Contributors

Crystal L. Coolbaugh
Biomedical Engineering Graduate Group, University of California Davis, Davis, California, United States of America

Ivan B. Anderson and Ezra A. Amsterdam
Division of Cardiovascular Medicine, Department of Internal Medicine, University of California Davis, Sacramento, California, United States of America

Machelle D. Wilson
Division of Biostatistics, Department of Public Health Sciences, University of California Davis, Davis, California, United States of America

David A. Hawkins
Biomedical Engineering Graduate Group, University of California Davis, Davis, California, United States of America
Department of Neurobiology, Physiology, and Behavior, University of California Davis, Davis, California, United States of America

Anne N. Thorndike, Sarah Mills, Deepak Palakshappa, Tian Gao, Cindy T. Pau and Susan Regan
Department of Medicine, Massachusetts General Hospital, Boston, Massachusetts, United States of America

Lillian Sonnenberg
Food and Nutrition Services, Massachusetts General Hospital, Boston, Massachusetts, United States of America

Mathieu B. Brodeur
Douglas Mental Health University Institute and Department of Psychiatry, McGill University, Montré al (Québec), Canada

Katherine Guérard
Department of Psychology, Université de Moncton, Moncton (New Brunswick), Canada

Maria Bouras
Department of Education, University of Sheffield, Sheffield (South Yorkshire), United Kingdom

Maria Pia Francescato, Giuliana Stel, Mario Geat and Sabina Cauci
Department of Medical and Biological Sciences, University of Udine, Udine, Italy

Yong-In Ju
Department of Health and Sports Sciences, Kawasaki University of Medical Welfare, Kurashiki, Okayama, Japan

Teruki Sone and Kensuke Tanaka
Department of Nuclear Medicine, Kawasaki Medical School, Kurashiki, Okayama, Japan

Kazuhiro Ohnaru
Department of Orthopedic Surgery, Kawasaki Medical School, Kurashiki, Okayama, Japan

Hidetaka Yamaguchi
Department of Sports Social Management, Sports Health Course School of Social Science, KIBI International University, Takahashi, Okayama, Japan

Masao Fukunaga
Kawasaki Medical School, Kurashiki, Okayama, Japan

Donvina Vaitkeviciute, Evelin Lätt, Jarek Mäestu, Toivo Jürimäe, Meeli Saar, Priit Purge and Jaak Jürimäe
Institute of Sport Pedagogy and Coaching Sciences, Faculty of Exercise and Sport Sciences, Centre of Behavioral, Social and Health Sciences, University of Tartu, Tartu, Estonia,

Katre Maasalu
Department of Traumatology and Orthopedics, Faculty of Medicine, University of Tartu, Tartu, Estonia

Agnieszka Zofia Burzynska, Laura Chaddock-Heyman, Chelsea N. Wong, Anya Knecht, Andrew Lewis, Jim M. Monti, Gillian E. Cooke and Arthur F. Kramer
The Beckman Institute for Advanced Science and Technology, University of Illinois, Urbana, Illinois, United States of America

Michelle W. Voss
Department of Psychology, University oflowa, Iowa City, Iowa, United States of America

Neha P. Gothe, Erin A. Olson, Thomas R. Wojcicki, Jason Fanning, Hyondo David Chung and Elisabeth Awick
Department of Kinesiology and Community Health, University of Illinois, Urbana, Illinois, United States of America

Edward McAuley
The Beckman Institute for Advanced Science and Technology, University of Illinois, Urbana, Illinois, United States of America
Department of Kinesiology and Community Health, University of Illinois, Urbana, Illinois, United States of America

Emma J. Adams and Mary Goad
British Heart Foundation National Centre for Physical Activity and Health, School of Sport, Exercise and Health Sciences, Loughborough University, Loughborough, United Kingdom

Shannon Sahlqvist
Centre for Physical Activity and Nutrition Research (C-PAN), School of Exercise and Nutrition Sciences, Deakin University, Geelong, Australia

Fiona C. Bull
Centre for the Built Environment and Health, School of Population Health, University of Western Australia, Perth, Australia

Ashley R. Cooper
Centre for Exercise, Nutrition and Health Sciences, School for Policy Studies, University of Bristol, Bristol, United Kingdom

David Ogilvie
Medical Research Council Epidemiology Unit and UKCRC Centre for Diet and Activity Research (CEDAR), University of Cambridge, Cambridge, United Kingdom

Nadia Lascar, Amy Kennedy and Parth Narendran
School of Clinical and Experimental Medicine, University of Birmingham, Edgbaston, Birmingham, United Kingdom
Department of Diabetes, Nuffield House, The Queen Elizabeth Hospital, Edgbaston, Birmingham, United Kingdom

Beverley Hancock and Robert C. Andrews
School of Clinical Sciences, University of Bristol, Bristol, United Kingdom

David Jenkins
Department of Diabetes, Nuffield House, The Queen Elizabeth Hospital, Edgbaston, Birmingham, United Kingdom

Sheila Greenfield
Primary Care Clinical Sciences, University of Birmingham, Edgbaston, Birmingham, United Kingdom

Erik Madssen
K.G. Jebsen Center of Exercise in Medicine, Department of Circulation and Medical Imaging, Faculty of Medicine, Norwegian University of Science and Technology, Trondheim, Norway
Department of Pulmonary Medicine, St. Olavs Hospital, Trondheim, Norway

Ingerid Arbo
K.G. Jebsen Center of Exercise in Medicine, Department of Circulation and Medical Imaging, Faculty of Medicine, Norwegian University of Science and Technology, Trondheim, Norway

Ingrid Granøien and Liv Walderhaug
Ålesund Hospital, Ålesund, Norway

Trine Moholdt
K.G. Jebsen Center of Exercise in Medicine, Department of Circulation and Medical Imaging, Faculty of Medicine, Norwegian University of Science and Technology, Trondheim, Norway
Women's Clinic, St. Olavs Hospital, Trondheim, Norway

G. Ruben H. Regterschot and Marieke J. G. Van Heuvelen
University of Groningen, University Medical Center Groningen, Center for Human Movement Sciences, Groningen, The Netherlands

Edzard B. Zeinstra
University of Groningen, University Medical Center Groningen, Center for Human Movement Sciences, Groningen, The Netherlands
Center of Behaviour and Neuroscience, Department of Molecular Neurobiology, University of Groningen, Groningen, The Netherlands

Anselm B. M. Fuermaier, Lara Tucha, Janneke Koerts and Oliver Tucha
Department of Clinical and Developmental Neuropsychology, University of Groningen, Groningen, The Netherlands

Eddy A. Van Der Zee
University of Groningen, University Medical Center Groningen, Center for Human Movement Sciences, Groningen, The Netherlands

Kevin Murach, Ulrika Raue, Brittany Wilkerson, Kiril Minchev, Bozena Jemiolo, James Bagley,

Nicholas Luden and Scott Trappe
Human Performance Laboratory, Ball State University, Muncie, Indiana, United States of America

Twan ten Haaf
Department of Nutrition & Dietetics, School of Sports and Nutrition, Amsterdam University of Applied Sciences, Amsterdam, The Netherlands

Peter J. M. Weijs
Department of Nutrition & Dietetics, School of Sports and Nutrition, Amsterdam University of Applied Sciences, Amsterdam, The Netherlands
Department of Nutrition & Dietetics, Internal Medicine, VU University Medical Center, Amsterdam, The Netherlands
EMGO+ Institute for Health and Care Research, VU University Medical Center, Amsterdam, The Netherlands

Gregory Kordas, George Lagoumintzis, Sotirios Sideris and Konstantinos Poulas
Department of Pharmacy, University of Patras, Patras, Greece

Socrates J. Tzartos
Department of Pharmacy, University of Patras, Patras, Greece
Department of Biochemistry, Hellenic Pasteur Institute, Athens, Greece

Mariana Yasue Saito Miyagi, Angela Castoldi, Danilo Candido de Almeida, Vinicius Andrade-Oliveira Yuri Hayashida, Meire Ioshie Hiyane, Niels Olsen Saraiva Camara and Mariane Tami Amano
Laboratory of Immunobiology of Transplants, Department of Immunology, Institute of Biomedical Sciences, University of Sao Paulo, Sao Paulo, SP, Brazil

Marilia Seelaender, Lucas Maceratesi Enjiu and Marcus Pisciottano
Cancer Metabolism Research Group, Department of Cell Biology, Institute of Biomedical Sciences, University of Sao Paulo, Sao Paulo, SP, Brazil

Aline Villa Nova Bacurau, Caroline and Patricia Chakur Brum
Laboratory of Molecular and Cellular Exercise Physiology, School of Physical Education and Sport, University of Sao Paulo, Sao Paulo, SP, Brazil

Ayman K. M. Hassan, Salwa R. Dimitry and George W. Agban
Department of Cardiovascular Medicine, Faculty of Medicine, Assiut University, Assiut, Egypt

Kåre Birger Hagen, Hanne Dagfinrud and Silje Halvorsen Sveaas
National Advisory Unit on Rehabilitation in Rheumatology, Department of Rheumatology, Diakonhjemmet Hospital, Oslo, Norway
Department of Health Sciences, University of Oslo, Oslo, Norway

Nina Vøllestad
Department of Health Sciences, University of Oslo, Oslo, Norway

Inge C. Olsen, Tore K. Kvien, Inger Jorid Berg, Sella Aarrestad Provan and Anne Grete Semb
Department of Rheumatology, Diakonhjemmet Hospital, Oslo, Norway

Camilla Fongen
National Advisory Unit on Rehabilitation in Rheumatology, Department of Rheumatology, Diakonhjemmet Hospital, Oslo, Norway

Annika Michelsen
Research Institute of Internal Medicine, Oslo University Hospital, Rikshospitalet, Oslo, Norway

Thor Ueland
Research Institute of Internal Medicine, Oslo University Hospital, Rikshospitalet, Oslo, Norway
Institute of Clinical Medicine, University of Oslo, Oslo, Norway

Pål Aukrust
Research Institute of Internal Medicine, Oslo University Hospital, Rikshospitalet, Oslo, Norway
Section of Clinical Immunology and Infectious Diseases, Oslo University Hospital, Rikshospitalet, Oslo, Norway
Institute of Clinical Medicine, University of Oslo, Oslo, Norway
K.G. Jebsen Inflammatory Research Center, University of Oslo, Oslo, Norway

Rogelio A. Coronado and Corey B. Simon
Department of Physical Therapy, University of Florida, Gainesville, Florida, United States of America

Carolina Valencia
Department of Applied Medicine and Rehabilitation, Indiana State University, Terra Haute, Indiana, Unites States of America

Jeffrey J. Parr
Department of Sports Medicine and Nutrition, University of Pittsburgh, Pittsburgh, Pennsylvania, United States of America

Paul A. Borsa
Department of Applied Physiology and Kinesiology, University of Florida, Gainesville, Florida, United States of America

Steven Z. George
Department of Physical Therapy, University of Florida, Gainesville, Florida, United States of America
Center for Pain Research and Behavioral Health, University of Florida, Gainesville, Florida, United States of America

Emma Harris and Karen M. Birch
Multidisciplinary Cardiovascular Research Centre, University of Leeds, Leeds, United Kingdom

Mark Rakobowchuk
School of Sport and Education, Brunel University, Middlesex, United Kingdom

Takashi Mizushima and Katsuya Yamauchi
Department of Rehabilitation, Hamamatsu University School of Medicine, Hamamatsu, Japan

Mayuko Morikawa, Yutaka Morishima and Hiroshi Nose
Department of Sports Medical Sciences, Shinshu University Graduate School of Medicine, Matsumoto, Japan
Jukunen Taiikudaigaku Research Center, Matsumoto, Japan

Shizue Masuki
Department of Sports Medical Sciences, Shinshu University Graduate School of Medicine, Matsumoto, Japan

Zhe-rong Xu, Zhong-ju Tan, Qin Zhan and Qi-feng Gui
Department of Geriatrics, First Affiliated Hospital, School of Medicine, Zhejiang University, Hangzhou, China

Yun-mei Yang
State Key Laboratory for Diagnosis and Treatment of Infectious Diseases, Department of Geriatrics, First Affiliated Hospital, School of Medicine, Zhejiang University, Hangzhou, China

Pernille Hojman, Jonas Fjelbye, Christine Dethlefsen, Claus Brandt and Bente Klarlund Pedersen
The Centre of Inflammation and Metabolism and the Centre for Physical Activity Research, Department of Infectious Diseases, Rigshospitalet, University of Copenhagen, Copenhagen, Denmark

Bo Zerahn
Department of Clinical Physiology and Nuclear Medicine, Copenhagen University Hospital Herlev, Herlev, Denmark

Jesper F. Christensen
Copenhagen University Hospital, The University Hospitals Centre for Health Care Research (UCSF), Copenhagen, Denmark

Camilla K. Lonkvist and Julie Gehl
Department of Oncology, Copenhagen University Hospital Herlev, Herlev, Denmark

Hanne Gissel
Institute of Biomedicine, University of Aarhus, Aarhus C, Denmark

Yan Zhang, Shengwen Dong, Hua Zhang and Yue Zhao
School of Nursing, Tianjin Medical University, Tianjin, China

Jianhua Zuo
Obstetrics and Gynecology Department, Wangdingdi Hospital, Tianjin, China

Xiangqin Hu
Tianjin Central Hospital of Gynecology and Obstetrics, Tianjin, China

Leeann M. Bellamy, Sophie Joanisse, Amanda Grubb, Cameron J. Mitchell, Bryon R. McKay and

Stuart M. Phillips
Department of Kinesiology, McMaster University, Hamilton, Ontario, Canada

Steven Baker
Department of Medicine, McMaster University, Hamilton, Ontario, Canada

Gianni Parise
Department of Kinesiology, McMaster University, Hamilton, Ontario, Canada
Department of Medical Physics and Applied Radiation Sciences, McMaster University, Hamilton, Ontario, Canada

Minako Wakasugi
Center for Inter-organ Communication Research, Niigata University Graduate School of Medical and Dental Sciences, Niigata, Japan

Junichiro James Kazama
Department of Clinical Nephrology and Rheumatology, Niigata University Graduate School of Medical and Dental Sciences, Niigata, Japan

Ichiei Narita, Kunitoshi Iseki, Toshiki Moriyama, Kunihiro Yamagata, Shouichi Fujimoto, Kazuhiko Tsuruya, Koichi Asahi, Tsuneo Konta, Kenjiro Kimura, Masahide Kondo and Tsuyoshi Watanabe
Steering Committee for "Design of the comprehensive health care system for chronic kidney disease (CKD) based on the individual risk assessment by Specific Health Checkups," Fukushima, Japan

Issei Kurahashi
iAnalysis LLC, Tokyo, Japan

Yasuo Ohashi
Department of Integrated Science and Engineering for Sustainable Society, Chuo University, Tokyo, Japan

Index